Anil Bhansali • Yashpal Gogate

Clinical Rounds in Endocrinology

Volume I - Adult Endocrinology

Springer

Anil Bhansali
Professor and Head
Department of Endocrinology
Postgraduate Institute of Medical Education and Research
Chandigarh
India

Yashpal Gogate
Harmony Health Hub
Nasik
India

ISBN 978-81-322-2397-9 ISBN 978-81-322-2398-6 (eBook)
DOI 10.1007/978-81-322-2398-6

Library of Congress Control Number: 2015942899

Springer New Delhi Heidelberg New York Dordrecht London

Printed on acid-free paper

Springer (India) Pvt. Ltd. is part of Springer Science+Business Media (www.springer.com)

Dedicated
to
My beloved mother late Smt Munna Kumari Bhansali,
the inspiring force in my life,
My father Shri M L Bhansali, the guiding light
of my life,
My wife Sandhya, my pillar of strength who always
stood by me and
My loving children Shipra, Shobhit and Akanksha.

Anil Bhansali

Foreword

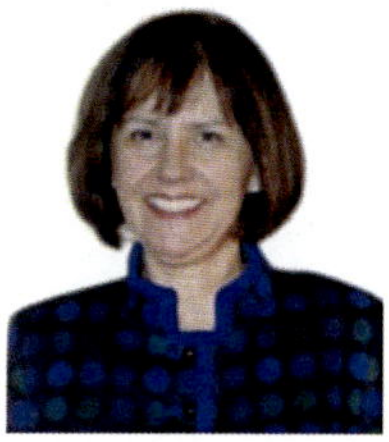

Clinical endocrinology is a wide-ranging, complex, and fast-moving medical discipline. The current volume of "Clinical Rounds in Endocrinology" captures the intricate nature of endocrinology by introducing case vignettes and discussing the steps how the diagnostic workup, differential diagnosis, and treatment modalities could lead to the best care of the patient. The succinct description of the case presentation is followed by short questions, each discussed in a paragraph summarizing the main points relevant for the management. This format is different from the usual handbook or textbook format and provides a unique insight and quick reference, not available elsewhere even in today's era of overwhelming information available on the Internet. This aspect makes this book unique and first of its kind in modern endocrinology.

Over the past years, much progress has been made in this field, with the introduction of better imaging and biochemical diagnostic tools and widening pharmacological treatments in addition to surgery and radiotherapy. This volume will help the practicing clinician to keep up to date with the novel diseases, diagnostic modalities, and management of these sometimes very rare diseases. The book comprises of 20 informative chapters. Five chapters are dedicated to pituitary-related diseases such as acromegaly and Cushing's syndrome, and there are four chapters discussing thyroid disorders including an informative section on pregnancy-related thyroid disease, three chapters on adrenal-related subjects, and three on bone and electrolyte household. The last five chapters cover type 1 and type 2 diabetes, diabetes complications, and management of pregnancy with diabetes. Fast advances in diagnostic modalities, such as PET scanning combined with novel isotope scannings or in genetics of endocrine diseases, such as the flurry of novel genes for pheochromocytoma and paraganglioma syndromes, are also expertly discussed in the relevant chapters.

The book covers most of the clinical endocrine field, they provide useful reference and practical tools for managing conditions that are relevant for clinicians involved in the care for patients with endocrine diseases, and I expect that it will be of interest not only for endocrinologists or under- and postgraduate students of endocrinology but also for internists, pediatricians, surgeons, radiologists, clinical geneticists, and radiotherapists active in this field.

The book provides excellent and often unique illustrative photographs and tables to facilitate the full understanding of the topic. The chapters are written by Prof Anil Bhansali, Head of Department of Endocrinology at the Postgraduate Medical

Institute (PGIMER), Chandigarh, India, and by Dr. Yashpal Gogate and their team members including Dr. Girish P. and Dr. Anuradha Aggarwal. This book shows the remarkable breadth and depth of their clinical knowledge, and this handbook will turn soon into a classic reference volume for students, trainee endocrinologists, and practicing endocrinologists worldwide.

London, UK Marta Korbonits, MD, PhD

Preface

Postgraduate Institute of Medical Education and Research (PGIMER), Chandigarh is one of the premier medical and research institutes in India. This tertiary health-care center, right from its days of inception, has always been at the forefront in the field of medical science. Endocrinology, as a super speciality department, was established way back in 1964 for the first time in India at PGIMER, Chandigarh.

This department has a long-standing tradition of academic rounds, with detailed discussions pertaining to every aspect of patient care, right from symptom analysis, demonstration and interpretation of signs, formulation of differential diagnosis, judicious use, and analysis of investigations and management strategies. This legacy of clinical rounds was inherited from my great teacher, Professor R.J. Dash, who had enormous knowledge of the subject with a great ability of critical analysis. Several thought-provoking questions are spontaneously generated during these interactive sessions with inputs and suggestions by residents and views and counter-views by faculty members. This continuous process of exchange of knowledge helps in providing the best possible medical care to our patients. Therefore, we had a thought to compile this information in the text that will facilitate dissemination of the knowledge to physicians and endocrinologists. Further, I had a long-cherished dream to write a book in endocrinology with precise information, comprehensive knowledge, and critical analysis of the facts.

One fine day, I expressed my desire to write a book to my student Yashpal, who not only appreciated this thought but also helped me in materializing the dream. It was decided to write a book in a "question and answer" format as this pattern not only simulates clinical rounds, but will also help the healthcare professionals in dealing with challenges in day-to-day practice. This book includes 20 chapters covering disorders of the pituitary, adrenal, thyroid, and parathyroid glands and diabetes and metabolic bone disease. Most chapters begin with a case vignette, followed by a stepwise analysis of the case including diagnosis and management and subsequently a series of question and answers. Another salient feature of this book is a multitude of clinical images, illustrations, tables, and algorithms for better understanding.

The framework of the book was created by me and helped by Dr. Yashpal over a period of 7 months. Later, my students, Dr. Girish Parthan and Dr. Anuradha Aggarwal, worked untiringly with me for the next 1 year in reviewing the literature, adding clinical images, tables, and illustrations and finally editing the text to final the book in its final shape. The whole process in itself was a great learning experience.

We hope this endeavor will help healthcare professionals to conceptualize the subject of endocrinology and will translate into better patient management.

Chandigarh, India — Anil Bhansali
Nasik, India — Yashpal Gogate

Acknowledgments

We are grateful to all those who have helped us in accomplishment of this endeavor. It is indeed difficult to name all who have contributed to the book, though a few names with a lion's share in the completion of the book are mentioned.

I, Dr. Anil Bhansali, would like to thank my colleagues Dr. Sanjay Kumar Bhadada, Dr. Pinaki Dutta, Dr. Rama Walia, Dr. Ashu Rastogi, and Dr. Naresh Sachdeva for their valuable suggestions and continuous support.

We sincerely appreciate the effort of Dr. Girish and Dr. Anuradha, for their immense contribution to this book. They have indeed inculcated "soul" to the book.

We thank all residents including Dr. Dheeraj Solanki, Dr. Soham Mukherjee, Dr. Mandeep Singla, Dr. Abhishek Hajela, Dr. Suja P Sukumar, Dr. Kushdev Jariyal, Dr. Vikram Shekhawat, and Dr. Rajneesh Mittal for their help and encouragement.

We also thank Prof. B.R. Mittal and Dr. Anish Bhattacharya from the Department of Nuclear Medicine, Prof. Paramjit Singh and Dr. Chirag Ahuja from the Department of Radio Diagnosis, and Prof. Uma Nahar from the Department of Histopathology for their suggestions and worthy contributions.

We are grateful to our family members for their continuous support and perseverance; without that it would have been impossible to fulfill this dream. I, Dr. Anil Bhansali, sincerely express my gratitude and appreciation to my wife Sandhya and my children Shobhit, Shipra, and Akanksha who have supported me throughout this long journey to accomplish this venture. I really admire my friends Justice Hari Pal Verma and Harish Singla for their continuous encouragement and support. I, Dr. Yashpal Gogate, sincerely thank my wife Dr. Ketki and my parents Dr. Vinita and Dr. Vikas Gogate.

We are also thankful to Mrs. Anjali Aggarwal and Sanjay Kumar for designing the beautiful diagrams and editing the images. We appreciate the kind help extended by Mr. Abhijeet for acquisition of the clinical images. We also thank Mrs. Rama Puri and Mr. Mahabir Singh for their uninterrupted assistance throughout the period of writing this book.

We are also grateful to all our patients who have helped us in learning clinical endocrinology.

We are also thankful to our publisher Springer and their team members Dr. Naren Aggarwal, Teena Bedi and Mr. Durai Gangapattla.

Finally, we are thankful to the Almighty for providing the wisdom, courage, and strength to complete this endeavor and for the fulfillment of this long-cherished dream.

Chandigarh, India Anil Bhansali
Nasik, India Yashpal Gogate

Contents

Authors

Anil Bhansali pursued his DM in endocrinology in 1989 from the Postgraduate Institute of Medical Research (PGIMER), Chandigarh, and is currently the Professor and Head of the department at the same institute. His areas of interest include adrenals, gonads, and type 2 diabetes mellitus. He is actively involved in research and clinical activities and has more than about 300 publications in various national and international journals. He also is the author of many chapters in various textbooks. He is the recipient of Prof. M.N. Sen ICMR Award, Prof. M. Vishwanathan Award, and Prof. Shurvir Singh Award, among others. He is also the Consulting Editor to the Indian Journal of Endocrinology and Metabolism and the past president of the Endocrine Society of India. Presently, he is actively involved in stem cell research and in establishing a state-of-the-art diabetic foot laboratory and facilities for clamp studies.

Yashpal Gogate completed his DM in Endocrinology from the Postgraduate Institute of Medical Research (PGIMER), Chandigarh. Currently, he is working as an Assistant Professor at Dr Vasantrao Pawar Medical College, Nasik, and is also a Consultant Endocrinologist at Harmony Health Hub, Nasik. He has a passion in teaching graduate and postgraduate medical students. He has been the recipient of the Jal Mehta Award in Community Medicine. His areas of interest include diabetes, thyroid disorders, and polycystic ovarian disease.

Acromegaly: Clinical Perspectives

1

1.1 Case Vignette

A 27-year-old male, presented with an episode of generalized tonic clonic seizures, altered sensorium, and rapid breathing. He was diagnosed to have diabetes mellitus about 6 months back and despite being on insulin had poor glycemic control. He had no family history of diabetes. There was history of acral enlargement for the past 8 years. He complained of intermittent episodes of headache, but did not have any visual disturbances. On examination, he was dehydrated, had a blood pressure of 100/60 mm of Hg, and was tachypneic. He had florid manifestations of acromegaly and had no goiter. There was diffuse hyperpigmentation. Although he was dehydrated, he had hyperhidrosis and seborrhea. At presentation, blood glucose was 550 mg/dl, HbA1c 17%, serum β-hydroxybutyrate 6.1 mmol/l, and arterial blood gas analysis revealed high anion gap metabolic acidosis. He was treated with intravenous saline and insulin infusion, with an insulin requirement around 200 units per day. Diabetic ketoacidosis gradually resolved, and he was switched to basal-bolus regimen with an insulin requirement of 100 units per day. His height was 176 cm and weight 80 kg with a BMI of 25.8 kg/m^2. Serum electrolytes, calcium profile, and renal and liver function tests were normal. Hormonal workup showed T_4 3.5 μg/dl (4.8–12.7), TSH 1.2 μIU/ml (0.27–4.2), 0800 h cortisol 592.6 nmol/L (171–536), ACTH 35 pg/ml (5–60), 0800 h serum cortisol after 1 mg dexamethasone 40 nmol/L (<50), prolactin 17.9 ng/ml (4.0–15), and testosterone 1.3 nmol/L (9.9–27.8). Serum insulin like growth factor 1 (IGF1) was 769.6 ng/ml (116–358), and growth hormone (GH) following glucose tolerance test was 120 ng/ml (<1 ng/ml). MR imaging showed a sellar–suprasellar mass of 4.8 × 3.2 × 3.5 cm abutting the optic chiasm, and his visual field examination confirmed bitemporal hemianopia. He was diagnosed as acromegaly due to macrosomatotropinoma, with secondary diabetes, diabetic ketoacidosis, secondary hypothyroidism, and hypogonadism. Genetic analysis for MEN1 and familial isolated pituitary adenoma (FIPA) was negative. He was started on levothyroxine and testosterone replacement therapy. He underwent transsphenoidal pituitary surgery uneventfully. He did not have

A. Bhansali, Y. Gogate, *Clinical Rounds in Endocrinology: Volume I - Adult Endocrinology*, DOI 10.1007/978-81-322-2398-6_1

CSF rhinorrhea, but had polyuria which resolved after 3 days. Postoperative day 2 serum GH was 4 ng/ml and cortisol was 450 nmol/L. His insulin requirement reduced substantially to 50 units per day. At 3 months he was reevaluated and had a serum IGF1 450 ng/ml and GH 3 ng/ml following glucose load suggestive of residual functioning somatotropinoma. Serum T_4 was 7.4 μg/dl and testosterone 7.0 nmol/L on levothyroxine and testosterone replacement and 0800 h cortisol 400 nmol/L. MR imaging showed a residual adenoma of size 1.2 × 1.1 × 0.8 cm, and he is planned for ϒ-knife therapy.

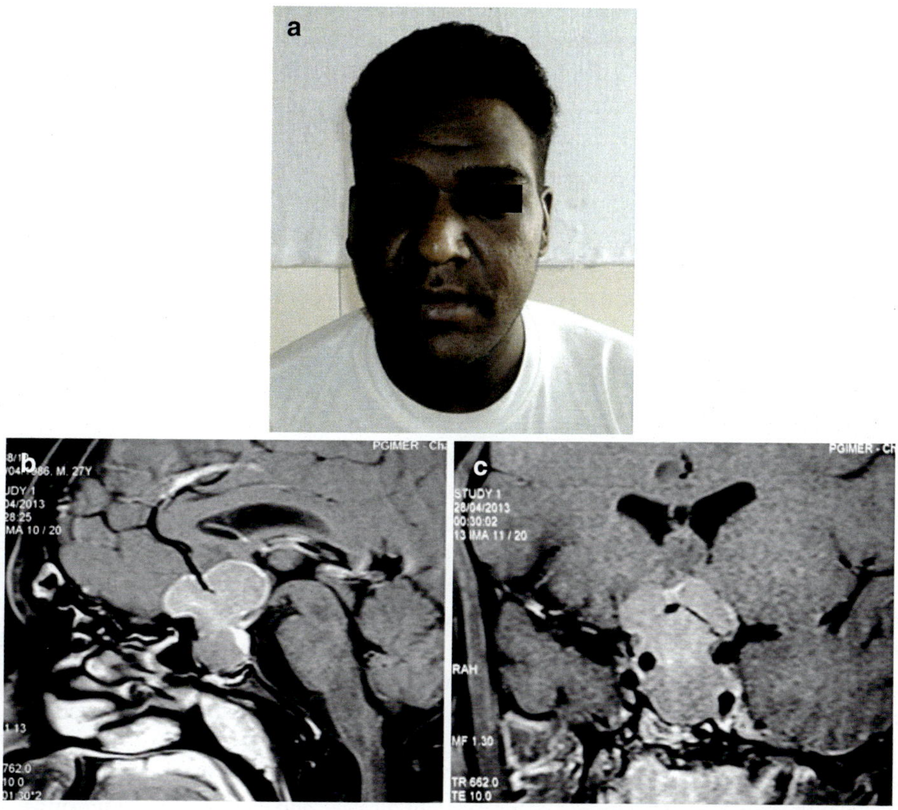

Fig. 1.1 (**a**) Patient with typical features of acromegaly along with hyperpigmentation. (**b**) Contrast-enhanced T1 MR sagittal image showing lobulated sellar–suprasellar mass abutting optic chiasm. (**c**) T1W CEMR coronal image showing pituitary macroadenoma with partial encasement of bilateral cavernous ICA segments without significant luminal compromise

1.2 Stepwise Analysis

This patient had history of acral enlargement for the past 8 years, suggestive of insidious onset of disease which is a usual feature of acromegaly. He had active acromegaly as suggested by the progressive worsening of headache, new-onset visual field defects, hyperhidrosis, seborrhea, and uncontrolled blood glucose. Dysglycemia in acromegaly occurs in 50% of patients, and 15–20% have overt diabetes. However, presentation as diabetic ketoacidosis is uncommon in patients with acromegaly and only a handful cases have been reported in the literature. Diagnosis of secondary diabetes should have been considered initially in this patient in view of young age at onset, lack of family history of diabetes, and severe and resistant hyperglycemia. It is not surprising to have such tremendous requirement of insulin in secondary diabetes associated with acromegaly. Seizure in the index patient may be due to cerebral dehydration as a result of diabetic ketoacidosis. In the presence of hyperglycemia, the estimation of serum GH and IGF1 for the diagnosis of acromegaly is debatable, as chronic hyperglycemia per se is associated with high GH and low IGF1 levels. Ideally, serum IGF1 and GH post-glucose load should be measured after optimal blood glucose control in patients of acromegaly with diabetes. However, high IGF1 (age and gender matched) in the presence of chronic hyperglycemia favors a diagnosis of active acromegaly. Diffuse hyperpigmentation in a patient with acromegaly can occur due to the direct effect of GH on melanocytes, GH, and ACTH co-secreting tumor and rarely diffuse acanthosis nigricans because of severe insulin resistance. Diffuse hyperpigmentation in the index case was due to the direct effect of GH on melanocytes. Majority of patients with acromegaly have macrosomatotropinoma as was seen in this case. In view of GH excess since adolescence, he was evaluated for familial causes of somatotropinoma like MEN1 and FIPA, which were negative. Polyuria after transsphenoidal surgery in patients with acromegaly may be due to central diabetes insipidus or passage of glycosaminoglycans in urine after reduction in circulating GH levels. Serum and urine osmolality was normal, thereby the diagnosis of diabetes insipidus was excluded in this patient. Postoperative day 1–7 fasting serum GH level <2 ng/ml predicts the cure. However in the index patient, postoperative fasting serum GH was 4 ng/ml suggestive of residual disease. Serum IGF1 should not be used for monitoring in the immediate postoperative period as it takes long time to normalize after curative adenomectomy. The treatment options available for residual disease in acromegaly are somatostatin analogues, cabergoline, pegvisomant and Υ-knife therapy. This patient was offered Υ-knife therapy for the treatment of his residual disease, and cabergoline 1 mg per day was administered during interim period.

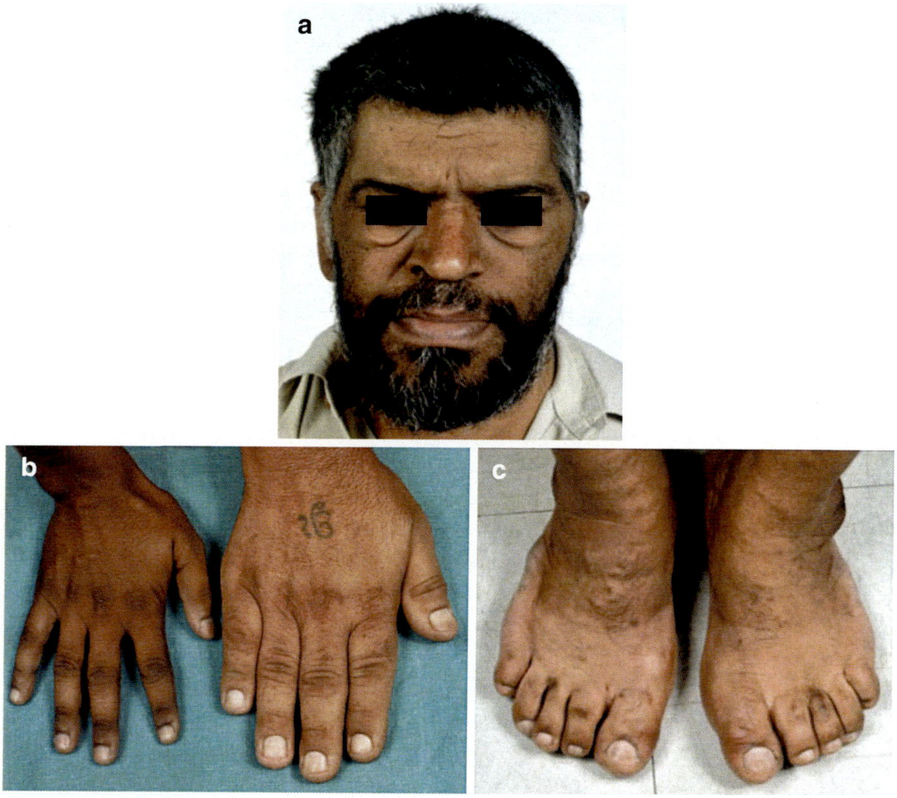

Fig. 1.2 (**a**) Coarse facial features, prominent supraorbital ridges, bulbous nose prognathism, and thick lips in a patient with acromegaly. (**b**) Enlargement of the hands in a patient with acromegaly (*left*) as compared to a normal individual (*right*). (**c**) Enlargement of the feet in the same patient with acromegaly

1.3 Clinical Rounds

1. **What is acromegaly?**

   Acromegaly is a Greek word meaning "akros" (extremity) and "megalos" (enlargement). Acral is a term pertaining to the outermost parts of the extremities (i.e., hands and feet) and face (i.e., supraorbital ridges, chin, nose, lips, and ears). It denotes enlargement of soft-tissue and osseous tissue in acral areas.

2. **What is "clinically active" acromegaly?**

   Acromegaly is said to be "clinically active" in the presence of worsening headache, hyperhidrosis, seborrhea, progressive soft tissue swelling, new-onset visual symptoms, arthralgia, compressive neuropathy, difficult to control hyperglycemia, and resistant hypertension.

3. **What are the causes of acromegaly with subtle facial features?**

Gradual alterations in facial features in a patient with acromegaly may not be appreciated for a long time, thereby causing a delay in diagnosis up to 8–10 years. By the time a diagnosis is made, facial features are too obvious. Disorders associated with subtle facial features of acromegaly are McCune–Albright syndrome (MAS), adolescent acromegaly (due to peripubertal growth spurt), mild acromegaly, concurrent thyrotoxicosis, fugitive acromegaly, and sarcopenia associated with poorly controlled diabetes or malignancy.

4. **What is fugitive acromegaly?**

Fugitive acromegaly is characterized by subtle features of acromegaly, predominantly raised prolactin, normal or mildly elevated GH, suppressible GH after glucose load, and marginally elevated insulin like growth factor 1 (IGF1). Intrinsic GH-like activity of prolactin along with marginally elevated IGF1 accounts for the subtle features of acromegaly. Fugitive acromegaly is commonly due to acidophil stem cell tumor which predominantly secretes prolactin along with small amounts of GH, with immunopositivity for both prolactin and GH in tumor tissue. These tumors are usually large, locally invasive, and resistant to dopamine agonist therapy.

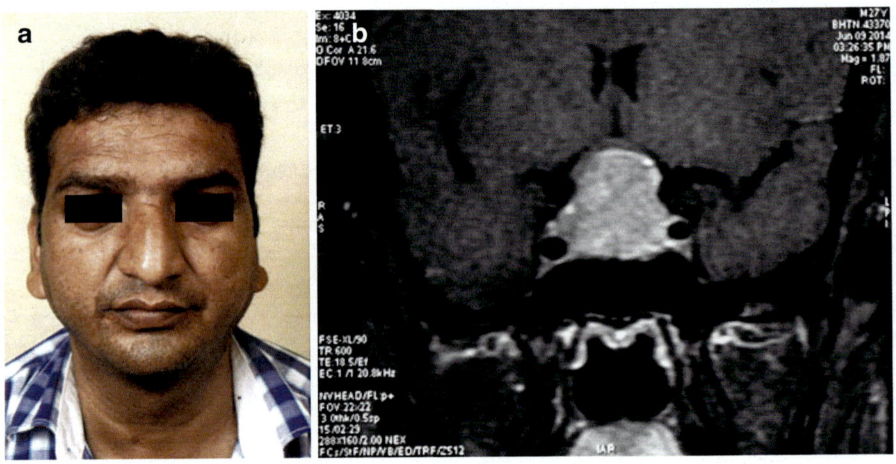

Fig. 1.3 (**a**) Coarse facial features in a patient with prolactinoma suggestive of fugitive acromegaly. (**b**) Coronal CEMR image showing homogenously enhancing sellar–suprasellar mass in the same patient ("figure of 8 appearance")

5. **What is pseudoacromegaly?**

Pseudoacromegaly is characterized by acromegaloid appearance without growth hormone excess. The causes include morbid obesity (severe insulin resistance), pachydermoperiostitis, hypothyroidism, insulin like growth factor 2 (IGF2)-

secreting tumors, insulinoma, and drugs like minoxidil and phenytoin. Pseudoacromegaly in patients with obesity and insulinoma due to the action of insulin on IGF1 receptor (specificity spillover). Presence of digital clubbing helps in differentiating pachydermoperiostitis from acromegaly. Minoxidil and phenytoin cause increased collagen growth and proliferation with abnormal cross-linking, resulting in an acromegaloid appearance. Pseudoacromegaly in patients with primary hypothyroidism is due to abnormal glycosaminoglycans (GAGs) deposition in the soft tissues.

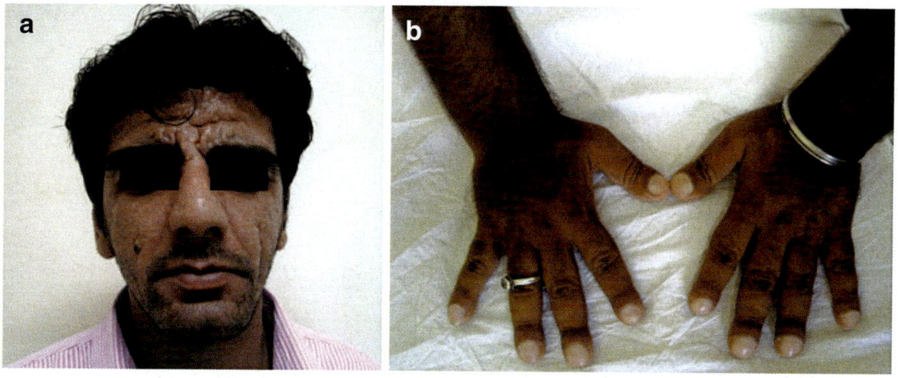

Fig. 1.4 (**a**) Pseudoacromegaly in a patient with pachydermoperiostitis. (**b**) Digital clubbing and broad hands in the same patient

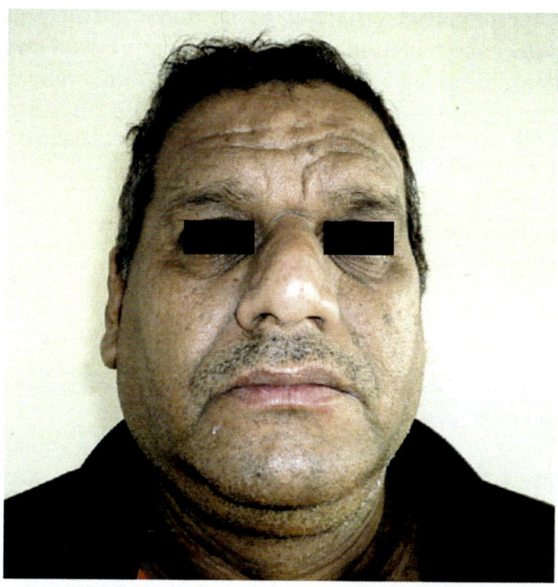

Fig. 1.5 Acromegaloid features in a patient with insulinoma

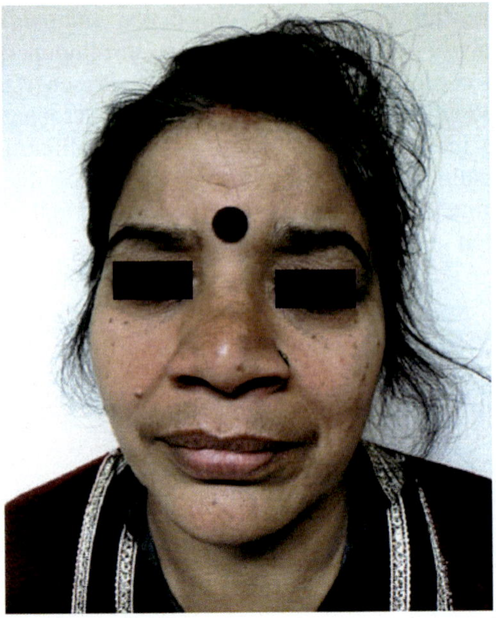

Fig. 1.6 Pseudoacromegaly due to phenytoin therapy

6. **What are the causes of acromegaly?**

   The most common cause of acromegaly is somatotropinoma (99%). The tumor is usually a macroadenoma (in nearly 80%) as the disease is insidious in onset. In addition, paracrine effect of GH–IGF1 on tumor growth and genetic abnormalities like AIP gene mutation and PTTG overexpression contribute to macroadenoma. The table given below enlists the causes of acromegaly.

Causes of acromegaly
Primary growth hormone (GH) excess
Somatotropinoma (99%)
Rarely GH-secreting pancreatic islet cell tumor and lymphoma
Primary growth hormone releasing hormone (GHRH) excess
Eutopic (<1%)
Hypothalamic hamartoma, choristoma, ganglioneuroma
Ectopic (<1%)
Bronchial carcinoid, pancreatic islet cell tumor, small cell lung carcinoma, adrenal adenoma, medullary thyroid carcinoma, pheochromocytoma

7. **Why is ectopic GHRH-secreting tumor more common than ectopic GH-secreting tumor?**

   GHRH has 44 amino acids and is a smaller peptide as compared to GH which has 191 amino acids. It is easier for dedifferentiated tumor cells to produce a peptide with a smaller number of amino acids; therefore, ectopic GHRH-secreting tumors are more common than ectopic GH-secreting tumors.

8. **When to consider the diagnosis of familial acromegaly?**

The diagnosis of familial acromegaly should be considered in acromegalic patients with younger age of onset (<30 years), aggressive tumor behavior, presence or subsequent development of multiple endocrine neoplasia, or family history of pituitary tumor. Causes of familial acromegaly with autosomal dominant inheritance are Carney's complex, familial isolated pituitary adenoma (FIPA), and multiple endocrine neoplasia (MEN1, MEN4). Rarely, paraganglioma-associated *SDH* mutations can be associated with acromegaly. McCune–Albright syndrome is not a cause of familial acromegaly as it is due to postzygotic somatic mutation and not due to germ line mutation.

9. **What are the characteristics of aryl hydrocarbon receptor-interacting protein (AIP) gene mutation-related acromegaly?**

Aryl hydrocarbon receptor-interacting protein (AIP) gene is responsible for ordered cell growth and proliferation in normal individuals. Loss-of-function mutation of the tumor suppressor gene AIP leads to dysregulation of the cell cycle and results in tumorigenesis. AIP gene mutation is responsible for 15–20% of cases of familial isolated pituitary adenoma (FIPA). Somatotropinoma and mixed GH- and prolactin-secreting tumor are the most common tumors associated with AIP mutations. The characteristics of AIP-related acromegaly are younger age of onset, family history of pituitary tumor, and aggressive and invasive adenoma refractory to treatment with somatostatin analogues. AIP-related mutations are also seen in prolactinoma, nonfunctioning pituitary adenoma, thyroid-stimulating hormone-secreting adenoma, and rarely corticotropinoma.

10. **Is there any correlation between clinical phenotype and histopathology of somatotropinoma?**

Clinical and histological correlation among various subtypes of somatotropinomas is summarized in the table below.

Histological subtype	Hormone secreted	Clinical correlation
Densely granulated	GH	Mild disease Good response to treatment
Sparsely granulated	GH	Rapidly progressive Poor response to treatment
Mammosomatotropinoma	GH, PRL	Usually in children Gigantism
Acidophil stem cell adenoma	PRL, GH	Fugitive acromegaly Predominantly hyperprolactinemia

11. **How to define acro-gigantism?**

Acromegaly is a disease of adults, but when GH excess occurs in children and adolescents before epiphyseal fusion, it results in acro-gigantism. It is defined as the height of an individual > 97th percentile or 3SD above normal mean height for age or height >2SD above the mid-parental height with features of acromegaly.

12. **What are the causes of acro-gigantism?**

Growth hormone excess associated with familial syndrome usually results in acro-gigantism and the causes include familial isolated pituitary adenoma, multiple endocrine neoplasia type 1 and Carney's complex. In addition, McCune–Albright syndrome can also lead to acro-gigantism.

13. **Why are all adolescent with GH excess not acro-giants?**

Prepubertal GH–IGF1 excess is expected to result in acro-gigantism. However, only one-third of patients with GH excess during adolescence are acro-giants. Patients who develop acro-gigantism have relatively higher GH–IGF1 levels, normal thyroid function, and concurrent hypogonadism as compared to those who do not develop acro-gigantism. Children with McCune–Albright syndrome with precocious puberty who are untreated, and subsequently develop GH excess may not have acro-gigantism. Further, patients with coexisting hypochondroplasia may not develop acro-gigantism.

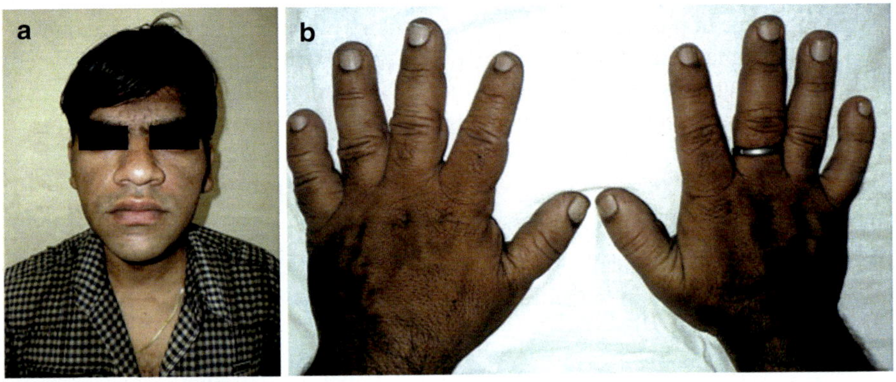

Fig. 1.7 (**a**) Characteristic facial features of acromegaly in an adolescent who had hypochondroplasia, but without acro-gigantism. (**b**) Short stout hands with soft tissue overgrowth in the same patient

14. **What are the characteristics of acromegaly associated with McCune–Albright syndrome?**

The characteristic features of acromegaly associated with McCune–Albright syndrome include younger age of onset, cafe-au-lait macule, fibrous dysplasia, hyperprolactinemia (70%), concurrent endocrinopathies, and lack of demonstrable pituitary adenoma in nearly half of the patients. Medical therapy is preferred in these patients as surgery is difficult, and radiotherapy is associated with an increased risk of osteosarcoma.

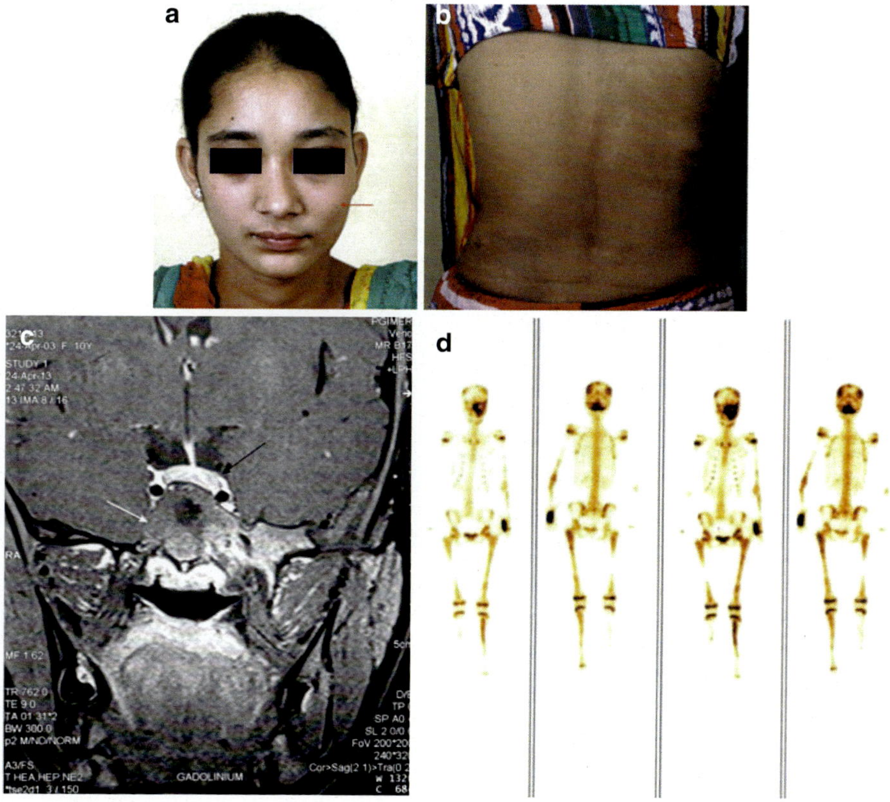

Fig. 1.8 (**a**) A 12-year-old girl with McCune–Albright syndrome who had precocious puberty, acro-gigantism, and hyperthyroidism. Facial asymmetry (*arrow*) due to fibrous dysplasia is also seen. (**b**) Cafe-au-lait macule in the same patient with McCune–Albright syndrome. (**c**) T1W CEMR coronal image showing normal pituitary gland (*black arrow*) in the same patient. Note upward convexity of sellar floor due to sphenoid bone fibrous dysplasia (*white arrow*). (**d**) ^{99m}Tc MDP bone scan showing increased tracer uptake in skull bones in the same patient

15. **What are the unusual presentations of acromegaly?**

    Majority of patients with acromegaly are either diagnosed incidentally or during evaluation for headache, visual symptoms, acral enlargement, arthralgia, and uncontrolled diabetes. The unusual presentations of acromegaly are malocclusion of jaw, diabetic ketoacidosis, pituitary apoplexy, CSF rhinorrhea, facial asymmetry (fibrous dysplasia in McCune–Albright syndrome), tonsillomegaly, recurrent nasal obstruction (nasal polyp), severe hirsutism, entrapment neuropathy, dilated cardiomyopathy, cutis verticis gyrata, and frontal lobe syndrome (antesellar extension of tumor or anterior cerebral artery spasm due to apoplexy).

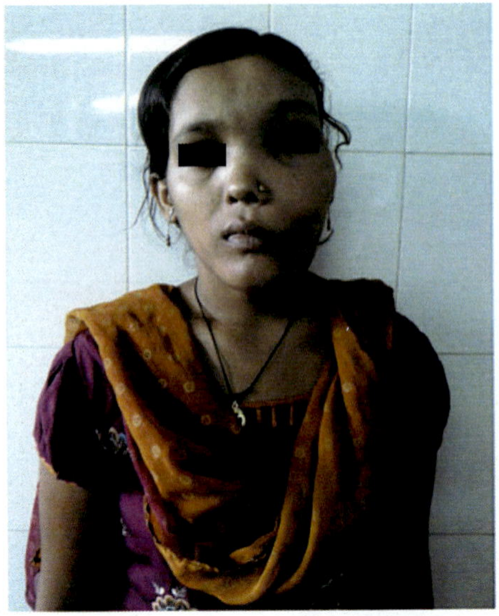

Fig. 1.9 Facial asymmetry (due to fibrous dysplasia) as a presenting manifestation of an acro-giant with McCune–Albright syndrome

16. **What are the emergencies in a patient with acromegaly?**

    Patients with acromegaly can present in emergency due to pituitary apoplexy, subarachnoid hemorrhage (rupture of intracranial arteriovenous malformations), status epilepticus (raised intracranial tension, hyponatremia, and cerebral invasion), paraplegia (intervertebral disc prolapse), accelerated hypertension, diabetic ketoacidosis, gastrointestinal bleed (colonic polyp/carcinoma), cardiac arrhythmias, and acromegalic cardiomyopathy.

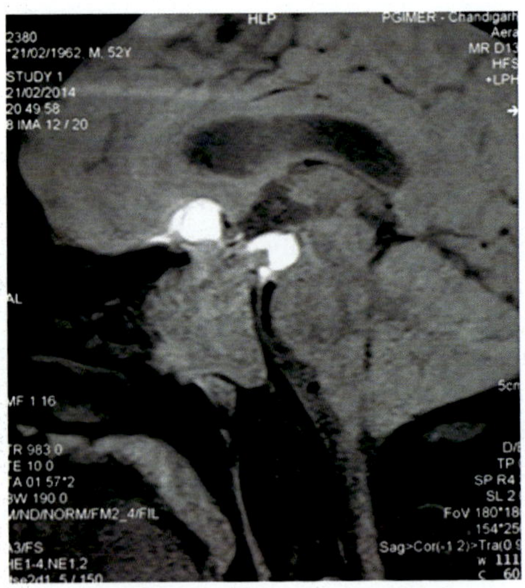

Fig. 1.10 T1W noncontrast sagittal MR image demonstrating pituitary macroadenoma with marked infra- and antesellar extension. Hyperintense areas are suggestive of hemorrhage within the tumor

17. **What are the unusual signs in patients with acromegaly?**

The unusual signs in patients with acromegaly include cutis verticis gyrata ("sulci and gyri"-like appearance on the scalp), facial asymmetry (fibrous dysplasia due to McCune–Albright syndrome and osteitis fibrosa cystica due to primary hyperparathyroidism, MEN1), tonsillomegaly, acromegalic rosary, orchidomegaly, gynecomastia, osteoma and tarsal tunnel syndrome.

18. **What are the causes of cutis verticis gyrata?**

Cutis verticis gyrata is not a specific feature of acromegaly, but is also seen in patients with neurofibroma, pachydermoperiostitis, melanocytic nevi, myxedema, and amyloidosis. The "cerebral convolution"-like appearance in acromegaly is an adaptive response to accommodate excessive soft tissue overgrowth in a limited space under the tight scalp fascia.

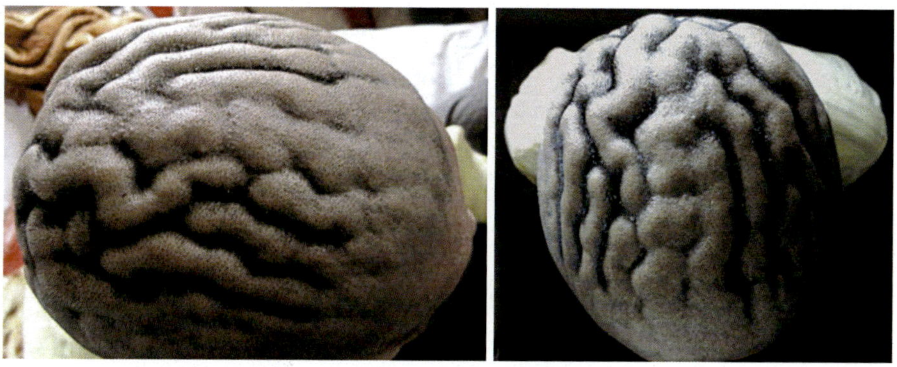

Fig. 1.11 Cutis verticis gyrata in a patient with acromegaly

19. **What are the causes of headache in acromegaly?**

Patients with acromegaly having microadenomas or macroadenomas can present with headache. In microadenomas, it is due to increased intrasellar pressure because of tumor growth in a closed space. In macroadenomas, headache is caused by stretching of the dura (supplied by ophthalmic division of the trigeminal nerve) due to suprasellar extension of tumor or direct involvement of the trigeminal nerve due to cavernous sinus invasion. Other causes of headache related to acromegaly per se, irrespective of tumor size, include calvarial thickening leading to periosteal stretch, osteomas, recurrent sinusitis, and secretion of putative algesic peptides by the tumor tissue. Causes of acute-onset severe headache in a patient with acromegaly include pituitary apoplexy, aneurysmal rupture, or rarely, raised intracranial tension due to hydrocephalus.

20. **What are the causes of macroglossia?**

Macroglossia is considered when the tongue extends beyond the alveolar ridge in the resting state. It is suggested by the presence of indentation marks on the tongue. Causes of macroglossia include acromegaly, primary hypothyroidism, Down's syndrome, amyloidosis, hemangioma, lymphangioma, and tongue neoplasms.

21. **What are the oral manifestations of acromegaly?**

Oral manifestations in a patient with acromegaly include prognathism, thick fleshy lips, increased spacing between teeth, malalignment of jaw, macroglossia and tonsillomegaly. In addition, thickened lamina dura may be present on imaging. Patients with acromegaly may have bony swellings in the oral cavity due to fibrous dysplasia or osteitis fibrosa cystica, when associated with McCune-Albright syndrome and MEN1, respectively.

22. **What are the cutaneous manifestations of acromegaly?**

The cutaneous manifestations in a patient with acromegaly include hyperhidrosis, seborrhea, hirsutism, acanthosis nigricans, skin tags (>3 correlates with the presence of colonic polyps), hyperpigmentation and cutis verticis gyrata. Patients with acromegaly may have cafe-au-lait macules when associated with McCune-Albright syndrome and lipoma, angiofibroma and collagenoma when associated with MEN1 syndrome.

23. **Why are hands warm and moist in patients with acromegaly?**

GH promotes peripheral deiodinase activity and increases T_4 to T_3 neogenesis. This is responsible for the increased adrenergic sensitivity manifesting clinically as warm and moist hands. The direct effect of GH per se, on sweat glands, also contributes. The effect of GH on pilosebaceous units explains the presence of seborrhea in patients with acromegaly.

24. **What are the causes of goiter in acromegaly?**

Goiter is present in 70–80% of patients with acromegaly. Thyroid enlargement may be diffuse or multinodular and is usually associated with normal thyroid function; however, 4–14% of patients may have hyperthyroidism. The causes of goiter in acromegaly include GH–IGF1-mediated growth and proliferation of thyroid follicular cells, McCune–Albright Syndrome, GH and TSH co-secreting adenoma, and medullary thyroid carcinoma with ectopic GHRH secretion. Solitary nodule in a patient with acromegaly should raise the suspicion of papillary thyroid cancer as it is one of the common cancers associated with acromegaly.

25. **What is the effect of GH on thyroid function?**

GH potentiates T_4 to T_3 neogenesis by the activation of 5′-monodeiodinase type 1, decreases thyroxine-binding globulin, and inhibits TSH. Suppression of TSH is mediated by increased somatostatin tone associated with GH excess.

26. **Why do patients with acromegaly have arthralgia?**

Arthralgia and osteoarthritis are common in patients with acromegaly with a prevalence of 50–70%. GH–IGF1 excess results in uneven articular chondrocyte proliferation and matrix production in a limited joint space followed by cartilage destruction leading to arthralgia and osteoarthritis. In addition, synovial hypertrophy and ligament laxity lead to joint instability.

27. **Why do patients with acromegaly have hypertension?**

Hypertension is present in 35–50% of patients with acromegaly. Causes of hypertension include extracellular volume expansion due to the anti-natriuretic action of GH–IGF1 on renal tubules, increased left ventricular mass, insulin resistance/hyperinsulinemia, production of digitalis-like substances, and altered sympathetic activity. Renin–angiotensin–aldosterone axis is suppressed in patients with acromegaly due to volume expansion. Concurrent obstructive sleep apnea also exacerbates hypertension. Diuretics are drug of choice for the management of hypertension in patients with acromegaly.

28. **Why do patients with acromegaly have diabetes?**

Dysglycemia is present in approximately 50% of patients with acromegaly (diabetes 10–15% and prediabetes 20–40%). It is more prevalent in those who have long duration of disease, higher GH levels, and family history of diabetes. Diabetes in acromegaly occurs despite GH-mediated β-cell hyperplasia. GH antagonizes the action of insulin at the liver, skeletal muscle, and adipocytes, and this results in increased hepatic glucose output due to augmented glycogenolysis and gluconeogenesis, reduced uptake of glucose into muscle and adipocytes, and increased lipolysis. Hyperglycemia associated with acromegaly is frequently severe and difficult to treat. Therefore, patients with resistant diabetes should be evaluated for acromegaly.

29. **What are the mechanisms for GH-mediated insulin resistance?**

Acromegaly is characterized by chronic GH and IGF1 excess, and these hormones have opposing effects on glucose metabolism; IGF1 has insulin like effects, whereas GH has insulin-antagonistic properties; the effects of GH predominates over IGF1. IGF1 acts on IGF1/insulin receptor and stimulates insulin-signaling pathway, while GH acts via its own receptor and interferes with the insulin-signaling pathway. Phosphatidylinositol 3-kinase (PI3K) and IRS-1 are involved in post-receptor insulin- signaling pathway. GH increases the p85 subunit of phosphatidylinositol 3-kinase (PI3K), which results in imbalance between p85 and p110 subunits of PI3K, and consequently reduced PI3K signaling. Further, GH increases the serine phosphorylation of IRS-1, thereby preventing its association with the insulin receptor. GH also induces suppressor of cytokine signaling (SOCS) pathway, which prevents tyrosine phosphorylation of IRS-1 and results in insulin resistance. GH also decreases the expression of insulin-sensitizing adipokines like adiponectin and visfatin. In addition, GH promotes lipolysis and increases the serum levels of non-esterified fatty acids, resulting in worsening of insulin resistance.

30. **What are the cardiovascular manifestations in acromegaly?**

Cardiovascular manifestations in acromegaly include cardiomyopathy, heart failure, asymmetrical septal hypertrophy, arrhythmias, and coronary artery disease. Diastolic dysfunction is the earliest abnormality in acromegalic cardiomyopathy, followed by systolic dysfunction and eventually heart failure which is characteristically associated with increased left ventricular muscle mass. Coronary artery disease in acromegaly is due to dyslipidemia, increased procoagulant activity and concurrent diabetes and hypertension. Arrhythmias are present in 40% of patients with acromegaly and include atrial fibrillation, supraventricular tachycardia, bundle branch block, and ventricular ectopy and are usually related to cardiomyopathy. In addition, bradycardia can occur in these patients with the use of octreotide.

31. **Why is there increased cardiovascular risk in acromegaly?**

Cardiovascular disease is the major cause of mortality (60%) in patients with acromegaly. Increased cardiovascular risk is due to hypertension, obstructive sleep apnea, increased left ventricular muscle mass, atherogenic lipid profile, hyperfibrogenemia, increased plasminogen activator inhibitor type 1 (PAI-1), and insulin resistance/hyperinsulinemia. These effects are mediated through GH–IGF1 excess and underscore the need for eusomatotropinemia in these patients.

32. **Why do patients with acromegaly have obstructive sleep apnea?**

Acromegaly is associated with obstructive sleep apnea (OSA) in 40–50% of patients. OSA is due to naso–pharyngo–laryngeal tissue overgrowth, nasal polyps, and macroglossia because of GH–IGF1 excess. In addition, direct effect of GH on the respiratory center causes central sleep apnea. OSA may not remit even after curative surgery.

33. **What are the possibilities when a patient with acromegaly presents with weight loss?**

Patients with acromegaly commonly present with weight gain due to increase in lean muscle mass because of the anabolic effects of GH. However, they may present with weight loss if associated with uncontrolled diabetes, thyrotoxicosis and malignancy. Thyrotoxicosis in acromegaly is due to GH excess per se (4–14%), GH and TSH co-secreting adenoma, or McCune–Albright syndrome. Acromegaly is associated with an increased risk of malignancy of colon, breast, and thyroid.

34. **What are the causes of hirsutism in acromegaly?**

Hirsutism is present in nearly half of the patients with acromegaly. It is due to direct effect of GH–IGF1 on pilosebaceous units and GH-mediated hyperandrogenemia. Hyperandrogenemia is due to decreased SHBG, insulin resistance/hyperinsulinemia, and increased ovarian steroidogenesis. In addition, hyperprolactinemia which is present in 30% of patients with acromegaly can also result in increased androgen production. Hirsutism in these patients is invariably accompanied with menstrual irregularities.

35. **Why do patients with acromegaly have hyperprolactinemia?**

Nearly 30% of patients with acromegaly have hyperprolactinemia. It can be due to stem cell adenoma, mammosomatotropinoma, mixed cell adenoma and stalk hyperprolactinemia. Lactotropes and somatotropes share a common origin during pituitary ontogenesis and this explains the development of stem cell adenoma and mammosomatotropinoma.

36. **What are the causes of menstrual irregularities in acromegaly?**

Menstrual irregularities are present in 40–80% of women with acromegaly and usually present as oligomenorrhea, secondary amenorrhea, and rarely menorrhagia. These manifestations are attributed to low gonadotropins due to mass effect, hyperprolactinemia, secondary polycystic ovarian disease, hyperandrogenemia and hypothyroidism. Despite hypogonadism, these women have endometrial hyperplasia due to the direct effect of GH on endometrial growth and proliferation.

37. **Can patients with acromegaly have menstrual irregularities and galactorrhea despite microadenoma and normal prolactin?**

Menstrual irregularities can occur even in patients with microadenoma and normal prolactin. This can be explained by the presence of hyperandrogenemia due to insulin resistance/hyperinsulinemia, direct GH–IGF1 effect on ovarian steroidogenesis, and decreased SHBG. GH is homologous to prolactin and has intrinsic "prolactin-like activity" (specificity spillover) which explains galactorrhea in some women with acromegaly despite normal prolactin.

38. **What are the causes of endometrial hyperplasia despite amenorrhea?**

The causes of endometrial hyperplasia (endometrial thickness >10 mm) despite amenorrhea are acromegaly, polycystic ovarian disease, and drugs like tamoxifen. Endometrial hyperplasia in acromegaly is due to the direct proliferative effect of GH–IGF1 on the endometrium, despite low gonadotropins.

39. **What is the difference in the pathogenesis of polycystic ovarian disease due to acromegaly from classical polycystic ovarian disease?**

Secondary polycystic ovarian disease (PCOD) is common in patients with acromegaly. PCOD related to acromegaly is due to the direct effects of GH–

IGF1 on ovary and is independent of LH as opposed to classical polycystic ovarian disease where LH plays an important role in thecal growth and proliferation.

40. **What are the peripheral neurological manifestations related to GH–IGF1 excess?**

Peripheral neurological manifestations associated with GH–IGF1 excess are entrapment neuropathy (eg., carpal tunnel and tarsal tunnel syndrome), peripheral neuropathy, compressive myelopathy (due to disc prolapse) and lumbar canal stenosis. Thickened peripheral nerve is also a feature of acromegaly and is due to perineural deposition of glycosaminoglycans (GAGs).

41. **Does brain size increase in acromegaly?**

Brain parenchymal tissue does not increase in size in response to GH–IGF1 excess. Nevertheless, patients with acromegaly have increased risk of cerebrovascular accidents, cerebral aneurysms, and radiation-induced brain damage (RIBD) due to detrimental effects of GH–IGF1 excess on cerebral vasculature.

42. **Do patients with acromegaly have increased prevalence of cerebral aneurysms?**

Yes. The available literature points to an increased prevalence of cerebral aneurysms (7–10%) in patients with acromegaly. Altered ratio of type-III to type-I collagen due to GH–IGF1 excess leads to degeneration of vessel wall and consequently results in the development of aneurysms. The cerebral aneurysms in patients with acromegaly are usually located in the internal carotid artery and rarely in the vertebrobasilar artery.

43. **Can patients with acromegaly have proximal muscle weakness?**

Yes. GH–IGF1 is required for the development and maintenance of lean muscle mass. However, acromegaly may be associated with proximal myopathy due to atrophy of type 2 muscle fibers with relative hypertrophy of type 1 fibers. In addition, hyperphosphatemia may also contribute to muscle weakness. Patients with acromegaly who have myelo-radiculopathy may also manifest proximal muscle weakness.

44. **What are the causes of anemia in acromegaly?**

GH plays a permissive role in erythropoiesis. Therefore, anemia in a patient with acromegaly is unusual and requires evaluation. The causes of anemia in acromegaly are gastrointestinal bleed due to adenomatous polyp, colonic carcinoma, acid peptic disease (MEN1, Zollinger–Ellison syndrome), and malabsorption due to megacolon and bacterial stasis (blind-loop syndrome). In addition, hypothyroidism, hypogonadism, and hypocortisolism may also contribute to the development of anemia.

45. **What are the causes of altered sensorium in a patient with acromegaly?**

The causes of altered sensorium in a patient with acromegaly are pituitary apoplexy, subarachnoid hemorrhage due to rupture of cerebral aneurysm, hypoglycemia (cortisol deficiency), and hyponatremia (cortisol and thyroxine deficiency). Further, generalized tonic clonic seizure (dyselectrolytemia, raised intracranial tension) and occasionally diabetic ketoacidosis can also result in altered sensorium in a patient with acromegaly.

46. **What are the alterations in calcium and phosphate metabolism in acromegaly?**

Hyperphosphatemia and hypercalciuria are the biochemical alterations in mineral metabolism in a patient with acromegaly. Hyperphosphatemia is a result of increased reabsorption of phosphate from proximal tubules as a consequence of GH excess. Serum calcium is normal in patients with acromegaly and the presence of hypercalcemia suggests MEN1-related primary hyperparathyroidism. Serum PTH levels may also be elevated in patients with acromegaly due to the direct stimulatory effect of GH and hyperphosphatemia on parathyroid cells. Hypercalciuria is the result of increased calcium absorption and decreased renal reabsorption of calcium due to elevated 1,25 dihydroxy vitamin D (as a consequence of GH-mediated increase in 1α- hydroxylase activity).

47. **What is the fracture risk in acromegaly?**

GH per se increases bone mineral density (BMD) at both hip and vertebrae, but this increase in BMD has been demonstrated only in eugonadal patients. The available literature regarding fracture risk in patients with acromegaly is conflicting; however, the data are inclined towards an increased fracture risk. Fracture in a patient with acromegaly, especially vertebral, is due to concurrent hypogonadism, secondary hyperparathyroidism (GH-mediated increase in PTH), and poor bone microarchitecture despite increased BMD on DXA. In addition, coexisting fibrous dysplasia (McCune–Albright syndrome) and osteitis fibrosa cystica (MEN1-related PHPT) may result in increased fracture risk.

48. **Is colonoscopy advised in all patients with acromegaly?**

Yes. Although there is no increase in the risk of colonic carcinoma in patients with acromegaly, most studies demonstrate an increased risk of adenomatous polyps and a higher risk of mortality with colonic carcinoma in patients with acromegaly as compared to those without acromegaly. Hence, a baseline screening colonoscopy is advised in all patients with acromegaly. Further, the risk of colonic neoplasia persist even after cure of acromegaly; therefore, periodic surveillance is recommended.

49. **What are the malignancies associated with acromegaly?**

Apart from colonic neoplasia, other malignancies associated with acromegaly are papillary thyroid carcinoma, infiltrating duct carcinoma of the breast, and melanoma. Although the risk of prostatic hyperplasia is increased, risk of prostatic cancer is uncertain. Prolonged exposure to GH–IGF1 excess leads to sustained activation of the MAP kinase pathway and oncogene overexpression, resulting in abnormal cell growth and proliferation.

50. **What are the organs which are devoid of growth-promoting effects of GH?**

Almost every organ in body requires GH–IGF1 for their growth and proliferation. The only exceptions are brain and eye, as their growth is GH–IGF1 independent.

Suggested Reading

1. Jameson JL, De Groot LJ. Endocrinology: adult and pediatric. Philadelphia: Elsevier Health Sciences; 2010.
2. Katznelson L, Atkinson JL, Cook DM, Ezzat SZ, Hamrahian AH, Miller KK. American Association of Clinical Endocrinologists medical guidelines for clinical practice for the diagnosis and treatment of acromegaly-2011 update. Endocr Pract. 2011;17:1–44.
3. Longo D, Fauci A, Kasper D, Hauser S, Jameson J, Loscalzo J. Harrison's principles of internal medicine. 18th ed. New York: McGraw Hill Professional; 2012.
4. Melmed S, Polonsky KS, Larsen PR, Kronenberg HM. Williams textbook of endocrinology: expert consult. London: Elsevier Health Sciences; 2011.

Acromegaly: Diagnosis and Treatment

2

2.1 Clinical Rounds

1. **A 42-year-old male presented with chronic and persistent headache. On examination, he was found to have acral enlargement with increased sweating. What to do next?**

   The best screening test for the diagnosis of acromegaly is serum insulin like growth factor 1 (IGF1), with a sensitivity of 97% and specificity of 90%. Serum IGF1 is chosen as a screening test because it is a measure of integrated GH secretion, has a long half-life (12–15 h) and is secreted in a non-pulsatile manner. In addition, serum IGF1 has a log-linear relationship with circulating GH levels.

2. **Who should be screened for acromegaly?**

   Screening is recommended in patients with typical signs and symptoms of acromegaly. In addition, patients having multiple comorbidities like type 2 diabetes mellitus, hypertension, sleep apnea syndrome, debilitating arthritis, carpal tunnel syndrome, and hyperhidrosis should be screened, even if they do not have typical features of acromegaly.

3. **What are the causes of low IGF1 in patients with acromegaly?**

   GH-mediated IGF1 generation is facilitated by T_4, insulin, testosterone, and low concentration of estrogen and is inhibited by cytokines. The causes of low IGF1 in patients with acromegaly include uncontrolled diabetes mellitus, hypothyroidism, hypogonadism, hepatic or renal failure, malnutrition, systemic illness, catabolic states, and oral estrogen therapy.

A. Bhansali, Y. Gogate, *Clinical Rounds in Endocrinology: Volume I - Adult Endocrinology*, DOI 10.1007/978-81-322-2398-6_2

4. **Why is IGFBP3 not used in the diagnosis of acromegaly?**

IGFBP3 reflects integrated GH secretion, has a long half-life and, as compared to IGF1, has lesser assay variability. However, IGFBP3 is less tightly regulated by GH as compared to IGF1 and the level of IGFBP3 in patients with acromegaly frequently overlap with those found in normal individuals; hence it is not used in the diagnosis of acromegaly.

5. **What are the alterations in GH dynamics in acromegaly?**

The circulating molecular variant of GH is 22 kD in normal individuals as well as in patients with acromegaly. A normal individual has 6–10 GH pulses in 24 h (5–6 pulses at night and 3–4 pulses at daytime). Nocturnal GH pulses begin 90 min after sleep and coincide with NREM sleep, while daytime pulses coincide with post-absorptive period. The amplitude of GH pulse extends from 0.5 to 20 ng/ml in healthy individuals. Patients with active acromegaly have increase in frequency and amplitude of GH pulses, non-suppressible GH after glucose load, and elevated levels of IGF1 and IGFBP3. The GH response to TRH, which is normally present only in infants, reappears in patients with acromegaly. This has been attributed to GHRH and TRH receptor fusion or GHRH receptor dedifferentiation on somatotropinoma.

6. **A patient with clinical features of acromegaly has an elevated serum IGF1. Is further testing required for confirmation of diagnosis?**

Yes, GH suppression test is required to confirm the diagnosis, as IGF1 is a screening test. GH suppression test after 75 g oral glucose load is considered as the "gold standard" for the diagnosis of GH excess. The inability to suppress serum GH to <1 ng/mL after oral glucose load is diagnostic of active acromegaly.

7. **What are the causes of non-suppressible GH after glucose load other than acromegaly?**

Uncontrolled diabetes, hypothyroidism, puberty, pregnancy, depression, chronic liver or renal disease, and anorexia nervosa are associated with non-suppressible GH after glucose load, in addition to acromegaly.

8. **How does glucose suppress growth hormone?**

Hypoglycemia is a potent stimulus for GH secretion, while acute hyperglycemia suppresses GH. In healthy subjects, acute glucose load increases somatostatin tone by its action on glucoreceptors on the hypothalamus, thereby resulting in suppression of GH. In addition, acute glucose load also suppresses ghrelin secretion. Ghrelin is an orexigenic peptide which stimulates GH secretion by potentiating the effect of GHRH. Therefore, decrease in ghrelin levels after acute glucose load also contributes to GH suppression. At the level of the hypothalamus, various neurotransmitters like opioids, GABA, serotonin, and cholinergic and $\alpha 2$-adrenergic systems are involved in the modulation of GH secretion, in response to glucose load. However, in patients with acromegaly because of autonomous secretion of GH from the adenoma, the suppressive effect of glucose on GH secretion is mitigated. On the contrary, in patients with chronic hyperglycemia (e.g., uncontrolled diabetes), the GH inhibitory effect of glucose is lost, via decreased IGF1-mediated feedback to the hypothalamus.

9. **A 37-year-old female presented with classical features of acromegaly. MRI of the sella revealed a macroadenoma of 34 × 21 × 20 mm. Is there a need to estimate IGF1 and GH after glucose load?**

   Estimation of serum IGF1 and GH after glucose load is required for confirmation of diagnosis of acromegaly and is also useful in differentiating active versus inactive disease. In addition, it can predict the outcome of pituitary surgery, as patients with GH levels >40 ng/ml are unlikely to achieve cure. GH and IGF1 estimation is also helpful in monitoring the disease during follow-up.

10. **What are the causes of discordant GH and IGF1 values in acromegaly?**

    Patients with clinically active acromegaly usually have concordant IGF1 and GH values, but it can be a diagnostic dilemma when the values are discordant. It needs to be confirmed that age-matched normative data is used for the interpretation of serum IGF1 levels. Some studies have shown that IGFBP3 may be useful in case of discrepancy between GH and IGF1. The table given below enlists the clinical situations that can have discordant GH and IGF1 values in patients with acromegaly.

Non-suppressed GH and low/normal IGF1	Suppressed GH and high IGF1
Poorly controlled DM	Mild acromegaly
Hypothyroidism	Immediate postoperative period
Oral contraceptive use	Post-radiotherapy
Liver failure	Hyperthyroidism
Renal failure	
Hyperthyroidism	
Early recurrence after surgery	
Somatostatin analogue therapy	
Dopamine agonist therapy	
Pegvisomant therapy	

11. **When is IGF1 more reliable than GH in acromegaly?**

    Patients with mild acromegaly and fugitive acromegaly usually have elevated IGF1 and suppressible GH. In patients with poorly controlled diabetes and in those who have received previous radiotherapy, IGF1 is more reliable than glucose-suppressed GH levels. Postoperatively, up to one-third of patients may have discordant results between IGF1 and glucose-suppressed GH levels. In this scenario, the normalization of IGF1 is more reliable than glucose-suppressed GH for monitoring of response to therapy as IGF1 is a better predictor of active disease than GH. Further, treatment with pegvisomant should be monitored only with IGF1.

12. **What are the alterations in the GH–IGF1 axis in patients of acromegaly with uncontrolled diabetes?**

Patients of acromegaly with poorly controlled diabetes have high basal GH, non-suppressible GH after glucose load and low IGF1 levels. Decreased IGF1 in patients with uncontrolled diabetes is due to relative hypoinsulinemia, as optimal levels of insulin are required for GH-mediated IGF1 generation. IGF1 has direct inhibitory effect on pituitary, while at the hypothalamus, it inhibits GHRH and increases somatostatin tone. Low levels of serum IGF1 result in loss of feedback inhibitory effect at pituitary gland and hypothalamus, thereby resulting in increased GH secretion.

13. **How to evaluate for GH–IGF1 excess in patients of acromegaly with uncontrolled diabetes?**

Ideally, patients should be evaluated for GH excess after optimizing blood glucose control (not necessary to normalize HbA1c) by estimation of serum IGF1 and GH response to glucose load. Nevertheless, the presence of an elevated IGF1 in the presence of uncontrolled blood glucose is highly suggestive of active acromegaly. In addition, the estimation of serum IGFBP3 may be helpful as it is not influenced by the degree of glycemic control.

14. **What are the investigations required in a patient with acromegaly after confirmation of diagnosis?**

After confirmation of diagnosis of acromegaly, serum calcium, phosphorus, blood glucose, and lipid profile should be estimated. Hormonal profile include T_4, TSH, 0800 h cortisol, testosterone/estradiol, and prolactin. Contrast enhanced MRI sella should be done to localize the source of GH excess. Computed tomography is required, especially in children to look for the pneumatization of the sella and fibrous dysplasia. The visual field and visual acuity need to be assessed. ECG should be done in all patients. Colonoscopy should be performed at baseline; multi-detector CT colonoscopy may be an alternative. X-ray spine should be done in patients with kyphoscoliosis, and DXA is necessary in hypogonadal subjects for evaluation of osteoporosis. Measurement of GHRH is indicated in patients with acromegaly when the cause is suspected to be ectopic.

15. **What are the possibilities to be considered when MR sellar imaging does not reveal an adenoma in a patient with acromegaly?**

The most common cause of acromegaly is somatotropinoma (99%) and is invariably visualized on sellar imaging. However, some patients with acromegaly may not have a pituitary adenoma on sellar imaging, and the causes include silent apoplexy, ectopic GHRH-secreting neuroendocrine tumors, McCune–Albright syndrome, and rarely ectopic pituitary adenoma (e.g., sphenoid sinus). Patients with ectopic GHRH-secreting neuroendocrine tumors and McCune–Albright syndrome may have diffuse pituitary enlargement. The following images show a classical case of acromegaly due to ectopic GHRH-secreting bronchial carcinoid, which was confirmed on immunohistochemistry.

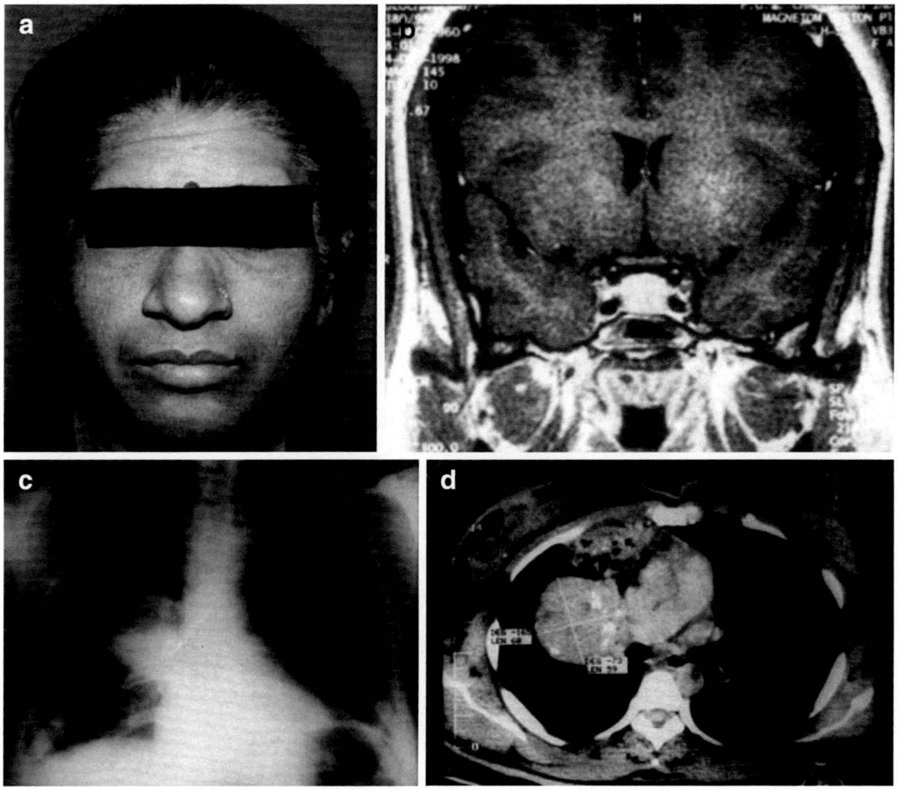

Fig. 2.1 (**a**) A patient with classical facial features of acromegaly. (**b**) T1W CEMRI coronal image showing diffuse pituitary enlargement due to ectopic GHRH secretion from a bronchial carcinoid. (**c**) X-ray chest PA view showing right hilar mass in the same patient. (**d**) CT chest showing a well-defined heterogeneous mass in the right lung

16. **How to prepare a patient with acromegaly for pituitary surgery?**

    Patients with acromegaly must have preoperative cardiac evaluation, airway assessment, adequate replacement therapy for pituitary hormone deficiencies, and optimal blood glucose and blood pressure control. Echocardiography should be done in those who have symptoms or signs of heart disease or abnormal ECG.

17. **What is the prevalence of microadenoma in patients with acromegaly?**

    The most common cause of acromegaly is somatotropinoma (99%). Majority of these patients have macroadenoma (75–80%), while the rest have microadenoma (20–25%).

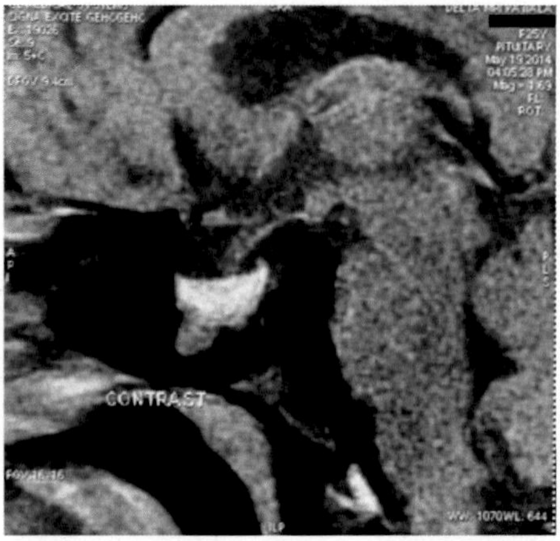

Fig. 2.2 T1W CEMRI sagittal image showing infrasellar polypoidal microadenoma in a patient with acromegaly

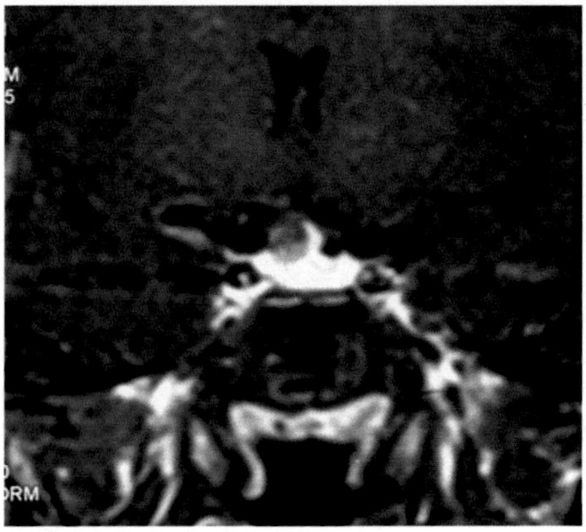

Fig. 2.3 T1W CEMRI coronal image showing pituitary microadenoma abutting infundibulum in a patient with acromegaly

18. **What is the primary modality of therapy in patients with acromegaly?**

    Transsphenoidal surgery is the primary modality of therapy in all patients with acromegaly, irrespective of tumor size. The surgical cure rate is 80–90% in patients with microadenoma and 50% in macroadenoma.

19. **What are the factors associated with poor response to treatment in acromegaly?**

    The factors that predict persistence of disease after surgery and/or medical therapy are younger age at onset, large and invasive tumors (e.g., cavernous sinus invasion), serum GH >40 ng/ml, AIP gene mutation, sparsely granulated tumors on histology (hyperintense on T2-weighted MR imaging), and overexpression of tumor proliferative indices like Ki67, p53, and pituitary tumor transforming gene (PTTG). In addition, reduced expression of somatostatin receptors subtype 2 and subtype 5 by the tumor is associated with poor response to therapy with somatostatin receptor analogues. The images illustrated below shows a young woman with acromegaly who is unlikely to be cured by surgery because of large invasive adenoma.

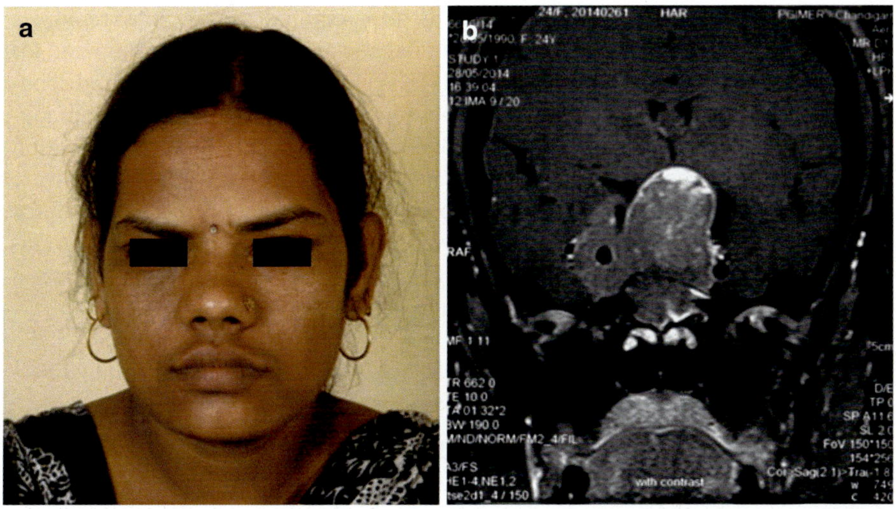

Fig. 2.4 (**a**) A 24-year-old female with classical facial features of acromegaly. (**b**) T1W CEMRI coronal image showing macroadenoma with suprasellar extension and right cavernous sinus invasion

20. **What is the immediate clinical response after curative surgery in acromegaly?**

    After curative surgery, the immediate clinical response includes polyuria (due to excretion of glycosaminoglycans), resolution of headache, decreased sweating and seborrhea, and reduction in the requirement of antihypertensives and antidiabetic medications.

21. **How to predict remission/cure in the immediate postoperative period in patients with acromegaly?**

    Immediate postoperative estimation of GH has been found to be useful in the prediction of remission in patients with acromegaly. A postoperative day 1 fasting serum GH level <2 ng/mL is predictive of clinical and biochemical remission at 5 years. GH–GTT can be performed as early as the 1st week postoperatively, and nadir GH level <1 ng/ml is predictive of remission in 98% individuals at 5 years. However, immediate postoperative assessment of GH (random or GH–GTT) may be influenced by surgical stress-induced increase in GH secretion; hence the current guidelines do not favor this approach.

22. **How to monitor a patient with acromegaly in the immediate postoperative period?**

    Monitoring of urine output and serum electrolytes is essential during the first postoperative week for the diagnosis of diabetes insipidus. Frequent monitoring of blood glucose and blood pressure is also required as they may require a reduction in antihypertensive and antidiabetic medications. Assessment for hypothalamo–pituitary–adrenocortical (HPA) axis should be done after discontinuation of hydrocortisone for 24 h between day 1–3 in those who were preoperatively on cortisol replacement, as there is rapid recovery of HPA axis within hours after surgery in patients with acromegaly. However, those who were eucortisolic preoperatively should also be reevaluated between day 1 and 3 for any corticotrope injury intraoperatively. Thyroid function test should be evaluated after 6 weeks of surgery as there is thyroid hormone reserve lasting for 6–8 weeks, and serum T_4 is the test of choice.

23. **What is the ideal time to assess disease activity and residual pituitary function in patients with acromegaly postoperatively?**

    Although immediate assessment of GH is useful to predict the success of surgery, the ideal time to assess disease activity is 3 months after surgery, as perioperative tissue edema and ischemia resolve by this time and allow the recovery of residual pituitary functions. The table enlists the parameters to be assessed at the end of 3 months.

Clinical assessment	Soft tissue regression
	Disease activity (e.g., hyperhidrosis, seborrhea, headache, arthralgia)
	Visual field and acuity
Biochemical assessment	IGF1 and random GH
	GH following glucose load if random GH >1 ng/ml
	T_4, 0800 h cortisol, prolactin, testosterone/estradiol
MR imaging	If disease is biochemically active

24. **How to define cure in acromegaly?**

    Resolution of symptoms and signs, normalization of age-adjusted IGF1, random GH <1 ng/ml and restoration of GH suppressibility after glucose load (<0.4 ng/ml), preservation of other pituitary hormone with complete removal/disappearance of the tumor is defined as cure in acromegaly. However, currently the term "cure" is not preferred as majority of patients with acromegaly harbor macroadenoma, which is less likely to be cured. Therefore, patients are classified as having either "controlled" or "active disease." Controlled disease is defined as resolution of symptoms and signs, normalization of age-adjusted IGF1, and random GH <1 ng/ml or nadir GH <0.4 ng/ml after glucose load. Elevated age-adjusted IGF1 and random GH >1 ng/ml or nadir GH after glucose load >0.4 ng/ml with or without clinical signs or symptoms of acromegaly are defined as active disease.

25. **Why does serum IGF1 normalization take a longer time?**

Serum IGF1 may take weeks to months to decline into the normal range despite cure of acromegaly. The slow decline in serum IGF1 is related to sustained hepatic sensitivity to GH and insidious decrease in IGFBP3 due to their long half-life.

26. **How to interpret discordant GH and IGF1 levels postoperatively in a patient with acromegaly?**

Assessment of GH–IGF1 axis should be done after 3 months of surgery. Normalization of serum IGF1 and random GH <1 ng/ml or nadir GH after glucose load <0.4 ng/ml suggests controlled disease. However, the results of GH and IGF1 can be discordant in one-third of patients. This is attributed to the disruption of neural or anatomical network of GH regulation after surgery. Patients with a normal age-adjusted serum IGF1 despite random GH >1 ng/ml /non-suppressible GH (>0.4 ng/ml) after glucose load are at a higher risk of recurrence and should remain under close follow-up. On the contrary, a patient with suppressed GH but elevated IGF1 levels should be considered as having active disease and be treated accordingly.

27. **What are the clinical features which are irreversible in a patient with acromegaly after curative surgery?**

Skeletal manifestations like prognathism, osteoarthritis, and kyphoscoliosis are usually irreversible in patients with acromegaly even after curative surgery. Further, hypertension, valvulopathy, and central sleep apnea may not improve. Soft tissue overgrowth usually regresses after curative surgery, although macroglossia and laryngeal hypertrophy may take a longer time to regress. However, in some patients even soft tissue changes may not regress, as long-standing disease results in soft tissue fibrosis consequent to deposition of glycosaminoglycans.

28. **When should primary medical treatment be considered in patients with acromegaly?**

Primary medical therapy should be considered in patients with acromegaly who are at high risk for surgery due to multiple comorbidities and those who refuse surgery. Primary medical treatment is also an option in patients with invasive macroadenoma (e.g., parasellar extension) without mass effects, as they are unlikely to be cured after surgery. In addition, primary medical therapy is preferred in patients with McCune–Albright syndrome either because of absence of tumor (constitutive activation of Gsα subunit) or difficult surgery due to cranial fibrous dysplasia. The available medical treatment options for acromegaly are somatostatin receptor ligands, dopamine agonists, and pegvisomant (GH receptor antagonist). The major disadvantage with medical therapy is that treatment is lifelong and expensive.

29. **When is medical treatment discouraged as a primary modality?**

    Medical treatment as a primary modality should be discouraged in patients with microadenoma, where the cure rate after surgery is 80–90%.

30. **What are the indications of preoperative medical therapy in patients with acromegaly?**

    Few studies have shown that preoperative use of somatostatin receptor ligands (for 3–6 months) particularly in patients with invasive macroadenoma was associated with higher remission rates after surgery as documented by normalization of serum IGF1. However, this has been debated, as normalization of IGF1 postoperatively may be a "carryover effect" of preoperative somatostatin therapy, rather than effective removal of tumor. Therefore, in the current scenario preoperative medical therapy is recommended only in those who have acromegalic cardiomyopathy or in those with obstructive sleep apnea syndrome.

31. **Does prior surgery influence the efficacy of somatostatin receptor ligand therapy?**

    Yes. Surgical debulking improves the efficacy of somatostatin receptor ligand therapy, possibly because of decreased tumor burden. In a prospective study, primary somatostatin receptor ligand therapy resulted in normalization of GH and IGF1 in 31 and 42% of patients, while after surgical debulking somatostatin receptor ligand therapy resulted in normalization of GH and IGF1 in 69% and 89%, respectively.

32. **How to manage patients of acromegaly with active disease after transsphenoidal surgery?**

    The options available to treat patients with acromegaly having active disease after TSS include repeat surgery, medical therapy and radiotherapy. Redo surgery should be considered in patients when the residual tumor is intrasellar as they are likely to be cured, while those with suprasellar extension and mass effects should undergo surgical debulking. However, redo surgery is technically more challenging due to distorted anatomy and is associated with a higher rate of complications. Further, tumors with parasellar extension are not amenable to redo surgery. Medical therapy for somatotropinoma include somatostatin receptor ligands, dopamine agonists and pegvisomant (GH receptor antagonist), either alone or in combination. Medical therapy is lifelong and expensive. Radiotherapy can be delivered as conventional fractionated therapy or stereotactic radiosurgery. However, a long lag time for normalization of GH–IGF1, need for medical management during interim period, and progressive development of hypopituitarism are the limitations of radiotherapy. Therefore, in clinical practice, redo surgery should be considered wherever it is feasible. Otherwise, radiotherapy with interim medical therapy should be offered to a patient with persistent disease.

33. **What is the preferred medical treatment in acromegaly?**

The preferred drugs in patients with acromegaly are somatostatin receptor ligands: octreotide and lanreotide. They have affinity for somatostatin receptor subtype 2 and subtype 5; however, their affinity for receptor subtype 2 is ten times higher, which is the predominant subtype expressed in somatotropinomas. Somatostatin receptor ligands suppress the release of GH via inhibition of cyclic AMP and exert antiproliferative action through cell cycle arrest, karyorrhexis, and impaired angiogenesis.

34. **What is the role of pasireotide in acromegaly?**

Pasireotide is a pan-somatostatin receptor ligand with high affinity for somatostatin receptor subtypes 1, 2, 3, and 5, with predominant affinity for subtype 5. A recent study compared pasireotide LAR and octreotide LAR in patients with acromegaly and showed higher rates of IGF1 normalization (38.6% vs. 23.6%) with pasireotide LAR, though GH normalization was similar (48.3% vs. 51.6%) in both the groups. This difference in GH and IGF1 response can be explained by the additional effect of pasireotide on hepatocytes (which express SSTR 1, 3, and 5 subtypes) and greater inhibitory effect on insulin secretion (as insulin also mediates IGF1 generation). However, hyperglycemia was more common in patients treated with pasireotide (28.7% vs. 8.3%). Pasireotide may also be useful in the management of patients with sparsely granulated somatotropinomas, who are commonly resistant to conventional SRL therapy, because these tumors predominantly express somatostatin receptor subtype 5.

35. **What is the dose schedule of somatostatin receptor ligands in patients with acromegaly?**

Octreotide LAR is given as an intramuscular injection once a month. The initial dose is 20mg monthly. If serum IGF1 does not normalize within 3 months, dose can be increased to 30–40mg per month. Lanreotide-sustained release is administered at a dose of 30mg every 7–14 days intramuscularly. Lanreotide autogel or depot is administered at a dose of 60–120mg every 4 to 6 weeks deep subcutaneously. Side effects related to the use of somatostatin analogues include gastrointestinal discomfort, gallstone disease, and dysglycemia. If hyperglycemia develops on somatostatin receptor ligand therapy, pegvisomant is preferred. Daily therapy with short-acting somatostatin receptor analogue octreotide is advocated for initial 2 weeks to assess the response and systemic tolerability. However, this is seldom followed in clinical practice.

36. **Why is there a dichotomy between clinical and biochemical response in patients during treatment with somatostatin receptor ligands?**

    There is a dichotomy in the clinical and biochemical response in patients with acromegaly who are treated with somatostatin receptor ligands (SRL), both in terms of onset and frequency of response. Clinical improvement in symptoms like headache, sweating, soft tissue swelling, and sleep apnea occurs rapidly, despite delayed normalization of GH (3–6 months) and IGF1 levels (6–12 months). Further, improvement in symptoms occurs in more than 80% of patients, while GH and IGF1 are normalized in 44% and 34%, respectively, when used as primary therapy and in 57% and 67%, respectively, when used after TSS. The reason for this dichotomy is that even minor reduction in GH and IGF1 levels leads to improvement in clinical profile.

37. **What is the efficacy of different available treatment modalities in the management of acromegaly?**

    The efficacy of different treatment modalities available in the management of acromegaly is summarized in the table given below.

Parameters	Surgery	Radiotherapy (conventional or stereotactic radiosurgery)	SRL Drug naive	SRL Adjuvant therapy (after TSS)	Pegvisomant	DA
GH <2.5 ng/ml	Microadenoma 80–90%, Macroadenoma 50%	35% at 10 years	44%	57%	Initial rise, followed by plateau	<15%
Normalization of serum IGF1	Microadenoma 80–90%, Macroadenoma 50%	30% at 10 years	34%	67%	90–97%	<15%
Reduction in tumor size (% of patients)	–	50% at 10–20 years	52%	21%	No change, may increase	30%
Tumor progression[a]	0–10%	0.3%	<1–2.2%	<1–2.2%	2–3%	NA

[a]Denotes tumor regrowth after surgery or radiotherapy and tumor progression during medical management

It is noteworthy that treatment-naive patients with acromegaly respond poorly to SRL therapy in terms of GH and IGF1 normalization but have a higher response in terms of tumor shrinkage, while SRL therapy when used as an adjuvant to surgery, biochemical response rate is higher, but the tumor reduction is poor.

38. **How to define "somatostatin receptor ligand resistance" in acromegaly?**

"Somatostatin receptor ligand resistance" in acromegaly is defined as failure to reduce serum GH and IGF1 levels to <50% or tumor shrinkage <20% or increase in tumor size despite optimal treatment with somatostatin ligands for at least 1 year.

39. **Dopamine agonists (levodopa) are useful to assess GH reserve in a short child and are also effective as treatment (cabergoline) in acromegaly. Why is it so?**

Cabergoline is the most effective dopamine agonist for the treatment of acromegaly. Dopamine, through its action on the hypothalamus, causes GH release by increasing GHRH and, through its action on the pituitary gland, inhibits GH release. In the physiological state, hypothalamic action of DA predominates, thereby increasing GH secretion, which is exploited in testing GH reserve. However, in patients with acromegaly, D_2 receptors are overexpressed on somatotropinoma, and DAs directly inhibit GH release through its action on the pituitary gland thereby overcoming the hypothalamic effects.

40. **What is the role of cabergoline in the management of acromegaly?**

Cabergoline normalizes GH and IGF1 only in <15% of patients, without significant reduction in tumor size. It is helpful in those with mildly elevated IGF1 as an adjunctive therapy after surgical debulking, during interim period following radiotherapy, or in those with suboptimal response to somatostatin receptor ligand therapy. Cabergoline is less expensive and orally administered, and the dose ranges from 0.5 to 1 mg per day. However, there is a greater risk of valvulopathy in patients with acromegaly as higher doses of cabergoline are used in these patients as compared to patients with prolactinoma.

41. **Does the concurrent hyperprolactinemia or prolactin immunostaining positivity predict the response to cabergoline?**

Hyperprolactinemia or prolactin immunopositivity on tumor tissue does not predict response to cabergoline in majority of the studies.

42. **What is pegvisomant?**

Pegvisomant is a GH receptor antagonist. GH molecule has two binding sites, site 1 and site 2, which bind with their corresponding sites on two GH receptors. Binding of native GH to both these receptor sites is necessary for the dimerization of receptors and activation of JAK–STAT pathway. Pegvisomant also has two binding sites, but only site 1 can bind with the receptor, whereas site 2 cannot bind with its receptor. Pegvisomant prevents binding of site 1 of native GH to its corresponding site on the receptor, thereby preventing the action of GH. This is illustrated in the figure 2.5. Pegvisomant is indicated in SRL therapy-resistant acromegaly and in patients of acromegaly with worsening of glycemic status on SRL therapy. The dose is 10–40 mg/day subcutaneously, and titration of doses is based on IGF1 levels. Normalization of IGF1 is achieved in >90% of patients with acromegaly.

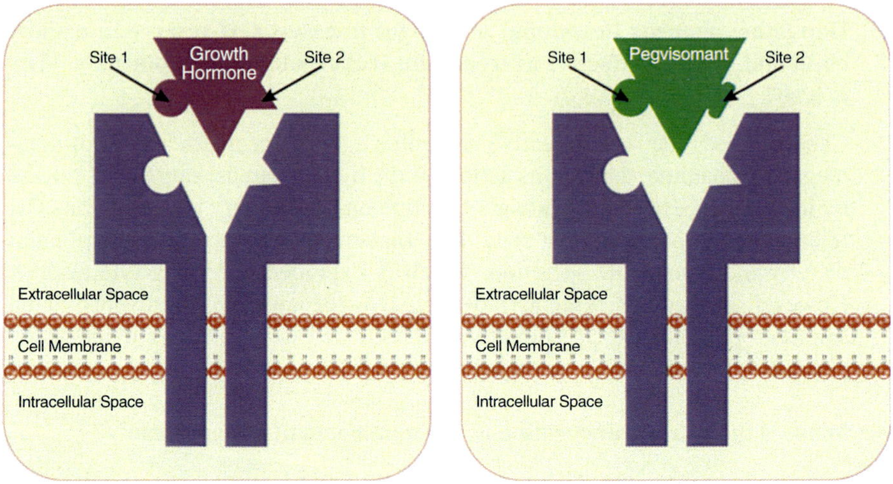

Fig. 2.5 (**a**) Binding of GH to its receptor through site 1 and 2 results in dimerization of receptor and activation of downstream pathways. (**b**) Binding of pegvisomant to GH receptor through site 1 blocks the binding of GH to its receptor

43. **What are the adverse effects of pegvisomant therapy?**

Adverse effects associated with pegvisomant therapy are hepatotoxicity and lipodystrophy. It is therefore recommended to monitor liver function test monthly for the initial 6 months after starting pegvisomant and biannually thereafter. Increase in size of tumor may occur in 3–5% of patients; however, it is not clear whether it is due to the natural history of the tumor or due to the decreased feedback effect of IGF1 on somatotropinoma. However, it is recommended to monitor tumor size by MRI biannually for a year and, if the tumor size is stable, then annually. Pegvisomant should be avoided in patients with large tumors abutting the optic chiasm or any other vital structures.

44. What is the advantage of combination of somatostatin receptor ligands with pegvisomant?

Combination of somatostatin receptor ligand and pegvisomant has the advantage of effective control of GH and IGF1 levels, decreased incidence of dysglycemia, lesser requirement of pegvisomant dose, and reduction in the risk of increase in tumor size. However, there is higher incidence of transaminitis with the use of combination therapy.

45. How to monitor a patient with acromegaly on different treatment modalities?

Treatment modalities	IGF1	GH dynamics	Remarks
Pituitary surgery	Yes	Random GH GH–GTT, if random GH >1 ng/ml	Random GH <1 ng/ml and normal IGF1 suggest disease control Nadir GH level <0.4 ng/ml on GTT and normal IGF1 suggest disease control
Somatostatin receptor ligand	Yes	Random GH	GH <1 ng/ml and normal IGF1 suggest disease control GH–GTT not recommended
Cabergoline	Yes	Random GH	GH <1 ng/ml and normal IGF1 suggest disease control GH–GTT not recommended
Pegvisomant	Yes	No	Normal IGF1 suggest disease control Random GH/ GH–GTT not recommended
Radiotherapy	Yes	Random GH GH–GTT, if random GH >1 ng/ml	Random GH <1 ng/ml and normal IGF1 suggest disease control Nadir GH level <0.4 ng/ml on GTT and normal IGF1 suggest disease control

Note: any discordance between GH and IGF1 levels need retesting and close follow-up

46. Which is the preferred test for assessing the efficacy of medical management in patients with acromegaly?

The preferred tests for the assessment of efficacy of somatostatin receptor analogue and dopamine agonist therapy are random GH and serum IGF1 levels. Glucose-suppressed GH is not recommended in this scenario because of the higher rate of discordance between GH and IGF1 levels. Discordance between GH and IGF1 levels has been reported in 48% of patients on SRL therapy and 18% on DA therapy. Non-suppressible GH with normal IGF1 is the predominant pattern of discordance seen with SRL therapy, while high IGF1 with suppressible GH is the predominant pattern of discordance seen with DA therapy. This is caused by alterations in the neuroendocrine regulations of GH secretion by SRL or DA therapy. Further, the additional effects of SRL therapy on hepatic IGF1 generation may contribute to this dichotomy. Patients on pegvisomant therapy should be monitored with serum IGF1.

47. **What is the preferred treatment for diabetes in acromegaly?**

Diabetes in acromegaly is refractory to therapy and requires high doses of insulin along with insulin sensitizers. SRLs are effective in controlling blood glucose by decreasing GH levels, but may worsen glycemic control in 20–30% of patients through its predominant inhibitory effect on β-cell (SSTR subtype 2 and 5) as compared to α-cell (SSTR subtype 2). As pegvisomant blocks GH receptors at hepatocytes and decreases hepatic glucose output, it is the preferred drug in this scenario. Addition of cabergoline to conventional treatment for preoperative control of blood glucose may be useful (unpublished observation). Cabergoline acts through dopamine subtype 2 receptor and resets the altered sympathetic tone leading to control of blood glucose level and decrease in GH–IGF1.

48. **What is dopastatin?**

Dopastatin is a chimeric analogue combining somatostatin (SSTR 2 and 5) and dopamine subtype 2 agonist. It may be available as a treatment modality in future, as somatostatin and dopamine subtype 2 receptors are known to be expressed on GH secreting adenoma.

49. **What are the advantages of stereotactic radiosurgery over conventional radiotherapy?**

The main advantages of stereotactic radiosurgery (SRS) as compared to conventional fractionated radiotherapy are single sitting delivery, targeted therapy to the tumor tissue (resulting in lesser probability of damage to surrounding brain parenchyma), and earlier achievement of remission. Although, there is no difference in response rate between SRS and conventional radiotherapy in the long run, mean time for the achievement of remission is 2 years after SRS, while it is 5–10 years with conventional radiotherapy.

50. **When is conventional radiotherapy preferred over stereotactic radiosurgery?**

Conventional radiotherapy is preferred over stereotactic radiosurgery when there is substantial residual tumor burden (tumor size >3cm) or the tumor is too close to the optic chiasm (within 5mm). The optic pathway is more sensitive to a single large dose of irradiation as used in SRS, compared to multiple small doses as used in conventional radiotherapy. The exposure of the optic chiasm to more than 8 Gy in a single dose is detrimental; therefore, SRS therapy is not preferred in tumors close to the optic chiasm.

51. **How to diagnose and manage acromegaly during pregnancy?**

It is difficult to make a diagnosis of acromegaly during pregnancy. Biochemical abnormalities like non-suppressible GH after glucose load and mildly elevated IGF1 occur in normal pregnancy due to placental production of GH. However, in patients of acromegaly with pregnancy, serum IGF1 is highly elevated and can help in establishing the diagnosis. Despite of active disease during pregnancy, signs and symptoms of acromegaly usually do not worsen because of a relative GH-resistant state due to rising estrogen levels during pregnancy. Tumor size does not increase during pregnancy despite higher estrogen levels. GH and IGF1 do not cross the placenta; therefore, it has no deleterious effect on neonatal outcome. However, GH–IGF1 excess-associated comorbidities like hyperglycemia and hypertension may influence the overall outcome and need to be aggressively treated. Treatment is not recommended in patients with acromegaly during pregnancy if they have microadenoma or macroadenoma without mass effects. However, visual field and acuity should be regularly monitored. The indications for therapy include patients with worsening headache or compressive symptoms, and the available treatment options include surgery or somatostatin analogues/cabergoline.

52. **What is radiation-induced brain disorder?**

Radiation-induced brain disorder (RIBD) is a clinical entity which manifests as seizures, cognitive dysfunction, rapid vision loss, altered sensorium, and rarely second malignancy, consequent to structural and/or functional alterations in the cerebral parenchymal tissue after exposure to irradiation. Patients with old age, having functioning pituitary tumors (e.g., acromegaly and Cushing's disease), and those who received external beam irradiation and radiation dose exceeding >2 Gy per fraction, are predisposed to RIBD. A high index of suspicion is required to make a diagnosis of RIBD particularly in a patient with pituitary tumor who presents with altered sensorium after pituitary irradiation. MR imaging findings are nonspecific and reveal shrinkage of brain volume, ventricular dilatation, periventricular hyperintense areas on T1WI, cerebral edema, and necrosis. EEG shows nonspecific changes. The mechanisms implicated in brain parenchymal tissue damage include free radical-mediated tissue injury, progressive vascular damage, and direct brain tissue injury by radiation. Treatment includes glucocorticoids, mannitol, and antiepileptics, if indicated. Periodic follow-up is required for ongoing parenchymal damage and regular monitoring for pituitary hormone deficiencies.

Suggested Reading

1. Jameson JL, De Groot LJ. Endocrinology: adult and pediatric. Philadelphia: Elsevier Health Sciences; 2010.
2. Katznelson L, Atkinson JL, Cook DM, Ezzat SZ, Hamrahian AH, Miller KK. American Association of Clinical Endocrinologists medical guidelines for clinical practice for the diagnosis and treatment of acromegaly-2011 update. Endocr Pract. 2011;17:1–44.
3. Katznelson L, Laws Jr ER, Melmed S, Molitch ME, Murad MH, Utz A, et al. Acromegaly: an endocrine society clinical practice guideline. J Clin Endocrinol Metab. 2014;99:3933–51.

4. Longo D, Fauci A, Kasper D, Hauser S, Jameson J, Loscalzo J. Harrison's principles of internal medicine. 18th ed. New York: McGraw Hill Professional; 2012.
5. Melmed S, Colao A, Barkan A, Molitch M, Grossman AB, Kleinberg D, Clemmons D, et al. Guidelines for acromegaly management: an update. J Clin Endocrinol Metab. 2009;94(5): 1509–17.
6. Melmed S, Polonsky KS, Larsen PR, Kronenberg HM. Williams textbook of endocrinology: expert consult. London: Elsevier Health Sciences; 2011.

3 Hyperprolactinemia

3.1 Case Vignette

A 28-year-old male presented with sudden onset of severe headache associated with projectile vomiting and dizziness for the last 7 days. There was no history of fever, altered sensorium, seizures, CSF rhinorrhea, or epistaxis. He had history of dull aching headache, visual deficits, and poor beard growth for the last 2 years. He did not have history of decreased libido or erectile dysfunction. He was married for the last 1 year, but had no children. There was no history of hypertension, head injury, or any recent surgery. On examination, he was conscious and oriented with pulse rate 78 min and BP 100/70 mmHg. He had sparse beard and mustache. He did not have ocular cranial nerve palsy, hemiparesis, or neck rigidity. There were no features of acromegaly, Cushing's syndrome, or any symptoms suggestive of diabetes insipidus. Ophthalmic evaluation revealed bitemporal hemianopia, normal visual acuity, and no papilledema. Noncontrast CT of head revealed a mass in the sellar–suprasellar region with hyperdense area suggestive of hemorrhage. MR imaging showed a sellar mass 4.4×3.5×2.5 cm with suprasellar extension abutting the optic chiasm along with parasellar and infrasellar extension with a hyperintense area on T1W images suggestive of hemorrhage. Biochemistry revealed serum sodium 142 mEq/L, potassium 4.6 mEq/L, creatinine 0.4 mg/dl, random blood glucose 76 mg/dl, corrected serum calcium 8.2 mg/dl, and phosphate 3.7 mg/dl. Hormonal workup showed serum prolactin 25,990 ng/ml (4–15), cortisol 216 nmol/L (>900), T_4 7.3 μg/dl (4.8–12.7), TSH 1.1 μIU/ml (0.27–4.2), LH 2.32 mIU/ml (1.7–8.6), FSH 3.36mIU/ml (1.5–12.4), testosterone 6.2 nmol/l (9.9–27.8), iPTH 41 pg/ml, and 25 (OH)D 6.6 ng/ml. With this clinical, radiological, and hormonal profile, he was diagnosed to have macroprolactinoma with apoplexy. He was started on dexamethasone 4 mg i.v. 6 hourly and tablet cabergoline 0.5 mg twice weekly. His vitals and neurological parameters were monitored closely. With treatment, headache and dizziness improved and there were no new-onset neurological deficits. Mutational analysis for MEN1 was negative. Dexamethasone was tapered after a week and he was advised oral hydrocortisone. At 4 weeks, his serum prolactin was 1,500 ng/ml and the dose of cabergoline was increased to 1 mg twice weekly.

A. Bhansali, Y. Gogate, *Clinical Rounds in Endocrinology: Volume I - Adult Endocrinology*, DOI 10.1007/978-81-322-2398-6_3

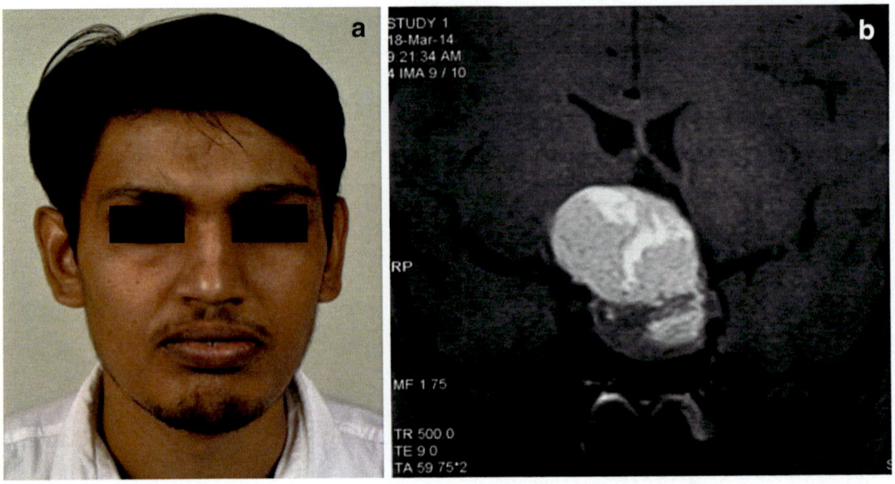

Fig. 3.1 (**a**) A 28-year-old male with macroprolactinoma having sparse beard and mustache. (**b**) T1W CEMR image of the same patient showing heterogeneously enhancing pituitary macroadenoma with supra-and infrasellar extension

3.2 Stepwise Analysis

Headache, bitemporal hemianopia, and symptoms of hypogonadism (poor beard growth) in the index patient suggest the presence of a mass in the sellar–suprasellar region. Acute worsening of headache along with symptoms of raised intracranial tension in this scenario indicates the development of pituitary apoplexy. The other differential which should be considered in this setting is subarachnoid hemorrhage, as intracranial aneurysms are present in up to 10% of patients with pituitary tumors. He had dizziness and low normal blood pressure which was suggestive of hypocortisolic state and was further confirmed by random serum cortisol <400 nmol/lL. A random serum cortisol <400 nmol/lL during critical illness suggests hypocortisolism, while a value >900 nmol/lL excludes abnormalities of the hypothalamo–pituitary–adrenal axis. The values between 400 and 900 nmol/lL require evaluation by ACTH stimulation test. Clinical examination did not reveal any stigma of acromegaly or Cushing's syndrome, but disclosed features of hypogonadism which indicates the presence of either nonfunctioning pituitary adenoma or prolactinoma in the index patient. Plain CT of head showed a sellar–suprasellar mass with an area of hyperdensity. The differential diagnosis of a hyperdense lesion in the sellar–suprasellar region on a noncontrast CT includes hemorrhage, meningioma, granuloma, lymphoma, and tumors associated with calcification like craniopharyngioma. However, the clinical profile in our patient suggested a diagnosis of pituitary apoplexy, and MRI findings were also consistent with pituitary macroadenoma with apoplexy. Serum cortisol and thyroxine levels are often estimated in patients suspected to have pituitary apoplexy; however, serum prolactin levels are inadvertently missed. Estimation of serum prolactin helps in differentiating prolactinoma from nonfunctioning pituitary adenoma. Further, low serum prolactin in this scenario denotes significant pituitary damage and low likelihood of recovery of residual pituitary function. High levels of serum prolactin despite tumoral bleed confirmed presence of prolactinoma in our patient. Low serum testosterone (<9 nmol/l) in the index patient may be the result of hyperprolactinemia or gonadotrope dysfunction due to mass effect or apoplexy. As the patient is young, evaluation for familial pituitary tumor syndromes like MEN1 and AIP mutations is mandatory. MEN1 was excluded by normal serum calcium profile and genetic analysis. However, AIP mutations could not be done. Pituitary decompressive surgery is indicated in patients with deteriorating level of sensorium or persistent/worsening/new-onset neuro-ophthalmic deficits or extravasation of blood into subarachnoid space. Our patient was conscious and had bitemporal hemianopia at presentation, and there was no deterioration in sensorium or neuro-deficit; therefore, he was offered conservative management. The patient was treated with intravenous dexamethasone as it has significant effect on peri-pituitary edema in addition to its glucocorticoid action. Cabergoline rapidly improves visual field defects within hours of its use. However, in a patient with apoplexy, use of cabergoline is fraught with the risk of worsening of apoplexy. In addition, CSF rhinorrhea may occur with the use of cabergoline in patients with infrasellar extension of tumor. Our patient was treated with cabergoline 0.5 mg twice weekly with close monitoring for CSF rhinorrhea and neurological status. Treatment with cabergoline progressively improves gonadal function in up to 60% of patients with macroprolactinoma after 4–6 months of therapy. In our patient, hypothalamo–pituitary–gonadal axis is less likely to recover because of the presence of giant adenoma (>4 cm) and concurrent apoplexy. If serum testosterone fails to normalize despite normalization of serum prolactin, testosterone therapy should be considered during follow up. However, treatment with testosterone may decrease the efficacy of cabergoline; therefore, prolactin levels should be monitored closely.

3.3 Clinical Rounds

1. What is the topographical distribution of cells in the pituitary gland?

Pituitary gland comprises of various cell types which include somatotropes (50%), lactotropes (10–30%), corticotropes (10–30%), gonadotropes (10–15%), and thyrotropes (5%). In addition, pituitary gland also consists of null cells, oncocytes, glial cells, and pituicytes. Somatotropes and lactotropes are laterally placed and corticotropes and thyrotropes in the mid-anterior and mid-posterior location, respectively, while gonadotropes are uniformly distributed.

2. What is the essential role of prolactin?

Prolactin is essential for galactopoiesis and plays a permissive role in mammogenesis. In addition, it also has an important role in immune system and gonadal function. Prolactin is a luteolytic hormone in all species, except in rodents where it is luteotrophic. Hypoprolactinemia is associated with impaired folliculogenesis and luteal phase defects in women and delayed puberty in boys.

3. **How does prolactin act?**

   Prolactin binds with its receptor, a member of cytokine receptor superfamily induces receptor dimerization and activates Janus kinase pathway. This stimulates **s**ignal **t**ransduction and **a**ctivators of **t**ranscription (STAT) protein which acts on target genes and mediates the effects of prolactin. Growth hormone also mediates its action through JAK–STAT pathway.

4. **What is hyperprolactinemia?**

   An elevated level of serum prolactin, above the gender-specific reference range, is called hyperprolactinemia (women >25 ng/ml and men >20 ng/ml). Because of the effect of estrogen, prolactin levels are higher in women as compared to men.

5. **What are the causes of hyperprolactinemia?**

   Hyperprolactinemia may be physiological, pathological or drug-related. The causes of hyperprolactinemia are summarized in the table given below.

Causes of hyperprolactinemia
Physiological
Exercise
Pregnancy Lactation
High protein diet
Breast stimulation
Venipuncture stress
Drug-related
Dopamine receptor antagonists (metoclopramide, domperidone)
Antidepressants (imipramine, amitriptyline)
Neuroleptics (haloperidol, chlorpromazine)
Estrogen
Anticonvulsants (phenytoin)
H_2 receptor blockers (cimetidine, ranitidine)
Pathological
Prolactinoma
Hypothalamo–pituitary disorders (sellar–suprasellar tumors, granulomatous disorders)
Primary hypothyroidism
Cranial irradiation
Polycystic ovarian disease
Chronic kidney disease, cirrhosis

6. **What are the non-tumoral causes of hyperprolactinemia?**

   Non-tumoral causes of hyperprolactinemia (HPRL) are more common than prolactinomas. Drugs are the most common non-tumoral cause of HPRL and include antidopaminergic agents (chlorpromazine, haloperidol, sulpiride, and domperidone), H_2 antihistamines (cimetidine), antidepressants (imipramine and amitriptyline), antihypertensives (α-methyldopa), phenytoin, estrogens, and calcium channel blockers like verapamil. Other causes include primary hypothyroidism, renal and liver insufficiency, polycystic ovarian disease, and chest/spine lesions. Serum prolactin level <100 ng/ml is a clinical clue to suspect non-tumoral causes of hyperprolactinemia.

7. **Why does hyperprolactinemia occur in primary hypothyroidism?**

   Approximatlely 25–30% of patients with primary hypothyroidism have hyperprolactinemia. The causes of hyperprolactinemia in primary hypothyroidism are lactotrope hyperplasia due to increased TRH drive, decreased prolactin clearance, and suppressed dopaminergic tone. Serum prolactin levels usually does not exceed >100 ng/ml. Treatment with levothyroxine normalizes prolactin levels in 6–12 weeks. However, the persistence of hyperprolactinemia mandates evaluation for concomitant prolactinoma.

8. **What are the causes of lactotrope hyperplasia?**

   The physiological causes of lactotrope hyperplasia are pregnancy and lactation and this effect is mediated through estrogen. The most common pathological cause of lactotrope(thyro) hyperplasia is primary hypothyroidism as TRH not only has a trophic effect on thyrotropes, but also stimulates lactotropes. Lactotrope hyperplasia can also occur due to pituitary stalk compression in patients with supra-sellar mass, as a result of impaired delivery of dopamine to lactotropes.

9. **What are the clinical features of hyperprolactinemia?**

   Clinical manifestations of hyperprolactinemia in women are menstrual irregularities, galactorrhea, and infertility, while men present with decreased shaving frequency, reduced libido, erectile dysfunction, and infertility. Galactorrhea is uncommon in postmenopausal women. Men rarely have galactorrhea because there is no glandular breast tissue, which is the prerequisite for galactorrhea.

10. **How does hyperprolactinemia cause gonadal dysfunction in women?**

    Prolactin inhibits GnRH pulse generator activity through inhibition of Kisspeptin neurons present in hypothalamus. In addition, prolactin directly suppresses gonadotropin secretion at the level of pituitary. Prolactin also impairs folliculogenesis, exerts inhibitory effects on granulosa cells (thereby decreasing estradiol production), and interferes with ovulation. It also causes luteal phase defects by its luteolytic action.

11. **A 20-year-old girl with a BMI 27 kg/m² presented with primary amenorrhea. On evaluation, she had Tanner stage $A_+P_3B_5$. Ultrasonography of pelvis showed small ovaries and atrophic uterus. Her serum prolactin was 2,387 ng/ml and MRI sella demonstrated a pituitary macroadenoma. How to explain the dichotomy between Tanner staging and presence of atrophic uterus?**

Development of secondary sexual characters is a gradual process due to progressive rise in gonadal steroids during puberty. Breast development requires lower levels of estrogens, while uterus and endometrium require higher level of estrogens. Hyperprolactinemia is associated with functional hypogonadotropic hypogonadism and therefore can result in delayed/arrested puberty in adolescents. The index patient with prolactinoma had normal breast development but atrophic uterus, which suggests that she has been exposed to estrogen, albeit at lower concentrations. The source of estrogen in this patient despite hyperprolactinemia includes increased prolactin-mediated adrenal androgen production which provides a substrate for synthesis of weaker estrogens in adipose tissue, increased aromatase activity due to obesity, and partial suppression of hypothalamo–pituitary–ovarian axis, thereby allowing measurable levels of FSH, which is required for induction of aromatase activity.

12. **How does hyperprolactinemia cause hypogonadism in men?**

Hyperprolactinemia causes hypogonadism in men by inhibiting GnRH pulse generator activity and gonadotropin secretion. Prolactin also leads to Leydig cell dysfunction thereby decreasing the production of testosterone. In addition, prolactin inhibits spermatogenesis by its direct effect on developing spermatogonia and indirectly through decreased intratesticular testosterone.

13. **What is Chiari–Frommel syndrome?**

Chiari–Frommel syndrome refers to postpartum amenorrhea, galactorrhea, and uterine atrophy persisting beyond 6 months after discontinuation of lactation. The exact cause is not known, but some patients may harbor prolactinoma.

14. **What is post-pill amenorrhea?**

Menstrual cycles commonly resumes within 3-6 months after discontinuation of combined oral contraceptive pills in most women. If amenorrhea persists beyond 6 months, it is called post-pill amenorrhea, and this may be due to estrogen-induced hyperprolactinemia.

15. **What are the precautions to be taken before sampling for prolactin?**

Sample for serum prolactin can be taken at any time of day. However, venipuncture stress, breast stimulation, strenuous exercise, and high protein meal should be avoided as this may result in inadvertent elevation of serum prolactin levels.

16. **Is a single value of prolactin enough to establish the diagnosis of hyperprolactinemia?**

Yes. But multiple measurements may be required in those with high clinical suspicion of hyperprolactinemia with normal prolactin, as hormone secretion is pulsatile. Reconfirmation is also necessary in those with mildly elevated prolactin.

17. **Does serum prolactin level help to establish the etiological diagnosis of hyperprolactinemia?**

Yes. Serum prolactin level helps in the differential diagnosis of hyperprolactinemia, as summarized in the table given below.

Prolactin level	Symptoms	Interpretation
>500 ng/ml	Yes	Macroprolactinoma
>250 ng/ml	Yes	Prolactinoma
100–200 ng/ml	Yes	Drugs like risperidone and metoclopramide Stalk compression
<100 ng/ml	Yes/no	Drug-induced hyperprolactinemia Stalk compression
<100 ng/ml	No	Macroprolactinemia

If prolactin levels are above the upper limit of detection of the assay, it should be measured in dilution to estimate the exact value. This is necessary in monitoring response to treatment. A low level of prolactin in a patient suspected to have hyperprolactinemia suggests "hook effect," which is a feature of immunoradiometric assays. Elevated serum prolactin levels, in the absence of symptoms of hyperprolactinemia, suggest a diagnosis of macroprolactinemia.

18. **A 28-year-old female presented with secondary amenorrhea, galactorrhea, and acromegaloid features. On evaluation, serum IGF1 levels were normal. What to do next?**

This patient had amenorrhea and galactorrhea with acromegaloid features suggesting a diagnosis of somatotropinoma. On evaluation, she had normal IGF1 and suppressible GH post-glucose load, thereby excluding the diagnosis of somatotropinoma. Further investigations revealed raised serum prolactin 450 ng/ml with normal T_4 and cortisol levels. Sellar MR imaging revealed a pituitary microadenoma (8 × 6 mm) and hence the diagnosis of microprolactinoma was made. Acromegaloid features in a patient with prolactinoma can be explained by intrinsic GH-like activity of prolactin because of its structural homology with GH. The patient was started on cabergoline and subsequently, prolactin levels normalized with regression of acromegaloid features.

19. **A 30-year-old woman presented with oligomenorrhea, galactorrhea, and infertility. On evaluation serum prolactin was 8 ng/ml on two occasions, and MRI showed 6 mm hypointense lesion in the right side of pituitary. What to do next?**

    The clinical profile of the index patient is strongly suggestive of hyperprolactinemia. However, normal serum prolactin on multiple occasions suggest the possibility of "hook effect". The "hook effect", also called as prozone phenomenon, is a falsely low estimation of high levels of prolactin due to saturation of antibodies used in immunoradiometric assay (IRMA). To rectify "hook effect," prolactin should be estimated in dilution. Her repeat serum prolactin in dilution (1:100) was 800 ng/ml, confirming the presence of "hook effect" in this patient.

20. **A 25-year-old female was incidentally found to have high prolactin level of 100 ng/ml. She has regular menstrual cycles and there is no galactorrhea. She is not on any medications. What is the possibility?**

    Asymptomatic hyperprolactinemia should raise a suspicion of macroprolactinemia. The circulating prolactin is predominantly (85%) monomeric and has a molecular weight of about 23 Kd. But, in certain individuals, prolactin exists as multimers forming big prolactin (48 Kd) or big-big prolactin (100 Kd). In addition, prolactin can bind with IgG and with anti-prolactin antibodies. These prolactin multimers, prolactin–IgG complex, and prolactin–anti-prolactin antibody complex constitute macroprolactin which has a molecular weight of >150 Kd. Macroprolactin interferes with prolactin assay and results in fallaciously high prolactin value. In the index case, estimation of prolactin by polyethylene glycol precipitation method revealed macroprolactinemia.

21. **A 20-year-old girl presented with oligomenorrhea. On evaluation she had a BMI 26 kg/m^2 and did not have hirsutism or galactorrhea. Her serum prolactin was 50 ng/ml, thyroid function tests were normal, and USG revealed bilateral polycystic ovaries. How to proceed further?**

    As the index patient is obese and has oligomenorrhea and polycystic ovaries on USG, a diagnosis of PCOS is likely. She has mild hyperprolactinemia which can occur in patients with PCOS. This is attributed to decreased dopaminergic and increased opioidergic tone in patients with PCOS. However, a possibility of secondary PCOS due to hyperprolactinemia should also be considered. As drugs are the most common cause of mild hyperprolactinemia, a detailed history for ingestion of related drugs was sought, but it was noncontributory in the index patient. She was advised lifestyle modification, following which she lost 5 kg weight and resumed her cycles. Serum prolactin decreased to 25 ng/ml, further substantiating the diagnosis of PCOS with associated hyperprolactinemia.

22. **A 30-year-old woman has persistent amenorrhea despite normalization of thyroid function after optimal levothyroxine treatment for primary hypothyroidism. What are the possibilities to be considered?**

After normalization of thyroid function with optimal levothyroxine treatment, majority of women with primary hypothyroidism resume their menstrual cycles within 3–6 months. However, if there is no resumption of cycles even after normalization of TSH, pregnancy should be excluded. Other possibilities include hyperprolactinemia due to residual thyro-lactotrope hyperplasia and secondary polycystic ovarian disease.

23. **A 28-year-old woman was evaluated for amenorrhea and galactorrhea. On investigation, she had a prolactin of 60 ng/ml. The MRI revealed an adenoma of size 4 mm. What to do next?**

Prolactinomas are usually associated with a serum prolactin >100 ng/ml and a level >250 ng/ml is virtually diagnostic of prolactinoma. Hence, in patients with serum prolactin <100 ng/ml despite the presence of microadenoma, other causes of hyperprolactinemia should be sought. In the index case, a detailed drug history revealed the use of domperidone. This was withdrawn for a period of 3 days and her repeat prolactin was 30 ng/ml. Therefore, the diagnosis of drug-induced hyperprolactinemia with non-functioning pituitary microadenoma was made. She discontinued domperidone and resumed her menstrual cycles.

24. **A 30-year-old female presented with oligomenorrhea and galactorrhea. On evaluation, she had a serum prolactin of 100 ng/ml. She was started on cabergoline 0.5 mg twice a week and a repeat prolactin after 4 weeks was 92 ng/ml. She was referred for further evaluation. What to do next?**

The index patient had oligomenorrhea and galactorrhea with elevated serum prolactin for which she was started on cabergoline but had suboptimal response. A detailed history revealed the ingestion of antipsychotic drug haloperidol. She was evaluated further; thyroid function tests and MR sellar imaging were normal. In any patient with mild hyperprolactinemia (<100 ng/ml), a thorough drug history must be elicited. Treatment of drug-induced hyperprolactinemia includes discontinuation of the offending drug if possible, substitution with alternative antipsychotics which does not cause hyperprolactinemia (aripiprazole or quetiapine), or use of oral contraceptive to relieve hypogonadal symptoms. Another option is initiation of DA therapy with antipsychotics. This may normalize serum prolactin in approximately 75% of patients but has a risk of worsening of underlying psychosis and hence is not recommended.

25. **A 34-year-old female on anti-psychiatric drugs presented with oligomenorrhea and galactorrhea. On investigation, serum PRL was 85 ng/ml. The anti-psychotic medications cannot be discontinued. What to do next?**

    In symptomatic patients of hyperprolactinemia, where withdrawal of incriminating drug is not possible and there is a probability of worsening of underlying disorder with the use of dopamine type 2 receptor agonists, gonadal steroids may be used to relieve the symptoms of hypogonadism. The other option after appropriate consultation with psychiatrist is to switch to atypical anti-psychotic drugs like quetiapine which has low antidopaminergic effect or change to anti-psychotic drugs having dopamine agonist and antagonist activity like aripiprazole, to minimize the effect on serum prolactin levels without worsening of disease.

26. **Is treatment necessary in asymptomatic patients with drug-induced hyperprolactinemia?**

    There is no need to treat asymptomatic patients with drug-induced hyperprolactinemia. Patients should be carefully evaluated for symptoms of hypogonadism, especially in men. Bone mineral density should be assessed in all patients.

27. **Which is the most common functioning pituitary tumor?**

    Prolactinoma is the most common pituitary tumor and contributes to 40–45% of all pituitary tumors. This is followed by somatotropinoma (15%), mamosomatotropinoma (3–5%), corticotropinoma (10%), and thyrotropinoma (1%). Clinically non-functioning pituitary tumors contributes to the rest and include gonadotropinoma (15%) and null cell adenoma (5–10%).

28. **Is there any gender difference in the presentation of prolactinoma?**

    Yes. Women usually present with menstrual irregularities, galactorrhea, and infertility and hence are detected earlier and commonly have microadenoma. On the contrary, men present with symptoms of mass effects in addition to features of hypogonadism and usually harbor macroadenoma. This probably reflects a delay in diagnosis because of nonspecific symptoms in men, which allows more time for tumoral growth. In addition, high tumor proliferative indices might contribute to the occurrence of macroadenoma in men.

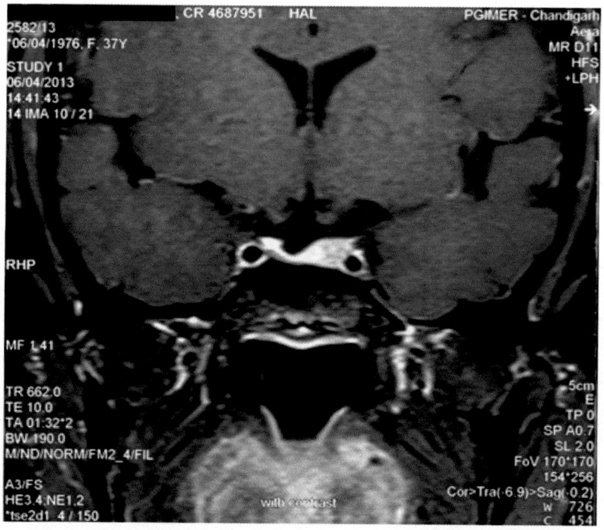

Fig. 3.2 T1W CEMRI coronal image showing hypointense lesion in the left half of pituitary in a 37-year-old female with hyperprolactinemia

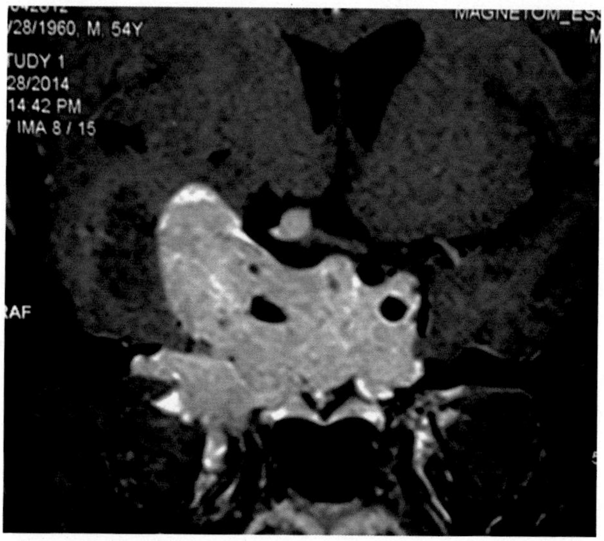

Fig. 3.3 T1W CEMRI coronal image showing a pituitary macroadenoma with bilateral parasellar, supra- and infrasellar extension with encasement of both carotid arteries in a 54-year-old male with hyperprolactinemia

29. **What is "giant" prolactinoma?**

Majority of prolactinomas are microadenomas (<10 mm) and occur more often in women, while macroprolactinomas (>10 mm) are more common in men. "Giant prolactinoma" is defined as an adenoma >4 cm in size or volume >10 cm^3 and is usually associated with serum PRL >1,000 ng/ml.

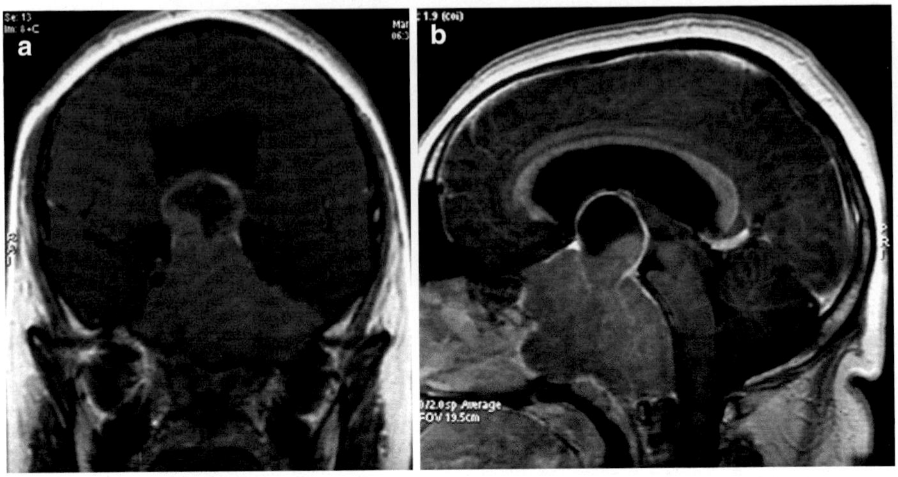

Fig. 3.4 T1W noncontrast MRI coronal (**a**) image and T1W CEMRI sagittal (**b**) image showing a "giant" pituitary macroadenoma with supra-, para-, and infrasellar extension and a hypointense area suggestive of necrosis in a 28-year-old male with prolactinoma

30. **What are the familial causes of prolactinoma?**

Prolactinomas are usually sporadic, but sometimes they may be familial. The familial syndromes associated with prolactinoma include multiple endocrine neoplasia type 1, familial isolated pituitary adenoma (AIP mutations), and rarely SDHB mutations (in association with paraganglioma). Patients with familial prolactinomas usually present at a younger age, have invasive adenomas, and are resistant to therapy.

31. **What is malignant prolactinoma?**

Malignant prolactinoma should be suspected in the presence of atypical clinical manifestation (e.g., third cranial nerve palsy at presentation), de novo resistance to DA therapy or appearance of DA resistance after initial response, aggressive tumor behavior , histological markers like cellular atypia, nuclear pleomorphism, and a high Ki-67 proliferative index (3%). However, the presence of distant metastasis is the only definitive evidence of malignant prolactinoma. Malignant prolactinoma has a male preponderance (2:1) and the mean age of presentation is 44 years. Seventy-five percent of patients have intracranial metastasis, while extracranial metastasis to spinal cord, bone liver, and lymph node is present in 40% of patients. Treatment options include surgery, high-dose cabergoline, temozolomide, and local radiotherapy.

32. **What are the unusual presentations of prolactinoma?**

    The unusual presentations of prolactinomas are primary amenorrhea, arrested puberty, pituitary apoplexy, CSF rhinorrhea, acromegaloidism, and rarely, galactorrhea in men.

33. **How does treatment of prolactinoma differ from other pituitary tumors?**

    Medical management is highly rewarding in patients with prolactinoma than in any other pituitary tumors. This is because of dense expression of dopamine type 2 (D_2) receptors on prolactinoma which makes it amenable to therapy with D_2 receptor agonists (DA). The other advantages of DA are lactotrope selectivity (sparing other pituitary cell lines), rapid improvement in visual field defects (usually within 12–16 h), normalization of serum prolactin in 90% (usually within 2–4 weeks), and reduction in tumor size by >50% in 70–90% of patients. Therefore, even the presence of visual field defects does not warrant immediate surgery in patients with macroprolactinoma and therapy with DA should be offered with close monitoring of visual field. In addition, there is always a possibility of recovery of residual pituitary function and drug discontinuation after optimal medical therapy.

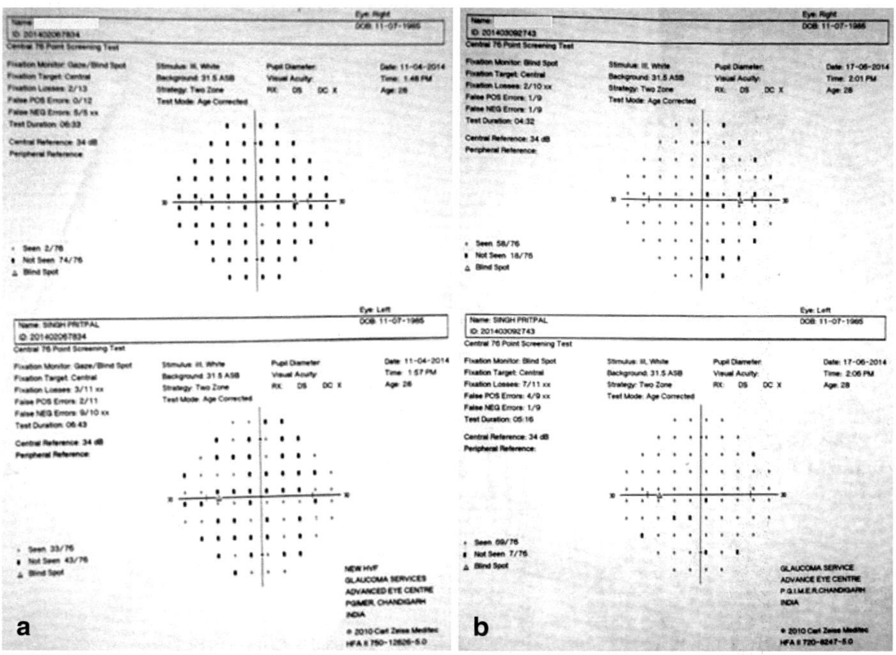

Fig. 3.5 (**a**) Visual field chart in a patient with giant prolactinoma showing almost complete field defects in right eye (*upper*) and field defects in all quadrants in left eye (*lower*). (**b**) Visual field chart of the same patient after 8 weeks of cabergoline therapy demonstrating marked improvement in visual fields of both eyes

34. **What are the types of D_2 receptor agonist?**

The D_2 receptor agonists are ergot and non-ergot derivatives. The ergot derivatives include bromocriptine, cabergoline, pergolide, and lisuride, while the non-ergot derivative includes quinagolide.

35. **Which is the preferred D_2 receptor agonist in patients with prolactinoma?**

All the available DAs are effective and safe, but efficacy in terms of prolactin normalization and tumor shrinkage is variable. The efficacy of different DAs in patients with macroprolactinoma is summarized in the table given below.

Drugs	Normalization of prolactin (%)	>50% reduction in tumor size (%)	Remarks
Bromocriptine	66	64	Short acting Daily administration GI side effects
Pergolide	68	86	Increased risk of valvulopathy (28%)
Cabergoline	90–100	96	Long acting Potent Better compliance Lesser side effects

Therefore, cabergoline seems to be the most effective among the available DAs.

36. **When to treat microprolactinoma?**

All microprolactinomas do not require treatment. The treatment indications are enlisted in the table below.

Clinical scenario	Treatment
Asymptomatic	Reassurance
Desire for fertility	D_2 receptor agonist
Troublesome galactorrhea	D_2 receptor agonist
Family completed but wishes regular cycles	D_2 receptor agonist or oral contraceptive pills
Concern for bone health (in women)	D_2 receptor agonist or oral contraceptive pills
Postmenopausal	No treatment/bisphosphonates for bone health
Men with hypogonadism and/or osteoporosis	D_2 receptor agonist

37. **How effective is the medical management in prolactinoma?**

The efficacy of medical treatment in terms of a composite endpoint including normalization of serum prolactin, restoration of gonadal function, and reduction in tumor size are listed in the table given below.

Drug	Microprolactinoma (%)	Macroprolactinoma (%)
Bromocriptine	80–90	70
Cabergoline	95	80

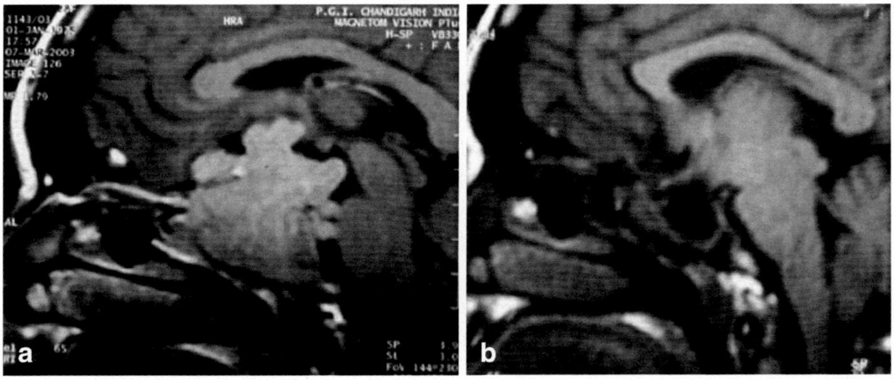

Fig. 3.6 (**a**) T1W CEMR sagittal image showing invasive giant prolactinoma in a 28-year-old lady. (**b**) T1W CEMR sagittal image of the same patient after 9 months of bromocriptine therapy showing complete disappearance of tumor with widened sella

38. **What are the adverse events associated with D_2 receptor agonist?**

    The major adverse events associated with the use of DA are gastrointestinal (nausea 30%, vomiting 20%), cardiovascular (postural hypotension, dizziness/syncope, and valvulopathy), and neurological (headache, drowsiness, and psychosis). Rarely CSF rhinorrhea, pituitary apoplexy, Raynaud's phenomenon, and retroperitoneal fibrosis have been reported.

39. **Is the risk of valvulopathy associated with D_2 receptor agonist therapy real in patients with prolactinoma?**

    Probably not. Patients with Parkinson's disease who are treated with cabergoline and pergolide have an increased risk of valvulopathy. This is due to action of DAs on serotonin type 2B receptors which are expressed on right-sided cardiac valves, resulting in tricuspid valvular tissue proliferation and dysfunction. The risk is dose dependent. In patients with prolactinoma the dose requirement is much less as compared to Parkinson's disease; hence the risk is likely to be minimal. However, some studies have shown increased risk of moderate tricuspid regurgitation with cabergoline in patients with prolactinoma. Therefore, regular surveillance with echocardiography is warranted.

40. **How to monitor a patient of prolactinoma on treatment with D_2 receptor agonist?**

Patients with microprolactinoma on treatment with D_2 receptor agonist (DA) require clinical evaluation and serum prolactin estimation every monthly. The dose of DA should be hiked up monthly in response to prolactin levels, till it normalizes. Serial MRI monitoring is not required but should be performed if planning withdrawal of therapy. Patients with macroprolactinoma require clinical monitoring, visual field analysis, and serum prolactin estimation monthly. In addition, MR imaging should be performed at an interval of 6 months. Prolactin usually normalizes by 2 weeks in majority of patients and precedes reduction in tumor size. Rapid increment of cabergoline (weekly) as against conventional increment (monthly or 2 monthly) offers no additional advantage.

41. **What are the causes of persistence of amenorrhea despite normalization of prolactin in a woman with prolactinoma on treatment?**

There is resumption of menses, usually within 2–3 months after initiation of treatment with DA. The causes of persistent amenorrhea despite normalization of prolactin include associated secondary polycystic ovarian disease, endometrial atrophy due to long-standing hypogonadism, and concurrent pituitary hormone deficiencies in macroprolactinoma. These patients require estrogen followed by progesterone supplementation.

42. **How to treat hypogonadism in men with prolactinoma despite normalization of prolactin?**

Normalization of serum prolactin usually occurs within 2–4 weeks in majority of patients. But, restoration of serum testosterone to normal range takes longer time (3–6 months) and may not recover in all patients as majority of men have gonadotrope dysfunction as a result of mass effect due to macroprolactinoma. These patients may be replaced with testosterone, and if fertility is a concern, treatment with hCG alone may be effective.

43. **When to withdraw cabergoline in a patient with prolactinoma?**

Criteria for withdrawal of cabergoline are similar in patients with micro- as well as macroprolactinoma. Those who have normalization of serum prolactin and disappearance of tumor (preferably) or >50% reduction in tumor size from baseline should be considered for withdrawal of cabergoline. After achieving these endpoints, treatment should be continued for another 12 months prior to discontinuation. Withdrawal of cabergoline should not be attempted in those with cavernous sinus invasion or tumor close to optic chiasm (distance <5 mm). However, other criteria which have been suggested for the withdrawal of cabergoline in patients with prolactinoma include normalization of serum prolactin with disappearance of tumor and at least 2 year of therapy with dopamine receptor agonists. Recurrence of hyperprolactinemia is seen in 32% of patients with microadenoma and 43% in macroadenoma, after 5 years of withdrawal of cabergoline, although tumor regrowth does not occur in these patients. Tumor size (>3.1 mm) and nadir prolactin levels (>5.4 ng/ml) during treatment with cabergoline are the predictors of recurrence of hyperprolactinemia after drug withdrawal. Therefore, patients should be followed up regularly after withdrawal of cabergoline.

44. **How to define D_2 receptor agonist resistance in prolactinoma?**

Failure to normalize prolactin or to reduce tumor size by >50% after 1 year of treatment with optimal doses of D_2 receptor agonist is termed as D_2 receptor agonist resistance. Though the optimal dose threshold for a particular DA is not well defined, the dose of cabergoline required to achieve both normalization of prolactin levels and tumor reduction in majority of patients is about 2 mg/week. However, before considering DA resistance, compliance to therapy should be ensured and concurrent gonadal hormone replacement must be excluded, as estrogen therapy decreases the efficacy of DAs by increasing serum prolactin. Overall, 24% of patients exhibit resistance to bromocriptine, 13% to pergolide, and 11% to cabergoline.

45. **Why do some patients with prolactinoma have D_2 receptor agonist resistance?**

D_2 receptor agonist resistance is reported in 10–20% of patients with prolactinoma. It may be related to lack of D_2 receptor expression, decreased affinity of D_2 receptors to DA, or altered post-receptor signaling pathway. In addition, density of D_2 receptor isoforms (short and long) also determine the response to DA therapy, as long isoforms are associated with better response.

46. **How to treat a patient of prolactinoma with D_2 receptor agonist resistance?**

Patients of prolactinoma with D_2 receptor agonist resistance should be managed by switching over to cabergoline (in those who are on bromocriptine) or escalating the dose of cabergoline up to 11 mg/week (maximum dose used in available literature) for those who are already receiving it. Patients with cabergoline resistance should be offered surgery and/or radiotherapy.

47. **What are the indications for surgery in macroprolactinoma?**

The indications for surgery in patients with macroprolactinoma are limited. They include DA resistance, drug intolerance, and invasive macroadenoma compromising vision which fails to improve after drug treatment. Other indications for surgery are pituitary apoplexy, concurrent CSF rhinorrhea, and macroprolactinoma in pregnancy not responding to drugs. Only 40% of patients with macroprolactinoma have normalization of PRL after surgery and 20% of these patients have recurrence of hyperprolactinemia within a year of surgery and about 50% within 5 years after surgery.

48. **A 35-year-old male presented with headache and erectile dysfunction. On evaluation, his visual fields were normal, he had a serum prolactin of 335 ng/ml, and MRI sella showed a 22×26×11 mm sellar–suprasellar mass. He was treated with cabergoline 1.5 mg twice weekly. Serum prolactin normalized after 3 months, but there was no reduction in tumor size even after 1 year of therapy. How to proceed further?**

    Treatment with cabergoline in patients with macroprolactinomas is associated with normalization of prolactin in 90–100% of patients and tumor reduction of >50% in 96% of patients. Normalization of prolactin usually occurs within 2–4 weeks, while tumor reduction takes a longer time, with maximum reduction by 3–6 months. Further increase in dose despite normalization of prolactin may cause additional reduction in tumor size, although modest. In the index case, dose of cabergoline was increased to 2.5 mg twice weekly and was continued for 1 year without any further reduction in tumor size. Therefore, a possibility of resistant prolactinoma or presence of double adenoma (nonfunctioning pituitary adenoma and prolactinoma) should be considered.

49. **What are the conditions which facilitate remission of hyperprolactinemia?**

    Pregnancy and menopause are associated with remission of hyperprolactinemia, in addition to dopamine agonists and surgery. During pregnancy, prolactinoma may undergo ischemic necrosis due to compromised vascularity of tumor as a result of concurrent lactotrope hyperplasia. In menopausal state, declining estrogen levels may result in remission of hyperprolactinemia.

50. **What are the experimental drugs used in the management of prolactinoma?**

    D_2 receptor agonists are the treatment of choice for the management of prolactinoma. However, some patients who do not respond to DAs require alternative therapies which include somatostatin analogues, nerve growth factor, interferon-α, and dopastatin.

51. **How to manage prolactinoma during pregnancy?**

    D_2 receptor agonist should be discontinued in patients with microadenomas after confirmation of pregnancy, while it should be continued in those having macroadenomas with suprasellar/parasellar extension. In case of development of new-onset visual symptoms and/or headache, MR imaging without contrast (gadolinium – category C agent) should be performed. The management of prolactinoma during pregnancy is summarized in the table below.

Prolactinoma	Clinical examination	Visual field	Serum prolactin	MR imaging
Microadenoma	Every trimester	Not required	Not required	Not required
Macroadenoma	Every monthly	Required (severe headache or visual deficits)	Not required	May be required

52. **When to discontinue D_2 receptor agonist (DA) treatment during pregnancy in a woman with macroprolactinoma?**

D_2 receptor agonist (DA) can be safely discontinued during pregnancy in a woman with intrasellar macroadenoma, as the risk of tumor expansion is marginally higher than with microadenomas. Withdrawal of DA is particularly safe in those who had already experienced significant tumor shrinkage (>50% shrinkage and preferably intrasellar) or had undergone surgery preconceptionally. However, patients having macroadenomas abutting optic chiasm or invasive macroadenomas, DA should either be continued throughout gestation or be planned for surgery during second trimester as the risk of tumor expansion is 15–30% in this scenario. Bromocriptine is preferred over cabergoline during first trimester of pregnancy as there is substantial evidence in favor of bromocriptine.

53. **How to plan lactation in a woman with macroprolactinoma?**

D_2 receptor agonists should be discontinued 7 days prior to expected date of delivery, with close monitoring of symptoms related to mass effect and periodic assessment of visual fields and acuity. Serum prolactin should not be monitored as suckling increases prolactin. MRI sella should be done when indicated.

54. **What are the causes of hyperprolactinemia with secondary hypothyroidism?**

The most common cause of secondary hypothyroidism with hyperprolactinemia is macroprolactinoma followed by non-functioning pituitary adenoma with supra-sellar extension and lymphocytic infundibulitis.

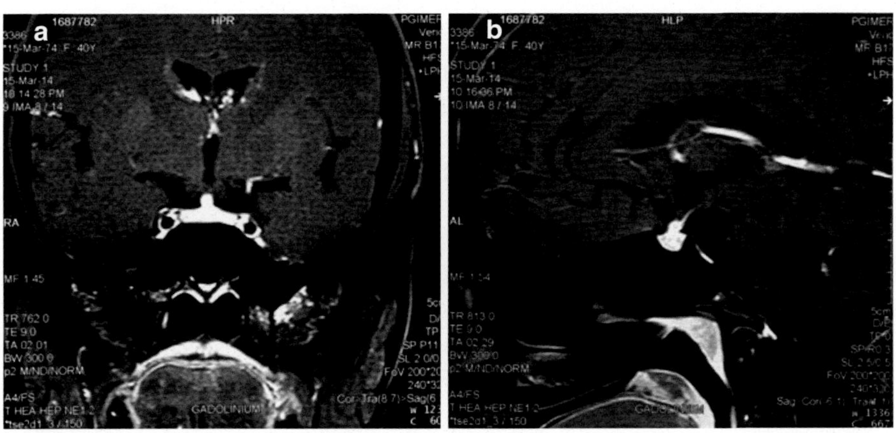

Fig. 3.7 T1W CEMR coronal (**a**) and sagittal (**b**) image showing diffusely enhancing pituitary with thickening of infundibulum (>4 mm) suggestive of hypophysitis

55. **What is pituitary apoplexy?**

The term apoplexy is derived from a Greek word *apoplexia* which means "a striking away" and usually connotes bleeding within internal organs. Pituitary apoplexy is a disorder due to hemorrhage or infarction of pituitary gland and is characterized by acute-onset headache, nausea, vomiting, visual impairment, altered sensorium, neuro-deficits, and seizures. Pituitary apoplexy may be clinically explosive or asymptomatic/silent which is appreciated only on imaging or histopathology by the presence of hemosiderin-laden macrophages.

56. **Who are predisposed for pituitary apoplexy?**

Hypertension, cardiac surgery, head injury, disseminated intravascular coagulation, and use of anticoagulants or dopamine receptor agonists predispose to pituitary apoplexy. In addition, dynamic tests for anterior pituitary functions using GnRH, TRH, CRH, and insulin-induced hypoglycemia may also trigger apoplexy. Therefore, pituitary apoplexy must be included in the differential diagnosis of any patient who develops headache and neuro-ophthalmic symptoms in the presence of these risk factors.

57. **Does pituitary apoplexy occur only in those with pituitary tumors?**

No. Pituitary apoplexy can occur even in a normal pituitary. This usually occurs in the setting of wide swings in systemic blood pressure as normal hypophyseal portal pressure is 15–25 cm of H_2O and is not able to withstand the frequent alterations in blood pressure particularly in a patient with shock. In addition, pregnancy, anticoagulant therapy, snake bite, and sickle cell anemia can be associated with apoplexy in a normal pituitary.

58. **Why is pituitary apoplexy common in prolactinoma?**

Nonfunctioning pituitary adenoma is the most common tumor associated with apoplexy in clinical practice. However, among the functioning tumors, prolactinoma is the most common tumor associated with apoplexy, followed by somatotropinoma. This is because lactotropes are laterally placed with a precarious blood supply.

59. **When to suspect pituitary apoplexy in an emergency setting?**

The diagnosis of pituitary apoplexy is straightforward when a patient known to harbor a pituitary tumor presents with acute-onset headache and neuro-ophthalmic deficits. The diagnosis should also be considered in a patient who presents with these symptoms and has clinical evidence of a functional tumor (e.g., acromegaly, Cushing's syndrome) even without a previous history of pituitary adenoma. In addition, history of acute-onset headache, worsening/new-onset visual deficits, presence of hypotension, optic atrophy, sparse facial hair in males, and pallor without anemia (feature of ACTH deficiency) in an unconscious patient even without a prior history of pituitary adenoma strongly suggest a diagnosis of pituitary apoplexy. The corroborating biochemical evidences for pituitary apoplexy include hyponatremia and hypoglycemia. Disorders which closely mimic pituitary apoplexy are meningitis, subarachnoid hemorrhage, and stroke.

60. **What are the unusual presentations of pituitary apoplexy?**

The unusual manifestations of pituitary apoplexy include epistaxis, meningitis, subarachnoid hemorrhage, hemiplegia, frontal lobe syndrome, status epilepticus, metabolic encephalopathy, and hypotension. The prerequisite for epistaxis in a patient with pituitary tumor is breach in the sellar floor. Hemorrhage in the tumor or erosion of surrounding vessels by tumor in the presence of breach in sellar floor leads to epistaxis. Meningitis is due to seepage of blood into the subarachnoid space which leads to meningeal irritation and causes chemical meningitis. Subarachnoid hemorrhage is due to extension of blood into subarachnoid space. Hemiplegia is due to internal carotid artery spasm as a result of extension of blood into parasellar area. Rarely, frontal lobe syndrome may be a presenting manifestation due to anterior cerebral artery spasm. Seizure is due to raised intracranial pressure, metabolic abnormalities (hyponatremia, hypoglycemia), and extension of blood into brain parenchyma. Metabolic encephalopathy occurs as a result of hyponatremia consequent to glucocorticoid and thyroxine deficiency and hypoglycemia due to cortisol and growth hormone deficiency. Hypotension is due to glucocorticoid deficiency. The figure illustrated below shows a patient with invasive pituitary macroprolactinoma who presented with epistaxis due to sphenoidal sinus extension and erosion of surrounding vessels. The patient did not have any tumoral bleed.

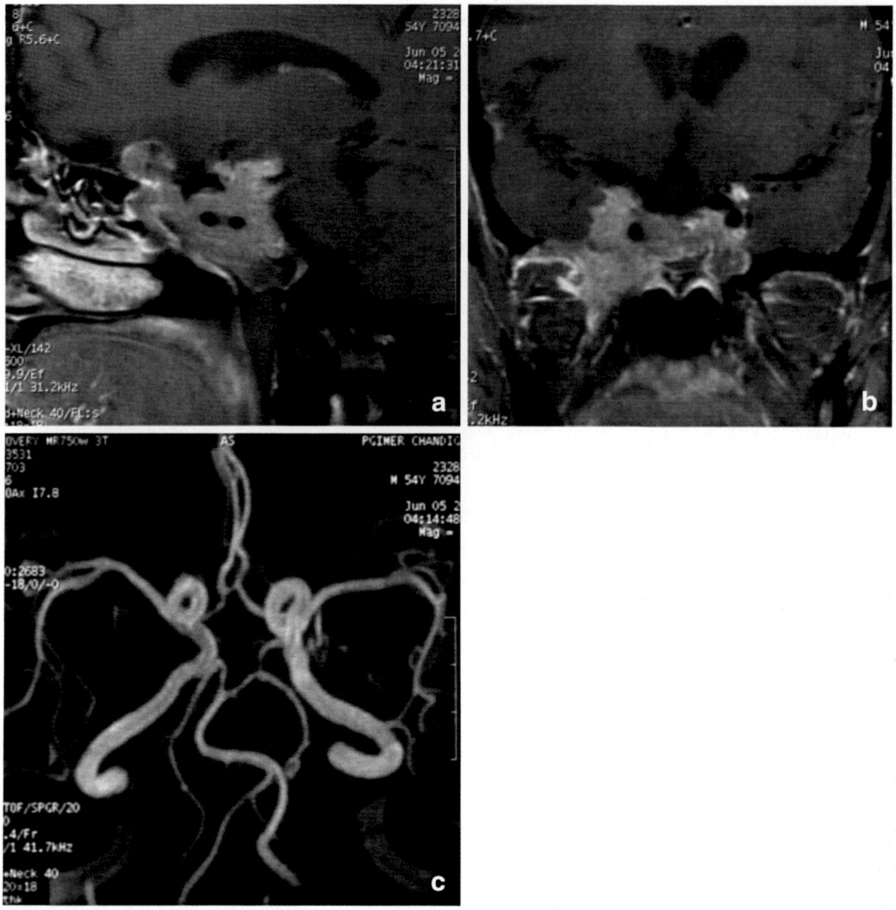

Fig. 3.8 (**a**) T1W CEMR sagittal image showing invasive pituitary macroadenoma with nasopharyngeal extension in a patient who presented with epistaxis. (**b**) T1W CEMR coronal image of the same patient showing pituitary macroadenoma with infra- and right parasellar extension. (**c**) MR angiography image of circle of Willis in the same patient did not demonstrate any vascular anomalies

61. **What are the causes of acute-onset headache in a patient with pituitary tumor?**

The most common cause of acute-onset headache in a patient with pituitary tumor is apoplexy. Ten percent of patients with pituitary tumor have coexisting intracranial aneurysms and its rupture may result in subarachnoid hemorrhage. In addition, cortical vein thrombosis, meningitis, and tension pneumocephalus, particularly in patients with postoperative Cushing's disease, may present with acute-onset headache.

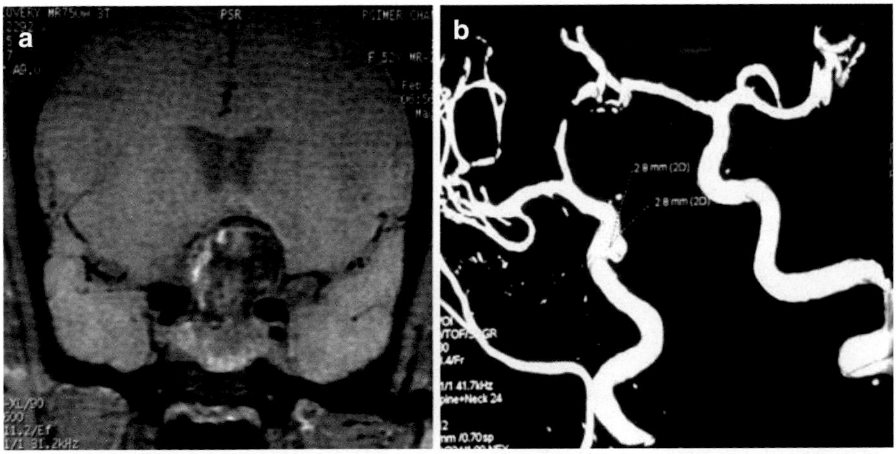

Fig. 3.9 (**a**) T1W noncontrast MR coronal image showing heterogeneous low (necrosis) and high signal intensity (hemorrhage) in a pituitary adenoma. The patient presented with acute-onset headache. (**b**) CT angiogram of the same patient showing a saccular aneurysm from cavernous segment of right internal carotid artery

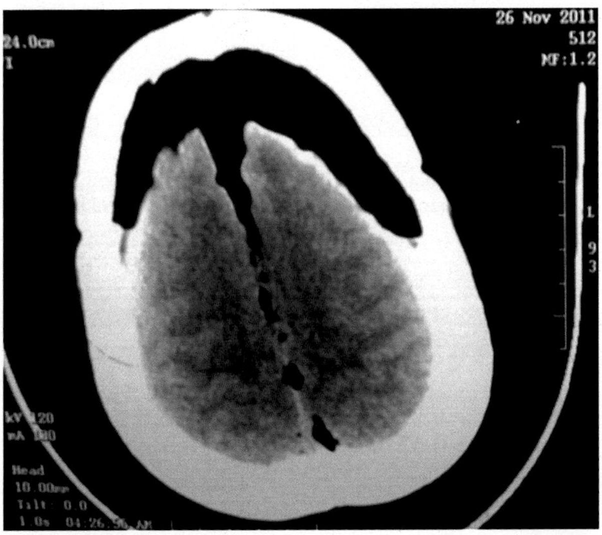

Fig. 3.10 Tension pneumocephalus causing compression of frontal lobes (Mount Fuji sign) in a postoperative (TSS) patient with Cushing's disease

62. **What are the endocrine disorders associated with ptosis?**

The differential diagnoses of ptosis from an endocrine perspective include diabetes mellitus, pituitary apoplexy, parasellar extension of pituitary tumor, rhinocerebral mucormycosis, myasthenia gravis in association with polyglandular endocrinopathies, and rarely, Graves' disease with superior orbital fissure syndrome.

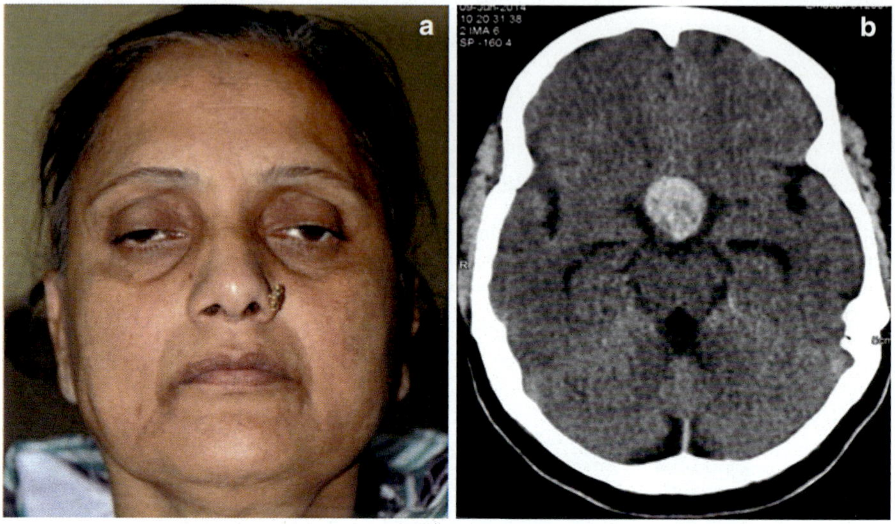

Fig. 3.11 (**a**) Ptosis of right eye in a 52-year-old female who presented with acute-onset severe headache. (**b**) NCCT head of the same patient showing hyperdense lesion in the sellar area suggestive of hemorrhage

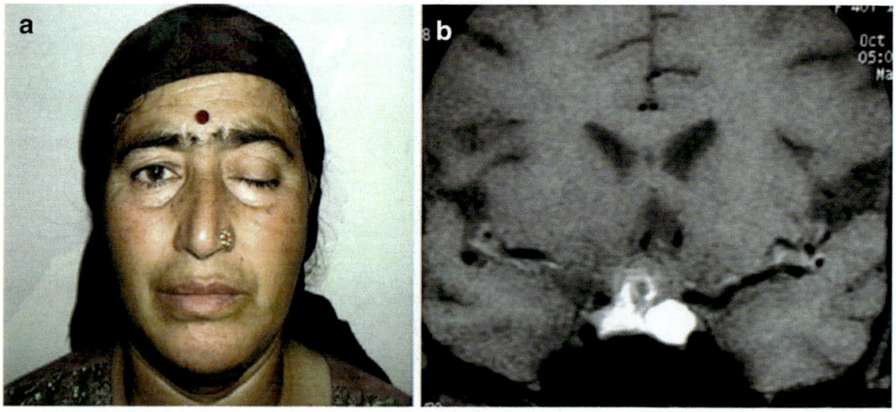

Fig. 3.12 (**a**) A 40-year-old female who presented with sudden-onset ptosis of left eye and headache. (**b**) T1W noncontrast MRI showing high signal intensity within a pituitary adenoma suggestive of hemorrhage

63. **What are the biochemical markers of pituitary apoplexy?**

Rapid development of hyponatremia, hypoglycemia, hypoprolactinemia, and hypocortisolemia is the surrogate biochemical evidence of pituitary apoplexy in a patient with pituitary tumor.

64. **What is the importance of low prolactin in a patient with pituitary tumor?**

Hypoprolactinemia, defined as serum prolactin below gender specific reference range, in a patient with pituitary tumor suggests pituitary apoplexy. Lactotrope contributes to approximately 30% of pituitary cell mass and substantial destruction is required to manifest as hypoprolactinemia. Therefore, patients with pituitary apoplexy who have hypoprolactinemia at presentation have very high intrasellar pressure and are unlikely to recover their pituitary function even after decompressive surgery.

65. **What is the preferred imaging modality for the diagnosis of pituitary apoplexy?**

MR imaging of sella is the preferred radiological investigation in a patient suspected to have pituitary apoplexy as it confirms the diagnosis in over 90%. If MR scan is contraindicated or not feasible, a dedicated CT scan of pituitary is advocated. However, the CT is diagnostic of apoplexy in only 21–28% of patients, though a sellar mass can be identified in up to 80%. MR angiography is required if there is a suspicion of aneurysm or extension of pituitary tumor bleed into subarachnoid space.

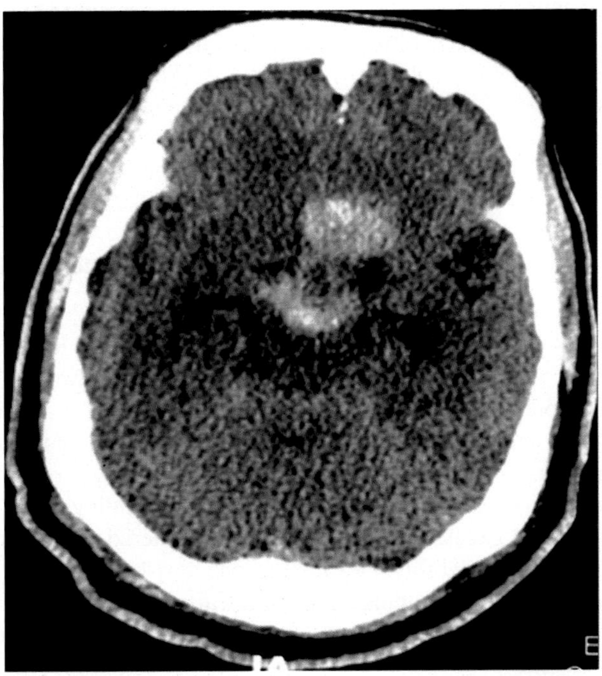

Fig. 3.13 NCCT head showing hyperdense area in the sellar region suggestive of hemorrhage in a patient with acromegaly

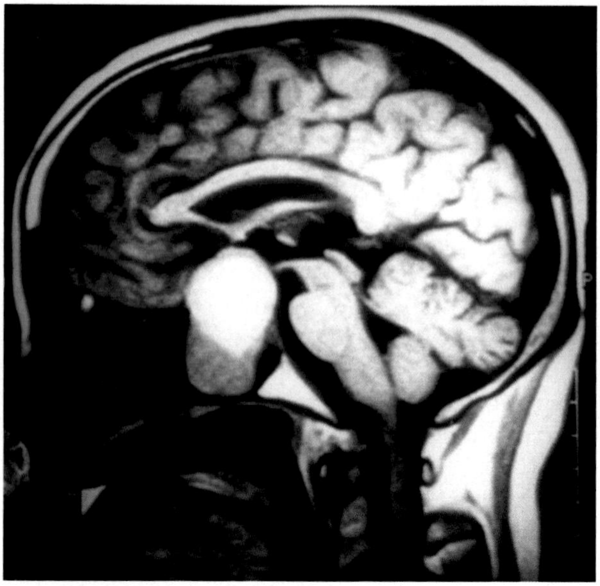

Fig. 3.14 T1W noncontrast MR sagittal image showing a sellar–suprasellar mass with a hyperintense area in the upper part, suggestive of hemorrhage

66. **What are the investigations required in a patient with pituitary apoplexy?**

All patients with pituitary apoplexy should have estimation of complete blood count, serum electrolytes, blood glucose, and hormonal profile which includes cortisol, T_4, TSH, and prolactin. Clinically, ACTH deficiency is most critical and is observed in 70% of patients whereas TSH and gonadotropin deficiencies are reported in 50 and 75% of patients, respectively. Serum LH, FSH, testosterone/estradiol, and IGF1 may also be included in the baseline evaluation; however, they may not influence immediate therapeutic decision.

67. **What are the indications for glucocorticoids in patients with pituitary apoplexy?**

Patients with pituitary apoplexy require glucocorticoids in the presence of hemodynamic instability, altered sensorium, or new onset/worsening of visual defects. The preferred glucocorticoid is hydrocortisone as it has immediate onset of action and innate mineralocorticoid activity. It is administered as 100–200 mg intravenous bolus followed by infusion at 2–4 mg per hour. Intermittent intravenous boluses should be avoided as cortisol-binding globulin is rapidly saturated; thereby, excess free cortisol is readily filtered across glomeruli leading to reduced bioavailability. Dexamethasone may be favored in patients with altered sensorium or visual defects as it may also reduce peri-pituitary edema. In addition, glucocorticoids should also be supplemented in those who have cortiosl deficiency.

68. **What are the indications of pituitary decompressive surgery in a patient with pituitary apoplexy?**

Any patient with deteriorating level of sensorium or persistent/worsening/new-onset neuro-ophthalmic deficits may be benefitted by surgical decompression. Patients who have extravasation of blood into subarachnoid space or develop hydrocephalus during the course of disease also warrant surgical intervention.

69. **Does surgical decompression improve outcome in patients with pituitary apoplexy?**

Because of the rarity of disease, there are no randomized controlled trials to compare surgical versus conservative management and the available data are only from case series/reports. The rationale of early surgical intervention is better visual and endocrine outcome. Decompressive surgery is associated with risk of CSF rhinorrhea, permanent diabetes insipidus, and loss of residual anterior pituitary function, while conservative management has a risk of worsening visual defects and sensorium. Therefore, from the available literature, it seems appropriate that any patient with deteriorating level of sensorium or persistent/worsening of neuro-ophthalmic deficits may be benefitted by surgical decompression. Patients who have extravasation of blood into subarachnoid space or develop hydrocephalus during the course of the disease warrant surgical intervention. However, patients with mild visual impairment or ocular palsy alone (III, IV, and VI cranial nerves) should be considered for conservative management as they may improve within days or weeks after initiating treatment. In addition, patients who demonstrate rapid involution of tumor or single hypodense area within tumor on imaging should also be considered for conservative management, as they show subsequent resolution of tumor.

70. **What is the cell of origin of nonfunctioning pituitary adenoma?**

Approximately two-thirds of nonfunctioning pituitary adenomas (NFPAs) originate from gonadotropes and the rest from null cells or oncocytes. These tumors present with symptoms of mass effect and hypogonadism. Tumors arising from gonadotropes show immunopositivity for LH and FSH, while null cell adenoma or oncocytoma lacks immunoreactivity for all anterior pituitary hormones. Oncocytoma and null cell adenoma are differentiated on electron microscopy by abundance of mitochondria in the former, while the latter is devoid of it.

71. **What is invasive pituitary adenoma?**

Invasiveness of a pituitary adenoma is assessed by the radiological and/or histological characteristics of tumor. Invasive pituitary adenoma is defined as tumors which invade surrounding structures like cavernous sinus (parasellar), sphenoid sinus (infrasellar), frontal lobe (antesellar), and brainstem (retrosellar). Pituitary tumors with suprasellar extension are not considered as invasive. Further, invasion of dura on histology also denotes invasion.

72. **What is aggressive pituitary adenoma?**

Aggressiveness of a pituitary adenoma is assessed by the clinical behavior of the tumor, which includes rapidity of tumor growth, poor response to conventional treatment, and high rate of recurrence after surgery. Unfortunately, there are no objective parameters to clinically define these characteristics. Histologically, aggressiveness of tumor can be assessed by high mitotic activity, Ki-67 ≥ 3%, or p53 immunopositivity. Some subtypes of pituitary tumors are known to be aggressive and include Crooke's cell corticotropinoma, sparsely granulated somatotropinoma, densely granulated prolactinoma, gonadotropinoma, thyrotropinoma, null cell adenoma, and silent adenoma. It is not necessary that all invasive adenomas are aggressive, and vice versa.

73. **What is pituitary carcinoma?**

Pituitary carcinoma is defined by the presence of extra-sellar cranial metastasis without anatomical contiguity with sellar mass or systemic metastasis in a patient with pituitary tumor. It is rare and contributes to 0.2% of all pituitary tumors. Two-thirds of the pituitary carcinoma are functional (prolactin secreting 36%, ACTH secreting 30%), while 23% are nonfunctioning. The most common site of metastasis is brain (35%) followed by spinal cord (17%), bone, lymph nodes, liver, and lungs.

74. **What is temozolomide?**

Temozolomide, an orally active alkylating agent, induces methylation of guanine base and leads to DNA damage. It easily crosses blood–brain barrier and is not cell cycle specific. It has been found to be useful in patients with aggressive pituitary tumors and carcinoma, irrespective of their functional status. The recommended dose schedule is 200 mg/m^2 given daily for 5 days PO every 28 days. If there is no response after 3 months of temozolomide therapy, it should be discontinued. However, if there is a response, it should be continued for 6–12 months, but no data is available regarding its long-term use. Unlike other alkylating agents, temozolomide is relatively safe, and the common adverse effect includes nausea, vomiting, fatigue, and myelosuppression.

Suggested Reading

1. Larry JL, De Groot LJ. Endocrinology: adult and pediatric. Philadelphia: Elsevier Health Sciences; 2010.
2. Longo D, Anthony F, Dennis K, Stephen H, Jameson J, Joseph L. Harrison's principles of internal medicine 18E EB. New York: McGraw Hill Professional; 2012.
3. Melmed S, Casanueva FF, Hoffman AR, Kleinberg DL, Montori VM, Schlechte JA, Wass JAH. Diagnosis and treatment of hyperprolactinemia: an Endocrine Society clinical practice guideline. J Clin Endocrinol Metab. 2011;96(2):273–88.
4. Melmed S, Polonsky KS, Larsen PR, Kronenberg HM. Williams textbook of endocrinology: expert consult. London: Elsevier Health Sciences; 2011.

4 Cushing's Syndrome: Clinical Perspectives

4.1 Case Vignette

A 45-year-old woman presented with weight gain, oligomenorrhea, easy bruising, and generalized weakness for the last 2 years. She was a known hypertensive for the last 8 years and diabetic for the past 2 years. On examination, she had BMI 30 kg/m^2, blood pressure 160/100 mm Hg, and had florid features of Cushing's syndrome including facial plethora, wide violaceous striae, cuticular atrophy, bruise, and proximal myopathy. She had hyperpigmentation of knuckles. Her Ferriman–Gallwey score was 20/36 and had no features of virilization. On biochemical evaluation, serum potassium was 4.8 mEq/L, and liver and renal function tests were normal. Fasting plasma glucose was 200 mg/dl, postprandial plasma glucose 260 mg/dl, and HbA1c 9.5%. Lipid profile revealed high triglycerides and low HDL-C. Cortisol dynamics showed 0800h cortisol 770 nmol/L, awake 2300h cortisol 667 nmol/L, 0800h ACTH 45 pg/ml, overnight dexamethasone suppression test (ONDST) 406 nmol/L, low-dose dexamethasone suppression test (LDDST) 375 nmol/L, and high-dose dexamethasone suppression test (HDDST) 127 nmol/L. Serum prolactin was 8.1 ng/ml, T_4 8 μg/dl, TSH 2.1 μIU/ml, testosterone 2.6 nmol/L, LH 1.1 μIU/ml, and FSH 2.1 μIU/ml. Compression ultrasonography of lower limb was normal, and DXA scan showed osteoporosis (T-score –2.6 and Z-score -3 at lumbar vertebra). Dynamic contrast-enhanced MRI of sella revealed 4.8 mm adenoma on right half of pituitary. She underwent bilateral inferior petrosal sinus sampling (IPSS) with AVP stimulation (10 IU i.v. infusion). IPSS localized the source of ACTH excess to pituitary gland and lateralized to right half of pituitary gland. As patient had right hypochondrial pain, CECT abdomen was done, which demonstrated a left adrenal mass measuring 2.5×2 cm and bulky right adrenal. As she had osteoporosis, she was treated with calcium, vitamin D, and zoledronic acid. She underwent transsphenoidal surgery after optimal blood glucose and blood pressure control. Postoperatively, her day 2 serum 0800h cortisol was 84 nmol/L. She did not have any complications after surgery. She was initiated on hydrocortisone replacement. Histopathology showed

A. Bhansali, Y. Gogate, *Clinical Rounds in Endocrinology: Volume I - Adult Endocrinology*, DOI 10.1007/978-81-322-2398-6_4

pituitary adenoma on ACTH immunopositivity. At 6 weeks, she had a weight loss of 6 kg, resolution of plethora, and reduction in the requirement of antihypertensives. She had normal plasma glucose profile without any medications. Her serum 0800h cortisol was 120 nmol/L after omission of hydrocortisone for 24 h, and serum T_4 was 6 μg/dl. At three months of follow-up, she is in remission and is doing well.

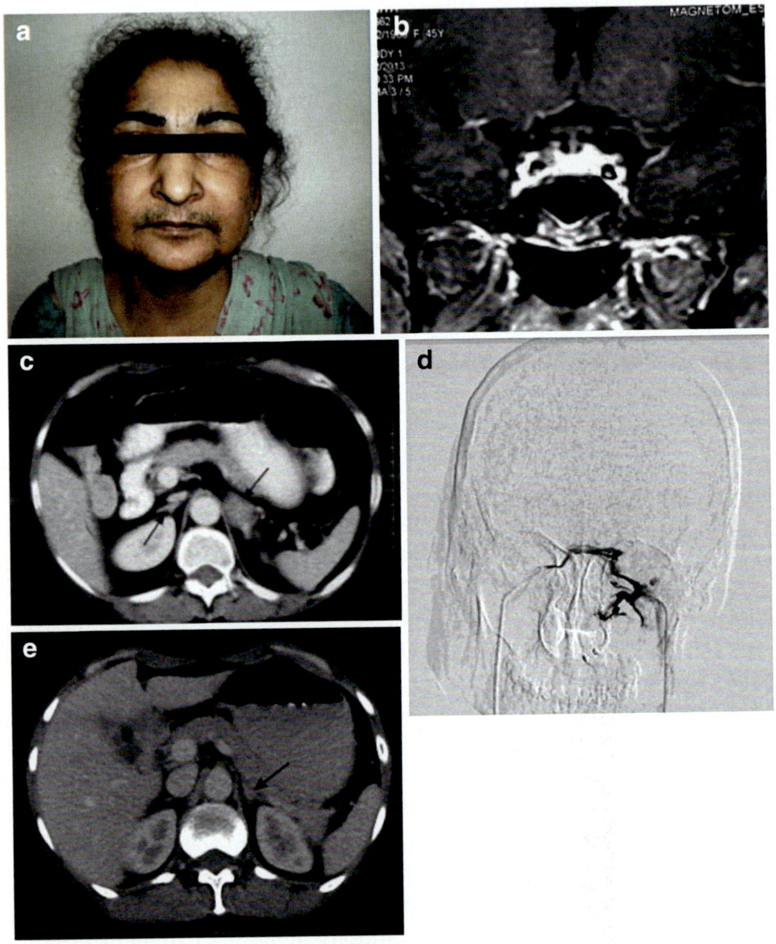

Fig. 4.1 (a) A 45-year-old lady with facial plethora, hirsutism, and thin scalp hair. (**b**) T1W dynamic CEMRI of sella showing hypointense lesion in right half of pituitary suggestive of micro-adenoma. (**c**) CECT abdomen showing enlarged right adrenal gland and left adrenal mass (2.5 × 2 cm) in the same patient. (**d**) DSA image showing catheterization of both inferior petrosal sinuses in the same patient. (**e**) CECT abdomen showing remarkable reduction in the size of left adrenal mass after curative surgery for Cushing's disease, as compared to previous scan

Results of inferior petrosal sinus sampling after AVP stimulation.

Time (Min)	Right central ACTH	Left central ACTH	Peripheral ACTH	ACTH ratio right central to periphery (right C:P)	ACTH ratio right central to left central (right/left)
−15	37.1	43.4	32.2	1.1	0.8
0	41.4	38.9	37.0	1.1	1.0
2	1717	75.4	43.7	*39.2*	*22.7*
3	1213	159.6	132.7	9.1	7.6
5	368.6	215	185.5	1.9	1.7
10	327.9	309.1	286.2	1.1	1.0
15	309.4	329	297.7	1.0	0.9
30	228.1	231	199.1	1.1	0.9
45	164.8	142.8	142.7	1.1	1.1
60	105.5	97.8	94.2	1.1	1.0

4.2 Stepwise Analysis

This patient presented with weight gain, oligomenorrhea, and hirsutism. On evaluation, she had features of protein catabolism in the form of striae, proximal myopathy, bruising, cuticular atrophy, and osteoporosis. Therefore, a diagnosis of Cushing's syndrome was considered. Presence of hyperpigmentation and features of androgen excess in index patient virtually excludes the possibility of exogenous Cushing's syndrome and strongly favors the diagnosis of ACTH-dependent Cushing's syndrome. Further, 0800h serum cortisol of 770 nmol/L excluded the diagnosis of exogenous Cushing's syndrome. Subsequently, she was subjected to the screening tests for the diagnosis of Cushing's syndrome. Her, ONDST was non-suppressible (406 nmol/L; normal <50 nmol/L). As the first screening test was positive, it requires further confirmation by either urinary free cortisol or late-night salivary cortisol. However, these two tests are not routinely available in our center; therefore, midnight awake serum cortisol was performed as a second screening test. High midnight serum cortisol of 667 nmol/L (normal <207 nmol/L) confirmed the loss of circadian rhythm of cortisol secretion and endogenous hypercortisolemia. LDDST was also non-suppressible; however, it did not offer any added advantage for the diagnosis of Cushing's syndrome in index case. Nevertheless, LDDST is preferred in place of ONDST as a screening test in patients with suspected pseudo-Cushing's syndrome.

Once the diagnosis of endogenous Cushing's syndrome was confirmed, 0800h plasma ACTH estimation was done to evaluate for the etiology of Cushing's syndrome. A 0800h plasma ACTH >20 pg/ml was suggestive of ACTH-dependent Cushing's syndrome. Subsequently, contrast-enhanced dynamic 3 Tesla MRI sella was performed as Cushing's disease contributes to 80% of ACTH-dependent Cushing's syndrome. MRI sella revealed an adenoma of size <6 mm, which has a high probability of being an incidentaloma, rather than corticotropinoma. Further, even a pituitary adenoma of size >6 mm has a sensitivity of only 40% to be a corticotropinoma, with a specificity of 98%. Therefore, the presence of a pituitary adenoma of 4.8 mm in the index case mandates IPSS to localize the source of ACTH excess. Hence, she underwent IPSS with AVP stimulation (as CRH was not available in our center). IPSS localized the source of ACTH excess to pituitary (right central to peripheral ratio 39.2) and lateralized to right side of pituitary (right central to left central ratio 22.7). A central to peripheral ratio, after stimulation (with CRH), >3 is suggestive of pituitary source of ACTH, and right central to left central ratio of >1.4 is suggestive of lateralization to that side. CECT abdomen revealed left adrenal mass and bulky right adrenal. This left adrenal mass was unlikely to be autonomous, as serum 0800h ACTH was >20 pg/ml and the other adrenal was bulky. High-dose dexamethasone suppression test not required in this patient, but it was performed as a part of Liddle's protocol followed at our institute. HDDST showed >50% suppression of 0800h cortisol (from 770 to 127 nmol/L) which suggests a pituitary cause. Osteoporosis in Cushing's syndrome is reversible with curative treatment particularly in children and young adults. However, our patient was in the perimenopausal age and had a T-score of –2.6, which is unlikely to recover completely; therefore, she was offered bisphosphonate therapy. After optimal blood pressure and glycemic control, she underwent transsphenoidal surgery uneventfully. She was monitored for signs and symptoms of adrenal insufficiency along with daily 0800h serum cortisol. Her postoperative day2 0800h serum cortisol was 84 nmol/L. She was started on hydrocortisone replacement and discharged. She had desquamation of skin in immediate postoperative period with progressive regression of features of protein catabolism, resolution of diabetes, and reduction in doses of antihypertensive drugs. At 3 months of follow-up, she continues to be in remission. The probability of cure is likely to be high in index case as she had a microadenoma without parasellar involvement on imaging, documented adenoma with ACTH immunopositivity on histopathology, immediate postoperative 0800h serum cortisol <140 nmol/L, and prolonged requirement of hydrocortisone supplementation. At 9 months of follow-up, she continues to remain in remission, and a CT abdomen showed marked reduction in size of left adrenal mass.

4.3 Clinical Rounds

1. **What is Cushing's syndrome**?

   Cushing's syndrome is a disorder of chronic glucocorticoid excess and is characterized by features of protein catabolism along with varying signs and symptoms. The most common cause of Cushing's syndrome is exogenous administration of glucocorticoids.

2. **What are the clinical features that best discriminate Cushing's syndrome**?

   The clinical features that best discriminate Cushing's syndrome are prototype manifestations of protein catabolism and include easy bruisibility, proximal muscle weakness, striae (especially if purplish and >1 cm wide), facial plethora, and cuticular/pulp atrophy. Features like obesity, hypertension, and diabetes are not discriminatory as they are highly prevalent in general population. However, onset of hypertension, diabetes, or vertebral osteoporosis at a younger age should raise a suspicion of Cushing's syndrome.

3. **What are the causes of endogenous Cushing's syndrome**?

The etiology of endogenous Cushing's syndrome is summarized in the figure given below.

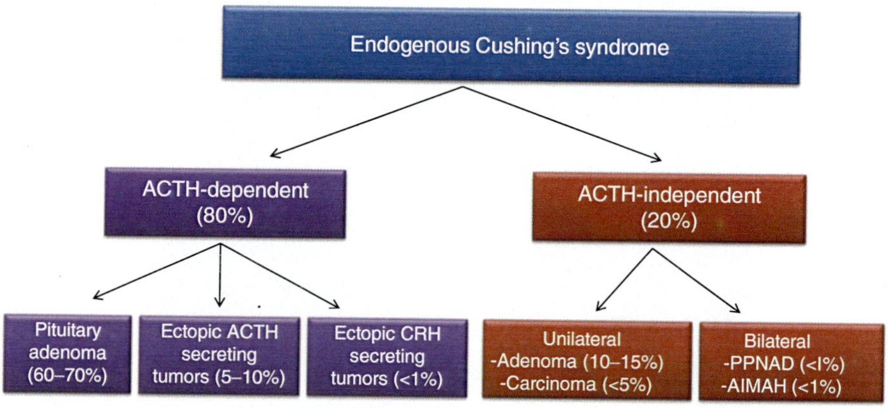

Fig. 4.2 Etiology of endogenous Cushing's syndrome

Cushing's disease is the most common cause of endogenous Cushing's syndrome. Approximately 90% of patients with Cushing's disease have microadenoma, while macroadenoma contributes to the rest.

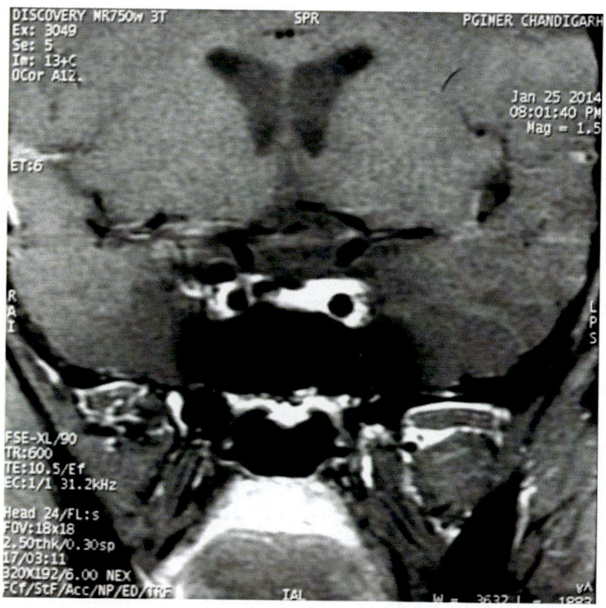

Fig. 4.3 T1W dynamic CEMR coronal image showing hypointense lesion in right half of the pituitary suggestive of microadenoma in a patient with Cushing's syndrome

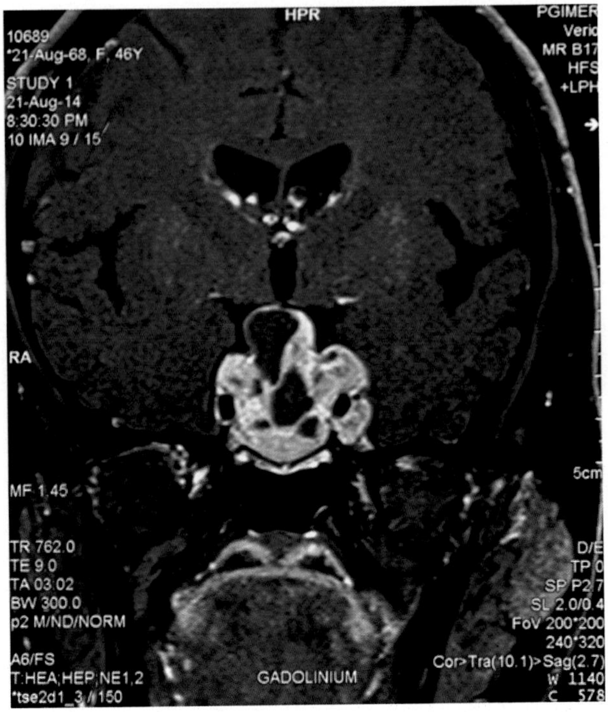

Fig. 4.4 T1W CEMR coronal image showing a sellar–suprasellar mass with cystic component and bilateral parasellar extension suggestive of macroadenoma in a patient with Cushing's syndrome

4. **What are the conditions associated with hypercortisolemia in the absence of clinical features of Cushing's syndrome?**

   Hypercortisolemia in the absence of clinical features of Cushing's syndrome may occur due to stress (hospitalization, surgery, and pain), intense chronic exercise, malnutrition, anorexia nervosa, and cortisol-binding globulin (CBG) excess states.

5. **What is pseudo-Cushing's syndrome?**

   Pseudo-Cushing's syndrome is a group of reversible disorders with subtle symptoms and signs of Cushing's syndrome and hypercortisolism with anomalous response to dexamethasone suppression tests. Morbid obesity, depression, alcoholism, metabolic syndrome, poorly controlled diabetes, and polycystic ovarian disease are associated with pseudo-Cushing's syndrome. Chronic stress is a common denominator in most of these disorders, which leads to increased cytokines and/or neurotransmitter overactivity resulting in hypercortisolemia by activation of the hypothalamo–pituitary–adrenocortical (HPA) axis. Resolution of the underlying disorder leads to amelioration of pseudo-Cushing's syndrome.

6. **What are the alterations in cortisol dynamics in obesity**?

Obesity is a pseudo-Cushing's state and is associated with loss of circadian rhythm of cortisol, normal total serum cortisol, mildly increased urinary free cortisol, and variability in response to overnight dexamethasone suppression test. Obesity is associated with increased cortisol turnover, with augmented synthesis as well as clearance of cortisol, resulting in a normal circulating level of cortisol. Increased cortisol secretion in obesity is due to IGF1-mediated inhibition of hepatic 11β-hydroxysteroid dehydrogenase type 1 (11β-HSD1) resulting in decreased peripheral conversion of cortisone to cortisol, thereby stimulating HPA axis due to loss of negative feedback. The augmented clearance of cortisol is due to enhanced A-ring reduction of cortisol leading to increased urinary excretion. Despite normal circulating levels of cortisol, some patients with morbid obesity may have cushingoid features which may be explained by increased 11β-HSD1 activity in adipose tissues leading to augmented local production of cortisol.

7. **What is cyclical Cushing's syndrome**?

Cyclical Cushing's syndrome is characterized by periods of waxing and waning symptoms and signs of hypercortisolemia and anomalous results of cortisol dynamic tests. It is biochemically defined as presence of three peaks and two troughs of cortisol secretion over a period of time (usually weeks to months). These patients require frequent monitoring with urine free cortisol or late-night salivary cortisol to establish the diagnosis, as cycle length varies from days to months. Spot urine cortisol to creatinine ratio and measurement of scalp hair cortisol may also be useful. Dexamethasone suppression test (DST) is not preferred for the diagnosis. Cyclical Cushing's syndrome can occur with pituitary (54%), ectopic (26%), or even with adrenal Cushing's (11%). The mechanism of cyclicity are elusive; however, periodic hormonogenesis is a commonly purported mechanism; periodicity in hormone biosynthesis may be due to recurrent hemorrhage in the tumor or early programmed tumoral cell death.

8. **What is subclinical Cushing's syndrome**?

Subclinical Cushing's syndrome is characterized by lack of specific symptoms and signs of Cushing's syndrome, but with evidence of autonomous glucocorticoid secretion. However, majority of these patients have obesity, hypertension, and type 2 diabetes. They are commonly diagnosed during evaluation for an adrenal incidentaloma. The diagnostic cutoff for subclinical Cushing's syndrome following 1 mg overnight dexamethasone suppression test (ONDST) is 0800h cortisol >135 nmol/L (5 μg/dl), with a specificity of 100%, instead of 50 nmol/L (1.8 μgm/dl) as in overt Cushing's syndrome. Suppressed dehydroepiandrosterone sulfate (DHEAS) and ACTH are surrogate evidences for the presence of subclinical Cushing's syndrome.

9. **What are the causes of weight gain in a patient with Cushing's syndrome**?

Causes of weight gain in a patient with Cushing's syndrome are increased appetite, enhanced adipogenesis, fluid retention, and decreased physical activity. Increased appetite is because of stimulatory effect of cortisol on feeding center through augmented adenosine monophosphate kinase activity, insulin resistance, decreased corticotrophin-releasing hormone, and increased neuropeptide Y. Enhanced adipogenesis is attributed to cortisol-mediated diversion of primitive mesenchymal stem cells to adipocytes and increased activity of lipoprotein lipase and glycerol-3-phosphate dehydrogenase. Fluid retention also contributes to weight gain and is due to action of excess cortisol on mineralocorticoid receptor (specificity spill-over). Decreased physical activity resulting from proximal muscle weakness or neuropsychiatric manifestations is also a cause of weight gain.

10. **Why is central obesity common in Cushing's syndrome**?

Nearly 45% of patients with Cushing's syndrome have central obesity as against 55% with generalized obesity. Central obesity is due to increased expression of glucocorticoid receptors and elevated 11β-HSD1 activity in omental fat as compared to subcutaneous adipose tissue. However, children with Cushing's syndrome usually have generalized obesity, probably due to lesser omental fat.

11. **When is Cushing's syndrome associated with weight loss**?

Weight gain is a hallmark feature of Cushing's syndrome; however, some patients may present with weight loss. The causes include adrenocortical carcinoma, ectopic Cushing's syndrome, uncontrolled diabetes, concurrent infections like tuberculosis, and endogenous depression. Rarely, concurrent thyrotoxicosis either due to ACTH and TSH co-secreting adenoma or McCune–Albright syndrome may also present with weight loss.

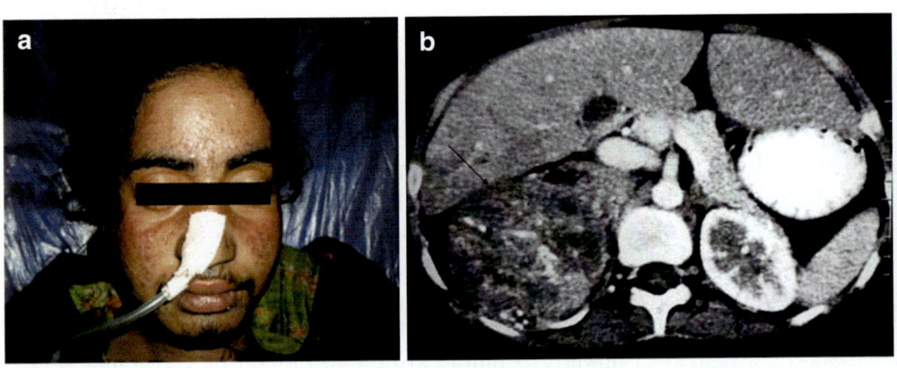

Fig. 4.5 (**a**) Severe acne, hirsutism, frontal recession of hair, and facial plethora in a patient with Cushing's syndrome due to adrenocortical carcinoma. She also had weight loss as a presenting manifestation. (**b**) CECT abdomen of the same patient showing large heterogeneous adrenal mass abutting inferior vena cava with areas of necrosis suggestive of adrenocortical carcinoma

12. **What are the causes of headache in a patient with Cushing's syndrome?**

Headache is an uncommon symptom of Cushing's syndrome. Headache in patients with Cushing's syndrome can be due to adenoma per se, sinusitis, cortical vein thrombosis, benign intracranial hypertension, and glaucoma.

13. **Why do patients with Cushing's syndrome have striae?**

Striae are one of the classical features of Cushing's syndrome and are present in 60–70% of patients. Striae in Cushing's syndrome are violaceous-purple, dehiscent, >1 cm wide and are commonly present over abdomen, thighs, buttocks, arms, and inframammary region. Wide and purplish striae are due to venular dilatation and thinned out dermis, which in turn occurs as a result of loss of perivascular collagen support and dermal collagen breakdown, respectively. Striae may be absent in patients with childhood Cushing's syndrome, adrenocortical carcinoma, ectopic Cushing's syndrome, and hypercortisolemia associated with androgen excess. Causes of striae in the absence of Cushing's syndrome include rapid weight gain during puberty, pregnancy, and pseudo-Cushing's states.

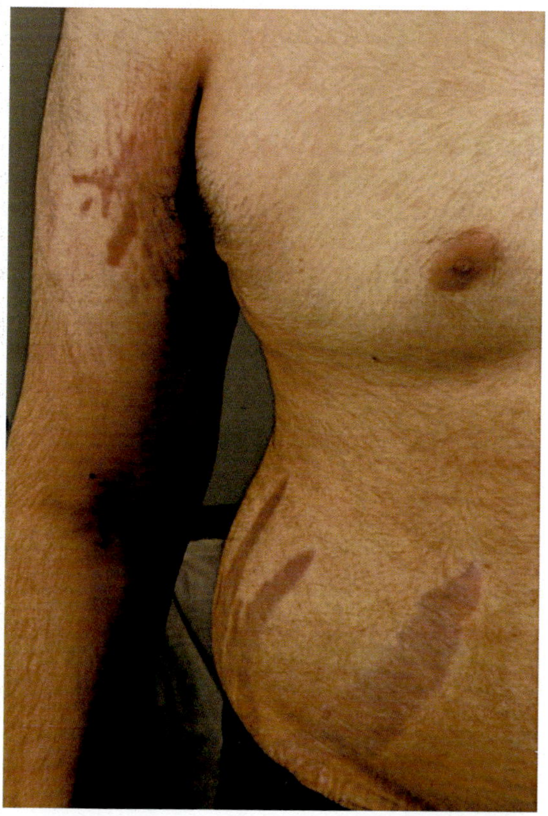

Fig. 4.6 Wide and purplish striae over abdomen and arm of a patient with Cushing's syndrome

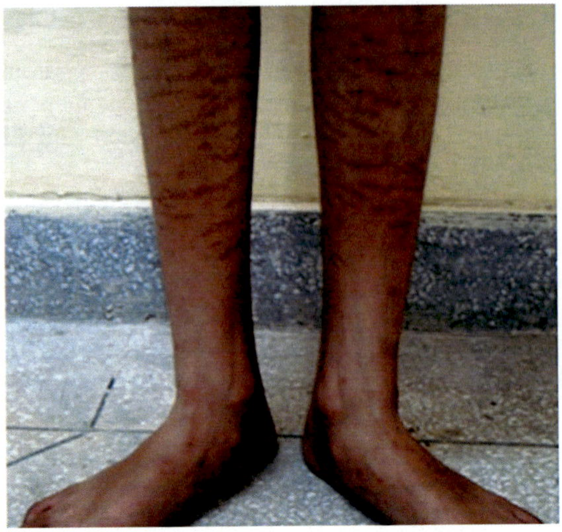

Fig. 4.7 Thin purplish striae over both legs in a child with Cushing's syndrome, giving the appearance of "tiger skin"

14. **What are the cutaneous manifestations of Cushing's syndrome?**

Cutaneous manifestations of Cushing's syndrome are bruise, striae, plethora, cuticular atrophy ("cigarette paper" appearance – Liddle's sign), and fungal infections. Bruise, striae, and plethora are due to loss of dermal collagen, while cuticular atrophy is a result of atrophy of stratum corneum. Rarely, purpura can be associated with Cushing's syndrome due to qualitative abnormalities in platelet function. In addition, patients with Cushing's syndrome can have hyperpigmentation when associated with ACTH excess and hirsuitism/acne due to androgen excess.

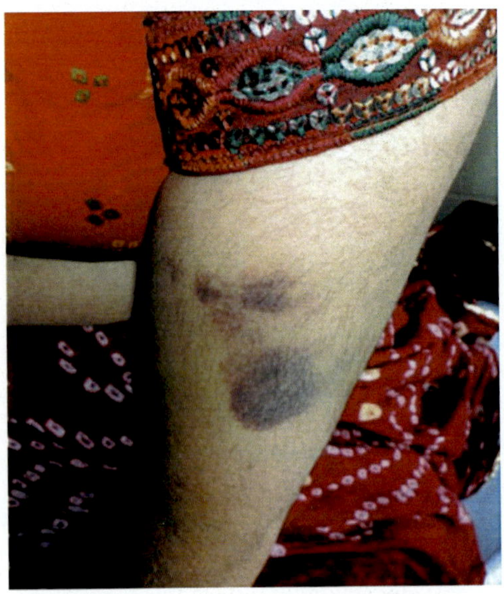

Fig. 4.8 Spontaneous bruise in a patient with Cushing's syndrome

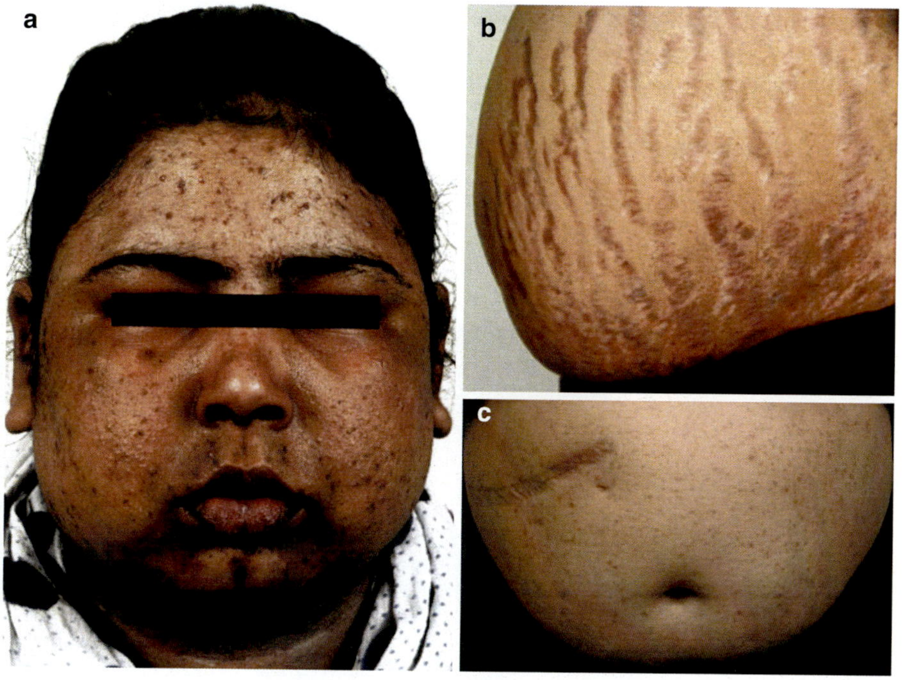

Fig. 4.9 (**a**) Hyperpigmented nodular and cystic acne in a patient with Cushing's disease. (**b**) Wide and purplish striae over the abdomen in the same patient. (**c**) Purpuric spots and hyperpigmented scar (post cholecystectomy) over the abdomen in a patient with Cushing's disease. Note the absence of striae

15. **Why do patients with Cushing's syndrome have proximal myopathy**?

    Proximal myopathy in patients with Cushing's syndrome is due to decreased muscle protein synthesis, increased muscle protein catabolism, and myocyte apoptosis. These are due to the direct effect of excess cortisol. In addition, cortisol suppresses muscle protein synthesis by inhibiting IGF1 and Akt1 signaling in myocytes. Histologically, it is characterized by atrophy of type II muscle fibers and relative hypertrophy of type I muscle fibers. Concurrent hypokalemia, hypophosphatemia, hypomagnesemia, vitamin D deficiency, and hypogonadism further contribute to muscle weakness in patients with Cushing's syndrome.

16. **Why do some patients with Cushing's syndrome lack features of protein catabolism**?

    The features of protein catabolism, also called as specific features, are present in 60–70% of patients with Cushing's syndrome. However, these features may not be present in patients with mild Cushing's syndrome, cyclical Cushing's syndrome, childhood Cushing's syndrome, and hypercortisolemia associated with androgen excess. The catabolic effects of hypercortisolemia are counteracted either by physiologically higher IGF1 (as in childhood Cushing's) or coexisting hyperandrogenemia. Patients with adrenocortical carcinoma and ectopic Cushing's syndrome may lack features of protein catabolism due to short lag time between onset of hypercortisolemia and diagnosis.

17. **Why do patients with Cushing's syndrome have plethora**?

Plethora is considered as a specific sign of Cushing's syndrome and is due to dermal collagen breakdown and increased erythropoiesis because of hypercortisolemia.

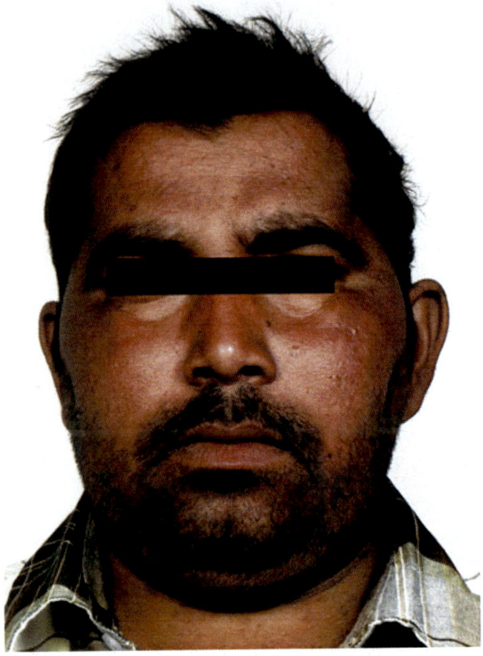

Fig. 4.10 Facial plethora in a patient with Cushing's syndrome

18. **Why do patients with Cushing's syndrome have hirsutism**?

Hirsutism is present in 60–80% of patients with Cushing's syndrome and is more common in ACTH-dependent Cushing's syndrome than in adrenal adenoma, while it is not present in exogenous Cushing's syndrome. The causes of hirsutism are increased adrenal androgen production either under increased ACTH drive or due to concurrent cortisol and androgen-producing neoplasm, secondary polycystic ovarian disease, hyperinsulinemia/insulin resistance, and decreased sex hormone-binding globulin. Hyperprolactinemia seen in 20–30% of patients may also contribute to increased adrenal androgen production. Further, patients with Cushing's syndrome may also have increased fine hair (vellus hair), especially on the forehead, back, and extremities due to a direct effect of cortisol on pilosebaceous units.

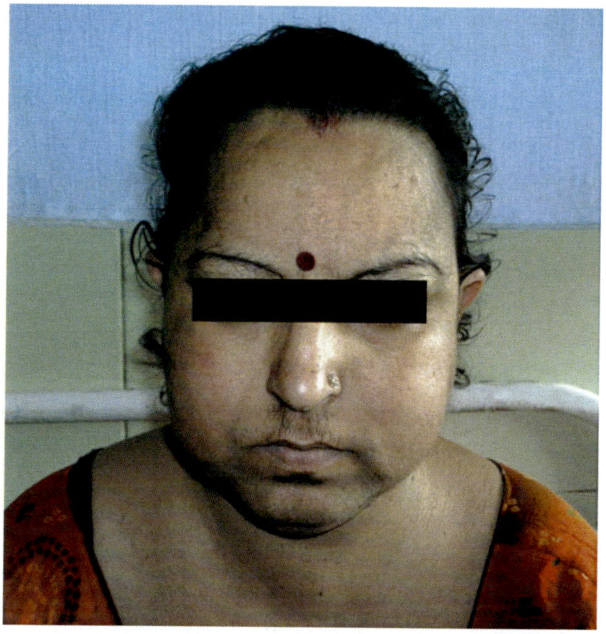

Fig. 4.11 Hirsutism in a patient with Cushing's syndrome. Also note androgenic alopecia as well

19. **What are the causes of menstrual irregularities in patients with Cushing's syndrome?**

    Menstrual irregularities are seen in 70–80% of women with Cushing's syndrome; the most common being oligomenorrhea followed by secondary amenorrhea. The causes of menstrual irregularities are cortisol-mediated inhibition of GnRH–gonadotropin axis, hyperandrogenemia, insulin resistance/hyperinsulinemia, secondary polycystic ovarian disease, and hyperprolactinemia.

20. **What are the causes of hypertension in patients with Cushing's syndrome?**

    Hypertension is seen in 75% of patients with endogenous Cushing's syndrome as against 20% in exogenous Cushing's syndrome. The mechanisms implicated in the development of hypertension in Cushing's syndrome are:

- Increased vasoreactivity to circulating vasoconstrictors (e.g., catecholamines, endothelin 1, and angiotensin II)
- Action of excess cortisol on mineralocorticoid receptor (glucocorticoid receptor type 1) due to saturation of renal tubular 11β-HSD2 activity
- Decreased endothelial nitric oxide synthase activity
- Insulin resistance-/hyperinsulinemia-mediated sodium and water retention
- Augmented renin substrate production in liver

- Accelerated catabolism of renal vasodilatory prostaglandins (prostacyclin)
- Increased intravascular fluid volume
- ACTH-mediated increase in deoxycorticosterone acetate

The lower prevalence of hypertension in patients with exogenous Cushing's syndrome is possibly due to minimal mineralocorticoid activity of the commonly used synthetic steroids. Spironolactone is the drug of choice for hypertension in patients with Cushing's syndrome, especially in those with recalcitrant hypokalemia. Hypertension can persist even after curative surgery due to permanent vascular remodeling or coexisting "essential" hypertension.

21. **How does hypercortisolemia cause diabetes?**

Hypercortisolemia is associated with glucose intolerance in nearly 37% of patients and overt diabetes in 10–15%, especially those with a family history of type 2 diabetes. The causes of hyperglycemia in Cushing's syndrome include increased hepatic glucose output, decreased glucose uptake in muscle/adipocytes, and impaired β-cell function. Increased hepatic glucose output is due to enhanced gluconeogenesis which occurs as a result of excess substrate availability (free fatty acids and alanine) and facilitated phosphoenol pyruvate carboxy kinase (PEPCK) activity. Paradoxically, glycogen synthesis is stimulated by glucocorticoids. Decreased peripheral glucose uptake is attributed to impaired GLUT4 expression, decreased protein kinase C activity, and reduced non-insulin-mediated glucose uptake (NIMGU) as a direct effect of glucocorticoids and free fatty acids. Further, glucocorticoids may interfere with GLUT2 expression in β-cells resulting in decreased insulin secretion as shown in mice.

22. **Why do some patients with Cushing's syndrome have edema?**

Patients with hypercortisolemia usually do not have edema, as cortisol causes diuresis by increasing GFR, inhibiting AVP release, and antagonizing its action at the renal tubule. However, 10–20% of patients with Cushing's syndrome can have edema due to the effect of glucocorticoids on mineralocorticoid receptor.

23. **Why is there osteoporosis in patients with Cushing's syndrome?**

Glucocorticoids predominantly affect trabecular bone as compared to cortical bone because trabecular bone is metabolically more active. Glucocorticoids decrease bone formation and increase bone resorption, thereby leading to osteoporosis. The factors leading to decreased bone formation are increased osteoblast and osteocyte apoptosis, diversion of primitive mesenchymal stem cells to differentiate into adipocytes rather than osteoblasts, impaired collagen synthesis, and decreased generation and action of local IGF1. The causes of increased bone resorption include enhanced osteoclastogenesis, decreased osteoprotegerin, and increased RANKL synthesis. Other contributory factors for the development of osteoporosis include glucocorticoid-mediated alterations

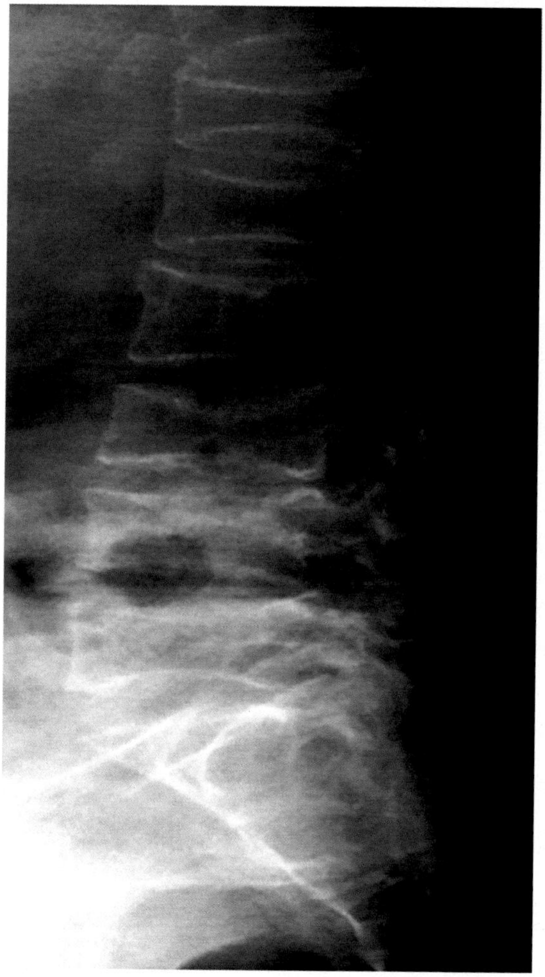

Fig. 4.12 Plain radiograph lateral view of LS spine showing diffuse osteopenia with multiple vertebral body collapse in a patient with Cushing's syndrome

in calcium and vitamin D homeostasis such as reduced intestinal calcium absorption and hypercalciuria, resulting in secondary hyperparathyroidism. Further glucocorticoid-mediated hypogonadism also contributes to osteoporosis. Hypercortisolemia-related osteoporosis is usually reversible after curative surgery as microarchitecture of bone remains intact, as opposed to postmenopausal osteoporosis.

24. **What are the ocular manifestations of hypercortisolemia?**

The ocular manifestations of hypercortisolemia are proptosis (increased retro-orbital fat), chemosis, posterior subcapsular cataract (usually bilateral), glaucoma, and rarely central serous retinopathy.

25. **What are the emergencies in a patient with Cushing's syndrome**?

Patients with Cushing's syndrome may present to emergency with accelerated hypertension, hyperosmolar nonketotic coma or diabetic ketoacidosis, cortical vein thrombosis, acute pulmonary thromboembolism, deep vein thrombosis, or life-threatening sepsis. In addition, they may also present with paraplegia (compressive myelopathy or spinal epidural lipomatosis), pancreatitis, fragility fracture, pituitary apoplexy, and recalcitrant hypokalemia. In post-transsphenoidal surgery, patients can present with meningitis and tension pneumocephalus.

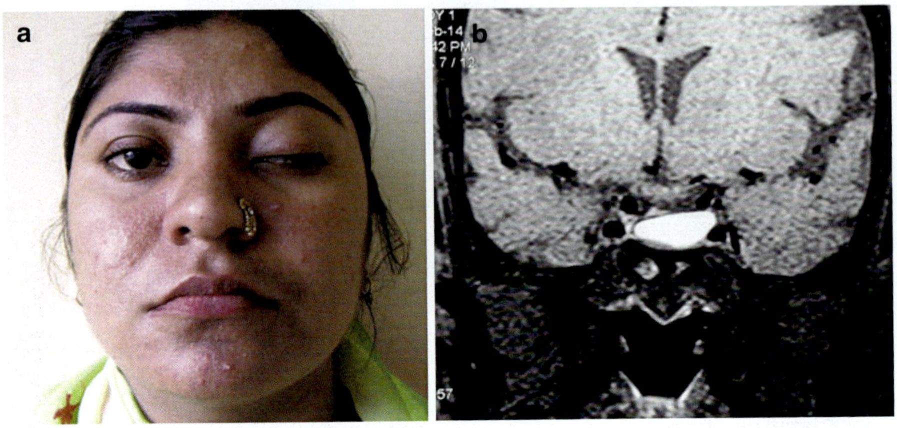

Fig. 4.13 (**a**) Acute-onset ptosis of the left eye in a patient with Cushing's syndrome due to pituitary apoplexy. (**b**) T1W noncontrast coronal MR image showing hyperintense signal suggestive of hemorrhage within pituitary adenoma in the same patient

26. **How do clinical features help in determining the etiology of Cushing's syndrome**?

History of administration of glucocorticoids, presence of florid manifestations of protein catabolism, absence of hyperpigmentation, and lack of virilization are classical of exogenous Cushing's syndrome. Insidious onset of disease, female gender, young age, presence of hyperpigmentation, and features of cortisol and androgen excess suggest a diagnosis of pituitary ACTH-dependent Cushing's syndrome. Rapid onset of disease, middle age, male gender, severe proximal muscle weakness, hyperpigmentation, hypokalemia, metabolic alkalosis, lack of features of protein catabolism, and signs of underlying disease favor a diagnosis of ectopic Cushing's syndrome. However, bronchial carcinoids usually behave like pituitary Cushing's syndrome but may have additional features like flushing, diarrhea, and bronchospasm. Rapid onset of disease, extremes of age (either <10 or >50 years), lack of hyperpigmentation, and presence of hirsuitism/virilization are seen with adrenocortical carcinoma. However, children with adrenocortical carcinoma usually present with isosex-

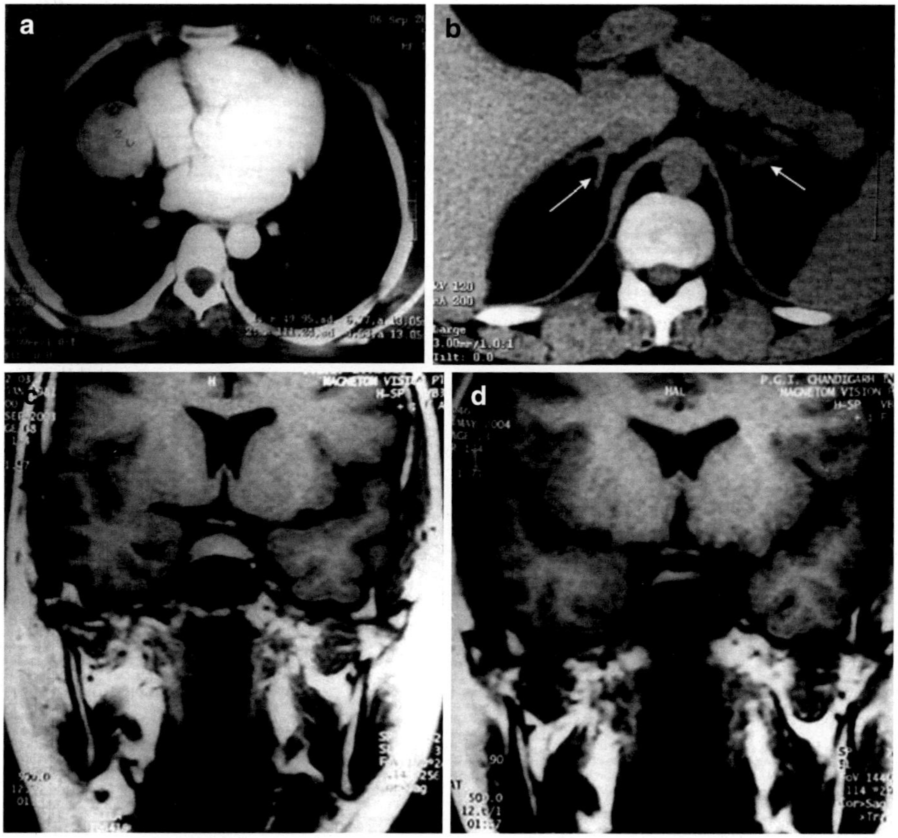

Fig. 4.14 (**a**) CECT chest showing right lower lobe mass abutting pericardium in a patient with Cushing's syndrome. (**b**) CECT abdomen of the same patient showing mildly enlarged adrenals and increased retroperitoneal fat. (**c**) T1W CEMR coronal image showing bulky pituitary gland with homogenous enhancement suggestive of hyperplasia. (**d**) T1W CEMR coronal image showing regression of pituitary hyperplasia after curative surgery

ual/heterosexual precocity. The following images depict a patient with ectopic Cushing's syndrome due to CRH-secreting bronchial carcinoid. The patient had pituitary hyperplasia and mildly enlarged adrenals. After excision of bronchial carcinoid, there was resolution of cushingoid features along with regression of pituitary hyperplasia.

27. **What are the intra-abdominal causes of ectopic Cushing's syndrome**?

    Various intra-abdominal neuroendocrine tumors have been shown to produce ACTH/CRH and result in ectopic Cushing's syndrome. These include pancreatic islet carcinoids, pheochromocytoma, paraganglioma, and rarely intestinal and ovarian carcinoids.

28. **What are the characteristic features of exogenous Cushing's syndrome?**

Exogenous Cushing's syndrome is characterized by florid manifestations of protein catabolism, absence of hyperpigmentation, and lack of features of androgen and mineralocorticoid excess. Features of protein catabolism are florid in patients with exogenous Cushing's syndrome due to use of more potent glucocorticoids. The manifestations which are more prevalent in patients with exogenous Cushing's syndrome include posterior subcapsular cataract, glaucoma, pancreatitis, panniculitis, avascular necrosis of head of femur, spinal epidural lipomatosis, and benign intracranial hypertension. Hyperpigmentation and features of androgen excess are absent in patients with exogenous Cushing's syndrome because of inhibition of endogenous ACTH drive. Hypertension is present only in 20% of patients with exogenous Cushing's syndrome as compared to 75% in endogenous Cushing's syndrome. Besides this, depressive disorders are more common in endogenous Cushing's, while euphoria/elation is more frequent in exogenous Cushing's syndrome.

29. **Why is osteonecrosis of head of femur common in Cushing's syndrome**?

Osteonecrosis of the head of the femur, previously referred as avascular necrosis (AVN), is more common with exogenous Cushing's syndrome. The postulated mechanisms include end-artery supply to femoral head, increased marrow adipogenesis, venous outflow obstruction due to endothelial dysfunction, fat embolization, and accumulation of microfractures due to impaired bone remodeling. Treatment strategies include decompression, hip prosthesis, calcium and vitamin D supplementation, and bisphosphonates, if glucocorticoid replacement is to be continued.

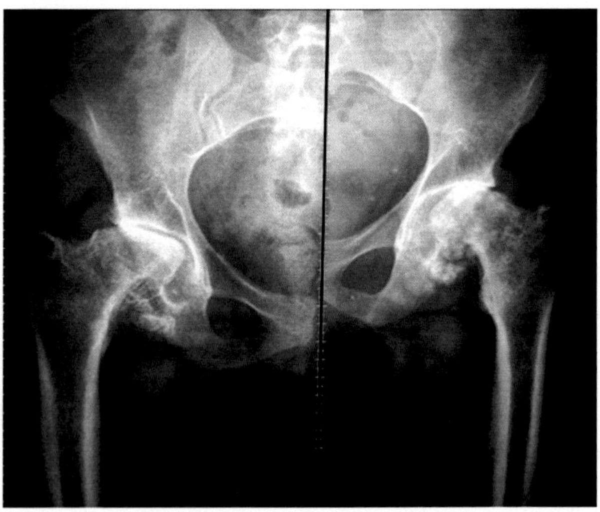

Fig. 4.15 Plain radiograph showing flattening of femoral heads with areas of lysis and sclerosis and reduced joint space suggestive of avascular necrosis in a patient with Cushing's syndrome

30. **What are the causes of "exuberant" callus formation?**

Exuberant callus formation is a characteristic of osteogenesis imperfecta (type VI). But it is also seen in patients with Cushing's syndrome, either exogenous or endogenous.

31. **Should all patients with type 2 diabetes be screened for Cushing's syndrome?**

No. When patients with type 2 diabetes are screened for Cushing's syndrome, the yield is only 3–4%. However, patients of diabetes with younger age of onset, difficult to control diabetes, muscle weakness disproportionate to peripheral neuropathy, or presence of features of protein catabolism need to be screened for Cushing's syndrome.

32. **What are the presentations of childhood Cushing's syndrome?**

The presenting manifestations of childhood Cushing's syndrome are short stature, obesity, and delayed puberty. Obesity is usually associated with accelerated growth rate velocity due to increased IGF1, while in children with Cushing's syndrome, obesity is associated with growth failure. In addition, the classical features of protein catabolism are less pronounced due to growing age and relatively higher IGF1 level in children. The unusual presentations of childhood Cushing's syndrome include precocious puberty, gait abnormalities (slipped femoral epiphyses, osteonecrosis), abdominal mass, and purpura.

33. **What are the distinctive features of childhood Cushing's syndrome?**

The distinctive features of childhood Cushing's syndrome, as compared to adult Cushing's, are male preponderance, less pronounced features of protein catabolism, presence of generalized obesity, and higher occurrence of features of androgen excess. As compared to adults, adrenal causes predominate (65%) in children. The other features of childhood Cushing's syndrome include normal neuroimaging even in those with Cushing's disease and excellent response to pituitary irradiation.

34. **How is hypercortisolemia associated with short stature?**

Hypercortisolemia, whether endogenous or exogenous, leads to decreased growth velocity and short stature. The causes of short stature include a direct effect of cortisol on the GHRH–GH axis, decreased pre-chondrocyte to chondrocyte differentiation, increased chondrocyte apoptosis, impaired local IGF1 generation, increased bone collagen breakdown, and concurrent hypogonadism. In addition the effect of excess cortisol on calcium–vitamin D homeostasis (e.g., inhibition of renal 1α-hydroxylase activity, decreased calcium absorption, and hypercalciuria) also contribute to short stature.

35. **What are the causes of childhood Cushing's syndrome**?

The causes of Cushing's syndrome are listed in the table given below. Cushing's disease is the most common cause of Cushing's syndrome after 5 years of age, and has a peak incidence at 14 years. Ectopic Cushing's syndrome is rare in pediatric population.

Age	Etiology
Infancy	McCune–Albright syndrome
1–5 years of age	Adrenocortical neoplasm
>5 years	ACTH-dependent pituitary Cushing's syndrome
	Primary pigmented nodular adrenocortical disease (PPNAD)
	Carney's Complex

36. **What are the causes of childhood Cushing's syndrome with normal/tall stature**?

Causes of childhood Cushing's syndrome with normal linear growth are PPNAD (mild hypercortisolemia and concurrent somatotropinoma if associated with Carney's complex), McCune–Albright syndrome with concurrent acro-gigantism, androgen co-secreting adrenocortical tumors, and rarely cyclical Cushing's syndrome.

37. **Why is there delayed puberty in childhood Cushing's syndrome**?

Majority of children with Cushing's syndrome present with delayed puberty. The causes include cortisol-mediated impaired GnRH pulse generator activity, direct inhibition of gonadotropins, and deleterious effect of cortisol on Leydig cells. However, despite delayed gonadarche, adrenarche may occur early.

38. **What are the causes of Cushing's syndrome with ACTH-independent adrenal hyperplasia**?

ACTH not only regulates adrenal steroidogenesis by its action on rate-limiting enzyme 20, 22 desmolase and StAR protein but also is responsible for adrenal growth and development. However, ACTH-independent adrenal hyperplasia occurs in ACTH-independent macronodular adrenal hyperplasia (AIMAH), McCune–Albright syndrome (Gsα mutation), and primary pigmented nodular adrenocortical disease (PPNAD).

39. **What is primary pigmented nodular adrenocortical disease**?

Primary pigmented nodular adrenocortical disease (PPNAD) is an ACTH-independent cause of Cushing's syndrome. The distinctive features of Cushing's syndrome due to PPNAD are young age of onset (< 15 years), subtle features of protein catabolism, obesity, normal growth velocity osteoporosis, suppressed ACTH, and paradoxical increase in serum cortisol/UFC following high-dose dexamethasone suppression test. Therefore, in patients with childhood Cushing's syndrome, a suppressed ACTH, normal adrenals on imaging, and paradoxical rise in serum cortisol after DST are suggestive of PPNAD. Occasionally, CT adrenal may demonstrate characteristic "beads on a string appearance." Multiple pigmented nodules (<5mm) with internodular atrophy is the characteristic histological feature of PPNAD. PPNAD is commonly (>90%) described in association with Carney's complex, an autosomal dominant disorder. The genes implicated in the pathogenesis of PPNAD are PRKAR1A, PDE11A, PDE8B, and MYH8, which upregulate cyclic adenosine monophosphate thereby facilitating tumorigenesis.

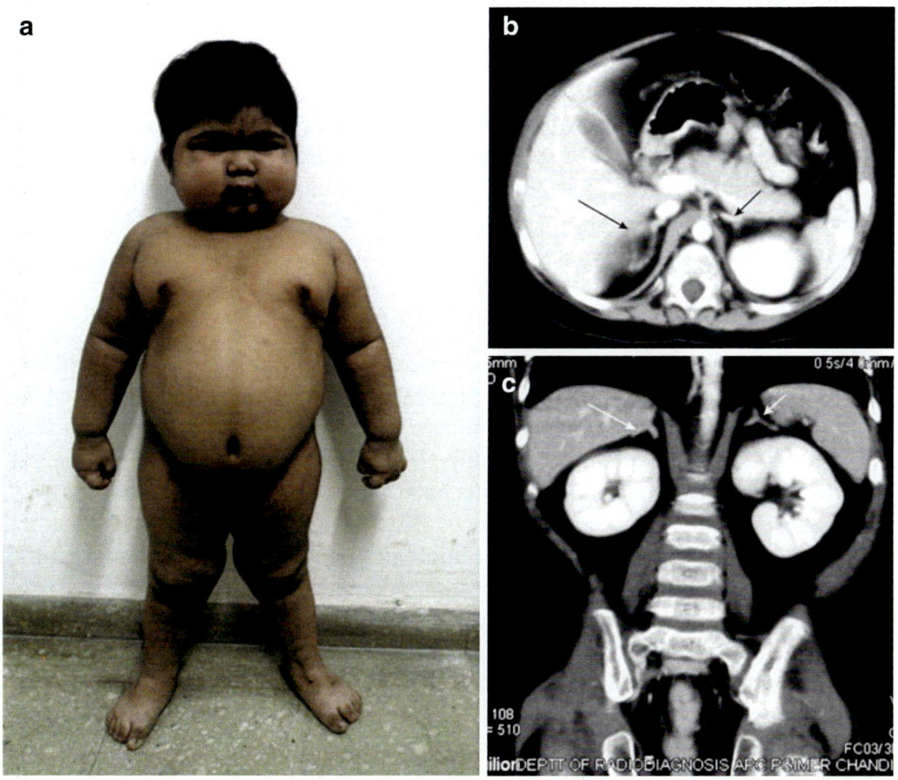

Fig. 4.16 (**a**) A 3-year-old boy with childhood Cushing's syndrome having generalized and truncal obesity, moon facies, and plethora. (**b**, **c**) CECT abdomen axial and coronal showing enlargement of right adrenal and normal left adrenal in the same child with PPNAD

40. **What are the atypical presentations of PPNAD**?

PPNAD may present as classical, subclinical or cyclical Cushing's syndrome. Rarely, some children with PPNAD may present with atypical Cushing's syndrome manifesting as asthenia, lean habitus, severe muscle wasting, osteoporosis, and short stature. Biochemically, 24 h urine free cortisol is usually normal. However, loss of normal diurnal cortisol rhythm and paradoxical increase in cortisol/UFC following HDDST point to diagnosis of PPNAD.

41. **What is paradoxical cortisol response to high-dose dexamethasone suppression test**?

In response to high-dose dexamethasone, more than 50% decline in serum cortisol from baseline (0800h) cortisol suggests suppressible HDDST, while failure to suppress serum cortisol by >50% indicates non-suppressible HDDST. The paradoxical response to dexamethasone is defined as more than 50% rise in serum cortisol from baseline (0800h) cortisol after HDDST during Liddle's protocol. PPNAD is the most common cause of paradoxical cortisol response to HDDST. Rarely patients with AIMAH and adrenocortical carcinoma may also have paradoxical response. The paradoxical increase in cortisol after HDDST is attributed to increased glucocorticoid receptor expression on adrenocortical cells or due to non-genomic effect of dexamethasone which is mediated via protein kinase A.

42. **What are the distinctive features of AIMAH**?

AIMAH contributes to <1% of all causes of Cushing's syndrome, and the characteristic features include familial predisposition, lack of gender predilection, and presentation at middle age. Patients may present with features of Cushing's syndrome or can be incidentally diagnosed due to bilateral adrenal nodules. Majority of patients have hypercortisolemia, while some may co-secrete androgens or aldosterone. Biochemical features are not distinct from Cushing's syndrome of other etiologies. Imaging shows bilateral multiple adrenal nodules with size >10 mm. Histopathology shows characteristic nodular hyperplasia with internodular atrophic/hypertrophic areas. AIMAH is due to the illicit stimulation of the adrenal gland by a wide variety of peptides. The treatment of choice is bilateral adrenalectomy in those with overt Cushing's syndrome.

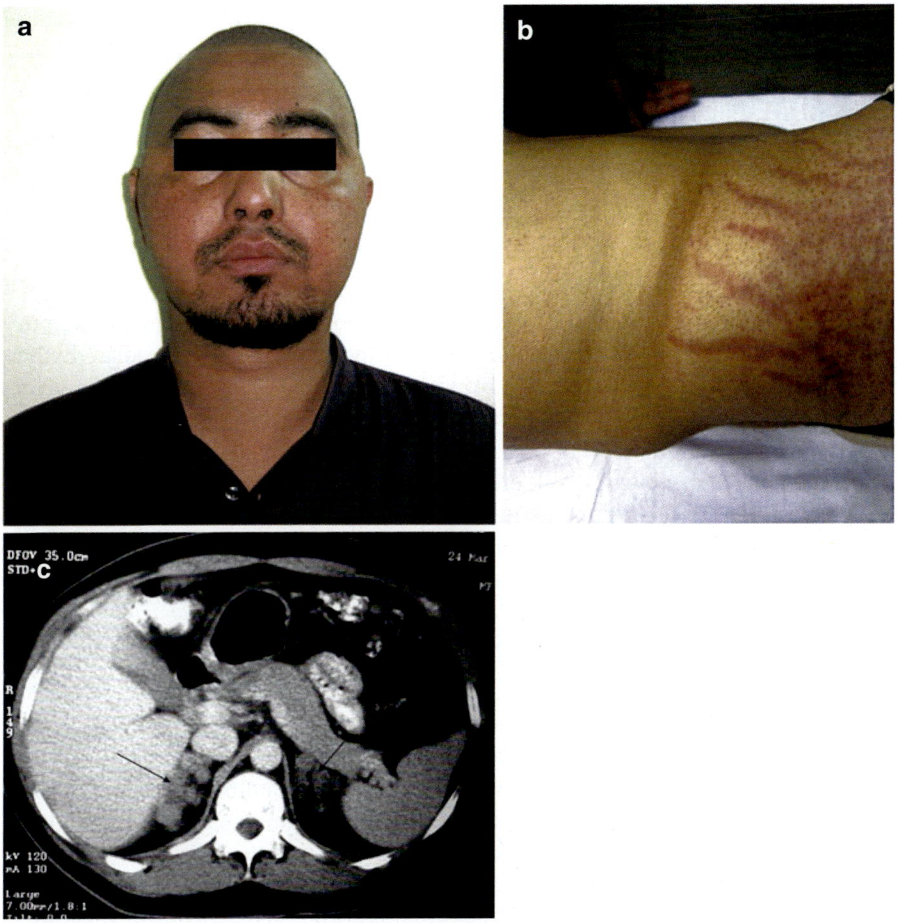

Fig. 4.17 (**a**) Moon facies and plethora in a patient with Cushing's syndrome due to AIMAH. (**b**) Wide purplish striae over the posterior aspect of lower thigh in the same patient. (**c**) CECT abdomen showing bilateral nodular adrenal enlargement classical of AIMAH

43. **What are the illicit stimulators in ACTH-independent macronodular adrenal hyperplasia**?

ACTH-independent macronodular adrenal hyperplasia (AIMAH) is a result of aberrant expression of receptors for peptide hormones/amines (illicit stimulators) on adrenocortical cells, leading to autonomous production of cortisol. The illicit stimulators include arginine vasopressin, glucose-dependent insulinotropic peptide, beta-adrenergic agonist, LH/hCG, serotonin, leptin, and angiotensin II. The exact pathogenesis is not known, but overexpression of eutopic receptors or expression of ectopic receptors of illicit stimulators with coupling of these receptors to steroidogenic pathway explains adrenal hyperplasia in few patients. Recently, intra-adrenal ACTH has also been incriminated in the pathogenesis of AIMAH. In addition, mutations of a putative tumor suppressor gene, armadillo repeat containing 5 (*ARMC5*), have been reported to cause AIMAH. Pituitary ACTH per se is unlikely to be involved in the pathogenesis of AIMAH as after bilateral adrenalectomy in these patients, Nelson's syndrome is rare.

44. **What are the alterations in cortisol dynamics during pregnancy**?

Pregnancy is associated with high serum cortisol, non-suppressible dexamethasone test, and mildly elevated UFC and ACTH, posing a challenge in the interpretation of diagnostic tests for Cushing's syndrome. However, the circadian rhythm of cortisol secretion is preserved during pregnancy, albeit at a higher level. Estimation of midnight serum cortisol is required to define the circadian rhythm; however, the cutoffs for the same during pregnancy are not defined. High serum cortisol in pregnancy is a result of estrogen-mediated increase in cortisol-binding globulin during the second and third trimesters. Non-suppressible dexamethasone test, mildly elevated UFC, and ACTH are due to activation of the maternal hypothalamo–pituitary–adrenal axis as a result of placental CRH.

45. **When to suspect Cushing's syndrome in pregnancy**?

Pregnancy mimics Cushing's syndrome as weight gain, striae, and easy bruisibility are frequently present during pregnancy. But the presence of distinctive features like proximal myopathy and maternal weight gain with fetal intrauterine growth retardation and worsening of glycemic control and hypertension should raise a suspicion of Cushing's syndrome. The diagnosis of Cushing's syndrome in pregnancy is established by measurement of urine free cortisol (UFC). Although modest elevations of UFC are common during pregnancy, a value more than three times the upper limit of normal is diagnostic of Cushing's syndrome.

46. **How to manage Cushing's syndrome during pregnancy**?

The common cause of Cushing's syndrome during pregnancy is adrenal adenoma (40–50%) followed by Cushing's disease. Even in patients with adrenal adenoma (which are ACTH independent), plasma ACTH levels are measurable during pregnancy. This is due to the stimulatory effect of placental CRH on maternal HPA axis. Surgical resection of the adenoma (adrenal/pituitary) during the second trimester is the preferred treatment. If surgery is deferred, medical management with metyrapone is recommended as it is non-teratogenic. Ketoconazole, although known to be teratogenic in animals, has been used successfully in selected cases.

47. **What is an adrenal incidentaloma**?

Adrenal "incidentaloma" is an adrenal mass >1 cm, detected incidentally on imaging during evaluation for a reason unrelated to adrenal disorder. It excludes those detected while staging for cancer.

48. **How to biochemically evaluate a patient with adrenal incidentaloma**?

Detailed history and physical examination are necessary to identify the functional status of adrenal incidentaloma. If the diagnosis of myelolipoma is obvious (low CT attenuation of –10 to –20 Hounsfield units due to lipid content), biochemical evaluation is not warranted, unless clinically indicated. The workup required in a patient with adrenal incidentaloma is 1 mg overnight dexamethasone suppression test and plasma free metanephrines/normetanephrines or 24-h urinary metanephrines/normetanephrines. Those with bilateral adrenal incidentaloma should also be evaluated for adrenal insufficiency. The ratio of plasma aldosterone concentration (PAC) to plasma renin activity (PRA) is indicated only in those with hypertension. Screening for adrenal androgen excess (dehydroepiandrosterone sulfate, DHEAS) is indicated only in those with obvious clinical manifestations. Low DHEAS indicates autonomous functioning adrenal mass or adrenal insufficiency, and high DHEAS suggests adrenocortical carcinoma.

49. **How does imaging phenotype help to evaluate an adrenal incidentaloma**?

The characteristics of an adrenal mass on imaging—"the imaging phenotype" is helpful in establishing the etiological diagnosis of an adrenal incidentaloma. Unilateral lesion with a size > 4 cm, irregular margins, heterogeneity, necrosis, hemorrhage or calcification, attenuation value >10 HU, delayed contrast washout (<50% at 10 min), and hyperintensity in relation to the liver on T2-weighted image favor a diagnosis of adrenocortical carcinoma (ACC) over adrenal adenoma. Metastasis to adrenal gland has similar features, but is usually bilateral and <3 cm in size. Imaging phenotype is unable to differentiate ACC from pheochromocytoma; however, the presence of heterogeneity with cystic areas and marked hyperintensity in relation to liver on T2-weighted images suggest pheochromocytoma. In addition, very low CT attenuation value (–10 to –20 HU) is characteristic of adrenal myelolipoma.

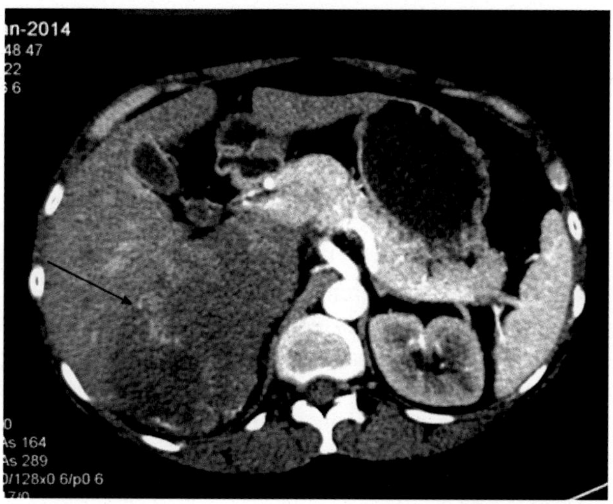

Fig. 4.18 CECT abdomen showing an heterogeneous mass in right adrenal region with hepatic invasion suggestive of adrenocortical carcinoma

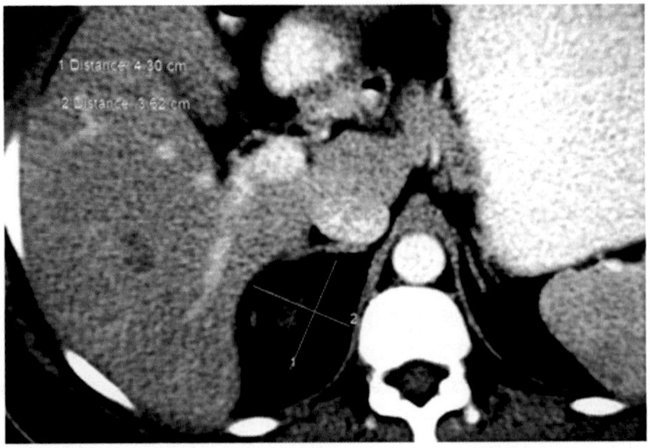

Fig. 4.19 CECT abdomen showing right adrenal mass with mixed fatty and soft tissue attenuation classical of myelolipoma

50. **What are the indications of fine-needle aspiration cytology in adrenal incidentaloma**?

Bilateral nonfunctioning adrenal incidentaloma, after careful exclusion of pheochromocytoma, should undergo fine-needle aspiration cytology (FNAC) to establish the diagnosis. The presence of nonfunctioning unilateral adrenal incidentaloma with features like fever, weight loss, lymphadenopathy, or adrenal insufficiency suggests systemic diseases like lymphoma, tuberculosis, or histoplasmosis and requires FNAC to establish etiological diagnosis. In patients with suspected inoperable adrenocortical carcinoma, FNAC should be performed to establish etiological diagnosis before initiating chemotherapy. In addition, FNAC is also indicated in patients with a known malignancy associated with an adrenal mass but without any obvious metastasis, as diagnosis of adrenal metastasis by FNAC may change the management of primary disease.

51. **How to manage adrenal incidentaloma**?

Hyperfunctioning adrenal incidentalomas (Cushing's syndrome, pheochromocytoma, or androgen excess) irrespective of size should be operated. However, patients of adrenal incidentaloma with subclinical Cushing's syndrome should be considered for surgery if age is <40 years with recent onset/worsening of diabetes, hypertension, or osteoporosis. Patients with suspected hyperaldosteronism need further evaluation. If aldosterone excess is established and age is >40 years, bilateral adrenal venous sampling is indicated. This is because of the fact that the incidence of adrenal incidentaloma increases with advancing age, and apparently normal looking contralateral adrenal gland may be functionally abnormal. Unilateral nonfunctioning adrenal incidentaloma with size >4 cm or imaging phenotype suggestive of adrenocortical carcinoma irrespective of size should be operated. Those with unilateral nonfunctioning adrenal incidentaloma <3 cm should undergo biochemical and radiological imaging annually, and a growth in size >1 cm/year or development of hyperfunction should undergo operative removal. Bilateral nonfunctioning adrenal incidentaloma after careful exclusion of pheochromocytoma should undergo fine-needle aspiration cytology to establish the diagnosis and be treated accordingly.

52. **What are the causes of bilateral adrenomegaly with adrenal insufficiency**?

The causes of bilateral adrenomegaly with adrenal insufficiency include infections (e.g., tuberculosis, histoplasmosis, cytomegalovirus adrenalitis), infiltrative disorders (e.g., amyloidosis, hemochromatosis, sarcoidosis), disorders related to adrenal steroidogenesis (e.g., congenital adrenal hyperplasia), malignant disorders (e.g., primary adrenal lymphoma, metastasis), and rarely adrenal hemorrhage. The figures given below illustrate a patient who presented with adrenal insufficiency and bilateral adrenal masses and was found to have adrenal histoplasmosis on laparoscopic adrenal biopsy.

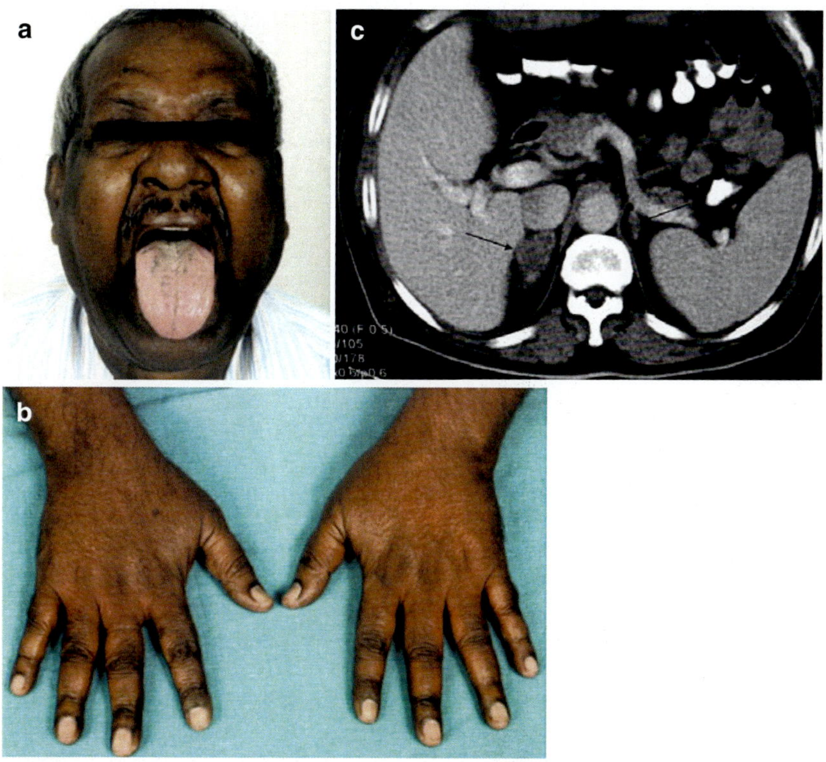

Fig. 4.20 (**a**, **b**) A patient of adrenal insufficiency with diffuse hyperpigmentation (face and knuckle). Note the sparing of pigmentation of the tongue mucosa. (**c**) CECT abdomen of the same patient showing bilateral asymmetrical adrenal enlargement (right > left)

Suggested Reading

1. Jameson JL, De Groot LJ. Endocrinology: adult and pediatric. Philadelphia: Elsevier Health Sciences; 2010.
2. Longo D, Fauci A, Kasper D, Hauser S, Jameson J, Loscalzo J. Harrison's principles of internal medicine. 18th ed. New York: McGraw Hill Professional; 2012.
3. Melmed S, Polonsky KS, Reed Larsen P, Kronenberg HM. Williams textbook of endocrinology: expert consult. London: Elsevier Health Sciences; 2011.

Cushing's Syndrome: Diagnosis and Treatment

5

5.1 Clinical Rounds

1. **What is the importance of diurnal variation of cortisol secretion?**

   Cortisol secretion peaks at 0400–0800h and troughs at 2300–2400h, and this diurnal rhythm is established by 2–3 years of age. Diurnal variation of cortisol secretion prevents sustained hypercortisolemia, which may be detrimental to neuronal function and sleep. Loss of diurnal rhythm of cortisol secretion is defined as a 1600h serum cortisol level more than 50% of 0800h serum cortisol or 2300h serum cortisol ≥207 nmol/L. This is the earliest abnormality of the hypothalamo–pituitary–adrenal axis in patients with Cushing's syndrome. Other causes of altered diurnal rhythm include pseudo-Cushing's syndrome, seizure disorder, depression, use of anticonvulsants, and shift workers. Pregnancy and glucocorticoid resistance syndrome are associated with preserved diurnal rhythm of cortisol secretion despite high serum cortisol.

2. **Does Liddle's protocol have a utility in ACTH-independent Cushing's syndrome?**

   Liddle's protocol was first described in 1960 and is also called as "adrenal suppression tests." It includes sequential low-dose dexamethasone suppression test (LDDST) followed by high-dose dexamethasone suppression test (HDDST) in patients with suspected Cushing's syndrome. It helps to establish endogenous hypercortisolemia (LDDST) and to differentiate between pituitary Cushing's syndrome and ectopic Cushing's syndrome (HDDST). In addition, it helps in the diagnosis of ACTH-independent Cushing's syndrome due to primary pigmented nodular adrenal hyperplasia (PPNAD), where a paradoxical increase in serum cortisol/UFC is seen after HDDST.

A. Bhansali, Y. Gogate, *Clinical Rounds in Endocrinology: Volume I - Adult Endocrinology*, DOI 10.1007/978-81-322-2398-6_5

3. **Why is dexamethasone used for cortisol dynamic tests?**

   Dexamethasone is the most potent glucocorticoid in suppressing hypothalamo–pituitary–adrenal axis (17 times more potent than hydrocortisone). It easily crosses the blood–brain barrier as it does not bind to cortisol-binding globulin (CBG). In addition, it has no cross-reactivity to hydrocortisone and other metabolites; therefore, it does not interfere with cortisol assay. Hence, dexamethasone is the preferred glucocorticoid for cortisol dynamic tests.

4. **What is the dose of dexamethasone for cortisol suppression test in children?**

   The dose of dexamethasone for overnight suppression test (ONDST) in children is 15 μg/kg at 2300h and for LDDST 30 μg/kg/day in four divided doses daily for 2 days. For HDDST, the dose is 120 μg/kg/day in four divided doses daily for two days. Children weighing >40 kg should receive similar doses as adults. However, the diagnostic cutoffs of suppression tests are same as in adults.

5. **How to perform overnight dexamethasone suppression test?**

   Overnight dexamethasone suppression test (ONDST) comprises administration of 1 mg dexamethasone between 2300 and 2400h and sampling for serum cortisol between 0800 and 0900h the next day. The use of higher dose (e.g 1.5 mg) in patients weighing >90 kg does not improve diagnostic accuracy of the test. Dexamethasone is administered between 2300 and 2400h to inhibit the ACTH secretion, which starts at 0300h and peaks by 0700h. The cutoff for diagnosing endogenous hypercortisolemia is ≥1.8 μg/dl (50 nmol/L) with a sensitivity of 95% and a specificity of 80%. The HPA axis recovers within 24 h after the administration of a single dose of 1 mg dexamethasone.

6. **What are the causes of false-positive overnight dexamethasone suppression test?**

   The causes of false-positive ONDST are disorders associated with pseudo-Cushing's syndrome, pregnancy, chronic kidney disease, glucocorticoid resistance syndrome, and acute stress. Also, drugs that either increase dexamethasone metabolism like rifampicin, phenytoin, phenobarbitone, carbamazepine, and pioglitazone or increase CBG like estrogen, mitotane, and tamoxifen are associated with false-positive ONDST. In addition, marked intra-individual variation in the absorption and metabolism of dexamethasone can also result in false-positive ONDST.

7. **What are the causes of false-negative overnight dexamethasone suppression test?**

   The causes of false-negative ONDST are cyclical Cushing's syndrome, exogenous Cushing's syndrome, and drugs that inhibit the metabolism of dexamethasone like ritonavir, itraconazole, cimetidine, fluoxetine, and diltiazem.

8. **What is the role of 0800–0900h cortisol in the diagnosis of Cushing's syndrome?**

The morning cortisol between 0800 and 0900h is helpful in differentiating exogenous Cushing's from endogenous Cushing's syndrome, as it is suppressed in patients with exogenous Cushing's syndrome. This is important because exogenous glucocorticoid administration is the most common cause of Cushing's syndrome. The other utility of morning cortisol is to establish the loss of circadian rhythm as compared to evening (1600h) cortisol. Baseline morning cortisol is also required for the interpretation of HDDST.

9. **What are the causes of normal/high 0800h cortisol despite exogenous Cushing's syndrome?**

Exogenous Cushing's syndrome is usually associated with 0800h cortisol <100 nmol/L. But the level can be normal/high in patients on exogenous hydrocortisone/ACTH treatment or during the recovery phase of axis following glucocorticoid withdrawal.

10. **What are the causes of low 0800h cortisol despite endogenous Cushing's syndrome?**

The causes of low 0800h cortisol despite endogenous Cushing's syndrome is glucose-dependent insulinotropic peptide (GIP)-mediated ACTH-independent macronodular adrenal hyperplasia, inactive phase of cyclical Cushing's syndrome, ketoconazole therapy, and pituitary apoplexy.

11. **A patient with PCOS screened for Cushing's syndrome was found to have high serum cortisol with a non-suppressible overnight dexamethasone suppression test. What to do next?**

A detailed history and examination revealed that the patient did not have any discriminatory feature of Cushing's syndrome, and hence a routine screening was unwarranted. Further, she was evaluated while on oral contraceptive pills (OCP). The estrogen content of OCPs increases CBG, which results in increased total serum cortisol, and non-suppressible ONDST in 50% of patients. Ideally, the patient should be reevaluated after discontinuing OCPs for 6 weeks. In addition, majority of women with PCOS are obese, and obesity per se may cause non-suppressible ONDST.

12. **What are the screening tests for diagnosis of Cushing's syndrome?**

After exclusion of exogenous Cushing's syndrome, screening tests recommended for the diagnosis of endogenous hypercortisolemia are urinary free cortisol (UFC; at least two consecutive measurements), late-night salivary cortisol (two measurements), and 1 mg overnight dexamethasone suppression test (ONDST)/low-dose dexamethasone suppression test (2 mg/day for

48 h) (LDDST). Out of these three, any one test can be performed initially and if positive needs subsequent confirmation with one of the remaining two tests. However, the time interval between the two screening tests is not clearly defined, particularly when LDDST is followed by measurement of late-night salivary cortisol or UFC. But it seems appropriate to have an interval of 7 days following LDDST, a period that corresponds to 5 half-lives of dexamethasone. ONDST as a screening test should be performed in those with specific features of Cushing's syndrome, while LDDST should be preferred in those with pseudo-Cushing's syndrome or subtle features of Cushing's syndrome. The advantage of salivary cortisol and UFC is that they estimate free cortisol; UFC, in addition, is an integrated measure of cortisol secretion. Midnight serum cortisol estimation can be used as an alternative screening test for the diagnosis of Cushing's syndrome in certain situations.

13. **How to approach a patient with suspected Cushing's syndrome?**

An approach to a patient with suspected Cushing's syndrome is depicted in the figure given below.

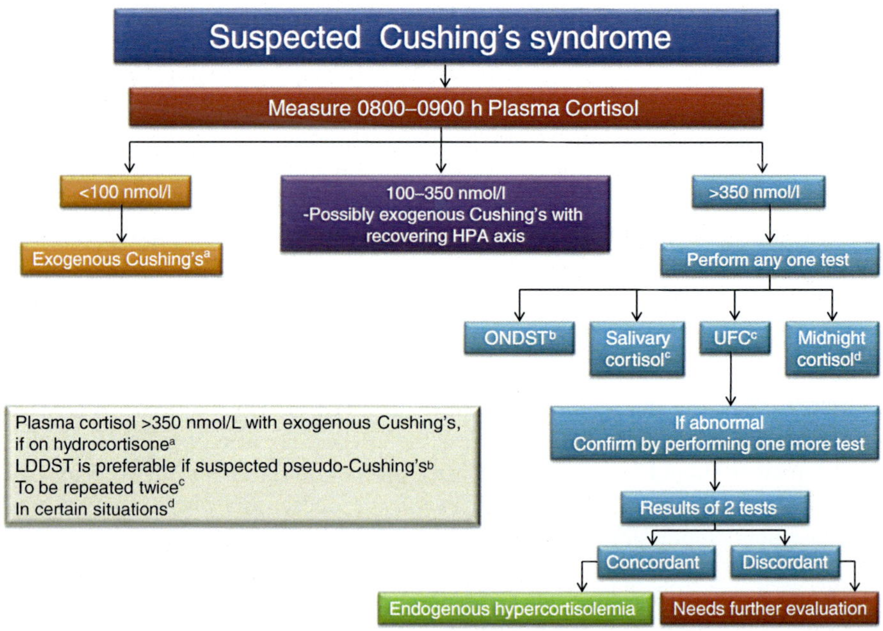

Fig. 5.1 Approach to a patient with suspected Cushing's syndrome

14. **What is the importance of midnight serum cortisol estimation in the diagnosis of Cushing's syndrome?**

Loss of circadian rhythm is the earliest biochemical abnormality in the evolution of Cushing's syndrome; thus, estimation of midnight serum cortisol may be used as an alternative screening test for the diagnosis of Cushing's syndrome in certain situations. These include:

- Patients with a high index of suspicion for Cushing's syndrome, but UFC/ONDST is negative.
- Patients with a low index of suspicion for Cushing's syndrome, but UFC/ONDST is positive.
- Patient on anticonvulsant medications with a non-suppressible dexamethasone suppression test.

In addition, midnight serum cortisol may also be useful when UFC or late-night salivary cortisol is not available. A sleeping midnight serum cortisol <50 nmol/L (1.8 μg/dl) or an awake midnight serum cortisol <207 nmol/L (7.5 μg/dl) effectively rules out the diagnosis of Cushing's syndrome in patients with low index of suspicion, while the cortisol values above these cutoffs increase the probability of Cushing's syndrome in patients with high index of suspicion. Late-night salivary cortisol could have been an alternative in place of midnight serum cortisol in the above mentioned situations, but the data is scanty.

15. **What is the sensitivity and specificity of various screening tests for the diagnosis of Cushing's syndrome?**

The sensitivity and specificity of different screening tests for the diagnosis of Cushing's syndrome are summarized in the table given below.

Biochemical tests	Diagnostic cutoffs	Sensitivity (%)	Specificity (%)
ONDST	≥50 nmol/L (1.8 μg/dl)	98–100	88
LDDST	≥50 nmol/L (1.8 μg/dl)	98–100	97–100
UFC	>ULN for the assay[a]	95–100	–
Late-night salivary cortisol	>5.5 nmol/L (2 ng/ml)	100	96
Sleeping midnight serum cortisol	≥50 nmol/L (1.8 μg/dl)	100	20
Awake midnight serum cortisol	≥207 nmol/L (7.5 μg/dl)	94	100

[a]Upper limit of normal

16. **What are the minimum tests required to establish the diagnosis of Cushing's syndrome in a resource constraint setting?**

In a patient with suspected Cushing's syndrome, the minimum battery of tests in a resource-constraint setting that will establish both endogenous hypercortisolemia and an etiological diagnosis are 2300h paired cortisol and ACTH and 0800h cortisol. A 2300h cortisol in an awake state ≥207 nmol/L (7.5 μg/dl) has a sensitivity and specificity >95% for the diagnosis of endogenous hypercortisolemia. A 2300h sleeping serum cortisol <50 nmol/L (1.8 μg/dl) virtually excludes the diagnosis of Cushing's syndrome. A 2300h ACTH > 22 pg/ml confirms ACTH-dependent Cushing's syndrome, and ACTH >90 pg/ml suggests ectopic Cushing's syndrome. A 0800h cortisol does not have a discriminatory value, but it is important to rule out exogenous Cushing's syndrome.

17. **How to differentiate between pseudo-Cushing's syndrome and Cushing's syndrome?**

The differentiation of pseudo-Cushing's from Cushing's syndrome is a clinical challenge as both share many clinical as well as biochemical similarities. Ideally, a patient of pseudo-Cushing's syndrome with known inciting cause like alcohol, or depression should be reevaluated, after resolution of primary disorder. However, in clinical scenario it is often impractical; hence, we need definite diagnostic tests to differentiate pseudo-Cushing's syndrome from Cushing's syndrome. The available tests are LDDST, loperamide challenge test, insulin-induced hypoglycemia, and LDDST with corticotrophin-releasing hormone (CRH) stimulation test. However, none of these tests have 100% specificity; hence, prospective follow-up is the best tool to discriminate between the two disorders. The tests which help in the differentiation of pseudo-Cushing's syndrome from Cushing's syndrome are summarized in the table given below.

Tests	Response in Cushing's syndrome	Response in pseudo- Cushing's syndrome	Remarks
LDDST	Non-suppressible	Suppressible	Specificity 70%
Loperamide challenge test	Non-suppressible	Suppressible	Loperamide is an opiate agonist which inhibits CRH–ACTH axis Specificity 95%
Insulin-induced hypoglycemia	Non-stimulable	Stimulable	Specificity 95%
LDDST with CRH test	Stimulable	Non-stimulable	Specificity 60%

18. **What are the tests available for establishing the etiological diagnosis of Cushing's syndrome?**

The measurement of 0800h cortisol helps in excluding exogenous Cushing's syndrome. The tests that help in differentiating ACTH-dependent from ACTH-independent Cushing's syndrome are 2300h/0800h ACTH and CRH stimulation test. The tests that differentiate between pituitary and ectopic Cushing's are plasma ACTH, HDDST, CRH stimulation test, and inferior petrosal sinus sampling (IPSS). A plasma ACTH >90 pg/ml, non-suppressible HDDST, lack of ACTH response to CRH, and absence of central to peripheral ACTH gradient to CRH on inferior petrosal sinus sampling (IPSS) support the diagnosis of ectopic Cushing's syndrome, while 0800h plasma ACTH >20 pg/ml or 2300h plasma ACTH>22 pg/ml, suppressible HDDST, ACTH response to CRH, central to peripheral ACTH ratio >3 following CRH on IPSS, and presence of adenoma on sellar imaging (>6 mm) favor the diagnosis of pituitary Cushing's syndrome.

19. **How to establish the etiological diagnosis of a patient with Cushing's syndrome?**

    The approach to a patient with Cushing's syndrome is summarized in the figure given below.

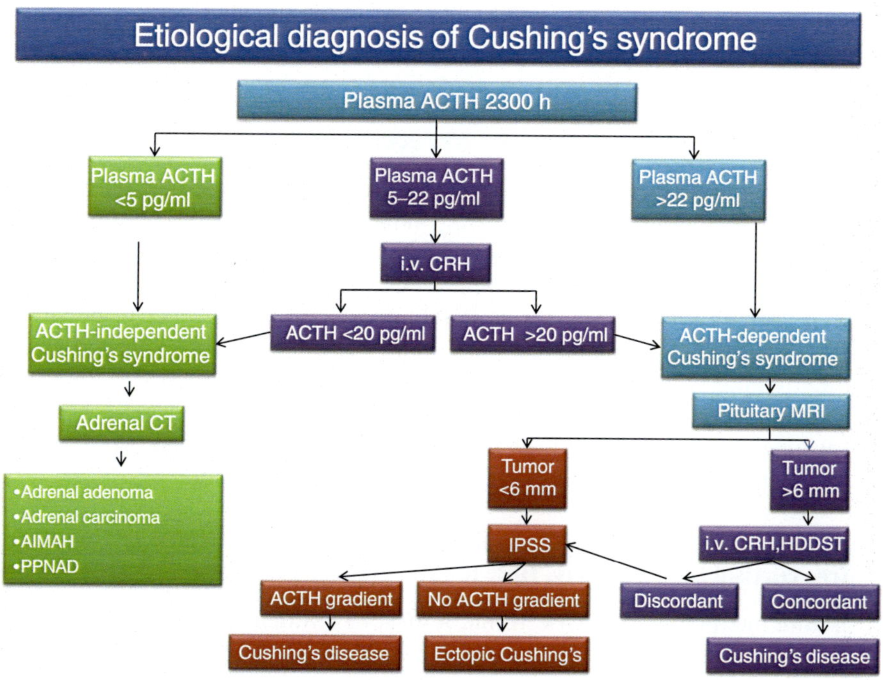

Fig. 5.2 Approach to a patient with Cushing's syndrome

20. **What does urinary free cortisol denote?**

    Approximately 90% of circulating cortisol is in bound form (cortisol-binding globulin and albumin), while the rest is in free form, and this fraction is freely filtered across glomerulus. Ninety percent of filtered cortisol is reabsorbed in renal tubules, and the rest is excreted in urine. In hypercortisolic states, the fraction of serum free cortisol increases, with consequent increase in urinary cortisol excretion. UFC measures the free form of cortisol and represents an integrated measure of cortisol secretion.

21. **What are situations where UFC is preferred?**

    UFC is preferred in patients with suspected Cushing's syndrome during pregnancy, cyclical Cushing's, in patients with adrenocortical carcinoma receiving mitotane therapy, and during postoperative (TSS) follow-up of patients with Cushing's disease. Pregnancy and mitotane therapy are associated with increase in CBG levels, and therefore, estimation of UFC is preferred. Patients with cyclical Cushing's syndrome exhibit periodic hormonogenesis, and "cycle" may vary from days to months; therefore, repeated measurements over a long duration are required for detection of hypercortisolemia. UFC and late-night salivary cortisol are preferred in this scenario as both are noninvasive and less cumbersome. UFC is also indicated in the follow-up of patients with Cushing's disease postoperatively to detect those with failed surgery or early recurrence.

22. **What are the fallacies with urine free cortisol estimation?**

    Adequate urinary collection is a prerequisite for the correct interpretation as under- or over-collection of urine may influence the results of UFC. UFC can be falsely negative in patients with adrenal incidentaloma (subclinical Cushing's), mild Cushing's, cyclical Cushing's, and renal insufficiency (eGFR < 60 ml/min). UFC can be falsely positive in the presence of polyuria, use of drugs like carbamazepine, fenofibrate, synthetic glucocorticoids (interference with immunoassays), and drugs that inhibit 11β-HSD2 (licorice, carbenoxolone). Further, a normal UFC level does not exclude the diagnosis of Cushing's syndrome as it may be normal in 8–15% of patients with proven Cushing's syndrome due to variability in cortisol metabolism.

23. **A 35-year-old woman with suspicion of Cushing's syndrome has urinary free cortisol of 150 μg/day. How to interpret the result?**

    Before interpretation of UFC result, it must be ensured that 24-h urine collection was adequate with appropriate precautions; proper refrigeration, but not frozen, avoidance of excess water intake, simultaneous measurement of urinary creatinine, and 2 consecutive UFC values are available. At least two values of UFC are recommended because of variability in cortisol metabolism. The index patient had only a single UFC measurement and, therefore, requires a repeat UFC. Any UFC value above the upper limit of normal should be considered abnormal and require a second test (other than UFC) for the confirmation of endogenous hypercortisolemia. Though any UFC value above the upper limit of normal (220–330 nmol/day or 80–120 μg/day) is considered abnormal, a UFC value fourfold higher than normal is rarely seen in disorders other than Cushing's syndrome.

24. **A 40-year-old man with suspicion of Cushing's syndrome has late-night salivary cortisol of 8 nmol/L. How do we interpret the result?**

    Poor oral hygiene, smoking and tobacco chewing may falsely elevate the late-night salivary cortisol; hence prior to estimation of late-night salivary cortisol estimation, it must be ensured that the patient has good oral hygiene and does not chew tobacco or smokes. Sample should be collected either with passive drooling or using a Salivette. Liquid chromatography – mass spectrophotometry is the best available assay; however, enzyme-linked immunosorbent assay is more commonly available and is equally sensitive. A cutoff of >5.5 nmol/L (2 ng/ml) is considered diagnostic of endogenous hypercortisolemia. A detailed history revealed that the index patient was a betel nut chewer, therefore, other screening tests should be advised for evaluation of Cushing's syndrome.

25. **A 35-year-old female, working in a call center on night shifts presented with specific features of Cushing's syndrome. What to do next?**

    The erratic sleep–wake cycle in shift workers can alter cortisol rhythm. Ideally, these subjects should be reevaluated after normalizing sleep pattern. But for practical purposes, they can be evaluated after stabilization of work schedule, with sleeping time considered as night and awake time considered as day. Nevertheless, UFC is the best screening test in such a scenario, and LDDST can be a second-line screening test.

26. **A 23-year-old female with specific features of Cushing's syndrome, has 0800h cortisol 540 nmol/L (20 μg/dl) but a normal urine free cortisol 90 μg/day and suppressible overnight dexamethasone suppression test. Is the diagnosis of Cushing's syndrome excluded?**

    No. In the index patient with a high clinical suspicion of Cushing's syndrome, a normal UFC and a suppressible ONDST does not rule out the diagnosis of Cushing's syndrome. A midnight serum cortisol should be performed in this scenario, as the earliest biochemical abnormality in Cushing's syndrome is loss of diurnal rhythm. If sleeping midnight serum cortisol is ≥50 nmol/L (1.8 μg/dl) or an awake value ≥207 nmol/L (7.5 μg/dl), the probability of mild Cushing's or cyclical Cushing's should be considered despite of negative screening tests.

In such circumstances, UFC should be reestimated to confirm the endogenous hypercortisolemia. If hypercortisolemia is confirmed, a search for etiological diagnosis should be made, or if the results are anomalous, these patients should be kept under surveillance.

27. **What are the precautions to be taken while sampling for midnight cortisol?**

    Midnight cortisol sample should be taken between 2300 and 2400h either in a sleeping or an awake state. Ideally, the patient should be admitted 24–48 h prior to sampling for adaptation to hospital environment. However, some studies have shown that prior hospitalization is not mandatory. A sample taken either during sleep or within 5–10 min of awakening is considered as a sleeping sample, while awakened sample is considered when the patient is kept awake till the sample is taken. The patient should be precannulated to avoid venipuncture stress.

28. **A 23-year-old female with specific features of Cushing's syndrome has 0800h cortisol 540 nmol/L (20 μg/dl), a urine free cortisol 590 and 620 μg/day, and non-suppressible low-dose dexamethasone suppression test. What to do next?**

    The patient has confirmed endogenous hypercortisolemia and the next step is to measure plasma ACTH to differentiate between ACTH dependent and independent causes of Cushing's syndrome. The ideal time to measure plasma ACTH is 2300h, when it is expected to be at nadir. But, some studies have shown that morning 0800h ACTH is equally rewarding in differentiating between ACTH-dependent and ACTH-independent causes of Cushing's syndrome. ACTH sample should be collected in a prechilled EDTA tube from a precannulated vein and immediately centrifuged and stored at –20°C, as it is a heat-labile protein and disintegrates rapidly. Plasma ACTH needs to be repeated twice. A 2300h plasma ACTH <5 pg/ml or 0800h plasma ACTH <10 pg/ml suggests ACTH-independent Cushing's syndrome, while 2300h plasma ACTH >22 pg/ml or 0800h plasma ACTH >20 pg/ml is suggestive of ACTH-dependent Cushing's syndrome. An 0800h ACTH value >90pg/ml suggests ectopic source of ACTH. A 2300h plasma ACTH between 5 and 22 pg/ml or 0800h ACTH value between 10 and 20 pg/ml is considered indeterminate, but probability of pituitary ACTH-dependent Cushing's syndrome is high.

29. **The above-described patient had a 0800h ACTH value 35 pg/ml. How to proceed further?**

    The patient had a plasma ACTH value of 35 pg/ml which suggests a likely diagnosis of pituitary ACTH-dependent Cushing's syndrome; hence, the patient should be subjected to CEMR imaging of pituitary gland to localize the source of ACTH excess. The sensitivity of conventional CEMRI to localize a pituitary microadenoma is around 50%. This can be improved by the use of either dynamic MRI or spoiled gradient recalled acquisition (SPGR) sequence. The principle of dynamic MRI is to take advantage of a relatively oligo-perfused microadenoma as compared to normal pituitary tissue. Therefore, by acquiring rapid sequential images, dynamic MRI helps in identifying hypointense microadenoma from normally enhancing pituitary tissue after contrast administration (differential enhancement). This increases the sensitivity to 67% as opposed to 50% with conventional MRI. The sensitivity can further be improved to 80% by use of SPGR technique. One millimeter thin section and the faster acquisition of images minimize artifacts from motion and vascular pulsation, resulting in improved sensitivity with SPGR. Although the sensitivity is improved, both these techniques are associated with higher false-positive rates.

30. **What are the causes of low ACTH in a patient with ACTH-dependent Cushing's syndrome?**

The most common cause of low ACTH in a patient with Cushing's syndrome is improper sample collection and transportation, because ACTH is a heat-labile peptide. The other causes include cyclical Cushing's syndrome, ACTH-dependent macronodular adrenal hyperplasia, and recent pituitary apoplexy.

31. **In a patient with confirmed ACTH-dependent Cushing's syndrome, if MRI sella reveals an adenoma of size 7mm, is diagnosis of pituitary Cushing's syndrome confirmed?**

A size ≥6 mm is likely to be corticotropinoma, but it should be further complemented by high-dose dexamethasone suppression test (HDDST) and corticotrophin (CRH) stimulation test, as the sensitivity of 6-mm microadenoma to be a corticotropinoma is 40% with a specificity of 98% (in patients with ACTH-dependent Cushing's syndrome). HDDST is suppressible in 90% of patients with microadenoma and non-suppressible in patients with ectopic Cushing's, pituitary macroadenoma, and adrenal Cushing's. A positive response with CRH stimulation test (defined as an ACTH increase of 100% or a cortisol rise of 50% over baseline values) effectively eliminates a diagnosis of ectopic Cushing's syndrome. CRH is not easily available; therefore, desmopressin or arginine vasopressin can be an alternative. In case of concordant results of these tests (size >6 mm, HDDST suppressible and positive CRH/desmopressin/AVP stimulation test), the diagnosis of Cushing's disease is confirmed, and patients can be subjected to surgery. However, when the results of these tests are discordant, IPSS is required to establish the etiological diagnosis of Cushing's syndrome.

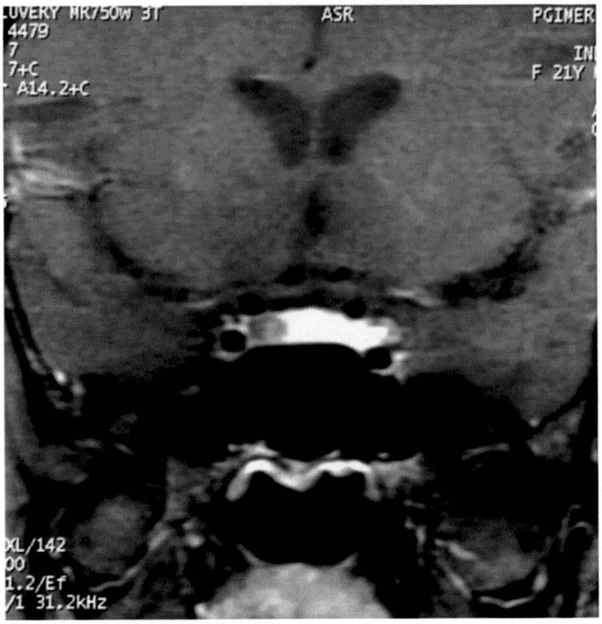

Fig. 5.3 T1W CEMR coronal image showing hypointense lesion in the right half of pituitary gland suggestive of microadenoma of size 7 mm

32. **In a patient with confirmed ACTH-dependent Cushing's syndrome, if MRI sella reveals an adenoma of 3-mm size, how to approach further?**

In a patient with confirmed ACTH-dependent Cushing's syndrome, if MRI reveals an adenoma of size 3-mm, the clinical possibilities are corticotropinoma or nonfunctioning pituitary microadenoma with ectopic ACTH-secreting Cushing's syndrome. These possibilities should be considered in all patients with ACTH-dependent Cushing's syndrome who have a pituitary adenoma size of <6 mm. In this clinical scenario, IPSS with CRH/AVP stimulation is required to substantiate the diagnosis of corticotropinoma. If IPSS is not available, HDDST and CRH/AVP stimulation may be complementary, but is not definitive. A third possibility, though rare, is the presence of a nonfunctioning pituitary microadenoma with a contralateral non-visualized corticotropinoma (double adenoma), which is suggested by localization to pituitary in IPSS but with lateralization to side opposite to visualized pituitary microadenoma. If IPSS does not reveal a gradient, a high-resolution and contrast-enhanced CT chest and CECT abdomen should be performed for localization of ectopic ACTH-secreting Cushing's syndrome.

33. **A patient with confirmed Cushing's syndrome, had a 0800h ACTH 35pg/ml and a normal MRI sella. How to proceed further?**

A normal MRI sella does not rule out a diagnosis of Cushing's disease as corticotropinomas are usually small and are frequently not visualized on MRI.

Further, the probability of pituitary Cushing's syndrome is high (90%) in a patient with ACTH-dependent Cushing's syndrome. In addition, the likelihood of ectopic Cushing's syndrome is low in the index patient as plasma ACTH is 35 pg/ml. Hence, in this scenario, the index patient should be subjected to IPSS.

34. **A 33-year-old female with specific features of Cushing's syndrome has an 0800h cortisol 675 nmol/L (25 μg/dl), a urine free cortisol 620 and 510 μg/day, and a non-suppressible low-dose dexamethasone suppression test. 0800h ACTH is 110 pg/ml. Is the diagnosis of ectopic ACTH-secreting Cushing's syndrome confirmed?**

No. Although a high ACTH value (>90 pg/ml) suggests ectopic source of ACTH, it does not exclude the diagnosis of pituitary Cushing's syndrome. In such a scenario, HDDST, CRH stimulation test, MRI sella, and if necessary, IPSS should be performed. This is because ectopic Cushing's syndrome accounts for only 5–10% of all patients with Cushing's syndrome. The differentiating features between ectopic and pituitary Cushing's syndrome are enlisted in the table given below.

Parameters	Pituitary Cushing's syndrome	Ectopic Cushing's syndrome
Clinical features	Insidious onset	Rapid onset (except for bronchial carcinoids)
		Presence of features related to underlying disease
Hypokalemia	Rare	Present
Metabolic alkalosis	Rare	Present
ACTH	High, >20 but <90 pg/ml	Very high, >90 pg/ml
HDDST	Suppressible	Non-suppressible
CRH stimulation test	Positive	Negative
IPSS (basal) Central/peripheral ACTH ratio	>2	<1.4
IPSS with CRH stimulation Central/peripheral ACTH ratio	>3	<3
MRI sella	Adenoma localized	Normal

35. **What is the rationale of high-dose dexamethasone suppression test?**

HDDST is helpful in discriminating varying etiologies of Cushing's syndrome. In normal individuals, ACTH is suppressed even by 1 mg of dexamethasone. However, in pituitary Cushing's syndrome, the negative feedback control of ACTH is set at a higher level than normal. Therefore, higher doses are required to suppress ACTH in pituitary Cushing's syndrome. Patients with ectopic Cushing's syndrome and large invasive pituitary macroadenoma do not show this responsiveness, even at higher doses of dexamethasone possibly because their threshold is set at a much higher level than in pituitary Cushing's syndrome.

36. **Has high-dose dexamethasone suppression test lost its value in the diagnosis of Cushing's syndrome?**

Possibly no. HDDST is a useful test in differentiating between pituitary and ectopic Cushing's syndrome. HDDST is considered suppressible if plasma cortisol is suppressed to >50% of the baseline 0800h cortisol. HDDST is suppressible in nearly 90% of patients with pituitary Cushing's syndrome, as opposed to 10% of patients with ectopic Cushing's syndrome. However, if a cutoff of >90% suppression of UFC from baseline is taken, HDDST has a specificity of 100% for the diagnosis of pituitary Cushing's syndrome. In current scenario, HDDST is a complementary test to i.v. CRH in a patient with ACTH-dependent Cushing's syndrome with a pituitary adenoma of size >6 mm on neuroimaging. Suppressible HDDST and stimulable ACTH/cortisol after CRH precludes the need for IPSS in such cases. However, if suppression of cortisol after LDDST is >30% from baseline, there may not be any added advantage with HDDST. Further, HDDST is also useful in patients with PPNAD, where paradoxical increase in cortisol following HDDST is observed.

37. **Why is inferior petrosal sinus sampling considered as the gold standard for the etiological diagnosis of ACTH-dependent Cushing's syndrome?**

Inferior petrosal sinus drains 80% of venous blood from pituitary and is thus the most appropriate site for ACTH sampling to localize the source of ACTH excess. Each half of pituitary drains into its corresponding inferior petrosal sinus, and in nearly 60% of individuals, venous drainage is symmetrical; thereby, it helps in lateralization of tumor. CRH-stimulated IPSS improves the specificity of test, and ovine CRH is preferred over human CRH, as it is more potent. The dose of ovine CRH is 1 μg/kg, but not exceeding 100 μg intravenously. The sensitivity of CRH-stimulated IPSS in localizing a pituitary corticotropinoma, even in the absence of visualization on imaging, is 85–88% as opposed to MRI which has a sensitivity of 70%. However, the accuracy of IPSS for lateralization of corticotropinoma is only 69%. Further, IPSS denotes both functional (localization) and structural (lateralization) localization of the tumor, while MRI only denotes structural presence of the tumor. The sensitivity and specificity of IPSS in localizing the source of ACTH excess are summarized in the table given below. However, the lateralizing ability of IPSS is only 69%, while in 31% IPSS lateralizes to contralateral side. If facility for IPSS is not available, then internal jugular vein sampling is an alternative, but the data available are not encouraging.

Parameters	Sensitivity (%)	Specificity (%)	Positive predictive value (%)
Basal: central vs peripheral ≥2	85	90	98
CRH stimulated: central vs peripheral ≥3	88	100	100

38. **What are the complications of IPSS?**

The most common complication associated with IPSS includes groin hematoma which occurs in 3–4% of cases and referred auricular pain. In addition, pulmonary thromboembolism, brainstem infraction, venous subarachnoid hemorrhage, and transient sixth-nerve palsy are uncommon adverse events associated with IPSS.

39. **What are the causes of false-positive localization during inferior petrosal sinus sampling?**

IPSS should only be performed in those who have specific features of Cushing's syndrome, definite biochemical evidence of hypercortisolemia, and demonstration of ACTH dependency. False-positive localization in IPSS can be observed in cyclical ectopic Cushing's syndrome (during inactive phase, e.g. bronchial carcinoid), and ectopic CRH-secreting tumor.

40. **What are the causes of false-negative localization during inferior petrosal sinus sampling?**

False-negative localization during IPSS are much more common than false-positive localization (rare). The causes of false-negative localization on IPSS are aberrant pituitary venous drainage, hypoplastic petrosal sinuses, incorrect bilateral IPSS technique (inability to cannulate each inferior petrosal sinus or dislodgement of cannula during the procedure), and the density of expression of CRH receptor on corticotropinoma.

41. **In a patient with Cushing's disease, when to suspect false-negative localization on IPSS?**

False-negative localization on IPSS in a Cushing's disease should be suspected when there is a peak CRH-stimulated value of central ACTH <400 pg/ml. False-negative causes due to faulty catheterization can be ascertained by estimation of basal central to peripheral gradient of prolactin. A central to peripheral prolactin ratio ≥1.8 is suggestive of successful catheterization. Prolactin is a reliable reference hormone, as it is the most abundant hormone secreted from pituitary gland and is the only anterior pituitary hormone not suppressed by hypercortisolemia. In addition, measurement of prolactin-corrected ACTH central versus peripheral ratio helps in overcoming the shortcomings associated with anomalous venous drainage. A prolactin-corrected ACTH central versus peripheral ratio of ≥1.3 is indicative of Cushing's disease, while a ratio of ≤0.7 suggests ectopic ACTH-secreting tumor.

42. **Why is there measurable ACTH level in the contralateral petrosal sinus during IPSS in a patient with localized pituitary microadenoma on one side?**

It is expected that in a patient with microcorticotropinoma, normal corticotropes are suppressed by hypercortisolemia; this is evidenced by the development of hypocortisolemia after curative adenomectomy. Therefore, ACTH levels are expected to be undetectable in the contralateral petrosal sinus during IPSS. However, this is usually not seen, and ACTH levels are measurable on the contralateral side. This can be explained by the fact that neither anatomically nor functionally pituitary gland behaves as right and left halves. Therefore, mixing of blood is expected within the gland and in cavernous sinuses (intercavernous venous mixing) resulting in measurable and stimulable ACTH on the contralateral side. The table given below shows the result of IPSS in a patient with a microadenoma on left half of pituitary and clearly shows detectable level of ACTH even in right petrosal sinus.

Time (min)	Right central ACTH	Left central ACTH	Peripheral ACTH	ACTH ratio Left central to periphery (Left C:P)	ACTH ratio Left central to right central (L:R)
–5	107	443.4	88.68	4.89	4.14
0	621	2,000	285.3	7.01	3.22
2	436	1,424	224.2	6.35	3.26
3	366.6	2,000	292.8	6.83	5.45
15	365	3,270	93.6	34.9	8.95
10	226.6	5,718	95.2	60.06	25.23
15	296.5	1,254	240.5	5.21	4.22
30	345.5	235	229.2	1.02	0.68
45	231.5	400.7	165.9	2.41	1.73

43. **A 40-year-old male presented with classical feature of Cushing's syndrome. He had biochemical hypercortisolemia and ACTH-dependent Cushing's syndrome. Dynamic MRI of the sella localized a –7 mm adenoma on the left half of the pituitary gland. IPSS localized the source of ACTH excess to the pituitary but lateralized to the right half of the pituitary gland. How to proceed further?**

This patient with ACTH-dependent Cushing's syndrome has a microadenoma on one side on imaging, while IPSS lateralized to the contralateral side. The sensitivity of dynamic MRI in localizing the source of ACTH excess is approximately 70% with a positive predictive value of 86% (as correlated with histopathology), which further increases to 92% if the tumor size is ≥4mm. The sensitivity of CRH-stimulated IPSS in localizing the source of ACTH excess is 88% with a positive predictive value of 100% (as correlated with histopathology). The sensitivity of CRH-stimulated IPSS in lateralizing the source of ACTH excess is 98% with a positive predictive value of only 69%. This dichotomy in lateralization between IPSS and MRI can be due to intercavernous venous mixing or dominance in pituitary venous drainage pattern (seen in 40% of healthy individuals) or presence of the epicenter of the tumor on one side with extension to the contralateral side. As right-sided dominance of pituitary venous drainage is common than left side, there is a higher rate of lateralization to right petrosal sinus with a lower accuracy and a higher rate of accuracy with left-sided lateralization. Rarely, there may be double adenoma; the one visualized on imaging being an incidentaloma, and the other adenoma, though non-visualized on MRI, is functional and is responsible for the gradient in IPSS. In the index case, as neuroimaging localized a tumor of >4 mm to left side, a decision was taken to explore the left half of the pituitary as pretest probability of tumor being on left side is 92% (based on MRI), while pretest probability of tumor being on the right side is only 69% (based on IPSS). At surgery, adenoma was confined to left half of pituitary and histopathology confirmed the same. The neuroimaging and IPSS data of the index patient is depicted below.

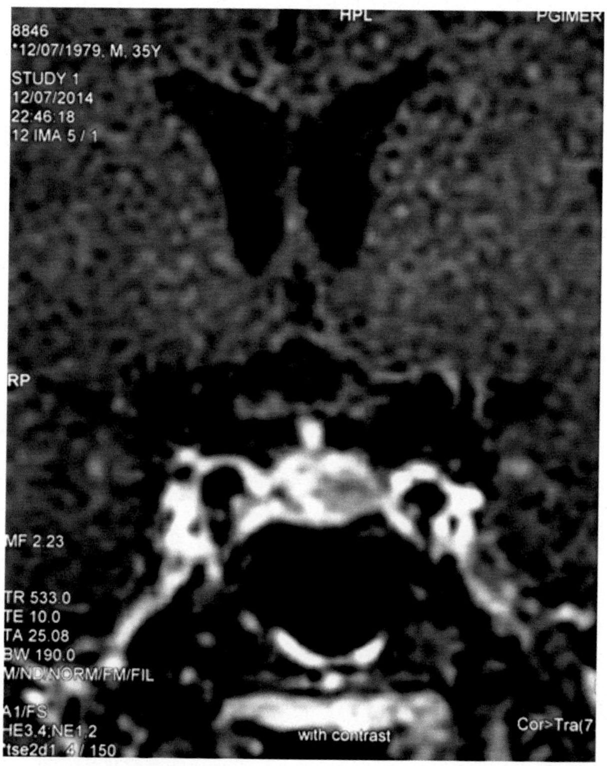

Fig. 5.4 T1W dynamic CEMR coronal image showing a hypointense lesion in the left half of pituitary in a patient with Cushing's syndrome

Time (min)	Right central ACTH	Left central ACTH	Peripheral ACTH	ACTH ratio right central to periphery (right C:P)	ACTH ratio right central to left central (R:L)
–5	1,212	133.2	107.7	11.25	9.09
0	13,160.0	228.1	561.3	23.44	57.69
2	661.8	418.2	482.5	1.37	1.58
3	607.9	473.8	540.7	1.12	1.28
5	546.4	501.0	621.6	0.87	1.09
10	456.1	354.8	369.9	1.23	1.28
15	355.7	366.8	312.5	1.13	0.96
30	272.4	193.0	271.5	1.03	1.03
45	223.1	168.2	194.7	1.14	1.32

44. **Is IPSS a must in all patients with ACTH-dependent Cushing's syndrome?**

    No. Patients with ACTH-dependent Cushing's syndrome with tumor size ≥6 mm on MR sellar imaging, suppressible HDDST, and positive CRH stimulation test do not require IPSS.

45. **What are the indications of IPSS in patients with ACTH-dependent Cushing's syndrome?**

    The indications for IPSS in patients with ACTH-dependent Cushing's syndrome are summarized in the figure given below.

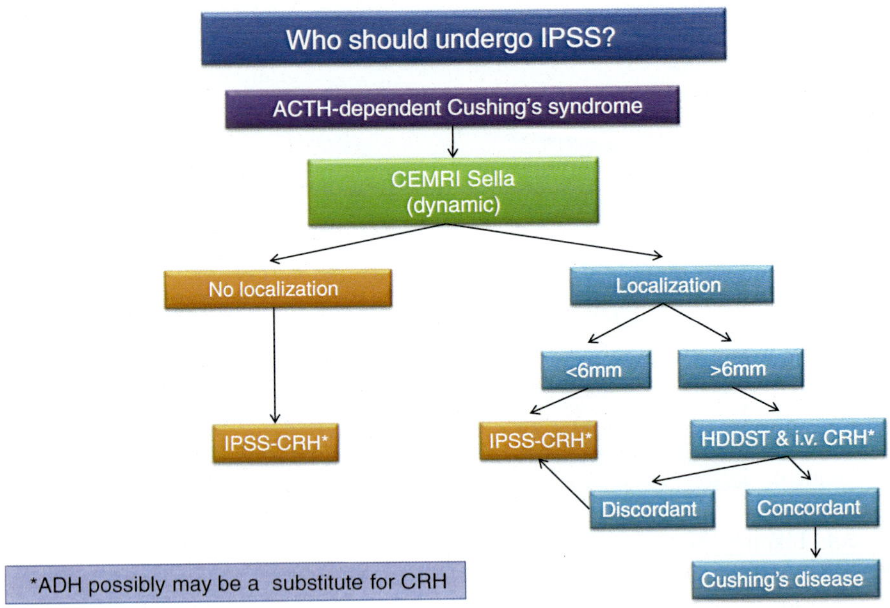

Fig. 5.5 Indications for IPSS in a patient with ACTH-dependent Cushing's syndrome

46. **A 32-year-old female with specific features of Cushing's syndrome has an 0800h cortisol 540 nmol/L (20 μg/dl), a urine free cortisol 640 and 666 μg/day, and a non-suppressible low-dose dexamethasone suppression test with an ACTH value 7 pg/ml. What to do next?**

    A 2300h plasma ACTH value between 5 and 22 pg/ml needs to be reconfirmed with adequate sampling technique. In case the second value is also indeterminate, CRH stimulation test should be performed. After CRH stimulation, if peak ACTH response is blunted (<20 pg/ml), an ACTH-independent cause is likely. If CRH is not available, HDDST is an alternative. A suppressible HDDST suggests pituitary ACTH-dependent Cushing's syndrome. Localization studies (e.g. MRI sella, CT chest and abdomen) should be performed only after biochemical confirmation of ACTH dependent/independent Cushing's syndrome. The index patient had repeat ACTH 8 pg/ml, and suppressible HDDST, which was suggestive of ACTH dependency. Subsequently, MRI revealed an adenoma of 3 mm and was further confirmed by ADH-stimulated IPSS.

47. **A 43-year-old male with specific features of Cushing's syndrome has an 0800h cortisol of 540 nmol/L (20 μg/dl), a urine free cortisol of 840 and 900 μg/day, and a non-suppressible low-dose dexamethasone suppression test with ACTH value of <1 pg/ml. Is the diagnosis of ACTH-independent Cushing's syndrome confirmed?**

    Yes. But ACTH needs to be reconfirmed on two occasions after following adequate sampling procedure. CECT adrenal should be performed to localize the source of hypercortisolemia. The presence of unilateral adrenal mass with a contralateral atrophic adrenal gland points to the diagnosis of adrenal adenoma or adrenal carcinoma. Bilaterally enlarged adrenal glands are suggestive of ACTH-independent macronodular hyperplasia (AIMAH), McCune–Albright syndrome, or rarely, bilateral adenoma. Bilaterally small/normal adrenals suggest PPNAD, which commonly presents in childhood but can also present during second to third decade of life.

48. **What are the specific precautions required for a patient with Cushing's syndrome prior to surgery?**

    Before subjecting a patient with Cushing's syndrome for surgery, the following measures should be ensured. Blood pressure and blood glucose should be optimized, and hypokalemia if present, should be corrected by oral potassium and spironolactone. Careful airway assessment is mandatory anticipating difficult intubation. Venous Doppler ultrasonography should be carried out to exclude deep vein thrombosis. Calcium and calcitriol should be supplemented and bisphosphonates administered, if indicated. Incentive spirometry should be advised to reduce postoperative morbidity. Gentle handling of the patient should be ensured during shifting, to avoid fragility fracture. Glucocorticoid should not be administered preoperatively in patients with Cushing's disease because it may interfere with postoperative monitoring of cortisol and may increase morbidity by exacerbating preexisting hypercortisolemia. However, in patients with adrenal Cushing's syndrome and in those with ectopic Cushing's syndrome, glucocorticoids should be administered perioperatively. Prior medical therapy with ketoconazole/metyrapone/pasireotide is indicated in those who are moribund and are at high risk for surgery, to achieve rapid eucortisolemia.

49. **What is the role of anticoagulation in the perioperative period in patients with Cushing's syndrome?**

    Patients with Cushing's syndrome are predisposed to thromboembolic diseases as cortisol excess is associated with procoagulant state due to increased factor VIII, von Willebrand factor, and fibrinogen, and decreased fibrinolytic activity due to increased PAI-1. The associated obesity, metabolic syndrome, and immobility further predispose to hypercoagulable state. In addition, patients with Cushing's syndrome having menstrual irregularities may be erroneously diagnosed to have polycystic ovarian disease and may be prescribed oral contraceptive, which greatly enhances the risk of thromboembolism. Therefore, every patient with Cushing's syndrome should be preoperatively evaluated for deep vein thrombosis. Perioperative complications related to hypercoagulability include pulmonary thromboembolism and cortical vein thrombosis. There are no definite guidelines regarding the use of anticoagulation in the perioperative period, but there seems to be a consensus that they are beneficial. The benefit of fractionated/unfractionated heparin/oral drugs and duration of anticoagulant therapy needs further evidence.

50. **How to define cure in patients with pituitary Cushing's syndrome?**

    Ideally, cure in patients with pituitary Cushing's syndrome should be defined as resolution of signs and symptoms, restoration of diurnal rhythm of cortisol secretion, normalization of UFC, suppressibility of cortisol after ONDST, and stimulability with 250 μg/1 μg ACTH without the need for glucocorticoid replacement and no evidence of other pituitary hormone deficiencies. But in clinical practice, development of new pituitary hormone deficiencies after surgery does not exclude cure. The term "remission" seems to be more appropriate than "cure" for patients with pituitary Cushing's syndrome, as they require long-term surveillance for years together (>10 years) to define cure.

51. **How to define cure in adrenal/ectopic Cushing's syndrome?**

    Cure in patients with ectopic Cushing's syndrome is defined as resolution of signs and symptoms of hypercortisolism, restoration of diurnal rhythm of cortisol secretion, suppressibility with overnight dexamethasone test and stimulability with 250 μg ACTH. However, this definition should not be applied to those who have undergone bilateral adrenalectomy. Pituitary hormone deficiencies also occur even in patients with ectopic Cushing's syndrome due to prolonged suppressive effects of cortisol on pituitary cells, particularly corticotropes and somatotropes. Patients with adrenal Cushing's syndrome attain cure after adrenalectomy. Those who have undergone unilateral adrenalectomy may require long term glucocorticoid therapy as there is a delay in recovery of HPA axis.

52. **What are the predictors of cure in Cushing's disease?**

The predictors of cure in Cushing's disease are well-localized microadenoma without parasellar extension, postoperative 0800h cortisol between day 1 and 7<50 nmol/L (1.8 μg/dl), plasma ACTH <20 pg/ml within 24 h of surgery, histological documentation of pituitary adenoma, positive ACTH immunostaining, and prolonged requirement of glucocorticoid replacement. Of these criteria, immediate postoperative hypocortisolemia is the best predictor of cure with a sensitivity of 85%.

53. **Is remission and cure in Cushing's disease synonymous?**

In clinical practice, the terms "remission" and "cure" are used interchangeably; however, they are not synonymous. Remission can be defined as resolution of clinical stigmata of Cushing's and achievement of eucortisolemia with recovery of hypothalamo–pituitary–adrenal axis or hypocortisolemia requiring long-term glucocorticoid replacement. However, patients in remission have a probability of recurrence of the disease anytime during surveillance; therefore, prospective follow-up for at least 10 years is required to consider the patient as cured, as the probability of recurrence is 10–20% at 10 years for microadenomas. Therefore, patients with sustained remission and not requiring glucocorticoid replacement at 10 years probably represent cure. Hence, all patients who are cured are in remission, while all patients in remission may not be cured.

54. **How to define persistence or recurrence of disease in pituitary Cushing's syndrome?**

There is no consensus on the definition of these terms. However, it is reasonable to define persistence of disease (failed surgery) if there is no resolution of clinical and/or biochemical hypercortisolemia 6–12 weeks postoperatively or if there is reappearance of clinical and/or biochemical hypercortisolemia within 1 year. Recurrence is as resurgence of clinical and/or biochemical hypercortisolemia after being in remission for at least 1 year postoperatively.

55. **What is the importance of immediate postoperative 0800h plasma cortisol?**

An immediate postoperative 0800h plasma cortisol <50 nmol/L is the best predictor of long-term remission with a recurrence rate of approximately 10% at 10 year. A 0800h plasma cortisol >140 nmol/L in the immediate postoperative period suggest lower probability of achieving remission. A 0800h cortisol between 50 nmol/L and 140 nmol/L also predicts long-term remission, as the recurrence rate in these patients appear similar to those with a 0800h cortisol <50 nmol/L. In addition, immediate 0800h cortisol also helps to decide the need for glucocorticoid supplementation; however, the cutoffs of serum cortisol for defining adrenal insufficiency are different from those to predict remission. Patients with a 0800h cortisol <100nmol/L require hydrocortisone supplementation irrespective of presence or absence of symptoms, whereas those with a serum cortisol >350 nmol/L can be followed up without any replacement. Patients with a 0800h cortisol between 100–350 nmol/L should be closely monitored for signs of adrenal insufficiency and be replaced with hydrocortisone in the presence of symptoms of adrenal insufficiency.

56. **How to perioperatively manage a patient with Cushing's disease after TSS?**

Timing	Monitor	Remarks
Intraoperative	Blood pressure Blood glucose Electrolytes	If hypotension, take sample for cortisol and start hydrocortisone supplementation
Immediate postoperative	Symptoms of adrenal insufficiency Blood pressure Blood glucose Electrolytes Urine output	0800h cortisol at least 2–3 samples, between day 1–7 **0800h cortisol < 100 nmol/L** Supplement hydrocortisone **0800h cortisol 100–350 nmol/L** Monitor closely for signs of adrenal insufficiency and replace with hydrocortisone if required **0800h cortisol > 350 nmol/L** Close follow-up

57. **How to follow up a patient with pituitary Cushing's syndrome after TSS?**

The follow-up protocol of a patient with pituitary Cushing's syndrome after TSS is shown in the figure given below. However, glucocorticoid supplementation should be continued based on 0800h cortisol and presence or absence of symptoms of adrenal insufficiency.

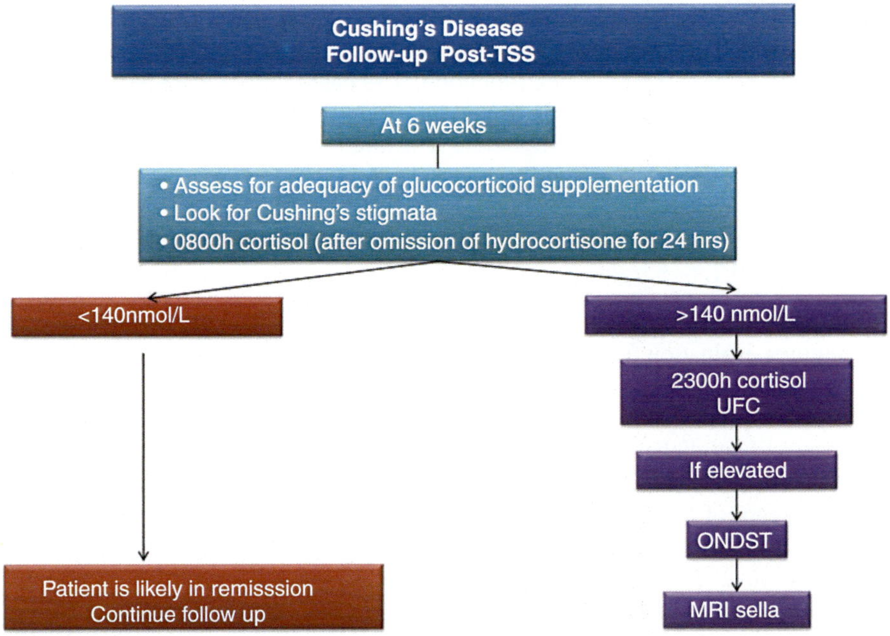

Fig. 5.6 Follow-up protocol of a patient with pituitary Cushing's syndrome after TSS

58. **A 23-year-old female with ACTH-dependent Cushing's syndrome has a pituitary adenoma of size 4 mm on MRI, with a central ACTH gradient on IPSS. She underwent transsphenoidal surgery. Her postoperative day 3 0800h cortisol value is 27 nmol/L (1 μg/dl). Is the patient cured?**

    A patient with immediate postoperative 0800h cortisol value <50 nmol/L has high likelihood of cure, with a recurrence rate of 10% at the end of 10 years. The index patient should be supplemented with glucocorticoids as her cortisol is <100 nmol/L. She needs reevaluation at 6 weeks (after withholding hydrocortisone for 24 h) to assess for remission and the need for glucocorticoid supplementation. If 0800h cortisol >140 nmol/L, patient requires further evaluation to rule out hypercortisolemia.

59. **A 28-year-old female with ACTH-dependent Cushing's syndrome has a pituitary adenoma of size 7 mm on MRI with a central ACTH gradient on IPSS. The patient underwent transsphenoidal surgery. Her postoperative day 3 0800h cortisol value is 210 nmol/L (7 μg/dl), and day 7 0800h cortisol value is 162 nmol/L (6 μg/dl). Should she be immediately reevaluated?**

    No. She should be reevaluated again at 6 weeks, as some patients may have a delayed remission. If 0800h cortisol remains >140 nmol/L (~5 μg/dl) even beyond 6 weeks, it needs further evaluation for persistence of disease. However, at 6 weeks if cortisol is <140 nmol/L (~5 μg/dl), then the patient is considered to be in remission and needs follow-up. The causes of delayed remission are partial adrenal autonomy due to previous long-term ACTH exposure and late necrosis of residual corticotropinoma. The index patient had a 0800h cortisol of 81 nmol/L (~3 μg/dl) at 6 weeks and she is under follow-up.

60. **How to evaluate further if at the end of 6 weeks 0800h cortisol is >140 nmol/L (~5 μg/dl)?**

A patient with 0800h plasma cortisol >140 nmol/L (~5 μg/dl) at 6 weeks requires evaluation for persistence of hypercortisolemia. The patient should be clinically evaluated for the resolution of symptoms and signs (weight loss, desquamation of skin, fading of striae) and reduction in doses of antihypertensives and antidiabetic medications. Biochemical evaluation includes measurement of 2300h cortisol and UFC. These tests are preferred to establish the persistence of disease, as the earliest biochemical abnormality is the reversal of diurnal variation in cortisol rhythm, and UFC is a measure of integrated cortisol secretion. ONDST should only be performed if 0800h cortisol is >350 nmol/L, as it is likely to be falsely negative at cortisol values below this level. A 0800h value of >350 nmol/L is suggested because it reflects the integrity of HPA axis as >95% of healthy individuals with 0800h cortisol >350 nmol/L will have an adequate cortisol response (>540 nmol/L) to insulin-induced hypoglycemia. If there is evidence of hypercortisolemia, the patient should undergo imaging and appropriate therapy. If there is no evidence of hypercortisolemia, the patient should be subjected to 1-μg or 250-μg ACTH stimulation test to assess adrenal reserve, and if the value <540 nmol/L (20 μg/dl), hydrocortisone should be supplemented during stress.

61. **What are the predictors of recurrence of disease?**

Even before the reappearance of clinical features, the earliest detectable biochemical abnormality for prediction of recurrence of disease is elevated 2300h cortisol.

62. **What is the outcome of transsphenoidal surgery in patients with pituitary Cushing's syndrome?**

Transsphenoidal surgery with selective adenomectomy is the preferred treatment for pituitary Cushing's syndrome. The remission rate for microadenoma is 65–90% with a recurrence rate of 5–10% at 5 years and 10–20% at 10 years. The remission rate for macroadenoma is low (50%), and the recurrence is higher (12–45%) and is earlier. Remission rate in patients with non-localization of adenoma who undergo total or partial (central core or hemi-) hypophysectomy is 70% with a higher rate of complications related to surgery and hypopituitarism. Complications after TSS include CSF rhinorrhea, diabetes insipidus, meningitis, sepsis, and cortical vein thrombosis.

63. **What are the causes of headache in a patient with Cushing's disease postoperatively?**

The causes of headache in a patient with Cushing's disease post-TSS are CSF rhinorrhea, meningitis, cortical vein thrombosis, sinusitis, suboptimal glucocorticoid replacement, and rarely, tension pneumocephalus. Patients with Cushing's disease are prone for CSF rhinorrhea, as sellar floor is thinned out due to hypercortisolemia.

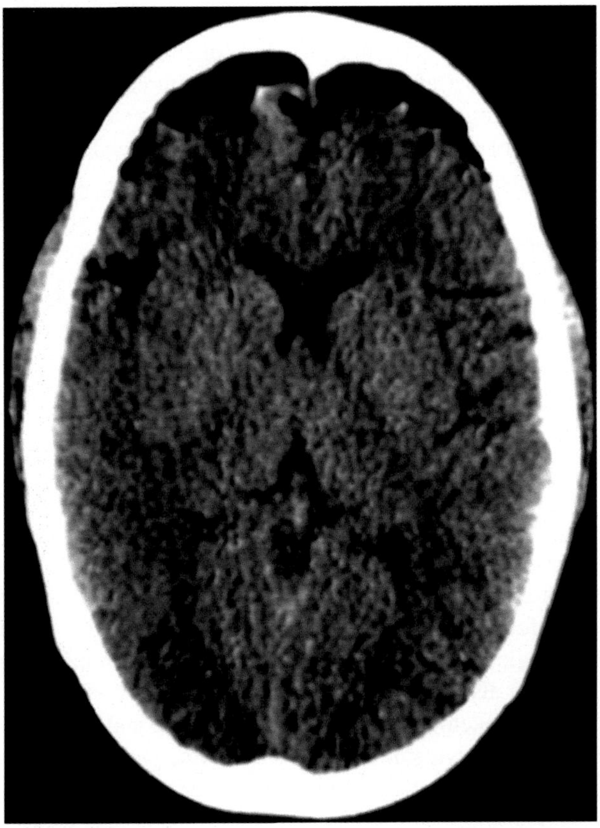

Fig. 5.7 NCCT head showing pneumocephalus in a patient with Cushing's disease after TSS

64. **What are the causes of weight loss after curative surgery in Cushing's disease?**

Gradual weight loss is a consistent feature after curative surgery in Cushing's disease. However, if there is a rapid weight loss after pituitary surgery, a possibility of new-onset multiple pituitary hormone deficiencies should be considered. In addition, subacute thyroiditis may manifest due to sudden decrease in cortisol after curative surgery.

65. **Why is there desquamation after curative surgery in Cushing's syndrome?**

    Desquamation represents increased epidermal cell turnover. Hypercortisolemia has an inhibitory effect on stratum corneum, thereby resulting in cuticular atrophy. After curative surgery, withdrawal of inhibitory effect of cortisol on the stratum corneum allows faster epidermal cell turnover manifesting as desquamation.

66. **What are the indications of medical therapy in Cushing's syndrome?**

    The role of medical therapy in Cushing's syndrome is limited because of its low efficacy, adverse side effects, and the need for lifelong therapy. However, it is indicated in patients with failure to localize the source of ACTH excess, persistent disease after surgery, preoperative preparation, interim period after radiotherapy, presence of concurrent comorbidities which renders patient at high risk for surgery, and patient refusal for surgery.

67. **How does ketoconazole act?**

    Ketoconazole is an imidazole derivative and inhibits cytochrome P450-dependent enzymes in adrenal steroid biosynthetic pathway; particularly side-chain cleavage, 17,20-lyase, and 11-β hydroxylase. It has a cytostatic effect with a t½ of 8–12 h. Ketoconazole is initiated at a dose of 400 mg/day in divided doses and the dose can be increased up to 1,200 mg per day.

68. **What is the advantage of ketoconazole over other adrenal cytostatic drugs?**

    The adrenal cytostatic drugs available to treat hypercortisolemia are ketoconazole, aminoglutethimide, and metyrapone. The advantage of ketoconazole is that it is a pan-enzyme inhibitor (except 3β-HSD) in the steroid biosynthetic pathway; therefore, rising ACTH is unable to overcome this inhibition, as opposed to single enzyme blockade with other adrenal cytostatic drugs. Ketoconazole has also been shown to have inhibitory effect on corticotropes in vitro. In addition, ketoconazole is easily available and inexpensive. However, medical therapy with cytostatic drugs is less effective in macronodular adrenal hyperplasia, ectopic Cushing's syndrome, and adrenocortical carcinoma.

69. **What are the adverse effects with ketoconazole?**

    The adverse effects associated with ketoconazole are transaminitis, hyperbilirubinemia, and adrenal insufficiency. Anorexia, nausea, vomiting, and hypotension in a patient on ketoconazole therapy should alert the physician to consider the possibility of adrenal insufficiency. Ketoconazole is a potent inhibitor of 17,20 desmolase leading to decreased testosterone production and can result in decreased libido and gynecomastia in males. It can also cause hypocalcemia especially in those with severe bone disease due to inhibition of renal 1α-hydroxylase, which is also a cytochrome P450-dependent enzyme. Further, preoperative use of ketoconazole may interfere with prediction of cure after pituitary surgery.

70. **What is pasireotide?**

Pasireotide is a somatostatin receptor analogue which acts on receptor subtypes $SSTR_1$, $SSTR_2$, $SSTR_3$, and $SSTR_5$, with the highest binding affinity for $SSTR_5$. Corticotropinoma predominantly expresses $SSTR_5$ receptor and hence the rationale for its use in patients with Cushing's disease. However, its limited efficacy precludes the use of pasireotide as a primary modality in patients with Cushing's disease, but it may be an option in those with residual or recurrent Cushing's disease. In a study, pasireotide was able to normalize urine free cortisol in 15 and 26% of patients at doses of 600 and 900 μg twice daily, respectively. Those who responded showed a reduction in UFC in the first 2 months, and this effect was sustained till 2 years. Reduction in tumor size was also noted at 1 year. The most common adverse event observed during the study was drug-induced hyperglycemia in 70%, due to inhibition of incretin secretion/effect. Further, pasireotide, being a pan-somatostatin receptor analogue, may inhibit the GH–IGF1 axis which can be particularly detrimental in children with Cushing's syndrome.

71. **Is there a benefit of preoperative medical therapy in patients with Cushing's syndrome?**

The aim of preoperative medical treatment in patients with Cushing's syndrome is to restore eucortisolemia and minimize immediate peri- and postoperative complications. The incidence of postoperative sepsis and wound dehiscence may decrease, but coagulation abnormalities have not been shown to improve with preoperative medical treatment. There is a possibility of early recovery of the hypothalamo–pituitary–adrenal axis leading to shorter duration of post-surgery adrenal insufficiency; however, this has not been well documented. But, preoperative medical treatment interferes with postoperative monitoring of serum cortisol and subsequent prediction of cure. This is particularly relevant in patients with pituitary Cushing's syndrome, where demonstration of low 0800h serum cortisol may be because of prior drug treatment rather than the curative surgery or measurable 0800h cortisol postoperatively because of early recovery of surrounding corticotropes rather than persistent disease.

72. **What is the role of combined medical therapy in patients with pituitary Cushing's syndrome?**

The need for combined medical therapy in patients with pituitary Cushing's syndrome arises due to high incidence of persistent/recurrent disease and the lack of an effective drug as monotherapy. The advantages with combined medical therapy are rapid achievement of eucortisolemia, reduction in doses of individual drug thus limiting the adverse effects, and the ability to target multiple sites, e.g., pituitary (somatostatin/dopamine type 2 receptor agonist), adrenal (ketoconazole/mitotane/metyrapone), and peripheral glucocorticoid receptors (mifepristone). A stepwise addition of three drugs including pasireotide, cabergoline, and ketoconazole has been shown to normalize UFC in almost 90% of patients. Glucocorticoid excess decreases the expression of somatostatin type 2 receptors in pituitary, and normalizing cortisol with combined medical therapy upregulates the expression of somatostatin type 2 receptors by nearly twelve-fold, thereby potentiating the effect of octreotide in corticotropinoma (which predominantly acts on $SSTR_2$). Hence, combined medical therapy effectively improves the clinical outcome.

73. **What are the indications for bilateral adrenalectomy in patients with Cushing's syndrome?**

    The definite indications for bilateral adrenalectomy in patients with Cushing's syndrome are AIMAH and PPNAD. However, patients with ectopic Cushing's syndrome with persistent hypercortisolemia despite removal of primary tumor, unresectable/metastatic tumor, or occult ectopic ACTH-secreting tumor are also benefitted with bilateral adrenalectomy. In patients with Cushing's disease, the indications for bilateral adrenalectomy are persistent disease after transsphenoidal surgery, presence of multiple comorbidities requiring rapid reversal of hypercortisolemia, and failure to localize adenoma in a patient where follow-up is not possible and probably, in women desiring fertility.

74. **Why not to prefer bilateral adrenalectomy in all patients with pituitary Cushing's syndrome?**

    Bilateral adrenalectomy is a definite, predictable, and rapid therapy of hypercortisolemia. Current use of laparoscopic adrenalectomy has decreased the procedure-related morbidity. There is no possibility of recurrence unless there is an ectopic adrenal tissue. In addition, preservation of pituitary hormones is an additional advantage, which is otherwise likely to be affected after pituitary surgery/radiotherapy. However, bilateral adrenalectomy itself is fraught with multiple risks like need for lifelong glucocorticoids, mineralocorticoid and DHEAS replacement, risk of adrenal crisis in poorly compliant patients, and lack of adrenomedullary response to stress. In addition, there is a future risk of Nelson's syndrome requiring regular ACTH monitoring and pituitary imaging, if indicated. Transsphenoidal surgery is curative in 65–90% of patients with microadenoma and 50% with macroadenomas. It is safe in experienced hands, without significant morbidity and mortality, and all patients may not need lifelong glucocorticoid replacement. Hence, bilateral adrenalectomy is not the treatment of choice in all patients with pituitary Cushing's syndrome.

75. **What is Nelson's syndrome?**

    Nelson's syndrome refers to growth of corticotropinoma after total bilateral adrenalectomy in a patient with pituitary Cushing's syndrome, regardless of previous pituitary surgery. The diagnosis should be considered if there is demonstration of expanding pituitary mass or 0800h serum ACTH of >500 pg/ml with 30% rise in ACTH from immediate post-adrenalectomy ACTH value. The prevalence of Nelson's syndrome is around 10–40% and is more common in children. The development of Nelson's adenoma is attributed to the aggressive histological subtype of corticotropinoma which progresses rapidly.

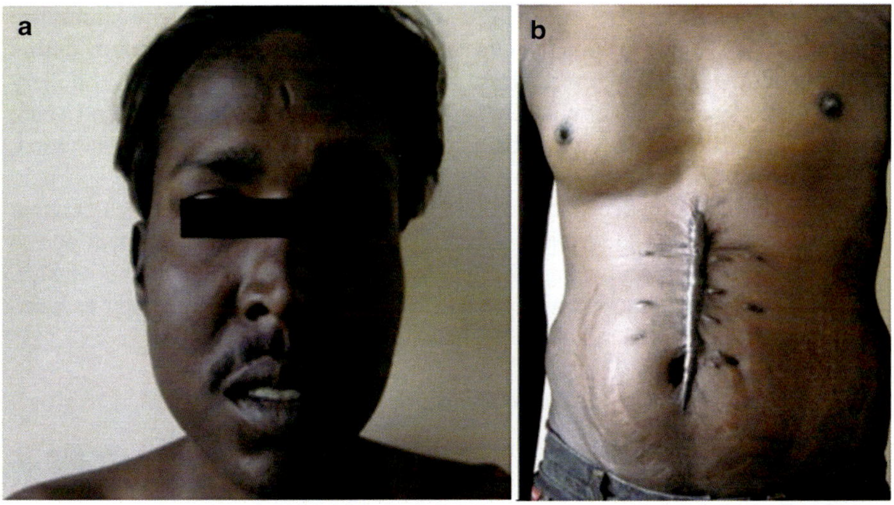

Fig. 5.8 (**a**) Diffuse cutaneous and mucosal hyperpigmentation in a patient with Cushing's disease after bilateral adrenalectomy. (**b**) Hyperpigmented scar in the same patient with Nelson's syndrome. Note the fading striae over the abdomen

76. **What are the predictors of Nelson's syndrome?**

    The predictors of Nelson's syndrome are presence of de novo or residual corticotropinoma prior to total bilateral adrenalectomy (TBA), increase in ACTH >100 pg/ml in the first year post TBA, aggressive histological variant of corticotropinoma, and lack of adjuvant radiotherapy after TBA. Some studies have demonstrated that lack of glucocorticoid receptor expression and greater tumor aggressiveness (as demonstrated by increased mitoses and Ki67-immunopositive nuclei) may contribute to the genesis of Nelson's adenoma. However, the available literature does not support the inadequacy of glucocorticoid treatment after TBA in causation of Nelson's syndrome.

77. **How to treat Nelson's syndrome?**

    Prophylactic radiotherapy after TBA may prevent the development of Nelson's syndrome, but it is not routinely recommended. The treatment of choice for Nelson's syndrome is transsphenoidal surgery, and in case of macroadenomas, transsphenoidal surgery followed by adjuvant radiotherapy is advocated. Medical treatment for Nelson's syndrome includes cabergoline, somatostatin analogues, temozolomide, and sodium valproate. Recently, the pan-somatostatin receptor analogue pasireotide has been shown to be effective.

78. **What is the role of radiotherapy in patients with pituitary Cushing's syndrome?**

    Radiotherapy is a second-line option in patients with pituitary Cushing's syndrome as it takes nearly 3–5 years to be effective, with a cure rate of 56–83%.

However, radiotherapy is associated with adverse effects like hypopituitarism and radiation-induced brain disorder and patients require medical therapy during the interim period. Nevertheless, radiotherapy in children with pituitary Cushing's syndrome is as effective as TSS with a short interim period, and a cure rate of 80–100% hence it can be considered as an initial therapy. In addition, TSS may be difficult in children due to poor pneumatization of the sphenoid sinus. However, the decision should be individualized taking into consideration the risks of growth failure and interference with pubertal development due to radiation. The reason for higher efficacy of radiotherapy in children is elusive. There seems to be no extra advantage with stereotactic radiotherapy as compared to conventional radiotherapy; however, literature is scanty.

79. **What is the role of anti-osteoporotic therapy in patients with Cushing's syndrome?**

    Bone mineral density usually improves following curative surgery in patients with Cushing's syndrome because of the preserved bone microarchitecture (trabecular pattern). Patients of Cushing's syndrome who are elderly, have osteoporosis/fracture or have a low probability of cure should be offered anti-osteoporotic therapy, whereas younger individuals who have osteopenia without fractures and have a high probability of cure do not need anti-osteoporotic therapy. All patients should be treated with calcium and vitamin D. Teriparatide may be preferred over bisphosphonates for the treatment of osteoporosis in patients with both endogenous as well as exogenous Cushing's syndrome.

Suggested Reading

1. Jameson JL, De Groot LJ. Endocrinology: adult and pediatric. Philadelphia: Elsevier Health Sciences; 2010.
2. Longo D, Fauci A, Kasper D, Hauser S, Jameson J, Loscalzo J. Harrison's principles of internal medicine. 18th ed. New York: McGraw Hill Professional; 2012.
3. Melmed S, Polonsky KS, Reed Larsen P, Kronenberg HM. Williams textbook of endocrinology: expert consult. London: Elsevier Health Sciences; 2011.
4. Nieman LK, Biller BMK, Findling JW, Newell-Price J, Savage MO, Stewart PM, Montori VM. The diagnosis of Cushing's syndrome: an endocrine society clinical practice guideline. J Clin Endocrinol Metab. 2008;93(5):1526–40.

Disorders of Androgen Excess

6

6.1 Case Vignette

A 24-year-old female presented with menstrual irregularity for the last 12 years. She had menarche at the age of 12 years, and soon after she started having menorrhagia. She received oral contraceptive pills (OCPs) for a period of 9 months. After discontinuation of OCPs, she had oligomenorrhea. She did not have thorough evaluation but continued to receive OCPs intermittently. However, for the last 6 months, she had secondary amenorrhea and did not have menstrual bleed on OCPs. She had progressive increase in hair growth all over the body along with weight gain of 10 kg for the past 3 years. There was no history of galactorrhea, striae, easy bruisibility, or proximal myopathy. She resorted to cosmetic measures including laser for her hirsutism without significant improvement. She was married for 1 year and had primary infertility. There was no history of hypertension or diabetes. She did not have family history of hirsutism or menstrual irregularity. On examination, her BMI was 24.4 kg/m^2, pulse rate 80/min, and BP 120/90 mm Hg with no postural drop. Her Ferriman–Gallaway score was 26/36. There was no acne, temporal recession, or low-pitch voice, but she had clitoromegaly and male torso without any features of defeminization. She did not have features of protein catabolism like striae, bruise, and proximal myopathy or any stigma of acromegaly. On investigation, serum sodium was 138 mEq/L, potassium 4.7 mEq/L, and creatinine 0.82 mg/dl. Hormonal workup showed serum T_4 8.0 μg/dl (4.8–12.7),TSH 2.5 μIU/ml, prolactin 10.4 ng/ml (4–23), 0800h cortisol 317 nmol/L (171–536), ONDST 24.5 nmol/L (<50), LH 9.9 mIU/ml (1.7–8.6), FSH 5.0 mIU/ml (3.5–12.5), estradiol 76.8 pg/ml (12.5–166), testosterone 10.2 nmol/L (0.2–2.9), DHEAS 944 μg/dl (148–407), and 17α-hydroxyprogesterone (17α-OHP) 2.2 ng/ml (<2). CECT abdomen revealed a well-defined mass of 4.3 × 3 cm arising from the medial limb of the left adrenal gland with no evidence of calcification, necrosis, or hemorrhage with absolute washout of 69% at 10 min suggestive of adrenal adenoma. In addition, there were bilateral bulky ovaries with multiple tiny cystic areas suggestive of polycystic ovaries. 24 h urinary metanephrines and normetanephrines were normal. She underwent laparoscopic left

A. Bhansali, Y. Gogate, *Clinical Rounds in Endocrinology: Volume I - Adult Endocrinology*, DOI 10.1007/978-81-322-2398-6_6

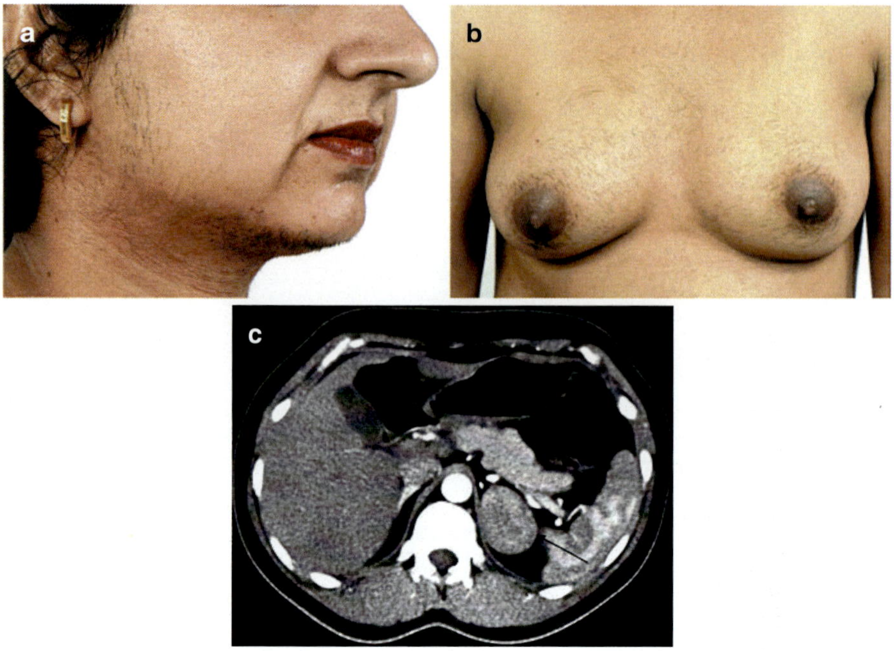

Fig. 6.1 (**a**, **b**) Excessive terminal hair growth over upper lip, chin, and chest in a 24-year-old lady. (**c**) CECT abdomen of the same patient showing 4.3 × 3 cm homogenous mass arising from left adrenal gland, without any area of calcification or necrosis

adrenalectomy uneventfully. Histopathology was consistent with the diagnosis of adrenal adenoma. Two weeks after surgery, hormonal profile showed serum LH 16.1 mIU/ml (1.7–8.6), FSH 4.7 mIU/ml (3.5–12.5), estradiol 115 pg/ml (12.5–166), testosterone 2.2 nmol/L (0.2–2.9), and DHEAS 174 μg/dl (148–407). At 6 weeks of follow-up, her hirsute score was same, but the frequency of cosmetic measures was reduced. She has not yet resumed her cycles.

6.2 Stepwise Analysis

Peripubertal menstrual irregularity is a usual feature in adolescent girls. However, if it persists beyond 2 years after menarche, it requires evaluation. Our patient had menstrual irregularity for the past 12 years, menorrhagia followed by oligomenorrhea, suggesting a clinical possibility of polycystic ovarian syndrome (PCOS) as it is the most common cause of menstrual irregularity in these adolescent girls. The other possibility which should be considered in an adolescent girl with menstrual irregularity is late-onset congenital adrenal hyperplasia (21α-hydroxylase deficiency, LOCAH); however, these patients usually present with hirsutism, acne, and sometimes virilization. Unfortunately our patient never had a thorough evaluation for the etiological diagnosis. Progressive increase in hair growth with severe hirsutism (>15/36) for the last 3 years and development of clitoromegaly and secondary amenorrhea indicate an additional cause of hyperandrogenism in the index case as patients with PCOS and LOCAH usually have a stable course, and hyperandrogenic signs and symptoms do not exacerbate with advancing duration of disease. The differential diagnosis in this scenario includes androgen-secreting adrenal or ovarian tumors, ovarian hyperthecosis, Cushing's syndrome, and use of androgens or androgenic progestins. Slow and progressive development of features of virilization without any defeminization and lack of palpable abdominal or pelvic mass virtually excludes the possibility of androgen-secreting ovarian or adrenal malignant tumors. Virilization with defeminization is usually seen with severe and rapid-onset hyperandrogenism and denotes the presence of androgen-secreting ovarian or adrenal malignant tumors. Ovarian hyperthecosis is unlikely as these patients commonly present in the postmenopausal period with severe manifestations of hyperandrogenism. Drug history was also not contributory. Possibility of Cushing's syndrome in our patient was low as she did not have any manifestations of protein catabolism. This patient was investigated as she had moderate to severe hirsutism (FG score 26/36), menstrual irregularities, and virilization. However, patients with isolated mild hirsutism (FG score <15/36) do not require further evaluation. Serum testosterone level was 10 nmol/L in our patient suggesting a diagnosis of adrenal or ovarian neoplasia; as even in patients with adrenal neoplasia, it is not only a high DHEAS, but higher levels of testosterone may also be present due to peripheral conversion of weaker adrenal androgens (androstenedione, DHEA, and DHEAS) to testosterone. Higher level of DHEAS in our patient (>700 μg/dl) further substantiates the diagnosis of adrenal neoplasia. CECT abdomen revealed a left adrenal mass without any evidence of malignancy and multiple cysts in both ovaries. The ovarian cysts seen in our patient are likely to be due to PCOS; however, secondary polycystic ovarian disease may also occur in the presence of androgen-secreting adrenal tumor. High LH and FSH level in our patient despite higher levels of androgens is possibly explained by inhibition of estrogen-mediated negative feedback by higher levels of testosterone that interfere with the binding of estrogen to its nuclear receptor at the hypothalamo–pituitary axis. She underwent laparoscopic adrenalectomy and had a remarkable decrease in serum testosterone and DHEAS levels. Size of the adrenal tumor was >4 cm in the index patient, and the probability of malignancy with a tumor size between 4.1 and 6 cm is 6%; however, histopathology did not reveal any features of malignancy. Nevertheless, she should remain under surveillance for any recurrence of disease. The biochemical improvement precedes clinical improvement by weeks to months as shedding of preexisting hair depends on the duration of hair cycle, as seen in our patient. Further resumption of menses occurs after restoration of endometrial thickness.

6.3 Clinical Rounds

1. **What is the source of androgens in a woman**?

   The source of androgens in a woman includes ovary and adrenal. Fifty percent of the circulating testosterone is directly produced by the adrenal and ovary, almost in equal proportions, and the rest is derived from the peripheral conversion of weaker androgens like androstenedione, dehydroepiandrosterone (DHEA), and dehydroepiandrosterone sulfate (DHEAS) secreted by the adrenal and ovary. The source of androgens in women is shown in the figure below.

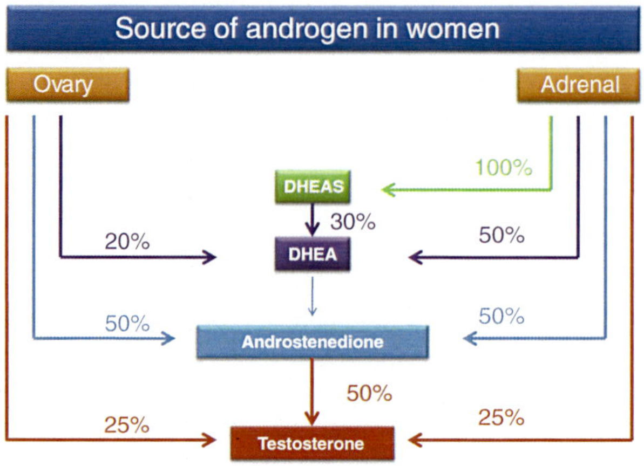

Fig. 6.2 Source of androgens in women

2. **What are the "disorders of androgen excess"?**

   Androgens are normally produced by the ovary and adrenals in women, but when it is associated with clinical features and/or biochemical evidence of androgen excess, they constitute "disorders of androgen excess." The common disorders associated with androgen excess are polycystic ovarian disease, late-onset congenital adrenal hyperplasia, idiopathic hirsutism, ACTH-dependent Cushing's syndrome, glucocorticoid resistance syndrome, hyperprolactinemia, and virilizing ovarian and adrenal neoplasm.

3. **What are the clinical manifestations of androgen excess?**

   The clinical manifestations of androgen excess are hirsutism, acne, androgenic alopecia, low-pitch voice, male torso, and clitoromegaly. It is usually associated with oligo- or amenorrhea and anovulation.

4. **What are the features of virilization?**

   The features of virilization in a woman include androgenic alopecia, acne, low-pitch voice, male torso, and clitoromegaly. These are the manifestations of severe androgen excess and are due to ovarian/adrenocortical malignancy or ovarian hyperthecosis. Hirsutism alone is usually not considered as a feature of virilization.

5. **What are the features of defeminization?**

   The features of defeminization include breast atrophy, oligomenorrhea/amenorrhea, and loss of gluteofemoral adiposity. These are the features of estrogen deficiency; however, they may be present with severe virilization, as androgen excess interferes with the binding of estrogen to its nuclear receptor. In a rapidly growing androgen-secreting tumor, features of defeminization precede virilization.

6. **What is hirsutism**?

Hirsutism is defined as excessive terminal hair growth in "male pattern" in an androgen-dependent area in a woman. The "male pattern" hair should not be considered synonymous with "hair in androgen-dependent areas" as axillary and pubic hair common to both men and women are also present in an androgen-dependent area but are not included in the "male pattern." Hirsutism should be differentiated from hypertrichosis which includes abnormal and excessive vellus hair all over the body.

7. **What are the types of hair**?

Hair are of two types: terminal and vellus. The terminal hair are thick, coarse, and pigmented and are present in androgen-dependent areas as opposed to vellus hair which are fine, thin, and unpigmented and are distributed all over the body.

8. **What are androgen-dependent hair**?

Hair present in almost all areas of the body is androgen dependent except eyebrows, eyelashes, nostrils, and lateral and occipital scalp hair (asexual hair). The axillary and pubic hair are common to both gender and are sensitive to low levels of androgen (ambosexual hair). However, hair on the upper lip, chin, chest, upper arms, abdomen, back, and thighs require a higher level of androgens and characterize the "male pattern" (sexual hair). On the contrary, scalp hair are the only exception where androgen excess results in regression. This is due to shortened anagen phase and possibly androgen receptor downregulation.

9. **What are estrogen-dependent hair**?

Most of the hair in women are androgen dependent, but some hair are estrogen dependent, e.g., scalp hair. This is evident by maximal scalp hair growth seen during pregnancy, and it occurs due to prolongation of the anagen phase because of estrogen. Further, despite normal adrenarche, pubarche is absent in patients with hypogonadotropic hypogonadism and Turner's syndrome as adrenal androgens act in concert with estrogen for the appearance of pubic and axillary hair.

10. **What are the determinants of hair growth**?

Hair growth depends on ethnicity (e.g., Hispanics, Mediterranean descent), genetic factors (number and density of pilosebaceous unit, CAG repeats in androgen receptor), and hormonal factors like testosterone and dihydrotestosterone (DHT). IGF-I, insulin, cortisol, thyroxine, and prolactin play a permissive role. Hair growth is testosterone dependent in almost all androgen-sensitive areas, while hair growth on face, chest, and upper abdomen is predominantly DHT dependent and requires higher level of androgens. This is evidenced by the absence of hair in these areas in patients with 5α-reductase deficiency. However, there is a poor correlation between hair growth and serum androgen levels as hair growth also depends on local growth factors and end-organ sensitivity. Estrogen also has a permissive effect on hair growth as girls with hypogonadism do not have pubarche despite having normal adrenarche, because estrogen is required for the conversion of DHEA to active androgen.

11. **What are the hormonal regulators of hair cycle**?

    Hair follicular growth is a continuous process characterized by a period of growth (anagen), transition (catagen), and rest (telogen). The anagen phase for scalp hair usually lasts for 2–6 years followed by the catagen phase lasting for 1–2 weeks and finally ends into the telogen phase for 4–6 weeks. The hormonal regulators of the hair cycle are androgen, estrogen, thyroxine, and IGF1. Estrogen regulates the anagen phase of the scalp hair and is responsible for longer hair in women.

12. **What are the causes of hirsutism**?

    Ovary and adrenal are the primary source of androgens, and adipose tissue is involved in the peripheral conversion of weaker androgens (e.g., androstenedione, DHEA, and DHEAS) to testosterone. Therefore, pathogenic abnormalities causing hirsutism involve ovary, adrenal gland or adipose tissue. Ovarian causes of hyperandrogenism include polycystic ovary syndrome (PCOS), HAIR-AN syndrome (hyperandrogenism, insulin resistance, and acanthosis nigricans), and ovarian neoplasm like hilus cell tumor and arrhenoblastoma. Adrenal causes of hirsutism include late-onset congenital adrenal hyperplasia (LOCAH), adrenal neoplasms, and glucocorticoid resistance syndrome. Other endocrine disorders associated with hirsutism include Cushing's syndrome, acromegaly, and hyperprolactinemia. Drugs causing hirsutism are phenytoin, minoxidil, cyclosporine, diazoxide, and androgens or androgenic progestins. Idiopathic hirsutism is the diagnosis of exclusion and is characterized by regular menstruation, normal androgen profile, and no ovarian or adrenal abnormalities.

13. **What are the lacunae of the modified Ferriman–Gallaway score**?

    Modified Ferriman–Gallaway score is an objective score to define hirsutism, and a score >8 is considered as significant. A score of 8–15 is classified as mild hirsutism and >15–36 as moderate to severe hirsutism. However, this data is derived from Caucasian women and has not been validated in other racial/ethnic groups. It is observer dependent as the grading from 0 to 4 is subjective and does not include hair growth on side burn, nape of the neck, and phalangeal and perianal region. In addition, a woman having significant hair growth over upper lip/chin but may still have a total score of <8; thus, this score does not reflect the cosmetic concern of the patient.

14. **How to define polycystic ovarian syndrome**?

    Polycystic ovarian syndrome (PCOS) is characterized by clinical and/or biochemical hyperandrogenism, menstrual irregularities, and polycystic ovaries. The classic syndrome originally described by Stein–Leventhal was based on the histomorphological description of the ovary. However, the term PCOS seems inappropriate as all women with PCOS may not necessarily have polycystic ovaries. Insulin resistance is the prime abnormality in the pathogenesis of PCOS; however, it is conspicuously missing in the definition. In other words, PCOS can be described as "testicularization" of the ovaries (structurally ovary but functionally testis).

15. **What are the clinical manifestations of PCOS?**

Menstrual irregularity is the most common manifestation of PCOS and is present in almost 80% of patients. The usual menstrual irregularities are oligomenorrhea or secondary amenorrhea and sometimes primary amenorrhea or menorrhagia. However, 20% of women may have apparently regular cycles despite anovulation. Hirsutism is present in 50–60%, acne in 15–20%, and androgenic alopecia in 5% of patients with PCOS. Approximately 30–75% of patients with PCOS are obese, and majority of them have an android distribution of fat, with features of insulin resistance like acanthosis nigricans and skin tags. Although patients with lean PCOS lack clinical features of insulin resistance, they may have biochemical evidence of insulin resistance (HOMA-IR or euglycemic–hyperinsulinemic clamp). Rarely, women with PCOS may have features of virilization like clitoromegaly and androgenic alopecia.

16. **What is the usual age of presentation of PCOS?**

PCOS is common during three phases of life, namely, peripubertal, peripartum, and perimenopausal; however, it is most common during peripubertal period. These phases in the life of a woman are characterized by maximum perturbations in GnRH pulse generator activity, increase in adipose tissue mass, and psychological disturbances. A slow GnRH pulse frequency preferentially stimulates FSH secretion, whereas fast GnRH pulsator stimulates LH. Due to fast GnRH pulsatility and insulin resistance (due to increased adipocyte mass) during these phases of life, LH is secreted more than FSH consequently resulting into thecal hyperplasia and anovulation, which are the characteristic features of PCOS.

17. **What are the unusual presentations of PCOS?**

The unusual presentations of PCOS include primary amenorrhea, menorrhagia, galactorrhea, and rarely virilization. Some adolescents with PCOS may present as primary amenorrhea with near-normal development of secondary sexual characters; however, these adolescents may have delayed pubarche, higher androgen levels, increased incidence of obesity/metabolic syndrome, and lack of withdrawal bleeding to progesterone as compared to those who present with oligomenorrhea/ secondary amenorrhea. Anovulation and poorly estrogenized endometrium are the causes for primary amenorrhea. Menorrhagia is a rare presentation which occurs due to endometrial hyperplasia and manifests as irregular breakthrough bleeding. It is a consequence of unopposed estrogen action and deficient progesterone production due to chronic anovulation/luteal phase defects. Hyperprolactinemia is present in 15% of women with PCOS and may manifest with galactorrhea.

18. **Is there an increased prevalence of PCOS in patients with type 2 diabetes mellitus?**

No. Insulin resistance is the prime abnormality in patients with PCOS, and they are at increased risk for the development of dysglycemia. However, patients with type 2 diabetes, where insulin resistance is the hallmark feature, do not have an increased prevalence of PCOS as compared to the general population.

19. **Why is there impaired folliculogenesis in PCOS?**

Folliculogenesis is a sequential, regulated, complex process and includes follicular recruitment, growth, and maturation that eventually result in ovulation. The initial primordial follicular recruitment up to the development of antral follicle is gonadotropin independent and is primarily regulated by anti-Mullerian hormone (AMH). AMH is a member of TGF-β superfamily and is produced by granulosa cells. The later process of growth and maturation of antral follicle to dominant follicle is FSH dependent and is finally in concert with LH surge, results in ovulation. These later events are facilitated by declining AMH levels. Therefore, progressively declining AMH along with increasing FSH acts in concert to allow normal folliculogenesis. In PCOS, decreased FSH and failure to decline in AMH result in impaired folliculogenesis. Decreased FSH is due to the fast pulsating GnRH pulse generator, which preferentially secretes LH instead of FSH, and increased inhibin B. The progressive decline in AMH during folliculogenesis does not occur in patients with PCOS because of hyperinsulinemia, increased intrafollicular androgens, and decreased follicular estradiol due to delayed acquisition of aromatase activity. Thus PCOS is a state of "increased folliculogenesis but arrested follicular growth."

20. **What are the causes of chronic anovulation in PCOS?**

Chronic anovulation is the hallmark of PCOS and is result of decreased FSH, increased intraovarian androgens, elevated AMH, and aberrant LH surges. Decreased FSH is due to hyperinsulinemia-mediated abnormality in GnRH pulse generator activity (fast pulsator which preferentially secretes LH), increased inhibin B, and selective negative feedback of estrone (peripheral aromatization of weaker androgens) to FSH. Increased intraovarian androgens are the consequence of hyperinsulinemia/insulin resistance-mediated increased 17,20 desmolase activity, LH-induced thecal hyperplasia, increased IGF1 (as a consequence of hyperinsulinemia), and probably acquired androgen biosynthetic defect (3β-hydroxysteroid dehydrogenase). Elevated AMH level is the result of increased selection of preantral follicles, increased intraovarian androgens, and lack of inhibition by decreasing follicular estradiol due to low FSH. The aberrant LH surge is the result of hyperinsulinemia-mediated abnormality in GnRH pulse generator activity and the positive feedback by estrone. All these events result in impaired folliculogenesis and chronic anovulation which clinically manifests as oligomenorrhea or amenorrhea. This is summarized in the figure given below.

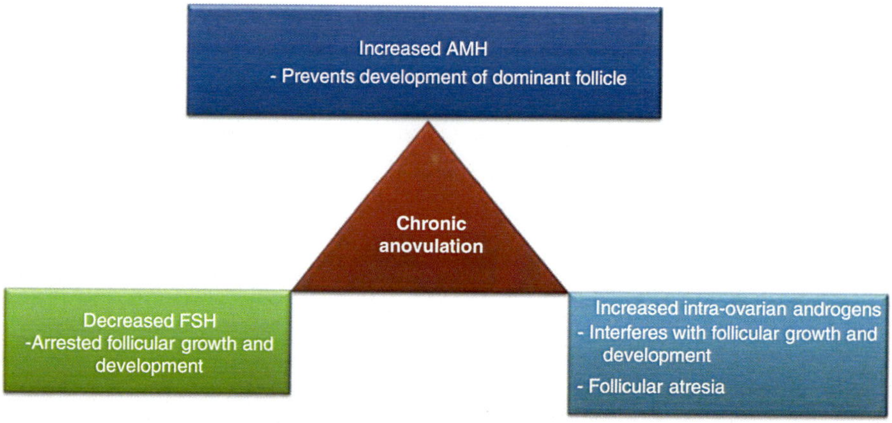

Fig. 6.3 Mechanisms of chronic anovulation in PCOS

21. **Why is obesity associated with hypogonadism in males and hyperandrogenism in females?**

A unique gender paradox of obesity is that it causes hyperandrogenism in females and hypogonadism in males. Obesity in women is associated with "differential insulin resistance" characterized by resistance to the metabolic actions of insulin but preserved sensitivity to proliferative actions in ovary. This results in thecal cell hyperplasia and overproduction of ovarian androgens. These effects are mediated through increased sensitivity to circulating LH, increased local IGF1 production, increased 17,20 desmolase (CYP17A1) activity, and decreased SHBG. Hence in obese women, structurally the gonad is ovary, but functionally it behaves like a testis. In addition, obesity is associated with increased 17β-hydroxysteroid dehydrogenase activity in adipose tissue, thereby promoting peripheral conversion of androstenedione to testosterone. On the contrary, obesity in men is associated with functional hypogonadism as insulin resistance has inhibitory effect on hypothalamo–pituitary–testicular axis. This effect is mediated through hyperinsulinemia, increased adipocytokines (TNF-α, IL-6), and enhanced aromatase activity. In addition, decrease in SHBG is associated with reduced total testosterone concentrations. But in morbidly obese men, due to markedly enhanced aromatase activity, free testosterone is also reduced, because of the inhibitory effect of estradiol on the hypothalamo–pituitary–testicular axis.

22. **What are the causes of bad obstetric history in patient with PCOS?**

Fetal loss is common in patients with PCOS. This is attributed to luteal phase defect, senescent ova fertilization, and dysglycemia. Luteal phase defect is due to impaired follicular growth and development resulting in defective corpus luteum and inadequate progesterone production, thereby leading to miscarriage. Senescent ovum is due to premature completion of the first meiotic division as a consequence of untimed LH surge, which is common in patients with PCOS. If these senescent ova are fertilized, it results in miscarriage. Dysglycemia is a common feature of PCOS due to high prevalence of insulin resistance and causes placental vascular insufficiency resulting in fetal wastage.

23. **What are the causes of infertility in PCOS?**

The causes of infertility in PCOS are chronic anovulation, presence of senescent ova, hostile cervical mucus, and unfavorable endometrial environment.

24. **How to establish a diagnosis of PCOS?**

Various guidelines advocate the diagnosis of PCOS based on clinical and biochemical hyperandrogenism, menstrual irregularity, and ultrasonography. The table enlists the various criteria proposed for diagnosis of PCOS.

Recommendations	Clinical or biochemical hyperandrogenism	Menstrual irregularity	Ultrasound criteria	Remarks
NIH	Must	Must	–	Only based on clinical and biochemical criteria
Rotterdam	May be	May be	May be	2 out of 3, more practical
Androgen Excess Society	Must	May be	May be	Focus only on hyperandrogenism
Endocrine Society Guideline	May be	May be	May be	2 out of 3, more practical

Rotterdam/Endocrine society criteria are most useful in clinical practice. Androgen Excess Society criteria underestimates the prevalence of PCOS as hyperandrogenism is a must for diagnosis. NIH criteria also have a poor sensitivity as it does not include imaging evidence in the diagnosis.

25. **What are the lacunae in diagnostic criteria used for defining PCOS?**

All guidelines essentially include clinical and/or biochemical hyperandrogenism and menstrual irregularities with or without polycystic ovaries on imaging. Ethnic variability in quantification of hirsute score, lack of assessment of tissue sensitivity to androgens, alterations in androgen levels with age, and non-standardization of androgen assays across the laboratories are the deficits associated with criteria based on clinical and/or biochemical hyperandrogenism. Ovulatory dysfunction is difficult to quantify, and 20% of women despite anovulation may have regular menses, thereby making it difficult to diagnose ovulatory dysfunction. Operator dependence, presence of similar sonologic features in other endocrine disorders, inability to perform transvaginal USG in adolescents, and lack of normative data across the different phases of the menstrual cycle are the limitations of USG criteria.

26. **How does adolescent PCOS differ from adult PCOS?**

Menstrual irregularities are the hallmark of PCOS. However, oligomenorrhea is a regular feature in peripubertal girls; hence, menstrual irregularity should not be considered as a diagnostic criterion of PCOS in adolescents unless it persists beyond 2 years after the onset of menarche. Hirsutism as assessed by Ferriman–Gallaway score is not validated in adolescents. Similarly, Rotterdam ultrasound criteria of PCOS are also not validated in adolescents. In addition, the transvaginal ultrasound is not practical in this age group. Therefore, diagnosis of PCOS in adolescents should be based on clinical and/or biochemical hyperandrogenism in the presence of persistent menstrual irregularities. Serum AMH may be useful as a noninvasive diagnostic marker for PCOS.

27. **How to differentiate between late-onset CAH and PCOS?**

Late-onset CAH (LOCAH) contributes to 10–15% of adolescent PCOS. LOCAH usually manifests as premature pubarche and peripubertal hirsutism. As opposed to PCOS, oligomenorrhea is less frequent (80% vs. 40–50%), and features of virilization may be present in LOCAH. These patients are usually lean with normal stature, and family history of hirsutism may be present. Diagnosis of LOCAH can be confirmed by stimulated 17 α-OHP >10 ng/ml. Treatment with glucocorticoids is less effective; therefore, antiandrogens and oral contraceptives are preferred for treatment of hirsutism and menstrual irregularities. However, glucocorticoids are in those with premature adrenarche and accelerated bone maturation.

28. **How does ovarian hyperthecosis differ from polycystic ovaries?**

Ovarian hyperthecosis, a variant of PCOS, is characterized by severe hyperandrogenism and insulin resistance and is seen primarily in postmenopausal women. Patients usually present with hirsutism, acne, and features of virilization. Prominent thecal hyperplasia and predominantly solid appearance of ovaries with few or no cysts are characteristic of ovarian hyperthecosis on imaging. On the contrary, patients with PCOS are usually young and present with mild hirsutism and menstrual irregularities and usually lack features of virilization. Multiple follicles (>12, size 2–9 mm) predominantly in the periphery (necklace pattern) and mild thecal hyperplasia, with or without increased ovarian volume (>10 ml), are classical imaging features of PCOS. Therefore, in a patient with suspected PCOS who has features of virilization, ovarian hyperthecosis should also be considered in the differential diagnosis in addition to virilizing adrenal or ovarian tumors. The case illustrated below shows severe virilization in a young girl with ovarian hyperthecosis.

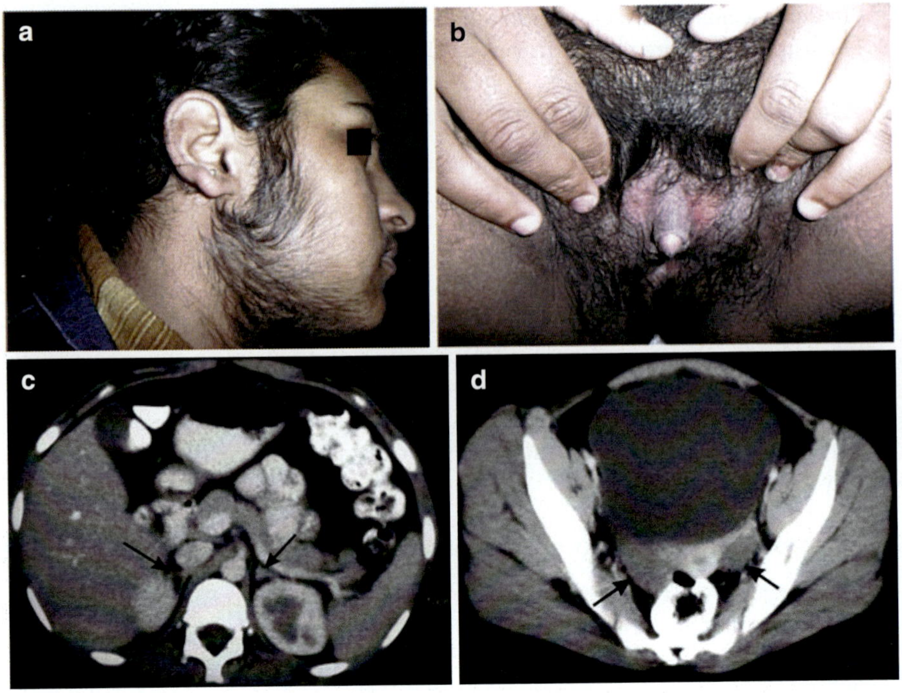

Fig. 6.4 (**a**) A 20-year-old girl with hirsutism and obesity. (**b**) Clitoromegaly in the same patient. (**c**) CECT abdomen of the same patient demonstrating normal adrenal glands. (**d**) CECT pelvis showing bilateral ovarian enlargement

29. **What are the causes of secondary PCOS**?

    Common causes of secondary PCOS are hypothyroidism, Cushing's syndrome, acromegaly, hyperprolactinemia, thyrotoxicosis, and late-onset CAH. These disorders are associated with androgen excess, variability in LH pulses, alterations in sex hormone-binding globulin (SHBG), and/or insulin resistance. Therefore, all patients with PCOS should have a baseline TSH, prolactin, and 17 α-hydroxyprogesterone to exclude secondary PCOS.

30. **Who should be investigated for disorders of androgen excess**?

    A detailed history and physical examination usually points to the diagnosis of hyperandrogenic disorders. Patients who require workup include those with hirsutism (score >8-15 with menstrual irregularities or isolated hirsutism with score >15), menstrual irregularities, virilization, rapidly progressive hirsutism, infertility, galactorrhea, and stigma of Cushing's syndrome.

31. **What are the minimum investigations required in a woman with disorder of androgen excess?**

Minimum investigations required in a woman with disorder of androgen excess include TSH, prolactin, 17α-hydroxyprogesterone, and testosterone. Estimation of TSH and prolactin may help in excluding the secondary causes of PCOS. Normal serum testosterone does not exclude the diagnosis of PCOS because of variable end-organ sensitivity, and the measurement of free testosterone or free androgen index (serum testosterone X SHBG/100) has no additive value because of poor standardization of assays. Routine estimation of LH and FSH is not useful, as characteristic LH/FSH ratio >2 is observed only in half of patients with PCOS; however, it must be estimated in patients with amenorrhea. Baseline 0800–0900h serum 17α -OHP <2 ng/ml in early follicular phase in a menstruating woman rules out the diagnosis of late-onset congenital adrenal hyperplasia due to 21α-hydroxylase deficiency (LOCAH). If it is >2 ng/ml, diagnosis needs to be confirmed with 250 μg ACTH stimulation test (17α -OHP >10-100 ng/ml at 60 min). Estimation of DHEAS may be useful in those with rapidly progressive hirsutism/virilization to exclude a diagnosis of adrenal neoplasia. The estimation of serum DHT is not helpful because of poor assay sensitivity and lack of correlation between circulating DHT levels and hirsutism (due to variations in 5α-reductase type 2 activity in pilosebaceous unit). In addition, patients with PCOS should undergo OGTT and fasting lipid profile as they are at high risk for future development of cardiovascular events. The estimation of serum AMH, fasting plasma insulin, and HOMA-IR are more of research interest.

32. **Does the level of androgen help in establishing the etiology of androgen excess?**

Majority of patients with PCOS have total testosterone level in the reference range. Serum total testosterone of >6.94 nmol/L is suggestive of ovarian/adrenal neoplasm, and serum DHEAS level >700 μg/dl is suggestive of adrenal neoplasm. However, some women with PCOS may have androgen levels in this range without any neoplasm.

33. **Why is the serum estradiol level normal in PCOS despite chronic anovulation?**

PCOS is a state characterized by "androgenization without defeminization." Normally, a growing follicle acquires aromatase activity at a size of 7mm under the effect of FSH and is a sustained source of estradiol till it matures into a dominant follicle. Theca cells produce a regulated quantum of androgens which are available as a precursor for estradiol biosynthesis in granulosa cells. In patients with PCOS, the follicular source of estradiol is reduced due to impaired folliculogenesis, but increased androgen production from theca cells (androstenedione) continues under the effect of aberrant LH drive and hyperinsulinemia resulting in uninterrupted delivery of androgenic precursors (androstenedione) for peripheral conversion to estrogen in adipocytes. Therefore, the ovary becomes a major source of androgens and adipose tissue for estrogen.

34. **What are the ultrasound criteria for the diagnosis of PCOS**?

    Transvaginal/pelvic ultrasound showing 12 or more follicles of size 2–9 mm predominantly in the periphery and/or increased ovarian volume (>10 ml) either unilaterally or bilaterally is suggestive of PCOS, and these criteria have a sensitivity and specificity of 75% and 99%, respectively. Incidentally detected polycystic ovaries in the absence of clinical features of PCOS do not merit further evaluation.

35. **When should USG be performed for the diagnosis of PCOS**?

    USG should be performed during early follicular phase (days 3–5) in a regularly menstruating woman, and at random/after 3–5 days of progesterone withdrawal bleed in a woman with oligomenorrhea or amenorrhea. The reason for performing USG during early follicular phase is that it represents a baseline status of hypothalamo-pituitary-ovarian axis in a woman.

36. **What are the clinical implications of progesterone withdrawal bleed**?

    Endometrial estrogenization, timely ovulation, and progesterone withdrawal are the prerequisites for normal menstruation. Lack of synchrony in these events results in menstrual irregularities. Patients with oligomenorrhea with clinical estrogen sufficiency (Tanner breast stages 4–5) should be subjected to progesterone challenge (medroxyprogesterone acetate 10 mg/day for 5–7 days) after ruling out pregnancy. If progesterone withdrawal results in bleeding, it suggests that the endometrium is adequately primed with estrogen, and the cause of oligomenorrhea is anovulation. Absence of bleeding after withdrawal of progesterone suggests inadequate endometrial priming with estrogen. Patients with PCOS are estrogen sufficient and usually do respond to progesterone challenge except adolescent PCOS who usually have thin endometrium. Patients with abnormalities in the hypothalamo–pituitary–ovarian axis like hypogonadotropic hypogonadism and hyperprolactinemia do not respond to progesterone withdrawal as they are estrogen deficient. Despite estrogen sufficiency, some women may not bleed with progesterone challenge and require further evaluation.

37. **In what situation a patient with secondary amenorrhea with estrogen deficiency may bleed on progesterone challenge test**?

    A patient with acromegaly may bleed on progesterone challenge despite secondary hypogonadism due to GH-IGF1-mediated endometrial hyperplasia. In addition, patients on progesterone therapy may have progesterone breakthrough bleed despite estrogen insufficiency.

38. **What are the predictors of ovulation**?

Predictors of ovulation help in timing the ovulation and in deciding the fertility period. They include thin, stretchy cervical mucus, ovarian follicular size of ≥16 mm, measurement of LH surge (serum/urine LH >50 IU/L), serum 17β-estradiol (>1,000 pg/ml), and increased vaginal blood flow on plethysmography.

39. **What are the markers of ovulation**?

The markers of ovulation indicate presence or absence of ovulation. The markers of ovulation are regularity in menstrual cycles, increased basal body temperature (0.5 °F), midluteal phase progesterone >10 ng/ml, and secretory endometrium in late luteal phase on endometrial curettage.

40. **What are the markers of ovarian reserve**?

The markers of ovarian reserve include serum levels of FSH during early follicular phase, serum estradiol, AMH, inhibin B, and ultrasound assessment of antral follicular count. Ovarian reserve helps in deciding the fertility potential of women.

41. **What are the treatment options in patients with PCOS**?

Treatment options depend on the need of patient and are listed in the table given below.

Primary concern	Must	First-line	Additive/ second line
Hirsutism	Lifestyle modification	Oral contraceptive pills	Antiandrogens
Menstrual irregularities	Lifestyle modification	Oral contraceptive pills	Metformin
Metabolic abnormalities (prediabetes/diabetes)	Lifestyle modification	Metformin	–
Ovulation induction	Lifestyle modification	Clomiphene citrate	Metformin

42. **Which is the preferred oral contraceptive in PCOS**?

Oral contraceptive pills (OCPs) consisting of optimal amount of ethinyl estradiol (30–35 μg) and non-androgenic/antiandrogenic progesterone like cyproterone acetate, drospirenone, desogestrel, norgestimate, or gestodene are preferred in the management of PCOS with hirsutism and/or menstrual irregularity.

43. **How do oral contraceptives help in PCOS**?

Patients with hirsutism and/or menstrual irregularities should be treated with oral contraceptives. OCPs help in regularizing menstrual cycles and decrease hyperandrogenemia. Ethinyl estradiol increases SHBG and results in decreased free testosterone levels. Further in conjunction with progesterone, ethinyl estradiol also decreases LH drive thereby resulting in reduced ovarian androgen production. In addition, some progestins have inhibitory effect on 5α-reductase activity and interfere with androgen action. Also, there is some evidence to suggest suppression of adrenal androgens with the use of OCPs, but the mechanism remains elusive.

44. **Why antiandrogens should not be used alone for treatment of PCOS**?

Antiandrogens are usually required as OCPs alone do not produce a rewarding outcome, especially in treating hirsutism. Lone use of antiandrogens is contraindicated as it may lead to menstrual irregularities (mid-cycle bleed due to deficient progesterone production/action) and can cause under-virilization in the male fetus, if conceived.

45. **Which is the preferred antiandrogen in PCOS**?

Spironolactone is the preferred antiandrogen, as its safety and efficacy are well established in clinical practice. It inhibits cytochrome P450-dependent enzymes in the androgen biosynthetic pathway and blocks the androgen receptor. The initial dose is 100 mg per day which can be increased slowly up to 200 mg per day in divided doses and is given for at least 12–18 months. However, low-dose spironolactone (25 mg) has also been shown to be effective. Other antiandrogens like cyproterone acetate, flutamide, and finasteride are mildly effective and fraught with adverse effects, hence are less preferred.

46. **A 20-year-old female presented with hirsutism and menstrual irregularity. Ultrasound showed characteristic radiological features of PCOS, and she was started on oral contraceptive pills. After 2 months she returned unhappy with the treatment response. What to do**?

The patient needs to be reassured that prolonged treatment is required to have an appreciable effect on hair growth, as hair cycle lasts 3–6 months. The efficacy of treatment is assessed by thinning of hair, decrease in hirsute score, resolution of acne, decrease in frequency of cosmetic treatment, and objective measurement of hair diameter. Further, treatment with OCPs does not target preexisting hair; therefore, cosmetic therapy for their removal is warranted.

47. **What are the possibilities when an adolescent girl with hirsutism who is on oral contraceptives shows suboptimal response or worsening of hirsutism with treatment**?

Suboptimal response or worsening of hirsutism to OCPs in an adolescent girl with hirsutism should raise the possibility of use of oral contraceptive with androgenic progestins, previously unrecognized simple virilizing classical congenital adrenal hyperplasia, or concurrent androgen-secreting adrenal/ovarian tumor.

48. **How is metformin useful in PCOS?**

Metformin is a biguanide which improves insulin sensitivity and reduces hyperinsulinemia by acting through AMP kinase pathway. This results in a decrease in ovarian hyperandrogenism, thereby provides a conducive milieu for follicular growth and development and regularizes menstrual cycles. The usual dose of metformin is 1–2 g/day. However, metformin is not effective for hirsutism. The current indications of metformin in patients with PCOS are dysglycemia, contraindications to OCPs, clomiphene-resistant ovulatory dysfunction, and during in vitro fertilization to prevent ovarian hyperstimulation syndrome. It was advised to continue metformin till the end of first trimester as it was thought to prevent fetal wastage (by facilitating timely oocyte maturation and improvement in luteal function), and possibly dysglycemia. However, the current guideline based on recent meta-analysis does not favor the continuation of metformin after the confirmation of pregnancy as its use is not associated with the improved outcome in terms of fetal loss, dysglycemia, and preeclampsia.

49. **Why is ovulation induction difficult in PCOS as compared to hypogonadotropic hypogonadism?**

Ovulation induction is difficult in patients with PCOS as there is an aberrant GnRH pulse generator activity (decreased FSH and increased LH) with impaired folliculogenesis. Patients with hypogonadotropic hypogonadism have GnRH deficiency, and therefore it is easier to induce ovulation with the use of exogenous gonadotropins. Continuous use of GnRH agonist in PCOS to knock-down the aberrant pulsatility improves fertility potential.

50. **What is the treatment of choice for ovulation induction in PCOS?**

PCOS contributes to about 20% of all causes of female infertility. Clomiphene alone or in combination with metformin is the preferred drug to treat infertility in PCOS. Clomiphene is a selective estrogen receptor modulator (SERM), which acts at the level of hypothalamus and resets the GnRH–gonadotropin axis. Disadvantages of clomiphene include multiple gestations, and its antiestrogen-like action at the endometrium which is unfavorable for blastocyst implantation. Use of hMG followed by hCG or GnRH agonist followed by hMG and hCG is recommended, if there is failure to induce ovulation with clomiphene and metformin.

51. **What are the complications associated with pregnancy in women with PCOS?**

Complications associated with pregnancy in PCOS may be due to disease per se or treatment-related. The complications related to disease are increased incidence of fetal loss, gestational diabetes, preeclampsia, and preterm delivery. Treatment-related complications are multiple pregnancies and ovarian hyperstimulation syndrome due to ovulation induction.

52. **What are long-term consequences of PCOS?**

PCOS is a state of insulin resistance and is associated with increased risk for future development of type 2 diabetes and cardiovascular diseases. The risk is higher even in those with lean PCOS. Other abnormalities associated with PCOS are dyslipidemia, increased prothrombotic activity, nonalcoholic fatty liver disease, and sleep apnea. In addition, there is an increased risk of endometrial carcinoma because of prolonged and unopposed estrogen action; hence, these women should remain under regular surveillance. Despite being a state of increased folliculogenesis and excessive follicular atresia, menopause does not occur at an earlier age in women with PCOS. Although oligomenorrhea/amenorrhea is common in PCOS, osteoporosis is not a feature due to combined impact of hyperandrogenism and estrogen sufficiency on bone mineral density.

53. **Why is there no defeminization despite hyperandrogenemia in a woman with PCOS?**

Mild androgen excess manifests as hirsutism, acne, or androgenic alopecia and is usually not accompanied with defeminization as seen in patients with PCOS. However, patients with severe androgen excess may have features of defeminization as seen in patients with adrenal or ovarian androgen-secreting tumors. Therefore, development of defeminization in a woman with androgen excess depends upon the severity of androgen excess and duration of androgen exposure.

Suggested Reading

1. Azziz R, Enrico C, Didier D, Evanthia D-K, Escobar-Morreale HF, Walter F, Janssen OE, et al. Criteria for defining polycystic ovary syndrome as a predominantly hyperandrogenic syndrome: an androgen excess society guideline. J Clin Endocrinol Metab. 2006;91(11):4237–45.
2. Carmina ENRICO. Diagnosis of polycystic ovary syndrome: from NIH criteria to ESHRE-ASRM guidelines. Minerva Ginecol. 2004;56(1):1–6.
3. Jameson JL, De Groot LJ. Endocrinology: adult and pediatric. Philadelphia: Elsevier Health Sciences; 2010.
4. Longo D, Anthony F, Dennis K, Stephen H, Jameson J, Joseph L. Harrison's Principles of Internal Medicine 18E EB. New York: McGraw Hill Professional; 2012.
5. Melmed S, Polonsky KS, Reed Larsen P, Kronenberg HM. Williams textbook of endocrinology: Expert consult. London: Elsevier Health Sciences; 2011.

7 Pheochromocytoma and Paraganglioma

7.1 Case Vignette

A 45-year-old lady presented with abdominal pain for the past 2–3 weeks. It was dull aching, continuous, and localized to right flank without any nausea, vomiting, bladder, or bowel complaints. Ultrasonography of abdomen revealed bilateral adrenal masses, and she was referred to endocrinology for further evaluation. She was a known hypertensive for the last 5 years and was on telmisartan 80 mg, amlodipine 10 mg, hydrochlorothiazide 25 mg, and metoprolol 50 mg per day. In addition, she was also on levothyroxine 125 μg/day. She had history of episodic palpitation not associated with headache or sweating. On evaluation, pulse rate was 108/min and BP 170/110 mm/Hg without any postural drop. There were no mucosal neuromas, cafe-au-lait macules, neurofibroma, bony lesion, retinal angiomas, Marfanoid habitus, or cutaneous lichen amyloidosis. She did not have any features of Cushing's syndrome or virilization. There was a scar in the neck, and on questioning she disclosed a history of neck surgery 15 years back. Past surgical records revealed that total thyroidectomy was contemplated for medullary thyroid carcinoma. There was no family history of hypertension, thyroid malignancy, or renal stone disease. On investigation, serum potassium was 3.4 meq/L, creatinine 1.1 mg/dl, corrected serum calcium 10.2 mg/dl, phosphorus 4.0 mg/dl, and alkaline phosphate 98 IU/ml. Fasting plasma glucose was 108 mg/dl and HbA1c was 6% and thyroid function tests were normal. Plasma-free metanephrine and normetanephrine were 1,000 pg/ml (<90) and 240 pg/ml (<180), respectively. Serum iPTH was 38 pg/ml (9–65) and 25(OH) D 22 ng/ml (>30). Serum calcitonin was 2 pg/ml (<5). CECT abdomen showed bilateral asymmetrical adrenal masses (right 5 × 3.5 cm and left 2 × 1.5 cm) without any areas of necrosis or calcification. With this clinical and biochemical profile, she was diagnosed to have multiple endocrine neoplasia type 2A with MTC and bilateral pheochromocytoma which was further confirmed on genetic analysis (RET proto-oncogene mutation). After adequate α-and β-blockade, she was subjected to bilateral adrenalectomy. Postoperatively, she was continued on oral hydrocortisone and fludrocortisone. The requirement of

A. Bhansali, Y. Gogate, *Clinical Rounds in Endocrinology: Volume I - Adult Endocrinology*, DOI 10.1007/978-81-322-2398-6_7

antihypertensive drugs was reduced after surgery, and BP was 140/90 on amlodipine 5 mg per day. After 2 weeks, plasma-free metanephrine and normetanephrine were estimated, and these were within the reference range suggestive of successful resection of catecholamine-secreting tumor. Estimation of serum calcitonin, calcium profile, and plasma-free metanephrine and normetanephrine were performed in the family members and were within normal reference range.

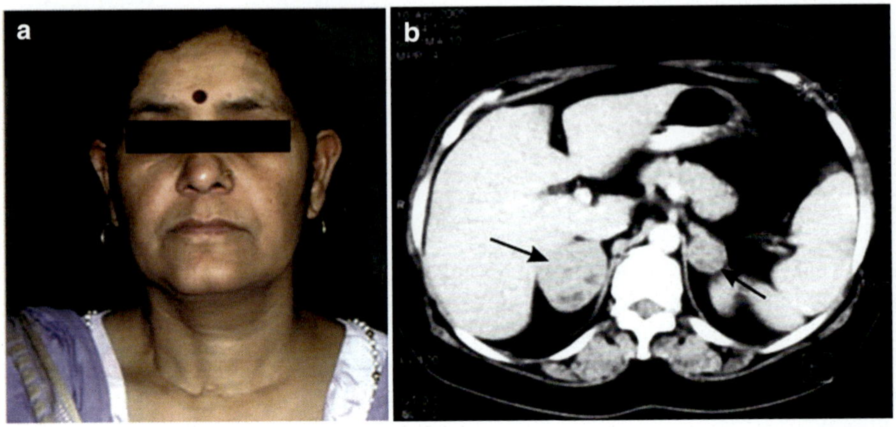

Fig. 7.1 (**a**) Post-thyroidectomy scar in a patient with MEN2A. (**b**) CECT abdomen showing well-defined adrenal masses bilaterally (right 5 × 3.5 cm and left 2 × 1.5 cm). Areas of necrosis are seen in both lesions

7.2 Stepwise Analysis

The index patient presented with abdominal pain and was found to have bilateral adrenal masses. Abdominal pain as a presenting manifestation of adrenal mass is unusual; however, it can occur due to stretching of the adrenal capsule, sudden hemorrhage into the tumor, or tumoral necrosis. The index patient had resistant hypertension, paroxysms, and bilateral adrenal masses. As she had uncontrolled blood pressure despite >3 antihypertensive drugs in optimal doses (including a diuretic), she mandates evaluation for secondary hypertension. The paroxysm in a patient with catecholamine-secreting tumor comprises of episodic hypertension with the classical triad of headache, tachycardia, and sweating. However, the presence of a single component of the triad should not be ignored especially if associated with hypertension, as the classical triad is present only in 30% of patients with pheochromocytoma. The most common cause of bilateral adrenal masses in the presence of hypertension with or without paroxysms is pheochromocytoma associated with familial syndromes. In addition, ACTH-independent macronodular adrenal hyperplasia, bilateral aldosteronoma, bilateral adrenocortical carcinoma, adrenal myelolipoma, and long-standing untreated congenital adrenal hyperplasia (11β-hydroxylase and 17α-hydroxylase deficiency) are the other differentials for hypertension with bilateral adrenal masses. The index patient had high levels of plasma free metanephrines (>3 times the upper limit of normal), which suggests presence of catecholamine-secreting tumor of adrenal origin. In addition, predominant secretion and very high level of metanephrine strengthen the possibility of MEN2-associated pheochromocytoma as opposed to sporadic pheochromocytoma, which preferentially secretes normetanephrines. Bilateral adrenal pheochromocytoma and past history of medullary thyroid carcinoma suggests a diagnosis of MEN2. In patients with MEN2, medullary thyroid carcinoma (MTC) is diagnosed concurrently with pheochromocytoma in 40%, while MTC precedes pheochromocytoma in 50% and follows it in 10%. In our patient, diagnosis of MTC preceded pheochromocytoma by almost 15 years. Absence of mucosal neuromas, lack of Marfanoid habitus, and late onset of disease diminute the possibility of MEN2B and favor the diagnosis of MEN2A. It is important to distinguish between these two entities because medullary thyroid carcinoma associated with MEN2B is more aggressive. In addition, de novo germ line mutations of RET proto-oncogene can occur in 50% of patients with MEN2B, which is rare in MEN2A. Genetic analysis further confirmed the diagnosis of MEN2A in the index patient. Primary hyperparathyroidism occurs in 20–30% and cutaneous lichen amyloidosis, a surrogate marker of MTC, in 5% of patients with MEN2A; however, both were absent in the index patient. Modestly elevated serum calcium in the index patient may be attributed to hemoconcentration because of intense vasoconstriction whereas hypokalemia is a result of transcellular shift of potassium by catecholamines. Mild dysglycemia as seen in our patient is common in patients with pheochromocytoma due to the inhibitory effect of catecholamines on insulin secretion as well as interference with post-receptor insulin-signaling mechanisms. These abnormalities are reversible after surgery. Patients with pheochromocytoma should be treated with α-blockers followed by β-blockers, to avoid hypertensive crisis due to unopposed α-adrenergic receptor action. Patients planned for bilateral adrenalectomy should be administered intravenous hydrocortisone infusion to prevent the development of adrenal crisis during surgery. Oral hydrocortisone should be supplemented lifelong in these patients, and the dose should be doubled during stress. In addition, fludrocortisone should be added to prevent postural hypotension and hyperkalemia. The presence of hypertension should not deter the use of fludrocortisone, and worsening of blood pressure can be managed with increased doses of antihypertensives.

7.3 Clinical Rounds

1. **What is secondary hypertension?**

   Patients with an underlying "identifiable" cause of hypertension are considered to have secondary hypertension. Hypertension is "essential or idiopathic" in nearly 85% of patients, while approximately 15% have secondary hypertension. Secondary hypertension commonly presents at a young age and is severe, multidrug resistant, and may be associated with target organ damage disproportionate to the degree and duration of hypertension. The probability of cure after definitive treatment merits evaluation for secondary hypertension.

2. **What are the causes of secondary hypertension?**

The common causes of secondary hypertension include renal (renal parenchymal or renovascular disease), vascular (e.g., coarctation of the aorta), and endocrine disorders. Many endocrine disorders are associated with hypertension and adrenal causes predominate. The adrenal disorders associated with hypertension are pheochromocytoma, primary aldosteronism, Cushing's syndrome, congenital adrenal hyperplasia due to 11β-hydroxylase or 17α-hydroxylase deficiency, glucocorticoid resistance syndrome (GRS), and apparent mineralocorticoid excess syndrome (11β-hydroxysteroid dehydrogenase type 2 defect). Other endocrine causes include acromegaly, paraganglioma, hypothyroidism, hyperthyroidism, and hyperparathyroidism. Majority of patients with type 2 diabetes and metabolic syndrome have hypertension and require multiple drugs to control blood pressure, but usually do not have an identifiable cause of hypertension and are thus classified as essential hypertension.

3. **Who should be evaluated for secondary hypertension?**

Young age of onset (<30 years), presence of paroxysms and hypokalemia in a patient with hypertension should prompt evaluation for secondary causes of hypertension. In addition, patients with labile hypertension, severe hypertension, resistant hypertension (uncontrolled blood pressure despite use of ≥3 antihypertensives of different classes in optimal doses, including a diuretic) and hypertension associated with clinical stigmata of a specific disorder (e.g., Cushing's syndrome, MEN2, NF1, GRS) or adrenal mass should also be evaluated.

4. **What are the clinical clues that help in defining the etiology of secondary hypertension?**

The clinical clues that point to the etiology of secondary hypertension are enlisted in the table given below.

Diagnosis	Clinical clues
Renovascular hypertension	Recurrent episodes of flash pulmonary edema
	Renal bruit
	Abnormal urine analysis
	Elevation in serum creatinine ≥30% after administration of angiotensin-converting enzyme (ACE) inhibitor or angiotensin II receptor blocker (ARB)
Pheochromocytoma/ Paraganglioma (PPGL)	Paroxysms of headache, palpitations, and sweating
	Postural drop in blood pressure
	Mucosal neuroma, Marfanoid habitus
	Neurofibromas, cafe-au-lait macules, retinal angiomas
Primary aldosteronism	Diastolic hypertension, hypokalemia-related symptoms, metabolic alkalosis
Cushing's syndrome	Classical stigma of Cushing's syndrome
	Hypertension with hypokalemia
Glucocorticoid resistance syndrome	Features of androgen excess
	Hypertension with hypokalemia

5. **What are the causes of labile hypertension?**

Labile hypertension is classically associated with pheochromocytoma/ paraganglioma. However, patients with autonomic neuropathy white coat hypertension, and acute emotional outbursts can also cause labile hypertension.

6. **What is pheochromocytoma?**

The term "pheochromocytoma" is derived from the Greek words *phaios* ("dusky"), *chroma* ("color") and *cytoma* ("tumor"); it refers to the dark staining that occurs when intracellular catecholamines are treated with chromium salts. Catecholamine-secreting tumors arising from the adrenal medulla (chromaffin tissue) are called as pheochromocytoma, and they constitute 85% of catecholamine-secreting tumors.

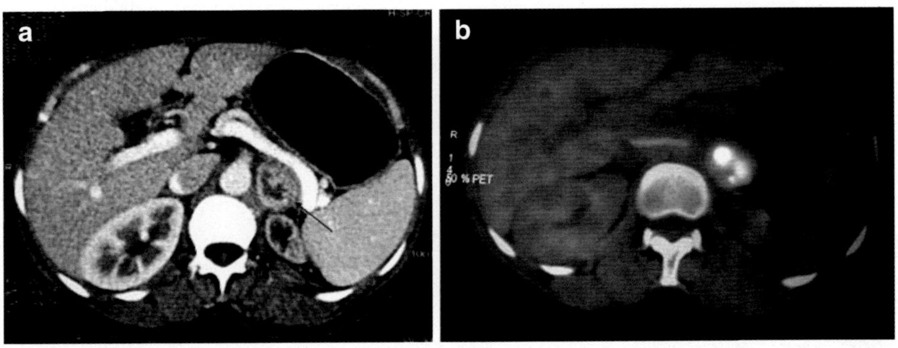

Fig. 7.2 (**a**) CECT abdomen showing heterogeneous lesion in the left adrenal gland in a patient with pheochromocytoma. (**b**) FDG PET–CT fusion image of the same patient showing FDG avidity of the left adrenal mass

7. **What is paraganglioma?**

Paragangliomas are extra-adrenal tumors arising from glomus cells or chromaffin tissue present in paraganglia, a tissue located in the vicinity of ganglia. Head and neck regions have parasympathetic paraganglia and consist of glomus cells, while chest, abdomen, and pelvis have sympathetic paraganglia and comprises of chromaffin tissue. Both glomus cell and chromaffin tissue are derivatives of neural crest cells. Head and neck paragangliomas arising from glomus cells of parasympathetic paraganglia are usually nonfunctional and include glomus caroticum, glomus jugulare, glomus tympanicum, and glomus vagale. Paragangliomas arising from chromaffin tissue of sympathetic paraganglia present in the chest, abdomen, and pelvis are usually functional (catecholamine secreting).

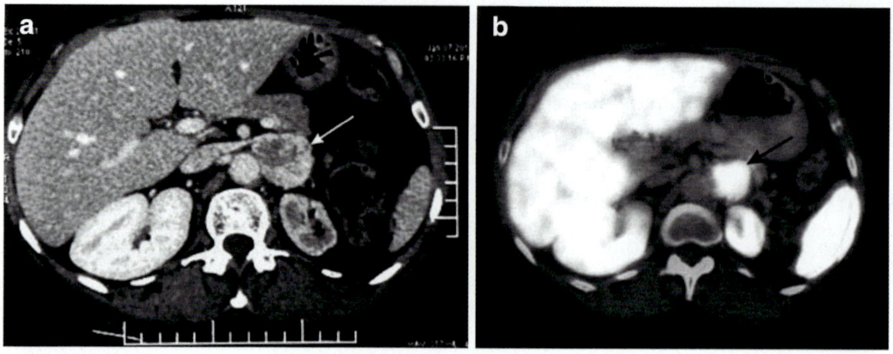

Fig. 7.3 (**a**) CECT abdomen showing heterogeneously enhancing left para-aortic mass suggestive of paraganglioma. (**b**) FDG PET–CT fusion image of the same patient showing increased FDG uptake in the mass

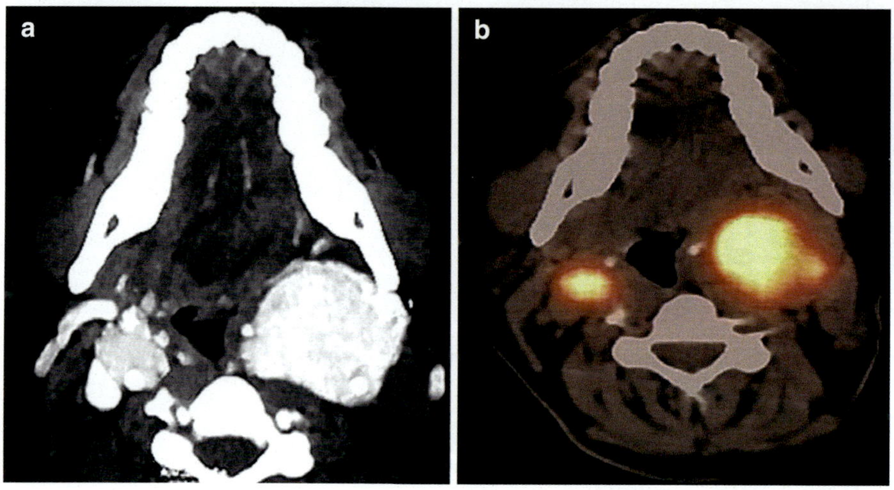

Fig. 7.4 (**a**) Cervical CECT axial section demonstrating heterogeneously enhancing bilateral neck masses at carotid bifurcation suggestive of cervical paraganglioma. (**b**) FDG–PET scan of the same patient showing FDG avidity of the cervical lesions

8. **What is the difference between "pheochromocytoma" and"paraganglioma"?**

   The table given below enlists the differences between pheochromocytoma and paraganglioma.

Characters	Pheochromocytoma	Sympathetic paraganglioma	Parasympathetic paraganglioma
Functionality	Usually functional	Usually functional	Rarely functional (<1%)
Location	Adrenal medulla	Mediastinum, abdomen, and pelvis	Head and neck
Inheritance	Commonly sporadic	Commonly familial	Commonly familial
Malignant potential	Low	High	High

9. **How does adrenal cortex and medulla interact with each other?**

   Conversion of norepinephrine to epinephrine in adrenal medulla is mediated by the enzyme phenylethanolamine N-methyltransferase (PNMT), which is induced by cortisol secreted from the adrenal cortex. The clinical implication of this fact is that all epinephrine-secreting tumors arise from the adrenal medulla, whereas all functioning paragangliomas secrete only norepinephrine, as they lack PNMT and its paracrine induction by cortisol.

10. **What is pseudopheochromocytoma?**

    Pseudopheochromocytoma is an entity characterized by a documented episode of hypertension and paroxysm but without any evidence of catecholamine-secreting tumors. The causes are panic disorders, hyperthyroidism, renovascular hypertension, tyrosine ingestion with monoamine oxidase inhibitors, perimenopausal syndrome, and rarely use of cocaine and lysergic acid diethylamide. Presence of emotional component or an inciting event, short duration of spell, variability in clinical manifestations, and presence of flushing favor a diagnosis of pseudopheochromocytoma.

11. **Why is it important to diagnose pheochromocytoma/paraganglioma?**

    It is important to diagnose pheochromocytoma/paraganglioma (PPGL) as it is a curable cause of hypertension, has malignant potential, lethal if not treated, and has strong familial predisposition. In addition, the patient may need further evaluation to detect coexisting endocrine neoplasia as a part of familial syndromes.

12. **Does the "rule of 10" still apply?**

    The "rule of 10" for catecholamine-secreting tumors is that 10% are extra-adrenal, 10% occur in children, 10% are familial, 10% are multiple or bilateral, 10% recur after surgical removal, 10% are malignant, and 10% are detected as adrenal incidentalomas. Although not accurate, it is still a good rule of thumb in routine clinical practice.

13. **What is the classical triad of pheochromocytoma/paraganglioma?**

    The classical triad of PPGL includes paroxysms of headache (usually pounding), tachycardia, and sweating. Paroxysm is stereotypical in a given patient and usually lasts for 15–20 min. Headache is present in 90%, sweating and tachycardia in 60–70%, and all three in only 30% of patients. The specificity of this triad is around 90%.

14. **Why do paroxysms occur in pheochromocytoma/paraganglioma?**

    Paroxysms occur in PPGL due to episodic release of catecholamines, variability in intra-tumoral metabolism of catecholamines, inconsistency in the binding of catecholamines with albumin in circulation, and rarely tumor infarction. In addition, precipitating factors like medications (e.g., metoclopramide, phenothiazines, methyldopa, tricyclic antidepressants, or glucocorticoids), postural changes, anxiety, and exercise may induce a paroxysm in these patients.

15. **What is the most common sign in pheochromocytoma/paraganglioma?**

    Hypertension is the most common sign in PPGL and is present in 90% of patients. Hypertension may be paroxysmal in 25–50% of patients, while the rest have sustained hypertension, and some may present with accelerated hypertension. Orthostatic hypotension is present in 50–75% of patients and is due to intense vasoconstriction leading to chronic volume depletion and impaired baroreceptor reflexes.

16. **Can hypotension be a presenting manifestation of PPGL?**

    Yes. Although hypertension is present in 90% of patients with PPGL, the presence of hypotension does not exclude the diagnosis. The causes of hypotension in these patients include tumors which secrete dopamine/epinephrine/adrenomedullin, severe volume depletion, catecholamine cardiomyopathy, ventricular arrhythmias, and tumor necrosis/ hemorrhage.

17. **What are unusual presentations of PPGL?**

    The unusual presentations of pheochromocytoma are catecholamine cardiomyopathy, hypotension, sinus bradycardia, micturition syncope, status epilepticus, lateral medullary syndrome, bad obstetric history, livedo reticularis, Raynaud's phenomenon, diabetic ketoacidosis, pancreatitis, and sudden death. Rarely, hypoglycemia can occur in a patient with pheochromocytoma due to catecholamine receptor downregulation, co-secretion of IGF2, and after curative surgery. The figure depicted below shows bladder paraganglioma in a patient who presented with classical paroxysm during micturition.

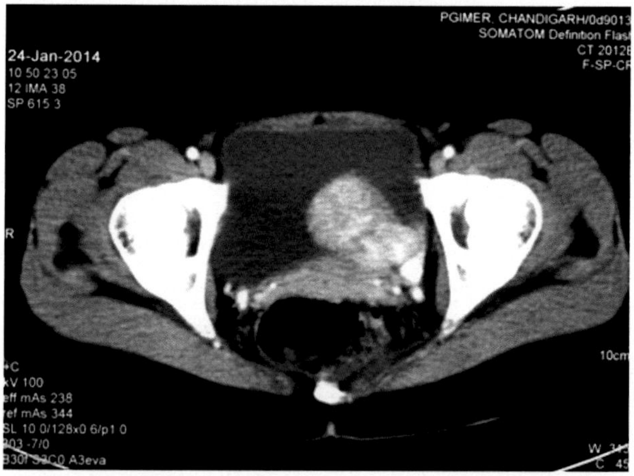

Fig. 7.5 CECT pelvis axial section showing heterogeneously hyperenhancing lesion arising from the posterior wall of urinary bladder on the left side in a patient who presented with classical paroxysms during micturition, suggestive of bladder paraganglioma

18. **What are the endocrine manifestations of PPGL?**

The endocrine manifestations of PPGL are due to co-secretion of other peptide hormones as these tumors are neuroendocrine in origin. The endocrine manifestations include Cushing's syndrome (ectopic ACTH production), SIADH (ADH), acromegaly (GHRH), hypoglycemia (IGF2), and hypercalcemia (PTHrP). In addition, patients may have mild hyperglycemia due to insulin resistance and impaired insulin secretion induced by catecholamines.

19. **What are the causes of dysglycemia in PPGL?**

Dysglycemia occurs in 50% of patients with PPGL. It is more commonly seen with epinephrine-secreting tumors than norepinephrine-secreting tumors due to high affinity of epinephrine to β_2-adrenergic receptors as compared to norepinephrine. Hyperglycemia is due to increased hepatic glucose output (increased glycogenolysis and gluconeogenesis) and decreased skeletal muscle and adipose tissue glucose uptake. This effect of catecholamines is mediated via β_2-adrenergic receptors. In addition, impaired insulin secretion mediated via α_2-adrenergic receptors also contributes to hyperglycemia.

20. **What are the causes of familial PPGL?**

The causes of familial PPGL are multiple endocrine neoplasia (MEN2A and 2B and rarely MEN1), von Hippel–Lindau disease, neurofibromatosis type 1, familial paraganglioma syndromes, ataxia telangiectasia, tuberous sclerosis, and Sturge–Weber syndrome. In addition, TMEM127 or MAX mutations are also associated with familial pheochromocytoma/paraganglioma.

21. **What are the causes of bilateral pheochromocytoma?**

The causes of bilateral pheochromocytoma are MEN2A and 2B, von Hippel–Lindau disease, and familial paraganglioma syndrome like SDHB and SDHD mutations. However, some familial syndromes are not associated with bilateral pheochromocytoma, e.g., NF1-related pheochromocytoma, which is usually unilateral. Bilateral pheochromocytomas may be metachronous (one after another) or synchronous in origin.

22. **What is the hormone secretory pattern of pheochromocytomas and paraganglioma?**

Catecholamine-secreting tumors originating from the adrenal gland can secrete epinephrine as well as norepinephrine, while functional paragangliomas can only secrete norepinephrine. The enzyme PNMT required for the conversion of norepinephrine to epinephrine is induced by high intra-adrenal cortisol concentration, which is lacking in paragangliomas. Therefore, paragangliomas do not produce epinephrine.

Etiology	Norepinephrine	Epinephrine	Dopamine
Sporadic pheochromocytoma	+++	++	±
Paraganglioma	+++	–	±
MEN-related pheochromocytoma	+	+++	±
VHL-related pheochromocytoma	+++	+	±
Malignant pheochromocytoma/ paraganglioma	+++	+	++

23. **What are the characteristic features of pheochromocytoma associated with multiple endocrine neoplasia type 2?**

MEN2-related pheochromocytomas are always adrenal, predominantly secrete epinephrine due to overexpression of PNMT and increased tyrosine hydroxylase activity, and are almost never malignant. Multiple endocrine neoplasia type 2 is an autosomal dominant disorder with gain-of-function mutation in RET proto-oncogene. The differences between the two subtypes of MEN2 are enlisted in the table given below.

Parameters	MEN2A	MEN2B
Gene defect	RET proto-oncogene in extracellular component	RET proto-oncogene in intracellular component
Medullary thyroid carcinoma	Virtually all	Virtually all
Pheochromocytoma	50%	50%
PHPT	20–30%	None
Mucosal neuromas	Absent	Present (98%)
Cutaneous lichen amyloidosis	5%	Absent
Intestinal ganglioneuromas	Absent	Present
Marfanoid habitus	Absent	Present

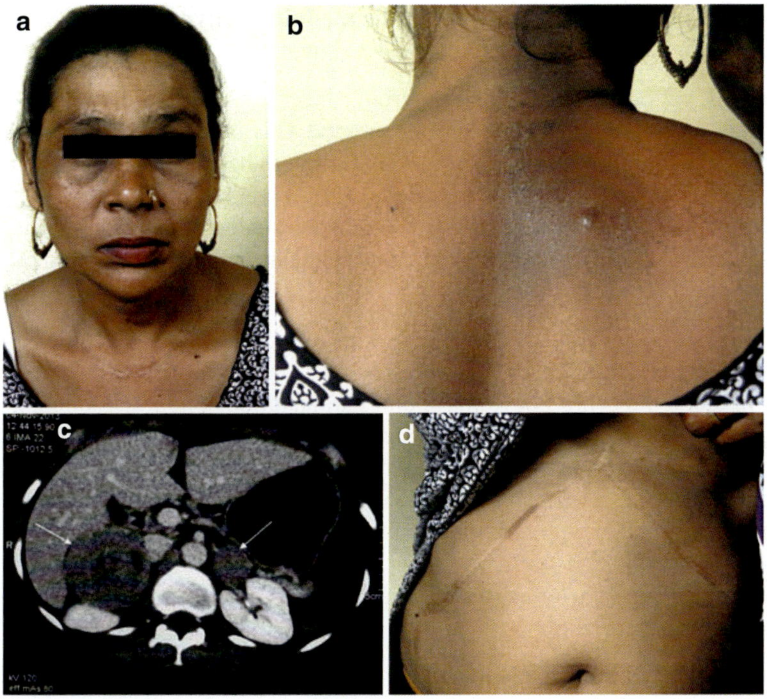

Fig. 7.6 (**a**) Post-thyroidectomy scar in a patient with MEN2A syndrome. She was operated for medullary thyroid carcinoma. (**b**) Cutaneous lichen amyloidosis in the same patient. (**c**) CECT abdomen of the same patient showing bilateral asymmetrical adrenal masses (with areas of necrosis in the right side) suggestive of familial pheochromocytoma. (**d**) Scar after bilateral adrenalectomy in the same patient

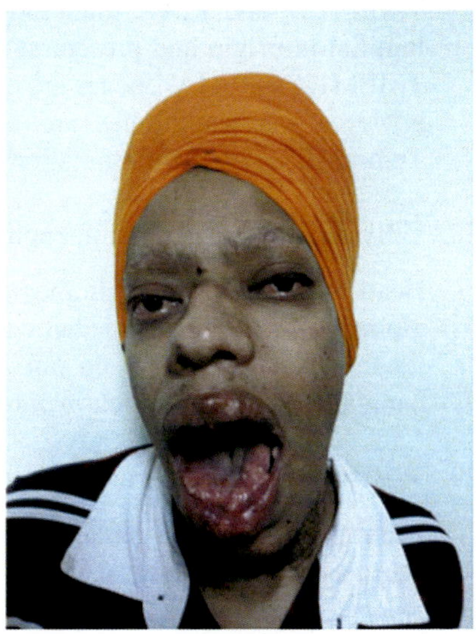

Fig. 7.7 Classical mucosal neuromas in a patient with MEN2B syndrome

24. **Do patients with apparently sporadic medullary thyroid cancer need evaluation for pheochromocytoma prior to surgery?**

    Yes. All patients with medullary thyroid cancer (MTC) should be evaluated for pheochromocytoma prior to thyroid surgery. This is because 6–8% of patients even with apparently sporadic MTC may harbor pheochromocytoma. Furthermore, absence of hypertension does not preclude the probability of concurrent pheochromocytoma as MEN2-associated adrenal medullary tumor preferentially secretes epinephrine, and these patients may only have palpitations.

25. **What is von Hippel–Lindau disease?**

    Von Hippel–Lindau disease is an autosomal dominant disorder characterized by bilateral pheochromocytoma and/or paraganglioma, nonfunctioning pancreatic islet cell tumor, hemangioblastomas of cerebellum, brainstem or spinal cord, retinal angiomas, and clear cell renal cell carcinoma. VHL gene expressed on chromosome 3 regulates hypoxia-inducible factor 1, and inactivation of this gene is associated with tumorigenesis.

26. **Why does pheochromocytoma associated with VHL predominantly produce norepinephrine?**

    Adrenal pheochromocytomas can secrete epinephrine as well as norepinephrine. However, patients with VHL having bilateral pheochromocytomas predominantly produce norepinephrine due to the under-expression of the enzyme PNMT.

27. **What are the characteristics of TMEM127 and MAX mutation-associated PPGL?**

    TMEM127 and MAX mutation-related catecholamine-secreting tumors are familial in origin and present at a later age (40–50 years). Mutations in both TMEM127 and MAX genes are associated with unilateral pheochromocytoma; however, paragangliomas are also described with MAX gene mutations. Tumors associated with mutation of these genes have low malignant potential.

28. **Why are head and neck paragangliomas nonfunctional?**

    Head and neck paragangliomas are usually nonfunctional as they arise from glomus cells of parasympathetic paraganglia. These paraganglia lack chromaffin tissue and therefore do not produce catecholamines, unlike sympathetic paraganglia which are rich in chromaffin cells.

29. **What are familial paraganglioma syndromes?**

    Patients with familial paraganglioma syndromes usually present in the fourth decade, have multicentric disease, and have tumors with high malignant potential.

Disease	Gene	Location	Remarks
Familial paraganglioma type 1	SDHD	Skull base and neck, occasionally adrenal medulla	Most common Usually parasympathetic Strong family history
Familial paraganglioma type 2	SDHAF2	Skull base and neck	Rare
Familial paraganglioma type 3	SDHC	Skull base and neck	Rare
Familial paraganglioma type 4	SDHB	Abdomen, pelvis, mediastinum, and occasionally adrenal medulla	High malignant potential Renal cell carcinoma, papillary thyroid carcinoma, pituitary adenoma

30. **What is succinate dehydrogenase, and how is it involved in tumorigenesis?**

Succinate dehydrogenase (SDH) is a mitochondrial enzyme which is involved in electron transport and oxidizes succinate to fumarate in tricarboxylic acid cycle; therefore, activity of this enzyme is essential for oxidative phosphorylation. The mutations in SDH gene result in accumulation of succinate which induces prolyl hydroxylase to produce hypoxia-inducible factor 1α (HIF1α), which promotes angiogenesis and extracellular matrix proliferation resulting in tumorigenesis.

31. **When to suspect familial pheochromocytoma/paraganglioma?**

Young age of onset of pheochromocytoma (<30 years), all cases of paraganglioma, bilateral adrenal pheochromocytoma, family history of pheochromocytoma, and presence of concurrent neoplasia like medullary thyroid cancer, pancreatic neuroendocrine tumor, parathyroid adenoma, or pituitary adenoma should raise the suspicion of familial pheochromocytoma/paraganglioma. These individuals require genetic analysis for further confirmation.

Phenotype	Mutation to be analyzed in sequence
Unilateral pheochromocytoma with age <30 years	VHL, RET, SDHB, SDHD
Bilateral pheochromocytoma	RET, VHL
Head/neck paraganglioma	SDHD, SDHC, SDHAF2
Abdominal paraganglioma	SDHB, SDHD, VHL, SDHC

32. **What does estimation of fractionated metanephrines signify?**

Catecholamines are metabolized within the tumoral cells to intermediate metabolites (epinephrine to metanephrine and norepinephrine to normetanephrine). Measurement of fractionated metanephrine denotes estimation of metanephrine and normetanephrines separately, either in plasma or in urine.

33. **What does estimation of fractionated plasma free metanephrines signify?**

Metanephrines and normetanephrines are present in circulation in free as well as in bound form (sulfate conjugates). Measurement of fractionated plasma-free metanephrines denotes estimation of free form of these metabolites separately in plasma.

34. **What does estimation of 24 h urine fractionated metanephrine signify?**

Metanephrines and normetanephrines are excreted only in conjugated form in urine. Therefore, measurements of 24 h urine fractionated metanephrines denote estimation of total (i.e., conjugated) metanephrine and normetanephrine separately.

35. **What are the biochemical tests that help in the diagnosis of PPGL?**

The measurement of either urine or plasma metanephrine and normetanephrine is preferred for the diagnosis of PPGL as intra-tumoral catecholamine metabolism is continuous and metanephrine and normetanephrine are intermediate products of catecholamine metabolism. A level >3 times the upper limit of normal is considered diagnostic. The available biochemical tests with sensitivity and specificity are listed in the table given below.

Tests	Sensitivity (%)	Specificity (%)
Plasma free metanephrine and normetanephrine	96–100	85–89
Plasma epinephrine and norepinephrine	84	81
24 h urinary metanephrine and normetanephrine	98	98
24 h urinary epinephrine and norepinephrine	86	88
24 h urinary VMA	66	94

Liquid chromatography with tandem mass spectrophotometry (LC–MS/MS) and liquid chromatography with electrochemical detection (LC–ECD) are the preferred methods for estimation of metanephrine and normetanephrines.

36. **How to collect sample for estimation of plasma metanephrines and normetanephrines?**

Sample for plasma metanephrines and normetanephrines should be taken in supine position, after being recumbent for 30 min. This is done as upright posture results in activation of sympathetic nervous system, thereby resulting in increased release, metabolism, and clearance of catecholamines. Sampling in upright position has been shown to increase the incidence of false-positive results by 2.8-fold. Further, if the sample is taken in supine position and interpreted with the reference range derived from blood samples drawn in seated position, there is a threefold increase in false-negative results.

37. **What are the medications to be discontinued prior to biochemical evaluation of PPGL?**

Tricyclic antidepressants, selective serotonin reuptake inhibitor (e.g., fluoxetine), decongestants, paracetamol, β-blockers and nonselective α-blockers (phenoxybenzamine), α-methyldopa, and labetalol should be discontinued 2 weeks prior to metanephrine or normetanephrine estimation. The antihypertensives that can be continued are calcium channel blockers, ACE inhibitors, ARBs, selective α-1 blockers, and diuretics. Discontinuation of clonidine should be avoided as it may lead to falsely elevated metanephrine.

38. **How to localize the source of catecholamine excess?**

Both anatomical and functional scans are used to localize the source of catecholamine excess. The anatomic imaging modalities include CT and MRI, while functional scans are ^{123}I-MIBG and ^{18}F-FDG–PET. Majority of catecholamine-secreting tumors are intra-abdominal in location; therefore, CECT abdomen and pelvis is the first imaging modality to be performed after biochemical confirmation. MRI abdomen has no additional advantage over CT in the localization of adrenal pheochromocytoma, but may be superior in localizing intra-abdominal paragangliomas. MRI is preferred for head and neck paragangliomas and for metastatic disease, whereas CT is preferred for thoracic paraganglioma. The sensitivity and specificity of different imaging modalities to localize the source of catecholamine excess are enlisted in the table given below.

Imaging modality	**Sensitivity (%)**	**Specificity (%)**
Ultrasonography	83–89	60
CT	98	92
MRI	93–100	50
^{123}I-MIBG	77–90	95–100
^{18}F-FDG–PET	89	96

39. **What are the indications for functional imaging in patients with pheochromocytoma/paraganglioma?**

The indications for ^{123}I-MIBG include adrenal pheochromocytoma >5 cm, all paragangliomas irrespective of size, multicentric disease, and recurrent disease. In addition, it is indicated in patients with metastatic disease when therapy with ^{131}I-MIBG is planned. The sensitivity and specificity of ^{123}I-MIBG for various indications are summarized in the table given below. ^{18}F-FDG–PET is the preferred functional imaging in those with metastatic disease with a sensitivity of 88%.

Parameters	Sensitivity (%)	Specificity (%)
Pheochromocytoma	85–88	70–100
Paraganglioma	56–75	84–100
Metastatic disease	56–83	–
Recurrent disease	75	–

40. **How does imaging help to differentiate between adrenocortical tumor and pheochromocytoma?**

Pheochromocytoma can be differentiated from adrenocortical adenoma on CT by size (>3 cm), texture (heterogeneity with cystic areas), high attenuation on NCCT (>25 HU), delayed washout of contrast (<50% at 10 min), and increased vascularity. The presence of markedly hyperintense lesion in relation to the liver on T2-weighted MR images favors pheochromocytoma. However, there are no definite pointers to differentiate between adrenocortical carcinoma and pheochromocytoma on CT; the presence of heterogeneous cystic lesion on CT favors a diagnosis of pheochromocytoma, while heterogeneity with mixed densities suggests adrenocortical carcinoma. Further, chemical-shift MR imaging helps in differentiating between benign and malignant adrenocortical tumors, taking the advantage of the higher lipid content of adrenocortical adenoma, but it does not differentiate between pheochromocytoma and adrenocortical carcinoma.

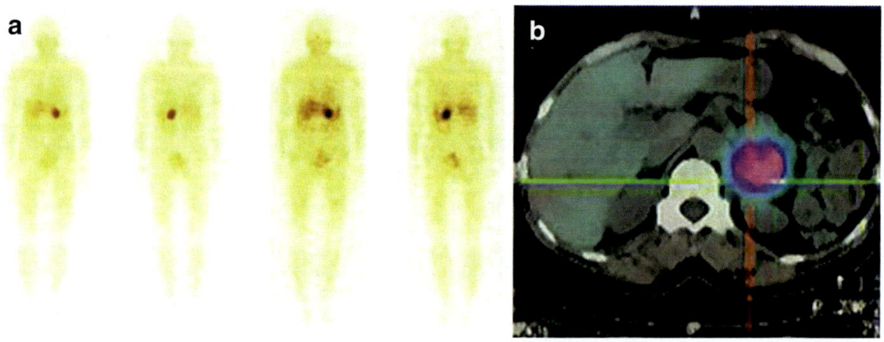

Fig. 7.8 (**a**) ^{131}I MIBG scintigraphy showing increased tracer uptake in the left upper quadrant of the abdomen. (**b**) SPECT/CT fusion image localized the mass to the left suprarenal region

41. **A 30-year-old female presented with hypertension and paroxysms. On evaluation she had elevated plasma free metanephrine and normetanephrine. CECT abdomen did not reveal any abnormalities. How to proceed further?**

The clinical probability of catecholamine-secreting tumor in the index case is very high as she is symptomatic and has elevated metanephrine and normetanephrine. The CECT abdomen has a sensitivity of 95–98% to localize the lesion. Failure to localize the lesion on CECT abdomen demands further investigation, and ^{123}I-MIBG scan may be the preferred choice as it has a sensitivity of 80–90%. If ^{123}I-MIBG fails to localize the source of catecholamine excess, ^{18}F-FDG–PET or ^{18}F-FDOPA-PET may be employed.

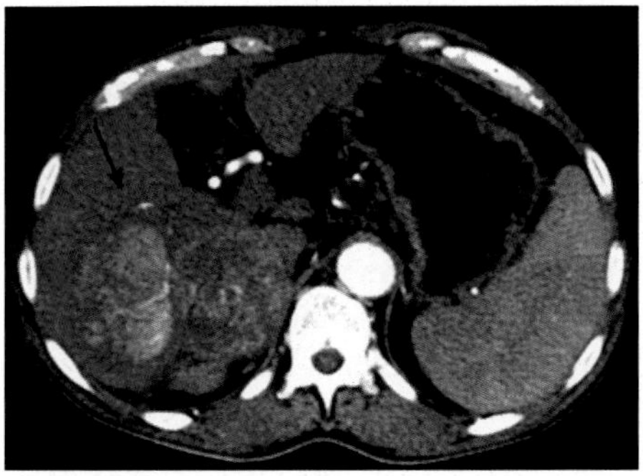

Fig. 7.9 CECT abdomen showing large heterogeneously enhancing mass in right subhepatic location suggestive of adrenocortical carcinoma

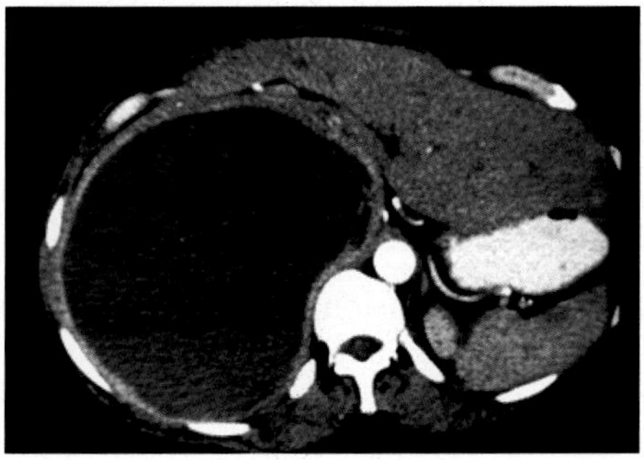

Fig. 7.10 CECT abdomen showing large cystic suprarenal mass with peripheral enhancement suggestive of pheochromocytoma

42. **What are the causes of false-negative ^{123}I-MIBG?**

    ^{123}I- metaiodobenzylguanidine is an analogue of norepinephrine and is actively taken up by the vesicular monoamine transporter. It has high specificity but low sensitivity. The causes of false-negative ^{123}I-MIBG scan are metastatic pheochromocytoma, paraganglioma (especially SDHB related), and necrotic tumors. This may be because of the lack of vesicular monoamine transporter either due to dedifferentiated cells (malignant) or nonfunctional cells (paraganglioma). In addition, drugs like calcium channel blockers, labetalol, tricyclic antidepressants, and sympathomimetics (e.g., decongestants) interfere with ^{123}I-MIBG uptake and may cause false-negative scan. Therefore, these drugs should be stopped at least 2 weeks prior to scan.

43. **What is the preoperative management of pheochromocytoma/paraganglioma?**

Preoperative management should focus on the control of blood pressure and appropriate volume expansion. Patients who are normotensive should also be administered α-blockers to prevent hypertensive crisis during surgery. Nonselective α-blocker, phenoxybenzamine, or selective α-1 blocker, prazosin, are used for preoperative α-blockade. Adequate α-blockade is suggested by nasal stuffiness, appearance/worsening of orthostatic hypotension, and tachycardia. After achieving adequate α-blockade, salt ad lib (>5 g/day) and β-blockers should be added to counteract the orthostatic hypotension and tachycardia induced by α-blockade, respectively. β-blockers should be used only after adequate α-blockade is achieved, as it might precipitate hypertensive crisis due to unopposed α-adrenergic action resulting in vasoconstriction. Effective β-blockade is considered when heart rate is 60–70 per minute (sitting) and 70–80 per minute (standing). Patients should receive α-blockade for at least 7 days prior to surgery to minimize hypertensive surges intraoperatively and to allow intravascular volume repletion with salt ad lib and fluid. Calcium channel blockers may be required if blood pressure is not controlled despite the use of α-and β-blockers. Target blood pressure of <130/80 mmHg (seated) and systolic blood pressure >90 mmHg on standing should be achieved prior to surgery. Labetalol should be avoided as it has more potent β-blocking activity than α-blocking activity (β: $\alpha = 5{:}1$).

44. **What are the disorders where salt ad lib is promoted despite the presence of hypertension?**

Despite the presence of hypertension, salt ad lib is advocated in patients with pheochromocytoma and primary aldosteronism. In patients with pheochromocytoma salt ad lib diet is required to replete the intravascular volume. Salt ad lib is also indicated in patients with primary aldosteronism to improve the sensitivity of the screening test (plasma aldosterone/plasma renin concentration), and it unmasks hypokalemia as well.

45. **What are the preferred anesthetic agents in PPGL?**

Propofol, etomidate, or barbiturates in combination with synthetic opioids are preferred. But preoperative use of atropine and anesthetics like fentanyl, ketamine, morphine, halothane, and desflurane should be avoided as they may precipitate hypertensive crisis in patients with PPGL.

46. **What is the treatment for pheochromocytoma?**

Surgical treatment is the preferred modality in patients with pheochromocytoma after adequate α and β blockade. Laparoscopic adrenalectomy is the treatment of choice for pheochromocytoma <6 cm; otherwise, open adrenalectomy is advocated. Cortical-sparing adrenalectomy is advised especially in case of bilateral pheochromocytoma. Intraoperative hypertension can be successfully treated with nitroprusside infusion and arrhythmias with short-acting β-blocker like esmolol or with lignocaine.

47. **How to monitor a patient of pheochromocytoma postoperatively?**

Pulse rate, blood pressure, and blood glucose should be monitored in the immediate postoperative period. Postoperative hypotension should be managed with fluids, whereas hypertension with diuretics. After curative surgery, there is a risk of hypoglycemia, because of sudden increase in insulin secretion. Biochemical testing for urine or plasma metanephrine and normetanephrine should be done after 2–4 weeks of surgery. If cured, then annual biochemical testing is recommended. In case of non-catecholamine-secreting tumors, not only biochemical monitoring but imaging is also advised.

48. **What are the causes of persistent hypertension despite curative surgery of pheochromocytoma?**

Hypertension resolves within a week in majority of patients after curative surgery; however, in few patients normalization of blood pressure may take a longer time. Persistent hypertension despite curative surgery may be due to resetting of baroreceptor tone, irreversible vascular alteration or structural changes in the kidney as a result of prolonged exposure to elevated levels of catecholamines. In addition, inadvertent ligation of renal artery or coexisting essential hypertension also results in persistent hypertension.

Suggested Reading

1. Jameson JL, De Groot LJ. Endocrinology: adult and pediatric. Philadelphia: Elsevier Health Sciences; 2010.
2. Longo D, Anthony F, Dennis K, Stephen H, Jameson J, Joseph L. Harrison's Principles of Internal Medicine 18E EB. New York: McGraw Hill Professional; 2012.
3. Melmed S, Polonsky KS, Reed Larsen P, Kronenberg HM. Williams textbook of endocrinology: Expert consult. London: Elsevier Health Sciences; 2011.

8 Disorders of Mineralocorticoid Excess

8.1 Case Vignette

A 24-year-old lady was incidentally diagnosed to have hypertension (BP 160/110 mmHg) 3 years back during a hospital visit for neck pain. She was started on amlodipine 10 mg and losartan 100 mg per day. In view of young-onset hypertension and uncontrolled BP despite medications, she was referred for endocrinology opinion. There was no history of paroxysms or periodic paralysis. Her family history was non-contributory. On evaluation, her body mass index was 22.4 kg/m^2, pulse rate 88/min, supine BP 152/90 mmHg, and standing BP 140/90 mmHg. She did not have any stigma of Cushing's syndrome or acromegaly. Investigations revealed hypokalemia with serum potassium ranging from 3.3 to 3.5 mEq/L on multiple occasions. Her serum creatinine was 0.9 mg/dl, fasting plasma glucose 110 mg/dl, and HbA1c 6.2%. Renal Doppler did not reveal renal artery stenosis. Diagnosis of primary aldosteronism was considered and antihypertensives were changed to prazosin and verapamil along with potassium supplementation. After 2 weeks, she was advised salt ad lib for 5 days, and with normalization of serum potassium, samples for plasma aldosterone concentration (PAC) and plasma rennin activity (PRA) were taken. The PAC was 57.5 ng/dl and PRA 0.04 ng/ml/h with a PAC/PRA ratio of 1,438 ng/dl/ng/ml/h. Subsequently, saline suppression test was performed and PAC at 0 min was 24.3 ng/dl and at 4 h 34.2 ng/dl. After biochemical confirmation of primary hyperaldosteronism, CECT abdomen was done which revealed hypodense nodular lesions in both adrenal glands, likely bilateral adrenal adenomas. Right-sided lesion (10 × 8 mm) was arising from the limb, with a washout of 70%, while the left one (14 × 10 mm) was arising from the body of adrenal gland with a washout of 60%. Other hormone profiles were as follows: serum cortisol 0800h 287 nmol/L (171–536), 0800h ACTH 10.3 pg/ml (5–60), T4 8.39 μg/dl (4.8–12.7), TSH 4.03 μIU/ml(0.27–4.2), TPO 21.3 IU/ml (<24), overnight dexamethasone suppression test 38 nmol/L, and 24-h urinary metanephrines and normetanephrines were normal. She did not have hypertensive retinopathy and 24-h urinary protein was within normal range. Echocardiography revealed regional wall motion abnormality in the right coronary artery territory, concentric left

A. Bhansali, Y. Gogate, *Clinical Rounds in Endocrinology: Volume I - Adult Endocrinology*, DOI 10.1007/978-81-322-2398-6_8

ventricular hypertrophy, and ejection fraction 45 to 50%. To lateralize the source for aldosterone excess, adrenal vein sampling was performed. After continuous ACTH infusion (50 μg/h) for 30 min, both adrenal veins were simultaneously catheterized. Samples were taken from both the adrenal veins for cortisol and aldosterone, with simultaneous sampling for cortisol from femoral vein at baseline (immediately after catheterization) and at 30 min. The source of aldosterone excess was lateralized to the left adrenal gland. Detailed results of the procedure are tabulated below. After investigations, she was started on spironolactone 100 mg per day and amlodipine 5 mg per day; verapamil and prazosin were withdrawn. She was subjected to laparoscopic resection of left adrenal gland and histopathology was consistent with aldosteronoma. PAC and PRA done on the second postoperative day showed PAC of 2 ng/dl and PRA of 0.04 ng/ml/h and blood pressure 130/80 mmHg without any antihypertensive drugs. She developed hyperkalemia on the third postoperative day and was advised salt ad lib, following which serum potassium normalized within 2 weeks. After 6 months of surgery, she continues to remain normotensive without any antihypertensive drugs.

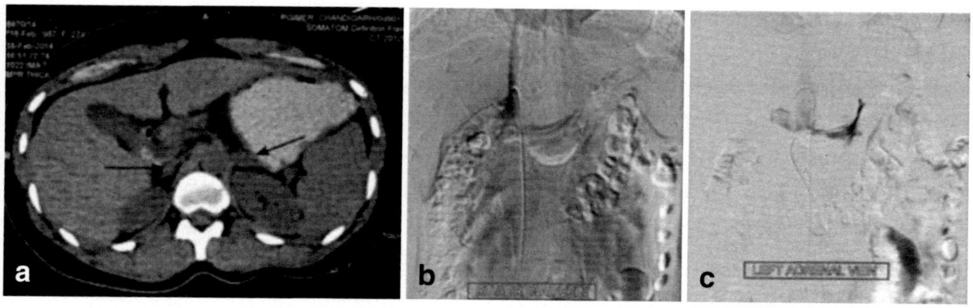

Fig. 8.1 (**a**) CECT abdomen showing bilateral adrenal masses (right 10×8 mm and left 14×10 mm) in a patient with hypertension and hypokalemia. (**b**, **c**) DSA images showing catheters in right (**b**) and left adrenal (**c**) veins during adrenal vein sampling

8.1.1 Adrenal Vein Sampling Profile

Time	**Cortisol (nmol/L)**				**Aldosterone (ng/dl)**	
	Right adrenal vein	Left adrenal vein	Femoral vein	**Cortisol: adrenal to periphery ratio**	Right adrenal vein	Left adrenal vein
0 min	38,320	8,944	789.6	Right—48.5 Left—11.3	414.7	12012.8
30 min	19,910	14,330	848	Right—23.4 Left—16.8	350.1	11528.7

Time	**Aldosterone : cortisol (A: C) ratios**		**Aldosterone ratio**[a]
	Right adrenal vein	**Left adrenal vein**	134
0 min	0.01	1.34	
30 min	0.02	0.8	40

[a]Left adrenal vein A: C ratio/right adrenal vein A: C ratio

8.2 Stepwise Analysis

Young age, severe hypertension (BP >160/100 mmHg), and hypokalemia are the clinical clues to suggest the presence of secondary hypertension in the index patient. Approximately 15% patients have secondary hypertension with an "identifiable" cause, and there is a possibility of cure after definitive therapy. Causes of secondary hypertension include renal (renal parenchymal or renovascular disease), vascular (coarctation of aorta), and endocrine disorders. The presence of hypokalemia along with hypertension narrows down the differential diagnosis to disorders associated with mineralocorticoid/cortisol excess. The index patient did not have any stigmata of Cushing's syndrome. Therefore, the diagnosis was further confined to disorders of mineralocorticoid excess. Spontaneous hypokalemia in a patient with hypertension strongly favors primary aldosteronism; however, diuretic-induced hypokalemia or presence of normokalemia does not preclude the diagnosis of mineralocorticoid excess. Hypokalemia can manifest as polyuria, periodic paralysis, metabolic alkalosis, or glucose intolerance; none of these were present in our patient except glucose intolerance. Presence of target organ damage (coronary artery disease) at young age and short duration of hypertension in the index case further suggest the diagnosis of aldosterone excess. For biochemical diagnosis, appropriate precautions should be taken before sampling for PAC and PRA. These include avoidance of antihypertensive drugs which interfere with renin–angiotensin–aldosterone system (RAAS), normalization of serum potassium, and salt ad lib. The index patient was on losartan which was stopped for 2 weeks prior to sampling for PAC/PRA. The preferred antihypertensive drugs in this scenario are prazosin and verapamil. Attainment of eukalemia is required to improve the sensitivity of screening test as hypokalemia suppresses aldosterone secretion. Salt ad lib for 3–5 days is recommended to maximally suppress RAAS, thereby improving the sensitivity. PAC >15 ng/dl is suggestive of aldosterone excess, but estimation of PRA along with PAC is essential to differentiate between primary and secondary hyperaldosteronism. PRA <1 ng/ml/h indicates suppressed renin activity and is classical of primary aldosteronism. A PAC/PRA ratio >20 ng/dl/ng/ml/h with a PAC >15 ng/dl has a sensitivity of 90%, while a ratio of >30 ng/dl/ng/ml/h with PAC >20 ng/dl has a sensitivity of 90% and specificity of 91% in diagnosing aldosteronoma. Our patient had a PAC of 57.5 ng/dl and a PRA of 0.04 ng/ml/h with a PAC/PRA ratio of 1,438 ng/dl/ng/ml/h, suggestive of primary aldosteronism. The diagnosis of primary aldosteronism was confirmed by saline suppression test which showed non-suppressibility of PAC (>10 ng/dl). Age<50 years, severe hypertension, spontaneous hypokalemia, and serum aldosterone >25 ng/dl in the index patient predict the likelihood of aldosterone-producing adenoma. However, CECT abdomen revealed bilateral adrenal masses which raised various possibilities: a) unilateral aldosterone-producing adenoma and contralateral nonfunctioning adenoma, b) idiopathic bilateral adrenal hyperplasia, and rarely c) bilateral aldosterone-producing adenoma. To resolve this dilemma, she was subjected to adrenal vein sampling (AVS). ACTH infusion was administered before and during the procedure to minimize the stress-induced fluctuation in aldosterone secretion and to maximize the aldosterone secretion from APA. Simultaneous sampling of cortisol from the respective adrenal and femoral vein was performed and an adrenal vein to femoral vein cortisol ratio >10:1 was suggestive of successful catheterization. Aldosterone : cortisol corrected ratio is preferred over plasma aldosterone levels, to minimize the dilutional effect during sampling, as catheter tip on left side is placed distal to the confluence of left inferior phrenic vein and left adrenal vein. Left adrenal vein AC ratio : right adrenal vein AC ratio of 134 at 0 min and 40 at 30 min (>4:1) lateralized the source of aldosterone excess to the left adrenal gland in the index patient. The sensitivity and specificity of AVS is 95% and 100%, respectively, for the lateralization of aldosteronoma. In the index patient, the baseline cortisol of 8,944 nmol/L in the left adrenal vein as opposed to 38,320 nmol/L in the right adrenal vein was possibly due to inadvertent displacement of catheter tip from the left adrenal vein during sampling for cortisol. However, after repositioning the catheter, the cortisol levels were comparable in both the adrenal veins. After complete evaluation, she was initiated on spironolactone to control blood pressure and maintain eukalemia and was subjected to laparoscopic left adrenalectomy. To document biochemical cure, estimation of PAC/PRA is recommended within 2–3 days after surgery. This is because contralateral adrenal gland remains suppressed during this period due to prolonged inhibition of RAAS, and undetectable aldosterone levels are expected in a patient who had undergone curative surgery. Delayed estimation of PAC/PRA may have a less discriminatory value because of the recovery of contralateral adrenal gland. Development of hyperkalemia postoperatively indicates curative surgery and is due to hypoaldosteronism resulting from chronic inhibition of RAAS. Salt ad lib is recommended during this period as excess sodium leads to kaliuresis, due to increased exchange of sodium for potassium at collecting ducts, counteracting hyperkalemia. Our patient had dysglycemia which reversed after curative surgery. The abnormality in glucose insulin homeostasis in patients with primary hyperaldosteronism is due to chronic hypokalemia-induced inhibition of insulin secretion and the adverse effect of excess aldosterone on insulin sensitivity.

8.3 Clinical Rounds

1. **What is hyperaldosteronism?**

   Hyperaldosteronism is defined as increased secretion of aldosterone which may result in hypertension and/or hypokalemia. Hyperaldosteronism may be primary or secondary. Primary hyperaldosteronism is due to autonomous production of aldosterone either by an adenoma or idiopathic adrenal hyperplasia and is associated with hypertension and/or hypokalemia. Secondary hyperaldosteronism is due to activation of renin–angiotensin–aldosterone system because of intravascular volume depletion as occurs in congestive cardiac failure and chronic liver disease. However, hypertension and hypokalemia are uncommon in these patients. Nevertheless, renovascular hypertension and reninoma are also causes of of secondary hyperaldosteronism, but are associated with hypertension and hypokalemia.

2. **What are the causes of hypertension with hypokalemia?**

   Hypertension with hypokalemia and metabolic alkalosis is a characteristic feature of mineralocorticoid excess, either due to aldosterone or deoxycorticosterone. In addition, action of excess cortisol on mineralocorticoid receptor (specificity spillover) can also mimic hyperaldosteronism. Further, constitutive activation of epithelial sodium channel (ENaC) in the collecting duct can cause hypertension with hypokalemia but without aldosterone excess. The causes of hypertension with hypokalemia are summarized in the table given below.

Pathogenesis	Disorders
Primary aldosteronism	Aldosterone-producing adrenal adenoma (35%) Bilateral idiopathic adrenal hyperplasia (60%) Unilateral idiopathic adrenal hyperplasia (2%) Familial hyperaldosteronism (2%)
Secondary aldosteronism	Renovascular hypertension Renin secreting tumors
Deoxycorticosterone-related	Congenital adrenal hyperplasia (11β-hydroxylase and 17α-hydroxylase deficiency) Deoxycorticosterone producing tumors Glucocorticoid resistance syndrome
11β-hydroxysteroid dehydrogenase type 2 (loss of function)	Congenital apparent mineralocorticoid excess syndrome Licorice administration
Specificity spillover due to cortisol excess	Cushing's syndrome
Gain-of-function mutation of ENaC in collecting tubule	Liddle's syndrome

3. **What are the causes of hypokalemia with metabolic alkalosis?**

Hypokalemia is commonly associated with metabolic alkalosis. However, the differential diagnosis can be narrowed down based on the presence or absence of hypertension.

Hypokalemia and metabolic alkalosis with hypertension	Hypokalemia and metabolic alkalosis without hypertension
Use of diuretics in a patient with hypertension Primary aldosteronism Glucocorticoid-remediable hypertension Cushing's syndrome Glucocorticoid resistance syndrome Apparent mineralocorticoid excess syndrome Congenital adrenal hyperplasia 11β-hydroxylase and 17α-hydroxylase Liddle's syndrome	Use of insulin, β_2-agonists, and amphotericin B Hypomagnesemia Bartter's syndrome Gitelman's syndrome Gastrointestinal loss (vomiting)

4. **Does normokalemia exclude primary aldosteronism?**

No. Hypertension is invariably present in all patients with primary aldosteronism, whereas hypokalemia is observed only in 30–40%. Hypokalemia is more frequent with aldosterone-producing adenoma (APA) as compared to idiopathic adrenal hyperplasia (IAH).

5. **Why is normokalemia more common in patients with primary aldosteronism?**

Prerequisites for the development of hypokalemia in a patient with primary aldosteronism are severe and prolonged exposure to aldosterone excess, significant depletion of body potassium stores, adequate sodium intake, and overriding of potassium homeostatic mechanisms. Aldosterone levels are relatively higher in APA as compared to IAH, which explains the higher prevalence of hypokalemia in APA. Potassium is predominantly an intracellular cation (normal intracellular levels 135–145 mEq/L); therefore, hypokalemia manifests only after severe depletion of body potassium stores. Adequate sodium intake is also necessary for the development of hypokalemia, as delivery of excess sodium increases the cellular exchange of sodium for potassium in the collecting tubule. Further, hypokalemia itself induces potassium reabsorption from the collecting duct as an adaptive response; therefore, these homeostatic mechanisms should be overcome to manifest hypokalemia.

6. **What is the cause of hypokalemia in primary aldosteronism?**

Hypokalemia in primary aldosteronism is a result of increased distal renal tubular exchange of sodium for potassium. The primary effect of aldosterone is the activation of luminal epithelial sodium channels (ENaC) in the collecting duct, thereby increasing the sodium reabsorption. The resultant increase in intracellular sodium concentration and aldosterone per se stimulate basolateral Na^+/K^+-ATPase channel, thereby promoting extrusion of sodium and intracellular shift of potassium. This increase in intracellular potassium concentration creates a favorable gradient for potassium secretion into the lumen. In addition, the negative luminal charge after sodium reabsorption further potentiates potassium excretion. This is illustrated in the figure given below.

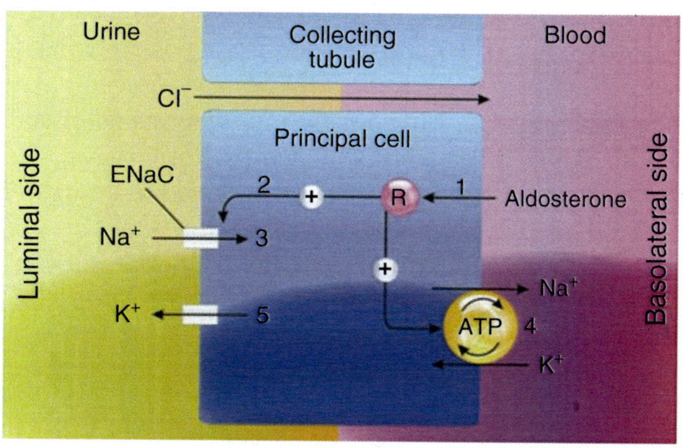

Fig. 8.2 The action of aldosterone in the collecting duct of kidney. (1) Aldosterone binds to its receptor in the principal cells (P cell) of collecting duct (on the basolateral surface). (2) This leads to activation of ENaC (in the luminal surface). (3) Sodium entry into P cell via ENaC. (4) Aldosterone-mediated activation of basolateral Na^+/K^+-ATPase, resulting in the transport of Na^+ into the blood and K^+ into P cell. (5) Extrusion of K^+ into the lumen to maintain electrochemical gradient of cell

7. **Is kaliuresis a direct effect of hyperaldosteronism?**

Possibly not. Kaliuresis in hyperaldosteronism is a consequence of increased K^+ excretion in response to increased Na^+ reabsorption. This is evidenced by the fact that blocking of ENaC by amiloride (K^+ sparing diuretic) abolishes hypokalemia and salt ad lib diet unmasks hypokalemia, suggesting that the predominant action of aldosterone is on sodium reabsorption and potassium wasting is consequent to it. However, aldosterone per se may have a modest direct effect on K^+ secretion.

8. **How does hypokalemia induce metabolic alkalosis?**

Metabolic alkalosis associated with hypokalemia is a consequence of increased H^+ excretion and enhanced bicarbonate reabsorption. Chronic hypokalemia upregulates luminal H^+/K^+-ATPase resulting in increased K^+ reabsorption in exchange of H^+, thereby resulting in increased H^+ excretion. Further aldosterone excess in patients with primary aldosteronism per se increases H^+ excretion by augmenting the activity of H^+-ATPase. Enhanced bicarbonate reabsorption is because of increased ammonium production due to binding of NH_3 with H^+. All these events occur at the intercalated cells of the collecting duct. Lastly, there is increased cellular shift of H^+ into potassium-depleted cells ubiquitously to maintain electrochemical neutrality, thereby worsening metabolic alkalosis.

9. **Why is hypernatremia not common in hyperaldosteronism?**

Hypernatremia is rare in hyperaldosteronism possibly due to the "escape effect" of aldosterone action at the collecting duct of renal tubule. Possible mechanisms of escape include inhibition of sodium reabsorption at proximal tubule and increased natriuresis mediated by atrial natriuretic peptide. Hyperaldosteronism results in intravascular volume expansion which leads to the inhibition of sodium reabsorption at the proximal tubule, and the resultant delivery of excess sodium to distal tubules overrides the action of aldosterone leading to urinary sodium loss. In addition, intravascular volume expansion stimulates atrial natriuretic peptide which counters hypernatremia. The escape effect also explains the absence of edema in patients with hyperaldosteronism. However, some patients may have hypernatremia due to polyuria and resetting of osmostat.

10. **What are the causes of edema in a patient with hyperaldosteronism?**

Edema is characteristically absent in patients with hyperaldosteronism due to the "escape effect" as discussed above. However, the presence of edema in a patient with aldosterone excess should lead to suspicion of congestive cardiac failure or renal failure.

11. **Should all patients with hypertension be screened for primary aldosteronism?**

Prevalence of primary aldosteronism in unselected hypertensive patients is around 5–13%. The recommendations of screening for primary aldosteronism include hypertension at a young age (<20 years), severe hypertension (BP >160/100 mmHg), drug-resistant hypertension (three antihypertensives in optimal doses including a diuretic), hypertension with spontaneous or diuretic-induced hypokalemia, and hypertension with adrenal incidentaloma. Further, a hypertensive patient with a family history of young hypertension or cerebrovascular accident (<40 years) or hypertensive first-degree relative of a patient with primary aldosteronism needs screening. Universal screening is not recommended as the available data do not support its benefit.

12. **What are the clinical manifestations of primary aldosteronism?**

The clinical manifestations of primary aldosteronism may either be due to the direct effect of aldosterone or as a consequence of hypokalemia. Aldosterone-related manifestations include severe diastolic hypertension with target organ damage (left ventricular hypertrophy, hypertensive retinopathy, and proteinuria) disproportionate to the duration and degree of hypertension. Hypokalemia-related manifestations are fatigue, muscle weakness, polyuria, polydypsia, periodic paralysis, and ventricular arrhythmias. Dysglycemia in patients with primary aldosteronism occurs due to impaired insulin secretion (hypokalemia) and reduced insulin sensitivity (aldosterone excess). The pathogenesis of hypokalemia-related manifestations are summarized in the table below.

Clinical feature	Pathogenesis
Fatigue, muscle weakness, periodic paralysis	Decreased activity of Na^+/K^+-ATPase leading to impaired contractility of actin–myosin complex
Polyuria and polydypsia	Due to impaired concentrating ability of distal convoluted tubule
Metabolic alkalosis	Hypokalemia-induced
Impaired glucose tolerance	Impaired β-cell function

13. **What are the endocrine causes of recurrent paraparesis?**

Any disorder associated with hypokalemia may present as paraparesis. The endocrine disorders accompanied with recurrent hypokalemia are thyrotoxic periodic paralysis, primary aldosteronism, ectopic ACTH-secreting tumors, and renal tubular acidosis. Besides this, Paget's disease of the bone can also present as recurrent paraparesis due to "steal phenomenon" as the bone lesions are highly vascular.

14. **Why is hypertension a feature of primary aldosteronism?**

Hypertension in primary aldosteronism is due to increased sodium reabsorption, extracellular volume expansion, and increased peripheral vascular resistance due to enhanced sensitivity to circulating vasoconstrictors like angiotensin

II and catecholamines. In addition, aldosterone excess causes endothelial dysfunction, reduced NO synthase activity, and vascular fibrosis, thereby aggravating hypertension.

15. **Why is target organ damage severe in primary aldosteronism?**

Target organ damage is severe in patients with primary aldosteronism and is disproportionate to the degree and duration of hypertension. Aldosterone induces the transforming growth factor β (TGF β), plasminogen activator inhibitor type 1 (PAI1), and collagen gene expression in vasculature and target organs, resulting in vascular damage (hypertensive microangiopathy) and myocardial/renal fibrosis, respectively.

16. **What are the differences between aldosterone-producing adenoma and idiopathic bilateral adrenal hyperplasia?**

The differences between aldosterone-producing adenoma and idiopathic bilateral adrenal hyperplasia are enlisted in the table given below.

Parameters	Aldosterone-producing adenoma	Idiopathic bilateral adrenal hyperplasia
Prevalence	35%	60%
Age of onset	Young	Middle-aged
Hypertension	Severe	Mild–moderate
Hypokalemia	50%	17%
Plasma aldosterone concentration	Very high	High
Plasma aldosterone concentration/plasma renin activity ratio (PAC/PRA)	Very high	High
Saline suppression	Non-suppressible	Usually intermediate
Adrenal imaging	Adenoma	Usually normal
Adrenal venous sampling	Unilateral gradient	No gradient
Effective treatment	Surgery	Medical management

Idiopathic unilateral adrenal hyperplasia (2%) may mimic aldosterone-producing adenoma; however, the disease is mild.

17. **What are the surrogate laboratory evidences for primary aldosteronism?**

The biochemical abnormalities associated with primary aldosteronism are hypokalemia, metabolic alkalosis, hypomagnesemia, mild hypernatremia, hyperglycemia, and proteinuria. Further, primary aldosteronism may be associated with U waves in ECG and left ventricular hypertrophy. The causes for development of these abnormalities are enlisted in the table given below.

Abnormality	Pathogenesis
Hypokalemia	Increased cellular exchange with sodium Potassium wasting
Metabolic alkalosis	Loss of H^+ into urine Shift of H^+ into potassium-depleted cells Increased bicarbonate reabsorption
Hypomagnesemia	Increased tubular secretion of magnesium
Mild hypernatremia	Increased sodium reabsorption
Hyperglycemia	Hypokalemia-induced β-cell dysfunction Aldosterone-mediated insulin resistance
Proteinuria	Hypertension-induced renal damage Direct effect of aldosterone
U waves	Hypokalemia related
Left ventricular hypertrophy	Hypertension Direct effect of aldosterone

18. **What are the precautions required prior to investigation in a patient with primary aldosteronism?**

Precautions to be taken before investigating a case of primary aldosteronism include selection of appropriate antihypertensives, salt ad lib, normalization of serum potassium, and adequate measures for blood sampling. The preferred antihypertensive drugs are prazosin and verapamil as they do not interfere with the renin–angiotensin–aldosterone system (RAAS). Salt ad lib is advocated to improve the sensitivity of screening test (plasma aldosterone concentration/plasma renin activity, PAC/PRA) as salt restriction leads to increased PRA resulting in false-negative test. However, salt ad lib unmasks hypokalemia which needs correction prior to the screening test, because hypokalemia leads to decreased aldosterone secretion. The following precautions should be ensured before sampling for PAC/PRA. Sampling is to be done in the morning and patient has to be ambulatory for at least 2 hours to ensure physiological activation of RAAS, followed by collection of blood after keeping the patient seated for 5–15 min. Use of tourniquet and fist clenching during sampling should be avoided as it will result in the shift of intracellular potassium to intravascular compartment and may interfere with the results of the screening test.

19. **How to evaluate a patient with suspected primary aldosteronism?**

The algorithm for evaluation of a patient with suspected primary aldosteronism is depicted in the figure given below.

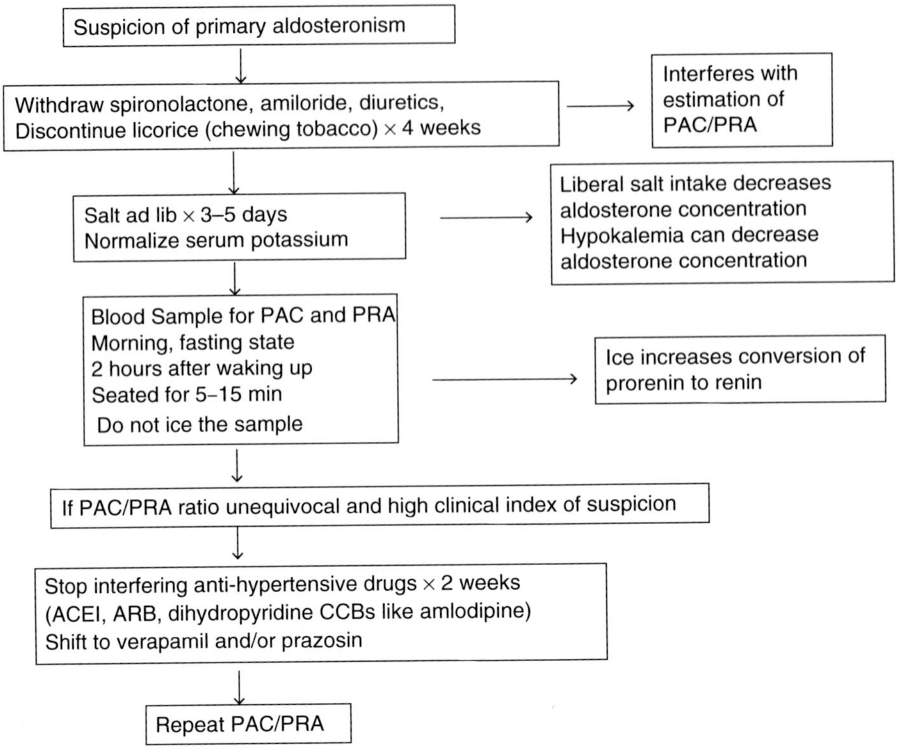

Fig. 8.3 Evaluation of a patient with suspected primary aldosteronism

20. How to interpret PAC/PRA ratio?

Before interpreting PAC/PRA ratio, it must be confirmed that PAC is expressed in ng/dL and PRA in ng/mL/h.

PAC (ng/dl)	PRA (ng/ml/h)	PAC/PRA ratio	Interpretation
↑	↑	<10	Renovascular hypertension Reninoma
↓	↓	–	Cushing's syndrome DOC-mediated hypertension Liddle's syndrome Apparent mineralocorticoid syndrome
↑ (>15)	↓(<1)	>20 favors >30 diagnostic	Primary aldosteronism

Interpretation of PAC/PRA should take into consideration PRA assay method and lower detection limit of the assay, as an assay with low detection limit could falsely elevate PAC/PRA ratio. PAC/PRA ratio should be cautiously interpreted in elderly individuals (>65 years) and patients with renal failure.

21. **What are the causes where plasma renin activity is not suppressed despite primary aldosteronism?**

    The causes of non-suppressible plasma renin activity despite primary aldosteronism are concurrent renovascular hypertension, malignant hypertension, salt-restricted diet, and use of ACE inhibitors/ARBs and diuretics.

22. **Is measurement of plasma renin concentration advantageous over plasma renin activity?**

    Estimation of plasma renin activity is a cumbersome process, has poor reproducibility, is performed manually, and requires special preanalytical precautions. The measurement of plasma renin concentration was devised to overcome these limitations. However, the available literature does not show an appreciable difference between the two tests.

23. **How to confirm the diagnosis of primary aldosteronism?**

    It is necessary to confirm the diagnosis of primary aldosteronism with any of the following tests: oral sodium loading, saline infusion, or fludrocortisone suppression test. Details of the commonly performed tests are summarized in the table given below.

Tests	Procedure	Cutoffs	Remarks
Oral salt loading test	6 g/day for 3 days Ensure eukalemia Measurement of 24-h urinary aldosterone on day 4	Urinary aldosterone > 12 μg/24 h	Cumbersome Poses a risk in patients with CHF/renal insufficiency Poor sensitivity of urinary aldosterone assay
Saline infusion test	Recumbent position 1 h prior to test 2 liters of 0.9% saline i.v. over 4 h Sampling at 4 h	PAC > 10 ng/dl diagnostic PAC 5–10 ng/dl probable PAC < 5 ng/dl excludes	Poses a risk in patients with CHF/renal insufficiency
Fludrocortisone suppression test	100 μg 6 hourly for 4 days Measure PAC and PRA on day 4 at 10 am	PAC > 6 ng/dl and PRA < 1 ng/ml/h	Cumbersome Most sensitive

24. **How to proceed in a patient with biochemically confirmed primary aldosteronism?**

After definite biochemical confirmation, a high-resolution contrast-enhanced computerized tomography (CECT) abdomen should be performed in all patients. APA are usually hypodense (HU <10) and are <2 cm in size while patients with IAH may have normal or bilateral adrenal masses on CT.

25. **What is the need for adrenal venous sampling in primary aldosteronism?**

Neither a normal CT excludes the possibility of APA/IAH nor the abnormal CT confirms the source of aldosterone excess. A normal CT adrenal may be seen with APA (as most are <1 cm) as well as with IAH. Even an abnormal CT in a patient with biochemically confirmed primary hyperaldosteronism has an accuracy of only 53%, as there is a poor correlation between structural defect/s and functionality of the apparent lesion. This is because the incidence of both adrenal incidentaloma and IAH increases with advancing age (>40 years). Therefore, adrenal venous sampling may be required to confirm the source of excess in either situations.

26. **Who should be subjected to adrenal venous sampling?**

Adrenal venous sampling (AVS) is indicated in patients with biochemically confirmed primary aldosteronism with a normal CT or bilateral adrenal masses on CT with a high probability of APA. High probability of APA should be considered in those who have severe hypertension, spontaneous hypokalemia, serum aldosterone >25 ng/dl, and age <50 years. In addition, even patients with localized single adenoma but age >40 years require AVS, as the probability of adrenal incidentaloma increases with advancing age. AVS is not indicated in those who have unilateral mass > 1 cm and age < 40 years and in those with normal CT or bilateral adrenal mass with a low probability of APA.

27. **How to interpret the results of adrenal vein sampling?**

The procedure and interpretation of the results of adrenal vein sampling are summarized in the following steps.

Step 1. Before adrenal vein catheterization, cosyntropin should be administered for 30 min at the rate of 50 μg/h to minimize the stress-induced fluctuations in aldosterone secretion and to maximize the aldosterone secretion from APA.

Step 2. After 30 min of initiation of ACTH infusion, procedure for catheterization of adrenal vein is started. Preferably, both the adrenal veins should be cannulated simultaneously to avoid variation in the results. The catheter tip is placed in right adrenal vein on the right side and distal to the confluence of left inferior phrenic vein and left adrenal vein on left side.

Step 3. Simultaneous sampling of cortisol from the respective adrenal vein and external iliac vein is performed to ensure the correct positioning of the catheter tip. An adrenal vein to peripheral vein cortisol ratio >10:1 is suggestive of successful catheterization.

Step 4. Aldosterone : cortisol corrected ratio is preferred over plasma aldosterone levels, to minimize the dilutional effect during sampling, as catheter tip is placed distal to the confluence of the left inferior phrenic vein and left adrenal vein on the left side.

Step 5. Aldosterone : cortisol corrected ratio (A : C ratio) is calculated by dividing the plasma aldosterone value by the respective adrenal vein plasma cortisol value. The interpretation of A : C ratio is summarized in the table below.

A : C ratio (high side/low side)	Interpretation	Etiology
>4:1	Unilateral aldosterone hypersecretion	Aldosterone-producing adenoma Unilateral primary adrenal hyperplasia
<3:1	Bilateral aldosterone hypersecretion	Bilateral idiopathic adrenal hyperplasia Bilateral adrenal adenoma

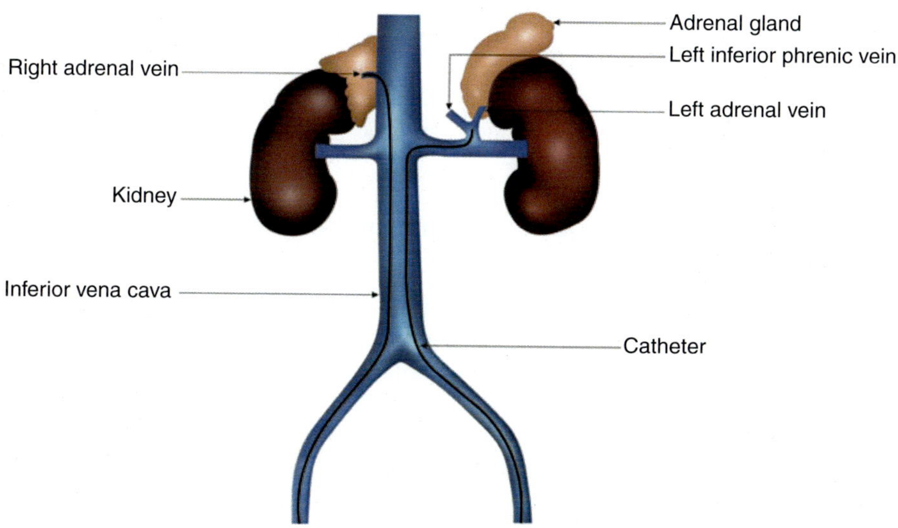

Fig. 8.4 Position of catheters during bilateral adrenal vein sampling

28. **What are the treatment options for patients with aldosterone-producing adenoma?**

The treatment of choice for aldosterone-producing adenoma is laparoscopic adrenalectomy, with a cure rate of 50% and a reduction in antihypertensive medications in almost all patients. Medical treatment with spironolactone is an option in patients who refuse surgery, but is less effective, requires lifelong therapy, and is fraught with adverse effects like gynecomastia, decreased libido, and erectile dysfunction in men and menstrual irregularities in women. An alternative drug devoid of these side effects is eplerenone, but is expensive. Overall, the surgical treatment is more cost-effective than medical management.

29. **What are the treatment options with idiopathic adrenal hyperplasia?**

Medical therapy with mineralocorticoid receptor antagonist spironolactone/eplerenone or ENaC blockers like amiloride/triamterene is preferred for bilateral idiopathic adrenal hyperplasia. Almost 50% of patients respond to spironolactone alone. The addition of thiazide, amiloride, or triamterene may reduce the dose of spironolactone. Surgery is not recommended as the disease is mild and even bilateral adrenalectomy does not cure hypertension possibly because of prolonged exposure to aldosterone, resulting in irreversible vascular damage.

30. **What are the advantages of eplerenone?**

Eplerenone is a newer, selective mineralocorticoid receptor antagonist without antiandrogenic and progesterone agonistic effects that are seen with spironolactone.

31. **How to manage a patient with aldosterone-producing adenoma postoperatively?**

Postoperatively, potassium supplementation and spironolactone should be discontinued and antihypertensive medications are tapered as appropriate. Salt ad lib is advocated to counteract hyperkalemia, which occurs due to hypoaldosteronism consequent to chronic inhibition of RAAS and suppression of contralateral zona glomerulosa. Occasionally, patient may have hypokalemia despite curative surgery due to severe depletion of body potassium stores. PAC/PRA ratio should be reestimated soon after surgery (within 2–3 days) to document biochemical cure.

32. **What is glucocorticoid resistance syndrome?**

Glucocorticoid resistance syndrome (GRS) is a familial disorder characterized by hypertension, hypokalemia, metabolic alkalosis, features of androgen excess, and hypercortisolemia without Cushing's stigmata. Affected females present in second or third decade with hirsutism, menstrual disturbances, and hypertension. Biochemically, GRS is characterized by high serum cortisol (0800h), preservation of circadian rhythm of cortisol, non-suppressible LDDST with suppressible HDDST, and increased dehydroepiandrostenedione sulfate (DHEAS) and deoxycorticosterone (DOC). Hypertension is due to increase in DOC and action of excess cortisol on mineralocorticoid receptor ("specificity spillover"), overwhelming the effect of 11β-HSD2. Although there is resistance to its action at glucocorticoid receptor (GC2), there is no resistance to its action at mineralocorticoid receptor (GC1), an example of differential resistance. Features of androgen excess are due to increase in DHEAS as a result of loss of negative feedback of cortisol on ACTH. As expected, bone mineral density is normal in these patients. Treatment with dexamethasone corrects most of these abnormalities.

33. **What is familial hyperaldosteronism?**

Familial hyperaldosteronism (FH) is a rare disorder with autosomal dominant inheritance and contributes to <3% of all causes of primary aldosteronism. The features of FH are enlisted in the table given below.

Disease	Genetic defects	Features
FH type I or glucocorticoid-remediable aldosteronism	11β-1/11β-2 hydroxylase chimerism resulting in ectopic aldosterone synthase expression in zona fasciculata	Hypertension Hypokalemia unmasked by thiazides Family history of young stroke Responds to glucocorticoids
FH type II	Chromosome 7p22	Most common form Familial occurrence of APA or IHA Glucocorticoid nonresponsive
FH type III	Potassium channel KCNJ5	Glucocorticoid nonresponsive

34. **What is "Cushing's disease of the kidney"?**

"Cushing's disease of the kidney" also called as apparent mineralocorticoid excess (AME) syndrome manifests as failure to thrive, polyuria, and hypertension. The biochemical abnormalities are hypokalemia, low PRA, low PAC, and normal plasma cortisol. It results from decreased activity of 11β-hydroxysteroid dehydrogenase 2 (11β-HSD2) in the collecting duct of kidney resulting in impaired conversion of cortisol to cortisone. The resultant accumulation of cortisol in the distal renal tubule acts on mineralocorticoid receptors (GC1) and is responsible for hypertension and hypokalemia, mimicking mineralocorticoid excess. This increase in intrarenal cortisol earns it the name "Cushing's disease of the kidney." AME syndrome may be congenital (autosomal recessive) or acquired. Congenital AME is due to loss-of-function mutation of 11β-HSD2 gene, while the acquired form is due to licorice use, which inhibits the activity of 11β-HSD2. Treatment options include mineralocorticoid receptor blocker or dexamethasone which suppresses hypothalamo–pituitary–adrenal axis thereby suppressing endogenous cortisol.

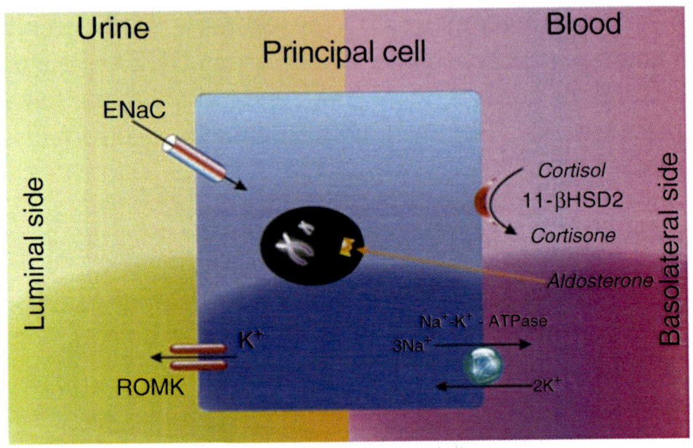

Fig. 8.5 Cortisol has similar affinity for mineralocorticoid receptor as aldosterone. However, 11β-HSD2-mediated inactivation of cortisol to cortisone in the collecting duct prevents action of cortisol on mineralocorticoid receptor. Inactivating mutations of 11β-HSD2 result in accumulation of cortisol in the collecting duct, which acts on mineralocorticoid receptor

35. **What are the causes of glucocorticoid-remediable hypertension?**

Glucocorticoid excess, whether endogenous or exogenous is associated with hypertension. On the contrary, in certain disorders hypertension associated with "mineralocorticoid excess/activity" resolves with glucocorticoids. These disorders include congenital adrenal hyperplasia (CAH) due to 11β-hydroxylase and 17α-hydroxylase deficiency, glucocorticoid resistance syndrome (GRS), familial hyperaldosteronism type 1 (glucocorticoid-remediable aldosteronism, GRA/FH type 1), and apparent mineralocorticoid excess syndrome (AME). The defects in these disorders include increased ACTH drive either due to cortisol deficiency (CAH) or resistance (GRS) or increased ACTH sensitivity (FH type1) or specificity spillover of cortisol action on mineralocorticoid receptor (AME).

36. **What is Liddle's syndrome?**

Liddle's syndrome is an autosomal dominant disorder characterized by hypertension, hypokalemia, metabolic alkalosis, low PAC and PRA, and normal serum cortisol. This occurs due to constitutive activation of ENaC involved in sodium reabsorption in the cortical collecting duct. ENaC is the final common pathway of aldosterone action for sodium homeostasis and tubular exchange of potassium. The biochemical features of Liddle's syndrome is identical to that of AME (inactivating mutation of 11β-HSD2). Failure to respond to spironolactone or dexamethasone but response to ENaC blockers like amiloride and triamterene suggests the diagnosis of Liddle's syndrome.

37. **What are the causes of hypertension with hyperkalemia?**

The most common cause of hypertension with hyperkalemia is renal insufficiency. Other causes include use of ACE inhibitors/ARBs or β-blockers for the management of hypertension. In addition, type IV renal tubular acidosis is associated with hypertension, hyperkalemia, and mild renal insufficiency; however, hyperkalemia is disproportionate to the degree of renal insufficiency in type IV RTA. The only cause of hypertension with hyperkalemia in the absence of renal insufficiency and drugs is pseudohypoaldosteronism type II (Gordon's syndrome).

38. **What is Gordon's syndrome?**

Gordon's syndrome also known as familial hyperkalemic hypertension is an autosomal dominant disorder characterized by low renin hypertension, hyperkalemia, and hyperchloremic metabolic acidosis with normal renal function. This syndrome is due to inactivating mutation of WNK 1 and 4 genes (**W**ith-**N**o-lysine **K**inase). These genes downregulate thiazide-sensitive sodium chloride co-transporter (NCCT) in the distal convoluted tubule, and their inactivating mutation results in increased activity of NCCT, thereby leading to enhanced sodium reabsorption and hypertension. Increased sodium and volume expansion inhibit RAAS resulting in low renin and aldosterone levels. Hyperkalemia is a characteristic abnormality which occurs as a result of hypoaldosteronism, decreased distal delivery of sodium to collecting tubules for potassium exchange, and possibly inhibition of renal outer medullary potassium channels (ROMK) due to WNK mutations. Salt restriction helps in abating hyperchloremic metabolic acidosis in addition to blood pressure control. Thiazide diuretics are the treatment of choice.

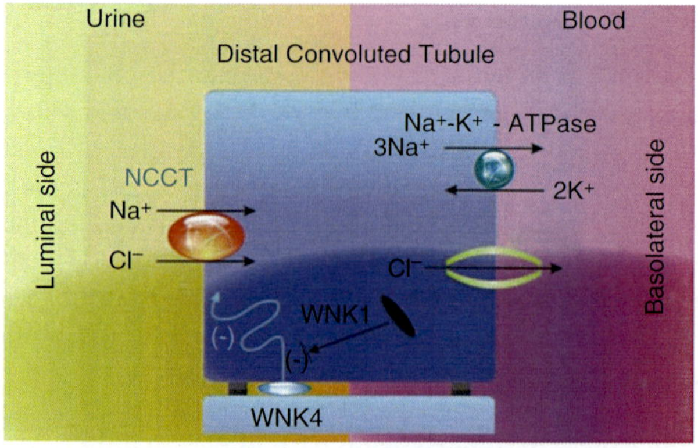

Fig. 8.6 WNK 1 and 4 genes downregulate NCCT in the distal convoluted tubule. Inactivating mutation of WNK 1 and 4 genes (Gordon's syndrome) results in increased Na^+ reabsorption and hypertension. Increased Na^+ reabsorption in the distal convoluted tubule inhibits the renin–angiotensin–aldosterone system and consequently results in hyperkalemia

39. **What is the difference between pseudohypoaldosteronism type I and pseudohypoaldosteronism type II?**

Pseudohypoaldosteronism is a disorder characterized by resistance to the action of aldosterone and manifests as hypotension, hyperkalemia, and metabolic acidosis. It is associated with increased plasma renin activity (PRA) and plasma aldosterone levels (PAC). However, pseudohypoaldosteronism type II is a misnomer as it has a normal or suppressed PAC/PRA. The differences between the two disorders are summarized in the table given below.

Parameters	Pseudohypoaldosteronism I	Pseudohypoaldosteronism II (Gordon's syndrome)
Inheritance	Autosomal recessive (AR) Autosomal dominant (AD)	Autosomal dominant (AD)
Age of presentation	Infancy	Adolescence or early adulthood
Clinical and biochemical features	Normo- or hypotension Renal salt wasting Hyponatremia Hyperkalemia Metabolic acidosis Elevated PAC and PRA Elevated Na^+ and Cl^- in sweat and saliva	Hypertension Normal or elevated sodium Hyperkalemia Metabolic acidosis Suppressed/normal PAC and PRA
Genetics	AR-ENaC channel (loss-of-function) AD-mineralocorticoid receptor (loss of function)	WNK-1 and WNK-4 mutations (gain-of-function)
Treatment	Salt supplementation Mineralocorticoid therapy	Salt restriction Thiazides

40. **What is Bartter's syndrome?**

Bartter's syndrome is an inherited disorder which is characterized by salt wasting, hypokalemia, metabolic alkalosis, hypomagnesemia, hypercalciuria, elevated prostaglandin E with normal to low blood pressure and elevated PAC and PRA. The disorder can manifest either during antenatal or postnatal period. Antenatal variant or hyperprostaglandin E syndrome is a severe form which manifests in utero with polyhydramnios and premature birth, and during neonatal period with severe salt wasting, failure to thrive, and polyuria. The classic variant (postnatal form) manifests in infancy or early childhood with polyuria, polydypsia, muscle weakness, growth retardation, and nephrocalcinosis and is a milder form of Bartter's syndrome. Bartter's syndrome results from defective epithelial transport of sodium and chloride in the thick ascending limb of loop of Henle (TALH) due to mutations in any one of the following transporter/channel/pump as summarized in the table given below.

Subtypes	Inheritance	Mutations	Remarks
Type 1 (antenatal variant)	Autosomal recessive	Inactivating mutations in Na^+–$2Cl^-$–K^+ co-transporter	Polyhydramnios
Type 2 (antenatal variant)	Autosomal recessive	Inactivating mutations in ROMK gene	Transient hyperkalemia at onset
Type 3 (classic variant)	Autosomal recessive	Inactivating mutations in CLC-Kb gene	Resembles Gitelman's syndrome
Type 4 (antenatal variant)	Autosomal recessive	Inactivating mutations in Barttin gene	Sensorineural deafness, Chronic kidney disease
Type 5 (classic variant)	Autosomal dominant	Activating mutations in calcium-sensing receptor	Chondrocalcinosis

Treatment includes liberal salt intake along with supplementation of potassium and magnesium. Non-steroidal anti-inflammatory drugs are of particular use in the management of Bartter's syndrome in view of elevated prostaglandins. Spironolactone or amiloride is also useful in the management of Bartter's syndrome.

41. **How to explain the biochemical abnormalities in Bartter's syndrome?**

Defective epithelial transport of sodium and chloride via sodium–potassium–chloride co-transporter (NKCC2) in the thick ascending limb of the loop of Henle results in salt wasting. Hypokalemia is due to increased delivery of sodium to the collecting ducts thereby enhancing the sodium reabsorption through ENaC and consequently potassium extrusion into lumen. In addition, intravascular volume depletion due to salt wasting results in secondary hyperaldosteronism which activates ENaC and further worsens hypokalemia. Reabsorption of Ca^{2+} and Mg^{2+} is a passive process and is coupled to Na + reabsorption in the thick ascending limb of the loop of Henle. Therefore, any defect in sodium reabsorption results in calcium and magnesium wasting. However, hypomagnesemia is mild as magnesium is predominantly absorbed in DCT. Elevation of prostaglandin E is a compensatory response to fluid and electrolyte loss and helps to maintain renal blood flow and glomerular filtration rate. This is illustrated in the figure given below.

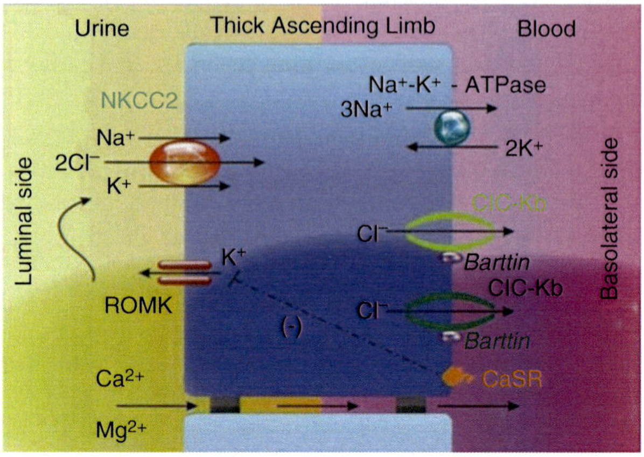

Fig. 8.7 Mechanism of different subtypes of Bartter's syndrome (type1 to type 5)

42. **What is Gitelman's syndrome?**

Gitelman's syndrome is an autosomal recessive disorder characterized by salt wasting, hypokalemia, metabolic alkalosis, hypomagnesemia, hypocalciuria and elevated PAC and PRA levels. It commonly presents during adolescence and young adulthood. The clinical manifestations include polyuria, weakness, and fatigue and are attributed to hypokalemia. Arthritis occurs due to chondrocalcinosis secondary to hypomagnesemia. Carpopedal spasms and muscle cramps can occur because of metabolic alkalosis and hypomagnesemia (even in the absence of hypocalcemia). The disorder is due to inactivating mutations in thiazide-sensitive sodium chloride co-transporter in the distal convoluted tubule (DCT), and hence, the clinical profile closely mimics chronic use of thiazide diuretics. Treatment includes salt intake with potassium and magnesium supplementation. Spironolactone and amiloride have been shown to be effective to normalize potassium.

43. **How to explain the electrolyte abnormalities in Gitelman's syndrome?**

Inactivating mutation of NCCT at distal convoluted tubular cell results in salt wasting. Hypokalemia, the cardinal biochemical abnormality, is due to the increased delivery of sodium to the collecting ducts, thereby enhancing the sodium reabsorption through ENaC and consequently potassium extrusion into the lumen. In addition, intravascular volume depletion due to salt wasting results in secondary hyperaldosteronism which activates ENaC and further worsens hypokalemia. Hypomagnesemia is a result of decreased expression of TRPM6 (transient receptor potential cation channel, subfamily M, member 6) which is the principal regulator of magnesium reabsorption in DCT. Hypocalciuria is due to the decrease in extracellular volume resulting in increased passive reabsorption of calcium in the proximal convoluted tubule. The other proposed mechanism for hypocalciuria is the activation of apical calcium channel as a result of hyperpolarization of the distal convoluted tubular cell consequent to decreased chloride reabsorption (NCCT mutations).

44. **What are the differences between Bartter's syndrome and Gitelman's syndrome?**

Parameters	Bartter's syndrome	Gitelman's syndrome
Inheritance	Autosomal recessive/dominant	Autosomal recessive
Site of defect in kidney	TALH	DCT
Age of presentation	Intrauterine to early childhood	Adolescence to young adulthood
Specific manifestations	Polyhydramnios, premature birth, failure to thrive, growth retardation	Carpopedal spasm, arthritis
Urinary calcium excretion	Increased	Low
Nephrocalcinosis	Present	Absent
Hypomagnesemia	Mild to moderate	Severe
Prostaglandin E	Increased	Normal
Treatment with NSAIDs	Effective	Not effective

45. **Why is blood pressure normal despite elevated plasma renin and aldosterone in patients with Bartter's and Gitelman's syndrome?**

The principal requirement for the development of hypertension due to elevated plasma renin and aldosterone is the optimal reabsorption of sodium in the renal tubular system. About 60–65% of filtered sodium is reabsorbed in the proximal convoluted tubule and is obligatory. Twenty-five to thirty percent of filtered sodium is actively reabsorbed in the thick ascending limb of the loop of Henle (TALH) via Na^{+}–K^{+}–$2Cl^{-}$ co-transporter, 5% in the distal convoluted tubule through Na^{+}-Cl^{-} co-transporter, and 1–2% in the collecting ducts through epithelial sodium channels (ENaC) under the influence of aldosterone, and only <1% of filtered sodium is excreted in urine. Therefore, for the development of aldosterone-mediated hypertension, sodium reabsorption (95–98%) proximal to ENaC is mandatory as sodium reabsorption via ENaC contributes only 1–2% of filtered sodium reabsorption. Therefore, patients with Bartter's syndrome and Gitelman's syndrome do not develop hypertension despite elevated PAC and PRA.

46. **What are the uses of spironolactone other than primary aldosteronism?**

Spironolactone is the drug of choice for managing hypertension in patients with primary aldosteronism. Other uses of spironolactone are summarized in the table given below.

Disorders	Rationale for use of spironolactone
Cushing's syndrome	Recalcitrant hypokalemia, hypertension
Glucocorticoid resistance syndrome	Hypertension, hypokalemia, and hirsutism (complementary to dexamethasone)
Apparent mineralocorticoid excess syndrome	Hypertension, hypokalemia, and metabolic alkalosis
DOC-producing tumor	Hypertension, hypokalemia, and metabolic alkalosis
Bartter's syndrome	Hypokalemia and metabolic alkalosis
Gitelman's syndrome	Hypokalemia and metabolic alkalosis
CHF	Myocardial remodeling, edema
Cirrhosis, nephrotic syndrome	Edema
Reninoma, renovascular hypertension	Hypertension, hypokalemia
Polycystic ovarian disease, idiopathic hirsutism	Hirsutism, acne

Suggested Reading

1. Funder JW, Carey RM, Fardella C, Gomez-Sanchez CE, Mantero F, Stowasser M, Young Jr WF, Montori VM. Case detection, diagnosis, and treatment of patients with primary aldosteronism: an endocrine society clinical practice guideline. J Clin Endocrinol Metab. 2008;93(9): 3266–81.
2. Jameson JL, De Groot LJ. Endocrinology: adult and pediatric. Philadelphia: Elsevier Health Sciences; 2010.
3. Longo D, Fauci A, Kasper D, Hauser S, Jameson J, Loscalzo J. Harrison's principles of internal medicine 18E EB. McGraw Hill Professional; 2012.
4. Melmed S, Polonsky KS, Larsen PR, Kronenberg HM. Williams textbook of endocrinology: expert consult. Elsevier Health Sciences; 2011.

9 Hypothyroidism

9.1 Case Vignette

A 28-year-old-lady presented with headache for the last 1 year. It was holocranial, continuous, mild in intensity, and not associated with vomiting, seizures, focal neurological deficits, or visual defects. There was history of weight gain, fatigue, and generalized bodyache for the last 2 years. She also had secondary amenorrhea of 1 year duration. She received treatment for migraine without any relief. Subsequently, neuroimaging revealed a sellar mass with suprasellar extension (26×18×15 mm) with a hypointense area. Her visual acuity and visual field examination did not reveal any abnormality. She was referred for surgical intervention. The preoperative workup included hormonal evaluation which revealed serum T_3 0.4 ng/ml (0.8–1.8), T_4 1.4 μg/dl (4.8–12.6), and TSH 328 μIU/ml (0.45–4.2), prolactin 112 ng/ml (5–25), 0800h cortisol 280 nmol/l (171–536), serum osmolality 270 mosm/kg, and urine osmolality 350 mosm/kg. She was diagnosed to have nonfunctioning pituitary tumor with hypothyroidism and was referred to endocrinology for opinion. On further evaluation, she had dry and coarse skin, periorbital puffiness, hoarse voice, delayed deep-tendon reflexes, and galactorrhea. She had no goiter. Additional investigations revealed antithyroid peroxidase antibody 600 IU/ml (<34), LH 11 mIU/ml (2.4–12.6), FSH 13 mIU/ml (3.5–13.5), and estradiol 30 pg/ml (12.5–166), and ultrasound pelvis showed bilateral polycystic ovaries. She was diagnosed to have autoimmune thyroid disease (Hashimoto's thyroiditis) with primary hypothyroidism, thyro-lactotrope hyperplasia, hyperprolactinemia, and secondary polycystic ovarian disease. She was started with levothyroxine 25 μg per day and the dose was escalated weekly to 150 μg per day. She was supplemented with hydrocortisone 20 mg per day in divided doses. After 6 weeks of therapy, she had resolution of symptoms, but did not resume menstruation. Her serum T_4 was 6.4 μg/dl, TSH 36 μIU/ml, prolactin 35 ng/ml, and 0800h cortisol after omission of hydrocortisone for 24 h 384 nmol/L; hence, hydrocoritosone was tapered and same dose of levothyroxine was continued. At 3 months of follow-up, she resumed her cycles and

A. Bhansali, Y. Gogate, *Clinical Rounds in Endocrinology: Volume I - Adult Endocrinology*, DOI 10.1007/978-81-322-2398-6_9

galactorrhea resolved. Repeat MRI showed regression of sellar–suprasellar mass (14×12×11 mm) with normalization of TSH and prolactin.

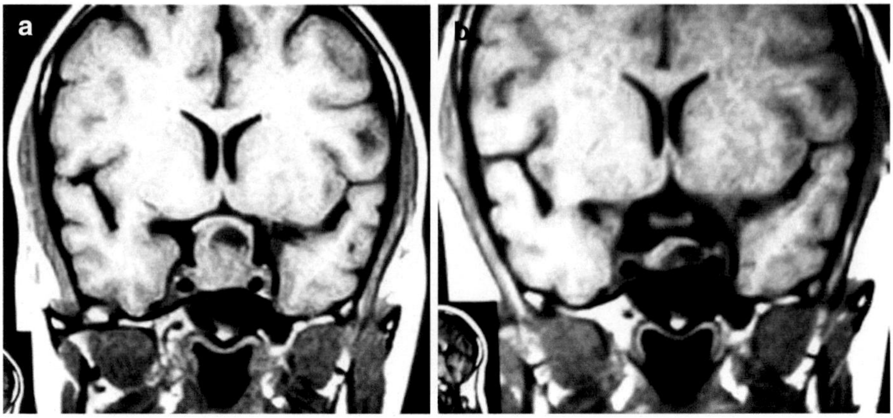

Fig. 9.1 (**a**) T1W CEMR coronal image showing sellar–suprasellar mass with hypointense area (necrosis) within it, suggestive of thyro-lactotrope hyperplasia. (**b**) T1W CEMR coronal image showing marked regression of sellar–suprasellar mass after levothyroxine therapy

9.2 Stepwise Analysis

Primary hypothyroidism presents with classical myxedematous features and the diagnosis is straightforward in most of the cases. However, at times the diagnosis is delayed for a long duration, particularly when patients have subtle features or present with unusual manifestations. The index patient presented with headache and was initially diagnosed to have nonfunctioning pituitary tumor with hypothyroidism. On analysis of complete profile of the patient, a diagnosis of primary hypothyroidism with hyperprolactinemia was considered, and the sellar–suprasellar mass was attributed to thyro-lactotrope hyperplasia, rather than nonfunctioning pituitary tumor with hypothyroidism. This was based on very high levels of TSH, which is characteristic of long-standing untreated primary hypothyroidism, while patients with nonfunctioning pituitary tumor usually have low or normal TSH. It is important to differentiate between these two disorders to avoid inadvertent surgical intervention in a patient with thyro-lactotrope hyperplasia, which usually responds to levothyroxine therapy. Thyro-lactotrope hyperplasia is commonly seen in young women (20–30 years of age) with long-standing, severe, and untreated primary hypothyroidism. Serum TSH levels are invariably high (100–1,000 μIU/ml) and is accompanied with low serum T_4. Although patients with TSH-secreting adenoma also have high TSH, with imaging features indistinguishable from thyro-lactotrope hyperplasia, presence of high serum T_4 favors the diagnosis of TSH-secreting adenoma. Thyro-lactotrope hyperplasia is due to increased TRH drive because of lack of T_4-mediated negative feedback on the hypothalamo–pituitary axis, which stimulates not only thyrotropes but also lactotropes. Hyperprolactinemia is seen in 23–50% of patients with primary hypothyroidism. The index patient had hypocortisolism which may be due to corticotrope dysfunction secondary to thyro-lactotrope hyperplasia or "lazy adrenal syndrome" because of hypometabolic state associated with primary hypothyroidism. Menorrhagia is the usual menstrual irregularity in patients with primary hypothyroidism, but amenorrhea is common in those with concurrent hyperprolactinemia, central hypogonadism due to mass effect, or secondary polycystic ovarian syndrome. The most common cause of primary hypothyroidism in majority of patients is Hashimoto's thyroiditis, as was evident in our patient. The treatment strategy in a patient of primary hypothyroidism with thyro-lactotrope hyperplasia includes levothyroxine supplementation either as conventional "step-up" protocol or uncustomary "step-down" approach. In the "step-up" protocol, levothyroxine is started at low dose and is escalated slowly. On the contrary, in "step-down" approach, high-dose levothyroxine (400–600 μg) is administered to achieve rapid reduction in thyrotrope hyperplasia; however, the results with this approach have been variable. Hydrocortisone supplementation is advised along with levothyroxine to avoid adrenal crisis in a patient with long-standing untreated hypothyroidism, as after initiation of levothyroxine there is an increase in metabolic clearance of cortisol which precedes the rise in cortisol synthesis. Serum T_4 returns to normal earlier than TSH and it requires 3–6 months for TSH to normalize. Regression of thyro-lactotrope hyperplasia usually occurs within 2–12 months; however, failure to regress after optimal therapy with normalization of TSH suggests either long-standing thyrotrope hyperplasia or the presence of double adenoma (e.g., thyrotrope hyperplasia with nonfunctioning pituitary adenoma).

9.3 Clinical Rounds

1. **How to define hypothyroidism?**

   Hypothyroidism is a disorder characterized by varied symptoms and/or signs related to decreased metabolism and/or increased glycosaminoglycans (GAG) deposition in soft tissue (myxedematous features) due to decreased production/action of thyroid hormones and/or thyroid-stimulating hormone (TSH) excess. Symptoms related to decreased metabolism are lethargy, fatigue, bradycardia, cold intolerance, and "aches and pains" and are primarily due to thyroxine (T_4) deficiency. Symptoms related to increased GAG deposition are periorbital puffiness, hoarse voice, nonpitting edema, and macroglossia and are predominantly due to thyroid-stimulating hormone (TSH) excess.

2. **Why are manifestations severe in primary hypothyroidism as compared to secondary hypothyroidism?**

The clinical manifestations are more pronounced in primary hypothyroidism as compared to secondary hypothyroidism. This is attributed to elevated TSH and severe T_4 deficiency in primary hypothyroidism resulting in overt myxedematous features. The increase in GAG is predominantly due to the stimulatory effect of TSH and lack of modest inhibitory effect of T_4 on hyaluronic acid, fibronectin, and collagen synthesis by fibroblasts. However, in secondary hypothyroidism, low–normal TSH and mild T_4 deficiency result in less severe myxedematous features. Mild T_4 deficiency in secondary hypothyroidism is due to TSH-independent T_4 synthesis which contributes to around 10–15% of circulating T_4. Also, the presence of concurrent multiple pituitary hormone deficiencies may mask the features of hypothyroidism.

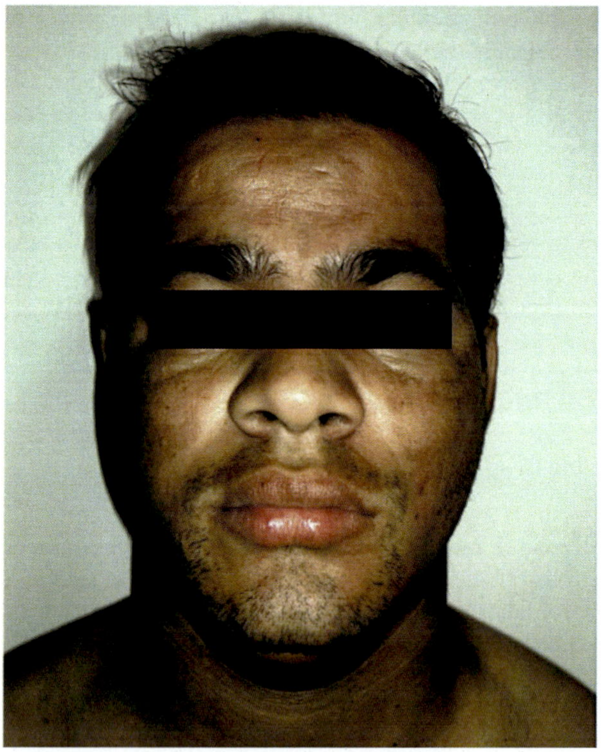

Fig. 9.2 Florid myxedematous manifestations in a patient with primary hypothyroidism

3. **What are the causes of hypothyroidism?**
The most common cause of primary hypothyroidism worldwide is environmental iodine deficiency, whereas in iodine-sufficient regions, the most common cause is Hashimoto's thyroiditis. Hypothyroidism is common in women and the incidence increases with advancing age. The causes of hypothyroidism are mentioned in the table given below.

Etiology of hypothyroidism
Primary hypothyroidism
Iodine deficiency
Hashimoto's thyroiditis
Post-ablative: thyroidectomy, radioiodine therapy, or external irradiation
Drugs—thioamides, iodides, lithium, amiodarone, interferon-α, interleukin-2, perchlorate, tyrosine kinase inhibitors
Transient hypothyroidism
Subacute thyroiditis
Postpartum thyroiditis
Congenital hypothyroidism
Ectopic thyroid
Thyroid dysgenesis
Thyroid dyshormonogenesis
Secondary hypothyroidism
Pituitary transcription factor defects
Pituitary tumors
Pituitary surgery
Hypophysitis
Infiltrative disorders of hypothalamo–pituitary region
CNS insults like head injury, subarachnoid hemorrhage, and radiotherapy
Resistance to thyroid hormone
Consumptive hypothyroidism
Hemangioma due to ectopic expression of type 3 deiodinase

4. **Does ectopic thyroid gland always present as congenital hypothyroidism?**

No. The development of hypothyroidism in a patient with ectopic thyroid gland depends upon the quantity of functioning thyroid tissue. Ectopic thyroid gland is usually devoid of lateral lobes and has a restricted proliferative capacity in response to TSH. Patients with ectopic thyroid gland usually present during childhood with hypothyroidism or obstructive symptoms; however, they may also present during adolescence with hypothyroidism, when thyroid gland fails to proliferate in response to increased metabolic demands. Rarely, autoimmune thyroiditis in an ectopic thyroid gland may lead to hypothyroidism in an adult.

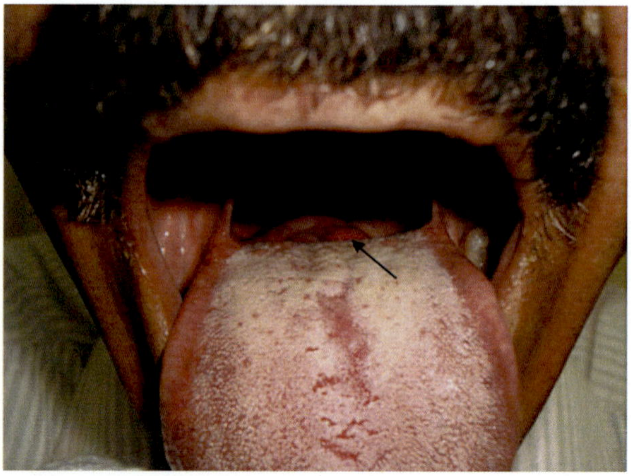

Fig. 9.3 Lingual thyroid in an adult with hypothyroidism

5. **What is subclinical hypothyroidism?**
Subclinical hypothyroidism is a biochemical abnormality characterized by normal serum free T_4 and elevated TSH above the reference range, irrespective of the presence or absence of symptoms. The reference range for normal TSH depends on sensitivity of the TSH assay, normative distribution of TSH, and iodine status of the study population. The most common cause of subclinical hypothyroidism is Hashimoto's thyroiditis. Approximately, 7–10% of elderly women have subclinical hypothyroidism. Before considering the diagnosis of subclinical hypothyroidism, thyroid function tests should be reconfirmed after 4 to 8 weeks to exclude the possibility of recovery phase of subacute thyroiditis or sick-euthyroid syndrome.

6. **What is the reason for normal free T_4 with an elevated TSH in subclinical hypothyroidism?**

A log-linear relationship exists between circulating free T_4 and TSH and is responsible for the characteristic biochemical profile of subclinical hypothyroidism. Log-linear relationship is explicited as a single-fold reduction in one variable (T_4) resulting in tenfold rise in the dependent variable (TSH). Hence, even a modest decrease in free T_4, although in reference range, leads to a log-linear rise in TSH.

7. **What are the causes of normal T_4 with elevated TSH apart from subclinical hypothyroidism?**

The causes of normal T_4 with elevated TSH apart from subclinical hypothyroidism include recovery phase of thyroiditis, convalescent phase of non-thyroidal illness, resistance to thyroid hormone, TSH receptor mutation, primary adrenal insufficiency, drugs (e.g., metoclopramide), and TSH assay interference by heterophile anti-mouse antibodies. In addition, patients on intermittent levothyroxine (LT_4) therapy with primary hypothyroidism may also have a biochemical profile similar to subclinical hypothyroidism. Hence, the diagnosis of subclinical hypothyroidism should only be considered after careful exclusion of these conditions.

8. **What are the long-term risks of subclinical hypothyroidism?**

   Long-term consequences of subclinical hypothyroidism are progression to overt hypothyroidism (3–8% per year) and increased risk of cardiovascular events, heart failure, dyslipidemia, nonalcoholic fatty liver disease, and possibly neuropsychiatric disorders. Treatment with levothyroxine delays the progression to overt hypothyroidism; however, the data regarding improvement in cardiovascular outcomes and nonalcoholic fatty liver disease with levothyroxine replacement are limited and conflicting.

9. **When to treat subclinical hypothyroidism?**

   Patients with subclinical hypothyroidism should be treated if TSH is > 10 μIU/mL because there is an increased risk for heart failure and cardiac events as shown in observational as well as in prospective studies. Patients with TSH between upper limit of normal and 10 μIU/mL, if accompanied with symptoms/signs suggestive of hypothyroidism or have a predisposition for progression to overt hypothyroidism (presence of goiter, positive antithyroid peroxidase antibody, personal history or family history of autoimmune disease) or on drugs (interferon, tyrosine kinase inhibitors, lithium and amiodarone) or have concurrent comorbidities like atherosclerotic cardiovascular disease, heart failure, dyslipidemia, infertility, and refractory anemia, also need to be treated. Those with nonspecific symptoms and neuropsychiatric disorders should be given a trial of levothyroxine for 3–6 months and further continuation of treatment should be based on clinical response.

10. **How to monitor patients with subclinical hypothyroidism?**

    Serum TSH should be monitored in patients with subclinical hypothyroidism, who are on treatment with levothyroxine. TSH should be targeted between 0.5 and 2.5 μIU/ml. This is based on normative distribution of TSH in healthy population and estimation of TSH by sensitive chemiluminescence assay. Overtreatment is to be avoided as it may result in decreased bone mineral density and increased risk of atrial fibrillation. Those who are not on treatment should undergo regular surveillance of TSH every 6 months.

11. **What are the monosymptomatic presentations of hypothyroidism in adults?**

    Monosymptomatic presentations of hypothyroidism in adults are weight gain, menorrhagia, infertility, galactorrhea, recurrent miscarriages, multicystic ovaries, pericardial effusion, sinus bradycardia, refractory anemia, dyslipidemia, carpal tunnel syndrome, dementia, ataxia, and depressive disorders. The index of suspicion should be high in these cases as treatment is rewarding.

12. **What are the causes of weight loss in a patient with hypothyroidism?**

Hypothyroidism is usually associated with weight gain (3–4 kg), but at times it may be associated with weight loss. The causes of weight loss in a patient with hypothyroidism include recovery phase of subacute thyroiditis, secondary hypothyroidism with multiple pituitary hormone deficiencies, hypothyroidism associated with polyglandular endocrine failure, and overtreatment with levothyroxine. In addition, children with concurrent type 1 diabetes or celiac disease may have weight loss despite hypothyroidism.

13. **What are the causes of tachycardia in a patient with hypothyroidism?**

Hypothyroidism is associated with sinus bradycardia in 10–20% of patients, while tachycardia is rare. The most common cause of tachycardia in patients with hypothyroidism is overtreatment with levothyroxine. The causes of tachycardia in treatment-naive patients are cardiac tamponade, congestive cardiac failure, and concurrent presence of anemia.

14. **What are the causes of anemia in hypothyroidism?**

Most common type of anemia in patients with hypothyroidism is normocytic and normochromic. The causes of anemia in hypothyroidism are menorrhagia, impaired absorption of micronutrients, and poor oral intake. Menorrhagia in patients with hypothyroidism is caused by coagulation abnormalities, platelet dysfunction, increased capillary fragility, and deficient progesterone secretion. Reduced gastric acid output and decreased gut motility contribute to impaired absorption of iron, vitamin, B_{12}, and folic acid. Erythropoietin deficiency as an adaptive response to decreased oxygen demand also contributes to anemia. Concurrent celiac disease, pernicious anemia (intrinsic factor deficiency), and blind loop syndrome may also result in anemia.

15. **What are the endocrine causes of pallor without anemia?**

The causes of pallor without anemia from endocrine perspectives are hypothyroidism, secondary hypocortisolism (ACTH deficiency), and hypogonadism. Although these disorders can be associated with anemia, they can cause pallor even without anemia. Cutaneous vasoconstriction in response to hypometabolic state in hypothyroidism, reduced melanin production from melanocytes due to ACTH deficiency in secondary hypoadrenalism, and decreased cutaneous vascularity due to testosterone deficiency in hypogonadism result in pallor without anemia, in these disorders.

16. **What are the neurological manifestations of hypothyroidism?**

Hypothyroidism is associated with dysfunction of central and peripheral nervous system. The most common neurological manifestation of hypothyroidism is "cerebral slowing" due to decreased cerebral blood flow, impaired glucose metabolism, and alterations in neurotransmitter activity. The uncommon neurological manifestations include dementia and movement disorders like ataxia, hemichorea, and pseudoparkinson like syndrome. Compressive neuropathies (carpal tunnel syndrome, tarsal tunnel syndrome), peripheral neuropathy with thickened nerves, and rarely autoimmune demyelinating neuropathies are other manifestations of peripheral nervous system involvement. In addition, "myxedema madness," a severe neuropsychiatric manifestation of long-standing untreated primary hypothyroidism, may also be seen rarely. Therefore, all patients with cognitive dysfunction, neuropsychiatric disorders, or entrapment neuropathy must have thyroid function tests.

17. **What are the musculoskeletal manifestations of hypothyroidism?**

Musculoskeletal involvement in patients with hypothyroidism includes delayed deep-tendon reflexes, proximal myopathy, calf hypertrophy (Kocher–Debre–Semelaigne syndrome in children and Hoffman syndrome in adults), arthralgia, and rarely myoedema. Myopathy is characterized by relative atrophy of type 2 and hypertrophy of type 1 muscle fibers and glycosaminoglycans deposition. These muscular dysfunctions are the result of abnormal glycogen metabolism, impaired mitochondrial oxidation, and defective sarcolemmal activity due to deficiency of thyroxine. Muscle enzyme creatine kinase is usually elevated and electromyogram may show polyphasic action potential. Patients with hypothyroidism are predisposed to rhabdomyolysis which may be precipitated by vigorous exercise or concurrent use of statin and fibrates.

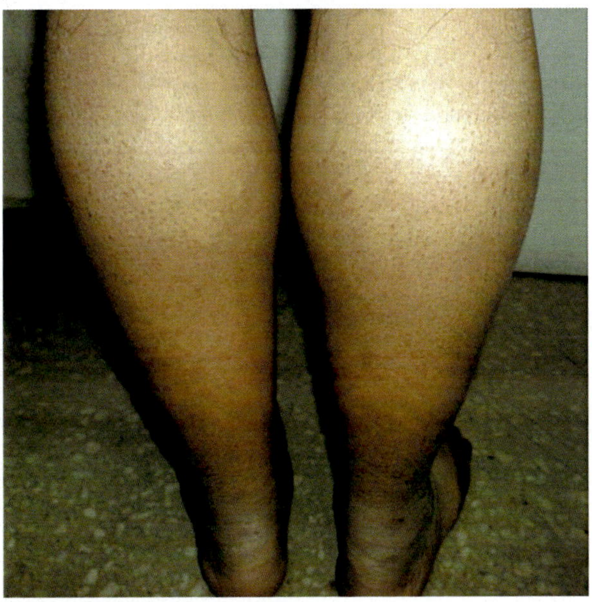

Fig. 9.4 Calf muscle hypertrophy in a patient with long-standing untreated primary hypothyroidism (Hoffman syndrome)

18. **Why are deep-tendon reflexes delayed in patients with hypothyroidism?**

    Deep-tendon reflexes are delayed in patients with hypothyroidism both during contraction phase and relaxation phase; however, the delay is more pronounced in relaxation phase and is myogenic in origin. Selective atrophy of type 2 and compensatory hypertrophy of type 1 muscle fiber (slow twitching), decreased Na^+/K^+-ATPase activity, reduced expression of myosin ATPase, impaired contractility of actin–myosin complex, and defective sarcolemmal depolarization are the underlying mechanisms for this phenomenon. The other causes of delayed deep-tendon reflexes are diabetes, obesity, pernicious anemia, iron deficiency anemia, hypothermia, and use of drugs (e.g., propranolol and chlorpromazine).

19. **What are the abnormalities of reproductive system in women with hypothyroidism?**

    Women with hypothyroidism may have various abnormalities of reproductive system at different phases of life. Girls in peripubertal period can present with delayed puberty, primary amenorrhea, or menorrhagia and rarely with large multicystic ovaries. Occasionally, these adolescent girls may present with acute abdomen due to ovarian torsion. In young women, hypothyroidism is associated with menstrual irregularities in about 23–30% of patients and these include menorrhagia, oligomenorrhea, and secondary amenorrhea. Premature ovarian failure may also occur in patients with primary hypothyroidism as a manifestation of polyglandular endocrine syndrome.

20. **How does hypothyroidism influence reproductive system in a woman?**

    Reproductive system abnormalities in a woman with hypothyroidism include oligo- or amenorrhea, menorrhagia, and infertility. The mechanisms for these abnormalities are enlisted in the table given below.

Clinical features	Mechanism
Oligo- or amenorrhea	Defect in GnRH pulsatility
	Impaired LH surge
	Hyperprolactinemia
	Secondary polycystic ovarian disease
	Decreased SHBG
	Altered estrogen metabolism
Menorrhagia	Estrogen breakthrough bleed
	Defect in hemostasis (factor VII, VIII, IX, XI)
	Platelet dysfunction
	Increased capillary fragility
Infertility	Defect in GnRH pulsatility
	Hyperprolactinemia
	Defect in oocyte maturation
	Luteal phase defect
	Impaired blastocyst formation (T_4 deficiency)

21. **Why is there hyperprolactinemia with hypothyroidism?**

Hyperprolactinemia is observed in 20–30% of patients with primary hypothyroidism. The causes of hyperprolactinemia in a patient with primary hypothyroidism include increased TRH-mediated prolactin secretion due to loss of negative feedback by T_4, decreased dopaminergic tone, and reduced prolactin clearance. If hyperprolactinemia does not resolve despite optimal dose and duration of levothyroxine therapy, a possibility of concurrent prolactinoma should be considered. Hyperprolactinemia can also be associated with secondary hypothyroidism in patients with macroprolactinoma with thyrotrope compression, lymphocytic infundibulitis, and stalk compression by nonfunctioning pituitary adenoma with thyrotrope dysfunction.

22. **When to suspect thyro-lactotrope hyperplasia in a patient with primary hypothyroidism?**

Patients with long-standing, severe untreated primary hypothyroidism are predisposed for the development of thyro-lactotrope hyperplasia. The presence of headache, visual field defects, amenorrhea–galactorrhea, and multiple pituitary hormone deficiencies in a patient with primary hypothyroidism should raise a suspicion of thyro-lactotrope hyperplasia.

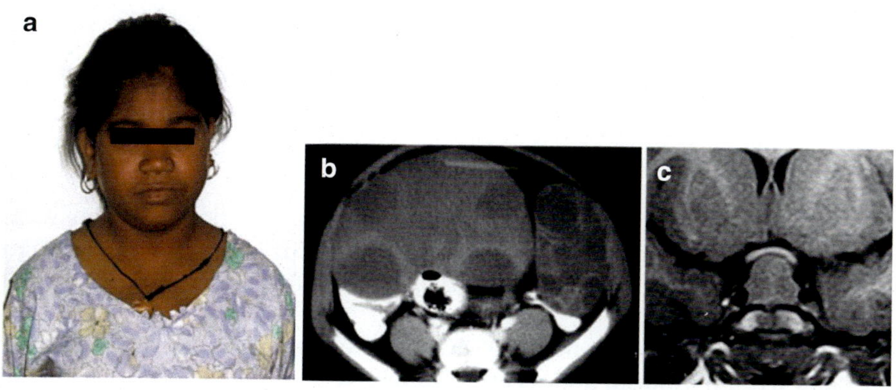

Fig. 9.5 (**a**) Adolescent girl with myxedematous appearance, multicystic ovaries, and thyro-lactotrope hyperplasia. (**b**) CECT pelvis showing bilateral huge multicystic ovaries in the same patient. (**c**) T1W CEMR coronal image showing sellar–suprasellar mass suggestive of thyro-lactotrope hyperplasia

23. **What are the emergencies in a patient with primary hypothyroidism?**

Emergencies in a patient with primary hypothyroidism are usually an outcome of undiagnosed or untreated long-standing disease. They may present with altered sensorium due to hyponatremia, hypoglycemia, myxedema coma, or Hashimoto's encephalopathy. The cardiac emergencies in patients with hypothyroidism are syncope due to sinus bradycardia, cardiac tamponade due to massive pericardial effusion, and congestive cardiac failure. They may also present as acute abdomen due to ovarian torsion, megacolon, paralytic ileus, and acute cholecystitis. Rarely, they may present as severe myoedema masquerading as tetanus, or rhabdomyolysis precipitated by use of statins or vigorous activity. In addition, hypokalemic periodic paralysis may rarely be a presenting manifestation.

24. **How was the normative data for TSH derived?**

Normative data for TSH were derived from the study of healthy subjects from iodine-sufficient region with no historical and ultrasonographic evidence of thyroid disease and negative thyroid autoantibodies. To derive the normative data, most of the studies have used third generation TSH assay. The upper limit of TSH reference range in self-reported "healthy" population in NHANES III was 4.5 μIU/ml and the lower limit was 0.45 μIU/ml. The upper limit of TSH was decreased to 4.12 μIU/ml after careful exclusion of subjects with TPO positivity, pregnancy, and use of various drugs that interfere with thyroid function. However, the National Academy of Clinical Biochemistry (NACB) reported the upper limit of TSH as <2.5 μIU/ml in >95% of study population without evidence of any thyroid dysfunction. Recent literature also supports that targeting TSH <2.5 μIU/ml is associated with better improvement in quality of life and lipid profile. Hence, for all practical purposes, serum TSH >4.12 μIU/ml suggests thyroid dysfunction and the treatment goal with LT4 should be targeted to TSH <2.5 μIU/ml. Serum TSH value rises with increasing age by 0.3 μIU/ml for each decade after the age of 40 years; hence, in elderly population, it should be interpreted cautiously.

25. **What is the screening test for hypothyroidism?**

Estimation of serum TSH is the primary screening modality in patients with suspected hypothyroidism. This is because rise in TSH is the earliest detectable abnormality due to log-linear relationship between free T_4 and TSH.

26. **Is there any correlation between severity of symptoms in patients with primary hypothyroidism and serum TSH levels?**

No. There is a poor correlation between severity of symptoms in patients with primary hypothyroidism and circulating TSH levels. Severity of symptoms of hypothyroidism depends upon serum free T_4 levels and the rapidity of development of hypothyroidism. The lack of correlation between serum TSH and symptomatology is due to increased secretion of TSH isomers by thyrotropes, which are immunoreactive but not bioactive and flattening of log-linear relationship at very low levels of serum free T_4.

27. **What are the limitations of TSH as a first-line test in patients with suspected thyroid dysfunction?**

Serum TSH as a first-line test can be misleading in patients with secondary hypothyroidism (normal TSH and low free T_4), non-thyroidal illness (normal TSH and low free T_4) and in the presence of anti-mouse antibodies (elevated TSH with normal free T_4). Further, it may be deceptive in the diagnosis of thyrotropinoma (elevated TSH and free T_4) and resistance to thyroid hormone (elevated TSH and free T_4).

28. **What are the causes of elevated TSH without thyroid gland dysfunction?**

The causes of elevated TSH without thyroid gland dysfunction include assay interference by heterophile antibodies, drugs (e.g., metoclopramide, ketoconazole), elevated rheumatoid factor titer, anti-TSH antibody, adrenal insufficiency, and immunoreactive but bioinactive TSH isomers.

29. **Who should be evaluated for hypothyroidism?**

Hypothyroidism is a common endocrine disorder with multifaceted presentation. In addition to those who have classical symptoms and signs of hypothyroidism, history of prior ablative therapy, or sellar-suprasellar mass evaluation for hypothyroidism should be performed in the disorders/conditions listed in the table given below.

Reproductive disorders	Menorrhagia, infertility, galactorrhea, multicystic ovaries, delayed puberty and recurrent fetal loss
	Pregnant women with risk factors for hypothyroidism[a]
Medical disorders	Dyslipidemia, refractory anemia, sinus bradycardia, unexplained pericardial effusion, hyponatremia, and hypoglycemia
Neuropsychiatric disorders	Mood disorders, entrapment neuropathy, ataxia, dementia
Autoimmune disorders	Type 1 diabetes, celiac disease, primary pulmonary hypertension
Drugs	Amiodarone, lithium, tyrosine kinase inhibitors, and interferon therapy
Special situations	Turner's and Down syndrome
	Women with type 2 diabetes aged >50 years
	Chronic kidney disease
	Past history of head injury

[a]Age >30 years, presence of goiter, TPO positivity, bad obstetric history, morbid obesity (BMI >40 kg/m^2), personal or family history of autoimmune thyroid disease or autoimmune disorders, presence of iodine deficiency, or prior thyroid surgery

30. **What is the rationale of screening for hypothyroidism in patients with depression?**

The prevalence of depressive symptoms in patients with subclinical hypothyroidism has been reported to vary from 13 to 63%. Neuropsychiatric symptoms have been correlated with levels of TSH, but treatment with levothyroxine alone does not remit the depressive symptoms. On the contrary, 8–20% of patients with depressive disorders have subclinical hypothyroidism and treatment with levothyroxine in these patients may augment the response to antidepressants. In addition, there are studies demonstrating the usefulness of liothyronine as well as levothyroxine in patients with refractory mood disorders, even with normal thyroid function; however, the data are inconsistent. Therefore, every patient with depression should be evaluated for hypothyroidism and particularly those who are resistant to anti-depressant therapy. However, the use of thyroid hormone supplementation is not recommended in euthyroid patients with depression.

31. **What is the appropriate time to measure TSH?**

Serum TSH can be measured at any time between 0800h and 1800h as the normative data for TSH has been derived during this period. However, it should preferably be estimated in the morning hours (0800–1000h) as TSH secretion peaks at midnight with nadir occurring between 1000h and 1600h, which approximate 50% of the peak value. Thus, the estimation of TSH in the morning hours may possibly detect higher number of patients with subclinical hypothyroidism as compared to TSH measurement later in afternoon.

32. **What are the investigations required for the diagnosis of hypothyroidism?**

Estimation of serum TSH and total T_4/free T_4 are required for the diagnosis of hypothyroidism. An elevated TSH with low total or free T_4 suggests the diagnosis of primary hypothyroidism. The measurement of antithyroid peroxidase antibodies helps in establishing the etiological diagnosis of autoimmune thyroid disease. Fine-needle aspiration cytology and USG are not required unless there is a thyroid nodule or thyroid gland is unusually firm. If serum T_4 is low with low/normal/mildly elevated TSH, then the diagnosis of secondary hypothyroidism should be considered and other pituitary hormones should be assessed. A mildly elevated TSH in a patient with secondary hypothyroidism suggests the possibility of concurrent ACTH deficiency, as glucocorticoids inhibit TSH secretion. MR imaging of sella should be performed after confirmation of diagnosis of secondary hypothyroidism to exclude hypothalamo–pituitary disorders.

33. **What is thyroid peroxidase?**

Thyroid peroxidase (TPO) is a microsomal enzyme involved in oxidation, organification, and coupling, required for thyroid hormone synthesis. TSH is the prime regulator of TPO activity, complemented by intrathyroidal iodine. Congenital deficiency of this enzyme results in thyroid dyshormonogenesis. Antithyroid drugs like carbimazole, methimazole, and propylthiouracil inhibit TPO, thereby suppressing the thyroid hormone biosynthesis. Anti-TPO antibody (also called as anti-microsomal antibody) is a surrogate marker of autoimmune thyroid disease and represents an "epiphenomenon" of thyroid autoimmunity but does not have a causative role.

34. **Why is estimation of serum T_3 not useful in the diagnosis of hypothyroidism?**

Serum T_3 estimation is not useful in the diagnosis of primary hypothyroidism, as it remains within normal range even in patients with overt hypothyroidism because of increased T_3 secretion by thyroid gland and augmented peripheral T_4 to T_3 conversion by peripheral deiodinase type 2 under intense TSH drive.

35. **What are the regulators of T_4 to T_3 neogenesis?**

Twenty percent of the circulating serum T_3 is secreted directly from thyroid gland, while the rest is derived by peripheral T_4 to T_3 neogenesis, which is regulated by type 2 and type 1 monodeiodinases. However, type 2 monodeiodinase contributes more (60%) to plasma T_3 than type 1 monodeiodinase (20%). The activity of type 2 deiodinase is increased by TSH and GH and inhibited by thyroxine and cytokines (TNF-α, IL-6). In addition, propranolol and glucocorticoids inhibit type 2 monodeiodinase, while propylthiouracil and amiodarone inhibit type 1 monodeiodinase.

36. **How does amiodarone cause hypothyroidism?**

Amiodarone consists of 37% iodine by weight; thus a 200 mg tablet of amiodarone contains 75 mg iodine, which far exceeds the recommended daily allowance of iodine (150 μg). Administration of amiodarone is associated with thyroid dysfunction in 20% of patients. Females, residents of iodine-replete area, and patients with TPO positivity or previous history of ablative treatment for Graves' disease are at risk for amiodarone-induced hypothyroidism (5–15%), and this is due to permanent "Wolff–Chaikoff's" effect. However, patients residing in iodine-deficient area are at increased risk for developing amiodarone-induced thyrotoxicosis (10%). Therefore, thyroid function should be performed prior to initiating amiodarone and monitored periodically. Despite normal thyroid function in majority of patients on amiodarone therapy, there is a "cardiac myxedema." This differential effect is due to amiodarone and its metabolite desethylamiodarone as both act as competitive antagonist to T_3 at cardiac cellular level.

37. **How to manage amiodarone-induced hypothyroidism?**

Amiodarone-induced subclinical/overt hypothyroidism should be treated with levothyroxine without discontinuation of amiodarone. Levothyroxine replacement does not increase the risk of cardiac arrhythmias in this scenario; however, thyroid function should be closely monitored to avoid iatrogenic thyrotoxicosis.

38. **What are the thyroid dysfunctions in a patient on lithium therapy?**

Lithium therapy is associated with development of goiter (4–60%), subclinical hypothyroidism (34%), and overt hypothyroidism (15%). Females and those with underlying autoimmune thyroid disease are predisposed for lithium-induced thyroid dysfunction. Lithium inhibits the release of thyroid hormones and consequently results in increased TSH, leading to the development of goiter. In addition, lithium therapy per se induces autoimmune thyroid disease. Lithium-induced autoimmune thyroid dysfunction and/or worsening of preexisting autoimmune thyroid disease results in subclinical/overt hypothyroidism. Thyroid function test should be done prior to initiation of lithium therapy and 6–12 monthly thereafter, as lithium-induced thyroid dysfunction can occur anytime during therapy. Lithium-induced hypothyroidism should be managed with levothyroxine without discontinuation of lithium.

39. **What is the importance of thyroid hormone-binding proteins?**

Circulating T_4 predominantly binds with thyroxine-binding globulin (70%) and a small fraction of it binds to albumin (20%) and prealbumin (10%), also known as transthyretin. These binding proteins act as circulating reservoir for thyroid hormones and maintain constant free thyroid hormone level. The role of these binding proteins is interchangeable as in case of thyroxine-binding globulin (TBG) deficiency, transthyretin predominantly binds with T_4.

40. **What are the disorders associated with altered TBG levels?**

Thyroxine-binding globulin (TBG) is an estrogen-dependent globulin. The disorders associated with altered TBG status are enlisted in the table. In all these states, total T_4 may be high or low depending on TBG status, but free T_4 levels are normal. It should be noted that TBG is increased in patients with hypothyroidism, whereas it is decreased in hyperthyroidism.

TBG increased	TBG decreased
Pregnancy	Active acromegaly
Chronic active hepatitis	Nephrotic syndrome
HIV infection	Familial TBG deficiency
Drugs—oral contraceptives, tamoxifen, and methadone	Drugs—androgens, glucocorticoids, and interleukins

41. **What are the common errors in the interpretation of thyroid function tests?**

Thyroid function tests	Clinical scenario	Usual interpretation	Correct diagnosis
Low TSH, low T_3 and T_4	Graves' disease on treatment	Hyperthyroidism	Hypothyroidism
Low TSH, high T_3 and T_4	Rapid weight loss and neck pain	Hyperthyroidism	Subacute thyroiditis
Low–normal TSH, low–normal T_3 and T_4	Systemic illness	Hypothyroidism	Non-thyroidal illness (sick euthyroid syndrome)
Normal TSH (T_3, T_4 low normal/low)	Pituitary disorder	Euthyroid	Secondary hypothyroidism
High TSH, normal T_3, T_4	Hypothyroid on optimal treatment, asymptomatic	Noncompliance with T_4	Heterophile antibodies
High TSH, high T_3, T_4	Euthyroid/ mildly toxic	Lab error	Thyrotropinoma Resistance to thyroid hormone

42. **How to differentiate between subclinical hypothyroidism and recovery phase of subacute thyroiditis?**

Thyroid hormone profile may be similar in patients with subclinical hypothyroidism and recovery phase of subacute thyroiditis. However, recent history of rapid weight loss, neck pain, and palpitations with or without tender goiter supports the diagnosis of subacute thyroiditis, while patients with subclinical hypothyroidism may be asymptomatic or may present with nonspecific symptoms. In clinical practice, many a time patients present with history of recent weight loss with elevated TSH and normal T_4; these patients are in the recovery phase of subacute thyroiditis.

43. **What is "fluctuating thyroid function"?**

"Fluctuating thyroid function" is a clinico-biochemical entity characterized by periods of hypothyroidism and hyperthyroidism in the background of autoimmune thyroid disease. This entity should only be considered after excluding overzealous treatment either with antithyroid drugs or levothyroxine, non-compliance to treatment, and factitious use of levothyroxine. Fluctuating thyroid function represents a spectrum of autoimmune thyroid disease, wherein a balance between TSH receptor-stimulating antibodies and TSH receptor-blocking antibodies determines the clinical presentation as thyrotoxicosis or hypothyroidism, respectively. The presence of goiter is a prerequisite for the development of "fluctuating thyroid function." These patients should be radio-ablated during the phase of hyperthyroidism to render them permanently hypothyroid, as it is easier to manage thereafter.

44. **How to treat primary hypothyroidism?**

The treatment of choice in patients with hypothyroidism is levothyroxine and is initiated at a dose of 1.6 μg/kg ideal body weight, particularly in younger individuals and in those who have undergone recent thyroid surgery. Lean body mass is the best predictor of daily requirements of levothyroxine. However, because of practical constraints in estimating lean body mass, the dose of levothyroxine is calculated based on ideal body weight. In patients with long-standing hypothyroidism, in those with cardiovascular disease, and in elderly individuals, it seems prudent to initiate levothyroxine therapy at a lower dose with gradual increment thereafter. Levothyroxine is preferred over liothyronine as levothyroxine is a prohormone and its supplementation ensures sustained and stable T_3 neogenesis. In addition, levothyroxine has a longer half-life (7 days) and is associated with lesser fluctuations in serum T_4 levels.

45. **Why should levothyroxine dose be escalated slowly?**

Long-standing hypothyroidism is a hypometabolic state and results in upregulation of thyroid hormone receptors; hence, administration of initial high doses of levothyroxine may cause palpitation, tremor, tachycardia, and angina.

Occasionally, initiation of high-dose levothyroxine therapy can precipitate adrenal crisis, due to accelerated cortisol catabolism in the backdrop of lazy adrenal syndrome. Therefore, levothyroxine therapy should be built up slowly in patients with long-standing hypothyroidism, in elderly subjects and in those with cardiovascular disease. Similarly, children and adolescents with long-standing hypothyroidism should also be replaced with levothyroxine slowly, as patients in this age group is susceptible for pseudotumor cerebri (due to fluid and electrolyte imbalance), hyperkinetic disorder, and poor scholastic performance with initial full-dose replacement. However, neonates, and pregnant women should be started with full doses of levothyroxine to normalize serum T_4 level faster.

46. **Who are predisposed for adrenal crisis on initiation of levothyroxine therapy?**

Patients with secondary hypothyroidism, long-standing isolated primary hypothyroidism, and primary hypothyroidism with polyglandular endocrine failure are predisposed for the development of adrenal crisis on initiation of levothyroxine therapy. Therefore, in these patients a 0800h sample for serum cortisol should be obtained and glucocorticoid replacement should precede levothyroxine supplementation. A 0800h serum cortisol <100 nmol/L confirms the diagnosis of adrenal insufficiency, while a value >550 nmol/L excludes it. Serum cortisol values in between 100–550 nmol/L require ACTH stimulation test later on. In patients with severe hypothyroidism who are critically ill, a random cortisol should be obtained and empiric intravenous hydrocortisone therapy should be initiated followed by administration of levothyroxine. A random serum cortisol <400 nmol/L suggest adrenal insufficiency, whereas a value >900 nmol/L suggest adequate adrenal reserve. Serum cortisol values in between 400–900 nmol/L requires ACTH stimulation test later on.

47. **When should levothyroxine be administered?**

Levothyroxine is commonly administered early morning in fasting state as its absorption is interfered by food intake. A few studies have shown that bedtime supplementation of levothyroxine was better in suppressing TSH, as compared to morning dose; however, the participants in these studies had an interval of several hours before the last meal and levothyroxine intake. Therefore, the time of administration in relation with food intake seems to be more important than the time of day. Hence, the appropriate time for levothyroxine administration seems to be 1 h prior to breakfast or 4 h after the last meal.

48. **How to assess the clinical response after levothyroxine therapy?**

The initial clinical response to levothyroxine therapy is polyuria, increase in heart rate, and weight loss, followed by improvement in appetite and amelioration of constipation (over weeks). Neuropsychiatric manifestations, hoarseness of voice, and cutaneous changes take a longer time to resolve (months). Hyponatremia, if present, is the earliest biochemical abnormality to ameliorate with treatment. Weight loss after optimal therapy with levothyroxine, even in patients with overt hypothyroidism, is around 3–5 kg and is due to excretion of GAG along with water. There is virtually no weight loss in patients with subclinical hypothyroidism with levothyroxine therapy.

49. **How to treat a patient with coronary artery disease and overt hypothyroidism?**

Treatment of overt hypothyroidism in a patient with concurrent coronary artery disease depends on whether the patient is planned for coronary revascularization procedure or not. If coronary revascularization procedure is planned, then it should be contemplated first followed by initiation of levothyroxine in low doses, with gradual titration over a period of time. However, if the patient is not planned for coronary revascularization, then optimal antianginal therapy including β-blockers should be initiated prior to institution of levothyroxine treatment.

50. **How to monitor a patient of primary hypothyroidism on levothyroxine therapy?**

In patients with primary hypothyroidism, serum TSH should be monitored after 6 weeks of initiation of levothyroxine therapy, with a target TSH between 0.45 and 4.12 μIU/ml or within laboratory reference range. However, recent literature shows that targeting TSH between 0.45 to <2.5 μIU/ml is associated with better improvement in quality of life and lipid profile. Failure to achieve TSH within target range requires dose adjustment. However, in elderly individuals, target TSH is higher and should be maintained in upper normal reference range, due to age-related increase in TSH. Sample for TSH should be taken in the morning hours and patient should not take levothyroxine tablet prior to sampling.

51. **What are the conditions where TSH is not useful in monitoring treatment of hypothyroidism?**

The clinical situations where TSH is not useful in monitoring treatment of hypothyroidism are secondary hypothyroidism and in few infants with congenital hypothyroidism during initial months of life (as hypothalamo–pituitary–thyroid axis is reset at a higher level). In addition, TSH is not useful in patients with Graves' disease who develop hypothyroidism while on antithyroid drugs or after radio-ablation, as TSH normalization takes a longer time. Therefore, in all these situations serum total/free T_4 should be monitored and maintained in the upper normal range.

52. **What are the causes of elevated TSH in a patient with primary hypothyroidism despite "optimal" LT_4 treatment?**

The most common cause of elevated TSH with normal T_4 in a patient with primary hypothyroidism on treatment is intermittent administration of levothyroxine, as normalization of serum T_4 occurs much faster than TSH. In addition, anti-mouse antibodies (heterophile antibodies) which interferes with TSH assay, presence of bioinactive but immunoreactive TSH, and occurrence of concurrent thyrotrope hyperplasia in a patient with long-standing hypothyroidism may also result in high TSH with normal T_4. Rarely, polymorphism in type 2 deiodinase may also lead to persistently high TSH despite optimal levothyroxine therapy. The causes of elevated TSH with low T_4 in a patient with hypothyroidism on levothyroxine therapy are poor compliance to treatment, inadequate spacing between the drug and food intake (1 h before breakfast or 4 h after the last meal), and concurrent administration of drugs interfering with levothyroxine absorption like iron, calcium, soya, and proton pump inhibitors. If these conditions have been excluded, then intake of high-fiber diet, celiac disease, inflammatory bowel disease, exocrine pancreatic insufficiency, and autoimmune gastritis should be excluded.

53. **Is weekly levothyroxine therapy better than daily levothyroxine therapy?**

The need behind weekly levothyroxine therapy is to improve compliance to treatment as 82% of hypothyroid patients report noncompliance with daily dose of levothyroxine. The reasons for noncompliance include need for daily administration in fasting state, recommended lag time of 30–45 min between ingestion of tablet and food intake, and the need to avoid commonly used medications like iron and calcium which interfere with absorption of levothyroxine. To improve compliance, weekly levothyroxine therapy has been suggested. The rationale behind weekly levothyroxine therapy is based on the fact that LT_4 has a half-life of 7 days. In a weekly regimen, seven times higher dose than the daily dose of levothyroxine is administered as a single dose once per week. Though administered once weekly, it is not a sustained release preparation of levothyroxine. In a recent study, there was no difference in serum TSH levels achieved with both the regimens, but free T_4 levels were significantly higher in the initial 4 h after administration of LT_4 with weekly regimen, but this was not accompanied with any symptoms of thyrotoxicosis or cardiac dysfunction. However, the data regarding nadir free T_4 levels prior to the administration was not available. Further, the long-term safety data are not available particularly in elderly individuals; therefore, weekly regimen is currently not recommended.

54. **What are anti-mouse antibodies?**

Heterophile antibodies are antibodies against specific animal immunoglobulins and human anti-mouse antibodies (HAMA) are the most common among them.

These antibodies are produced in humans due to contact with animals or vaccination containing animal immunoglobulins and are IgG in nature. Anti-mouse antibodies interfere with the TSH assays leading to falsely high TSH value in the absence of primary thyroid dysfunction. HAMAs are present in up to 10% of normal individuals and 0.5% have clinically significant titers to interfere with TSH assay. To overcome this interference, newer TSH assays have included blocking reagents like polymerized murine IgG.

55. **What is the role of iodine supplementation in patients with hypothyroidism?**

Iodine supplementation in patients with hypothyroidism on levothyroxine replacement has no added advantage in improving thyroid function. However, routine iodized salt intake should be continued as iodine has many extra-thyroidal advantages, which include improvement in pregnancy outcome, anti-oxidant and anticancer properties, and suppression of autoimmunity.

56. **How to treat a patient with hypothyroidism due to iodine deficiency?**

Levothyroxine is the treatment of choice for hypothyroidism due to iodine deficiency. In fact, therapeutic doses of stable iodine should be avoided in these patients because it may induce Jod–Basedow's phenomenon, as patients with long-standing iodine deficiency may harbor thyroid nodules. In addition, iodine deficiency-associated hypothyroidism may have concurrent Hashimoto's thyroiditis and stable iodine treatment in such a scenario may induce iodide myxedema due to permanent Wolff–Chaikoff's effect. Therefore, inadvertent use of stable iodine (e.g., Lugol's solution) in the management of hypothyroidism should be avoided. However, iodine supplementation in the form of iodized salt should be continued.

57. **How to supplement iodine for daily requirement?**

Iodine is an essential element for thyroid health. Iodine is present in alluvium soil and seawater. Therefore, vegetations grown in iodine-rich soil and food of marine origin are ample source of iodine. Because of recurrent floods and consequent soil erosion, iodine is leached away from the soil. Therefore, there is a need to provide iodine through a vehicle which is widely used by the people. This vehicle may be water, milk, salt, wheat flour, or bread. Common salt is universally and consistently consumed; hence, it is the preferred medium to deliver recommended daily allowance for iodine. Potassium iodate (KIO_3), the most stable iodine compound, is used to iodize the common salt. The usual concentration of iodide in salt is 15–20 ppm (1 ppm is equivalent to 1 mg per kg). To provide the RDA of 150 μg iodine with strength of 20 ppm, intake of 10 g salt per day is required. This will have 200 μg of KIO_3, which will be approximately equivalent to 150 μg of elemental iodine.

58. **What are the precautions required for the optimal delivery of iodine from iodized salt?**

The following precautions should be observed while using iodized salt. Salt should be purchased within 3 months of manufacturing date, and at time of purchase, it should be crystal clear and white. It should be stored in a dry airtight container along with plastic pack and should be kept away from the furnace. Once the pack is opened, it must be consumed within 4 weeks. Salt should preferably be added on the table rather than during cooking, as iodine quickly sublimates on exposure to heat.

59. **Does the treatment strategy differ in secondary hypothyroidism?**

In patients with secondary hypothyroidism, assessment of other pituitary hormones is mandatory and glucocorticoid replacement should be initiated prior to levothyroxine therapy, as there is a risk of precipitating adrenal crisis. Requirement of levothyroxine is usually lower in patients with secondary hypothyroidism, as TSH-independent thyroid hormone biosynthesis (15%) continues despite TSH deficiency. However, the requirement of levothyroxine increases with concomitant growth hormone or estrogen replacement. Serum T_4 should be monitored in patients with secondary hypothyroidism on levothyroxine therapy and targeted within the upper range of normal. After optimal replacement with glucocorticoids and/or levothyroxine, there may be unmasking of central diabetes insipidus, as both these hormones are counteractive to antidiuretic hormone.

60. **Is hypothyroidism a contraindication for emergency surgery?**

Hypothyroidism is not a contraindication for emergency surgery. These patients should be supplemented with levothyroxine and can be subjected to emergency surgery even without normalization of serum T_4. Perioperatively, these patients should be monitored for hypotension, hyponatremia, hypoglycemia, and paralytic ileus. Postoperatively, they may have difficulty in weaning from ventilator, bleeding diathesis, and central nervous system depression due to anesthetic agents. However, in patients with overt hypothyroidism planned for elective surgery, serum T_4 but not essentially TSH should be normalized as it is the circulating T_4 which determines the metabolic status and not the TSH. Patients with subclinical hypothyroidism can be taken up for surgery even without levothyroxine supplementation as circulating T_4 is normal in them. However, if treatment is indicated for subclinical hypothyroidism, levothyroxine should be initiated, but normalization of TSH prior to surgery is not warranted.

61. **What are the conditions which require higher doses of levothyroxine?**

Requirement of levothyroxine is increased by 30% in the second trimester of pregnancy and by 50% in third trimester. Similarly, patients on oral contraceptives/hormone replacement therapy also require higher doses. In addition, patients having malabsorption (e.g., celiac disease, jejunal bypass surgery) also need higher doses of levothyroxine. Concomitant use of drugs which are enzyme inducers like rifampicin, carbamazepine, phenytoin, growth hormone, and sertraline also mandates increment of levothyroxine dose. However, drugs interfering with levothyroxine absorption like iron, calcium, proton pump inhibitors, oral bisphosphonates, soya, sucralfate, orlistat, phosphate binders, and aluminum hydroxide need spacing for at least 4–6 h after levothyroxine administration.

62. **How to treat patients with persistent symptoms of hypothyroidism, despite optimal treatment with levothyroxine?**

All patients may not have complete resolution of symptoms despite optimal replacement with levothyroxine and TSH in the target range. These symptoms include lack of weight loss, fatigue, and mood-related disorders. This is usually because of false perception and undue expectations with levothyroxine therapy or rarely resistance to thyroid hormone predominantly at the peripheral level. Some of these patients may benefit with the combined use of levothyroxine and liothyronine, but the data is not supportive.

63. **What is the role of selenium in thyroid disease?**

Metallic elements act as a cofactor in most of the biological reactions, but selenium is an exception. Selenium is incorporated co-translationally into polypeptide chain as selenocysteine and forms selenoproteins. Thyroid gland contains more selenium per gram of tissue than any other organ. The important selenoproteins are iodothyronine deiodinases, glutathione peroxidase, and thioredoxin reductase; the latter two are antioxidants. Selenium deficiency contributes to malfunction of these selenoproteins and may contribute to the development of autoimmune thyroid disease, goiter, and endemic cretinism.

64. **Is routine supplementation of selenium advised?**

Although not robust, some data support that selenium supplementation may reduce anti-TPO antibody levels, decrease the incidence of postpartum thyroiditis, and may be beneficial in thyroid-associated ophthalmopathy. However, selenium use is associated with an increased risk of developing diabetes mellitus. Thus, routine supplementation of selenium is not advised.

65. **What is myxedema coma?**

Myxedema coma is a rare, life-threatening disorder usually seen in those with long-standing, untreated primary hypothyroidism. Rarely, patients with secondary hypothyroidism may also present as myxedema coma. It is characterized by altered mental state, hypoventilation, and hypothermia. Other characteristic features include hypotension, hypoxia, hypercapnia, hyponatremia, hypoglycemia, and heart failure. Myxedema coma is commonly seen in elderly women, especially during winter. Cold exposure, infection, drugs (e.g., diuretics, sedatives, and tranquilizers), trauma, stroke, heart failure, and gastrointestinal bleed are the usual precipitating factors. Euthermia in a patient with myxedema coma suggests the presence of infection. Free/total T_4 and T_3 are characteristically low and TSH is high, although it may not be grossly elevated because of severe systemic illness.

66. **How to treat myxedema coma?**

Recognition and rapid initiation of treatment is important as myxedema coma is associated with high mortality (20–30%). Maintenance of airway and ventilation, restoration of intravascular volume, and identification and treatment of precipitating events improve outcome. Intravenous T_4 is preferred, over oral administration of levothyroxine, as oral levothyroxine may be less effective due to impaired gastrointestinal absorption and paralytic ileus. However, some clinical studies have shown that the route of administration of levothyroxine (oral/intravenous) does not influence the outcome. A bolus of 300–500 μg T_4 intravenously followed by 50–100 μg daily is recommended, until oral medications can be initiated. If intravenous T_4 is not available, then a 500 μg oral loading dose of levothyroxine followed by 100 μg daily is an alternative option. Use of T_4 is advocated because it results in steady and smooth levels of serum T_4, but it has a slow onset of action and impaired T_4 to T_3 conversion in critical illness does not yield the optimal levels of T_3 required for metabolic action. Use of T_3 is suggested because of its greater biologic activity and rapid onset of action; however, it is associated with wide fluctuations in serum levels and increased risk of cardiovascular events. Because of these advantages and limitations, some prefer the combined use of T_4 and T_3. However, there is robust clinical data to suggest that use of T_4 alone is associated with favorable outcome. Intravenous hydrocortisone in stress doses (100 mg bolus followed by 4 mg/h infusion) should be supplemented in all patients anticipating adrenal crisis after T_4 therapy. Glucocorticoids also maintain water and sodium homeostasis. Other supportive measures include passive rewarming with blankets, correction of hypoglycemia, use of appropriate antibiotics, and use of vasopressors in fluid refractory hypotension. Digoxin, diuretics, hypotonic fluids, and active rewarming should be avoided. Poor prognostic factors include advanced age and associated comorbidities like heart failure and sepsis. Outcome is better in levothyroxine naive patients as compared to defaulters, as defaulters have no residual thyroid function.

67. **How is Hashimoto's encephalopathy different from myxedema coma?**

Myxedema coma is a complication of long-standing, untreated primary hypothyroidism and is invariably associated with low/undetectable T_4, whereas Hashimoto's encephalopathy (HE) is an immune-mediated cerebral disorder associated with autoimmune thyroiditis and high titers of anti-TPO antibody, usually with normal thyroid function. Hashimoto's encephalopathy (HE) is steroid responsive, while levothyroxine is the primary treatment of myxedema coma.

68. **What are the salient features of Hashimoto's encephalopathy?**

Hashimoto's encephalopathy is a disorder characterized by altered mental state, seizures, myoclonus, ataxia, memory loss, and hyperreflexia. It is more common in women and in those who have HLA-B8/DRw3 haplotype. These patients are usually euthyroid, but can either be hypothyroid or hyperthyroid. Presence of high titer of anti-TPO antibody and/or anti-thyroglobulin antibody is essential for diagnosis but the antibodies are neither involved in pathogenesis nor does the titer correlate with the severity of disease. The autoantibody against enzyme α-enolase is a specific marker for Hashimoto's encephalopathy. Elevated cerebrospinal fluid protein concentration and electroencephalographic changes like slowing of background activity, triphasic waves, and frontal intermittent rhythmic delta activity (FIRDA) are seen in 80–90% of the patients, but are not specific. MR imaging is usually normal but may demonstrate cerebral atrophy or nonspecific T2 signal abnormalities in the subcortical white matter. However, due to the lack of a sensitive and specific marker, Hashimoto's encephalopathy is a diagnosis of exclusion.

69. **How to treat Hashimoto's encephalopathy?**

Hashimoto's encephalopathy is steroid responsive and recently has been renamed as "steroid-responsive encephalopathy with autoimmune thyroiditis (SREAT)." Treatment includes glucocorticoid and in the presence of hypothyroidism, levothyroxine should be added. Other immunosuppressive drugs like azathioprine or cyclophosphamide may be used in patients who either do not respond to steroids or relapse during treatment. The recovery is rapid (days to weeks) and prognosis is usually good, if diagnosed early.

70. **What are the uses of levothyroxine in non-thyroidal diseases?**

Levothyroxine has been tried in the management of obesity, dyslipidemia, heart failure, and refractory depression even in patients without hypothyroidism. Use of levothyroxine in these non-thyroidal diseases was based on the fact that patients with hypothyroidism who had these abnormalities recovered on treatment with levothyroxine. However, no study has established the efficacy of levothyroxine in patients with these disorders who have normal thyroid function tests. On the contrary, over-replacement may be deleterious and may result in decreased lean mass, osteoporosis, and increased risk of atrial fibrillation.

71. **What are thyromimetics?**

Thyromimetics are designer drug molecules with tissue-specific actions based on their differential affinity to TRα or TRβ receptors. TRα receptor is expressed in heart and skeletal muscle and regulates heart rate and resting energy expenditure in muscle, respectively. TRβ1 receptor is predominantly expressed in liver and regulates cholesterol and lipoprotein metabolism and can be targeted in the treatment of dyslipidemia and nonalcoholic fatty liver disease. TRβ2 receptor in thyrotropes is involved in T_3-mediated feedback regulation and has prompted the use of thyromimetics in the management of resistance to thyroid hormone and in thyrotropinoma.

72. **Why are infections of thyroid gland uncommon?**

    Rich blood supply, profuse lymphatic drainage, adherent thick capsule, and high iodine content of thyroid gland are effective barriers which prevent the lodgment of microorganisms and consequently infection of the thyroid gland. However, tuberculosis and Pneumocystis jirovecii may affect thyroid gland, particularly in those who are immunocompromised.

73. **Do patients with primary hypothyroidism need screening for other autoimmune endocrine disorders?**

    No. The pretest probability of finding other autoimmune endocrine disorder in association with primary hypothyroidism is very low (3%); therefore, screening for other autoimmune endocrine disorder is not recommended.

Suggested Reading

1. Braverman LE, Cooper D. Werner & Ingbar's The Thyroid, 10e A fundamental and clinical text. Wolters Kluwer Health. Lippincott Williams & Wilkins; 2012.
2. Garber JR, Cobin RH, Gharib H, Hennessey JV, Klein I, Mechanick JI, Pessah-Pollack R, Singer PA, Woeber KA. Clinical practice guidelines for hypothyroidism in adults: cosponsored by the American Association of Clinical Endocrinologists and the American Thyroid Association. Endocrine Pract. 2012;18(6):988–1028.
3. Larry JJ, De Groot LJ. Endocrinology. Adult and pediatric. Philadelphia: Elsevier Health Sciences; 2010.
4. Longo D, Anthony F, Dennis K, Stephen H, Jameson J, Loscalzo J. Harrison's principles of internal medicine 18E EB. McGraw Hill Professional; 2012.
5. Melmed S, Polonsky KS, Reed Larsen P, Kronenberg HM. Williams textbook of endocrinology: expert consult. London: Elsevier Health Sciences; 2011.

Thyrotoxicosis 10

10.1 Case Vignette

A 23-year-old female presented with heat intolerance, anxiety, tremor, and palpitation for 4 years. She also complained of weight loss despite increased appetite for 3 years. There was history of proptosis with grittiness in eyes for the past 2 years. She had regular menstrual cycles. There was no family history of thyroid disorder or autoimmune disease. On examination, her pulse rate was 124/min and regular, blood pressure was 160/60 mm Hg, and she had fine tremors with warm and moist palms. She had grade II soft and diffuse goiter with presence of a bruit. Ophthalmic examination revealed proptosis (22 mm) with a clinical activity score of 0/7 and severity score was moderate to severe. There was no dermopathy or acropachy. On investigation, serum T_3 was 5.4 ng/ml (0.8–1.8), T_4 23.4 μg/dl (4.8–12.6), and TSH 0.001 μIU/ml (0.45–4.2). She was diagnosed to have Graves' disease with inactive thyroid-associated orbitopathy and treated with carbimazole 30 mg once a day and propranolol 40 mg thrice daily. She was also advised artificial teardrops, sunglasses with side cover, and head-end elevation while sleeping. After 6 weeks, she had improvement in clinical symptoms and her body weight stabilized. Repeat thyroid function test revealed T_3 2.4 ng/ml, T_4 16.2 μg/dl (4.8–12.6), and TSH 0.001 μIU/ml (0.45–4.2), and she was continued with 30 mg carbimazole and propranolol. Subsequently at 3 months, she had resolution of clinical symptoms and normalization of T_3 and T_4; however, TSH remained suppressed. The dose of carbimazole was decreased to 10 mg and continued for 2 years with 3 monthly monitoring of thyroid function tests. Later, she was subjected to decompressive eye surgery for severe proptosis. On follow-up she is doing fine.

A. Bhansali, Y. Gogate, *Clinical Rounds in Endocrinology: Volume I - Adult Endocrinology*, DOI 10.1007/978-81-322-2398-6_10

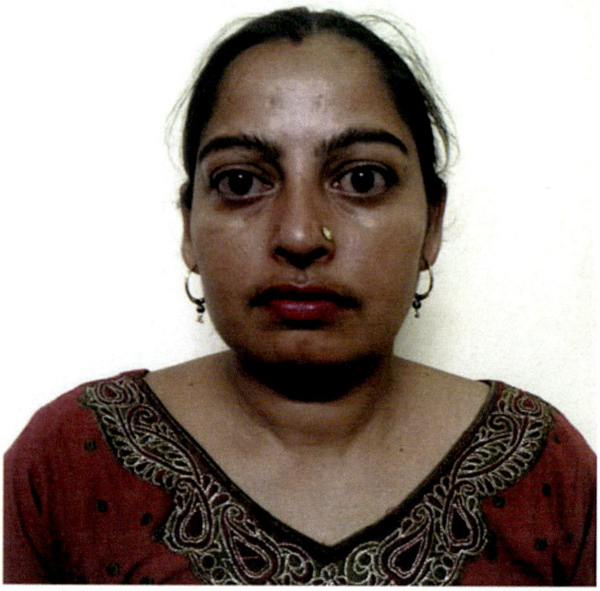

Fig. 10.1 Patient of Graves' disease with grade II goiter and bilateral proptosis

10.2 Stepwise Analysis

Long duration of symptoms of thyrotoxicosis, presence of diffuse goiter, and orbitopathy are consistent with a diagnosis of Graves' disease. In such a scenario, thyroid uptake/scan is not indicated to establish the diagnosis of thyrotoxicosis. However, thyroid scan should be performed in patients who present with short duration of symptoms without orbitopathy to exclude the possibility of subacute thyroiditis. A serum T_3/T_4 ratio >20 (ng/dl:μg/dl) suggests the presence of hyperthyroidism rather than thyroiditis; the index patient had a serum T_3/T_4 ratio of 23. TSH receptor antibody (TRAbs) estimation helps in confirming the diagnosis of Graves' disease, but is not recommended in routine clinical practice. As her serum T_4 was 23.4 μg/dl (i.e., >20 μg/dl), she was started on high-dose carbimazole therapy. β-blocker was added to rapidly ameliorate the adrenergic symptoms, alleviate anxiety, and inhibit peripheral T_4 to T_3 conversion. She had bilateral proptosis suggestive of thyroid-associated orbitopathy and the clinical activity score of 0/7 suggests inactive eye disease. Hence, immunosuppressive therapy was not offered and she was advised supportive measures. At 6 weeks, her symptoms improved, but as both serum T_3 and T_4 were high, she was continued on 30 mg of carbimazole. However, at 3 months as she had resolution of symptoms of toxicosis with normalization of T_3 and T_4, the dose was reduced to 10 mg and β-blocker was discontinued. Once serum T_3 and T_4 normalizes, the dose of antithyroid drugs should be reduced and β-blocker may be discontinued. She was continued with carbimazole for a period of 24 months to exploit the immunomodulatory effect of low-dose antithyroid drugs. She had moderate to severe thyroid-associated orbitopathy, which is unlikely to remit even after achievement of remission of Graves' disease. Therefore, she was subjected to orbital decompression surgery.

10.3 Clinical Rounds

1. **What is thyrotoxicosis?**

   Thyrotoxicosis is a disorder characterized by varied symptoms and signs related to increased metabolism and enhanced adrenergic sensitivity due to high circulating levels of thyroid hormones. The increased level of thyroid hormones may be due to increased endogenous production or release or overzealous exogenous administration of thyroxine.

2. **What is the difference between hyperthyroidism and thyrotoxicosis?**

   Thyrotoxicosis is a state associated with increased circulating levels of thyroid hormones with or without hyperfunctioning of thyroid gland whereas hyperthyroidism refers to increased circulating levels of thyroid hormones with hyperfunctioning of thyroid gland. Thus, "all patients with hyperthyroidism are thyrotoxic, while all patients with thyrotoxicosis are not hyperthyroid."

3. **What is Jod–Basedow phenomenon?**

   Iodine supplementation in an iodine-deficient area resulting in the development of hyperthyroidism is termed as Jod–Basedow phenomenon. The prerequisite for the development of this phenomenon is either the presence of autonomous nodule which is usually seen in elderly individuals or the presence of TSH receptor-stimulating antibodies with diffuse goiter as seen in younger subjects (latent Graves'). Iodine supplementation in these situations acts as a "fuel to fire" and consequently results in thyrotoxicosis. In the current scenario, use of agents with high iodine content like radio-iodinated contrast or amiodarone can induce Jod–Basedow phenomenon, in relatively iodine-deficient subjects with thyroid autonomy.

4. **What is Wolff–Chaikoff's effect?**

   Exposure to excess iodine resulting in transient inhibition of thyroid hormone synthesis is termed as Wolff–Chaikoff's effect. This is due to inhibition of oxidation and organification by excess iodine as a result of formation of organic iodo-compounds and suppression of thyroid peroxidase (TPO) activity. The minimum dose of organic iodide required to produce Wolff–Chaikoff's effect is 2,000 μgm. The inhibitory effect of iodine on thyroid hormone biosynthesis is transient and the gland usually "escapes" within few days. The "escape" is due to iodine-mediated downregulation of sodium–iodide symporter, which prevents further iodine influx into the gland.

5. **What are the causes of persistent Wolff–Chaikoff's effect?**

Wolff–Chaikoff's effect is usually transient and the thyroid gland escapes from this effect in few days in majority of individuals. Failure to escape results in permanent hypothyroidism and can occur in those with underlying thyroid disease, such as chronic autoimmune thyroiditis, past history of subacute or postpartum thyroiditis, and previous ^{131}I or surgical therapy for Graves' disease. Neonates are also predisposed for persistent Wolff–Chaikoff's effect. The persistence of Wolff–Chaikoff's effect is due to failure of downregulation of sodium–iodide symporter in response to excess iodine in these predisposed individuals.

6. **What is "iodide escape"?**

In addition to inhibition of oxidation and organification (i.e., Wolff–Chaikoff's effect), iodine also suppresses the release of thyroid hormones by inhibiting the proteolysis of thyroglobulin. This effect of iodine is exploited in the management of thyroid storm and preoperative preparation of patients with hyperthyroidism. However, after 5–7 days of its use, the gland escapes from this inhibitory effect of iodine on thyroid hormone release. This is called as "iodide escape."

7. **Why is there iodide escape?**

Iodide inhibits thyroglobulin proteolysis and results in inhibition of thyroid hormone release; escape from this effect usually occurs within 5–7 days and is termed as iodide escape. Thyroglobulin proteolysis is a TSH-dependent process. After iodide exposure, there is a rise in TSH due to inhibition of release of thyroid hormones. This increase in TSH restores proteolysis of thyroglobulin resulting in iodide escape. Therefore, when a normal thyroid gland is exposed to high doses of iodine, it exhibits iodide escape as well as escape from Wolff–Chaikoff's effect, whereas a diseased gland exhibits iodide escape but fails to escape from Wolff–Chaikoff's effect.

8. **Why do patients with thyrotoxicosis have adrenergic manifestations?**

Patients with thyrotoxicosis classically present with adrenergic manifestations like tachycardia, increased sweating, tremors, nervousness, and heat intolerance. Embryologically, the thyroid hormone regulates the ontogeny of adrenergic system, and both are involved in non-shivering thermogenesis in lower animals and in humans, to maintain core body temperature. Though adrenergic manifestations predominate the clinical feature of thyrotoxicosis, circulating level of catecholamines are normal. These adrenergic symptoms are due to increased β_1-adrenergic receptor number, affinity, and/or augmented post-receptor signaling mediated through thyroid hormone excess.

9. **Why do patients with thyrotoxicosis have tremor?**

Tremor in patients with thyrotoxicosis is fine, involuntary, and commonly involve hands, tongue, and eyelids. Tremor in thryotoxicosis is due to increased sensitivity and/or expression of β_2-adrenergic receptors on small muscles at these sites. This is evidenced by the rapid resolution of tremor after initiation of β-blockers.

10. **What are the monosymptomatic presentations of thyrotoxicosis?**

The monosymptomatic presentations of thyrotoxicosis include "lone" atrial fibrillation, pyrexia of unknown origin, malabsorption syndrome, hypokalemic or hyperkalemic periodic paralysis, and apathetic hyperthyroidism. Children may present with attention-deficit hyperactivity disorder and tall stature. Rarely hyperpigmentation, gynecomastia, and pruritus with hives can be a presenting manifestation.

11. **What is apathetic hyperthyroidism?**

Apathetic hyperthyroidism is characterized by absence of classical adrenergic manifestations like sweating, palpitations, and tremors, despite thyrotoxicosis. Patients usually present with monosymptomatic manifestations like generalized weakness, unexplained weight loss, "lone" atrial fibrillation, or congestive cardiac failure. Therefore, in clinical practice, a high index of suspicion is required to diagnose apathetic hyperthyroidism. The disorder is usually seen in males and occurs in 10–15% of older patients with hyperthyroidism. Adrenergic manifestations are "masked" due to age-related autonomic neuropathy and relative tissue resistance to thyroid hormone.

12. **What are the causes of loss of appetite in a patient with thyrotoxicosis?**

Patients with thyrotoxicosis commonly have increased appetite, but patients with thyrotoxic cardiomyopathy, apathetic hyperthyroidism, and thyrotoxicosis-induced hypercalcemia may have loss of appetite.

13. **Why is it important to examine the hands in a patient with thyrotoxicosis?**

Examination of the hand in a patient with thyrotoxicosis offers very useful information and can help in differential diagnosis. Tachycardia, tremors, palmar erythema, warm and moist hands are characteristic findings in thyrotoxicosis. Patients with anxiety neurosis can have many of these features; however the presence of cold and moist hands differentiate it from thyrotoxicosis. These manifestations in thyrotoxicosis are due to increased basal metabolic rate, enhanced adrenergic activity, and relative hyperestrogenemia. Thyroid acropachy and onycholysis can also be appreciated. Rarely knuckle hyperpigmentation, vitiligo, and thyroid-associated dermopathy can be seen on the dorsum of the hands.

14. **What are the common cardiac manifestations in thyrotoxicosis?**

Sinus tachycardia is invariably present in patients with thyrotoxicosis, both at rest (90%) and during sleep. Other common arrhythmias include atrial fibrillation (2–15%) and supraventricular tachycardias. Ventricular arrhythmias are extremely rare and if present suggest coexisting hypokalemia or underlying cardiac disease. Congestive cardiac failure is commonly seen in elderly patients with atrial fibrillation or in those with underlying heart disease. Occasionally, younger patients may also present with heart failure even in the absence of rhythm disorders or preexisting heart disease. This is due to thyrotoxic cardiomyopathy which is usually reversible with the achievement of euthyroid state. In addition, patients with thyrotoxicosis can have valvular heart disease, e.g., mitral valve prolapse, which is seen in 5–15% patients and is usually reversible. Lastly, patients with preexisting coronary artery disease may have worsening of their symptoms with the onset of thyrotoxicosis.

15. **Why are supraventricular arrhythmias common in thyrotoxicosis?**

    In patients with thyrotoxicosis, supraventricular arrhythmias like sinus tachycardia (>90%) and atrial fibrillation (5–15%) are more common than atrial premature beats, atrial flutter, and paroxysmal atrial tachycardia, whereas ventricular premature contractions and other ventricular arrhythmias are rare. The predominance of atrial arrhythmias is due to the effect of thyroid hormones on atrial ion channels and atrial enlargement related to volume expansion. The reason for rarity of ventricular arrhythmias is still unclear.

16. **What are the causes of bradycardia in a patient with thyrotoxicosis?**

    The most common cause of bradycardia in patients with thyrotoxicosis is the use of β-blockers. Rarely, sick sinus syndrome has been reported in association with thyrotoxicosis, which is reversible on achievement of euthyroidism.

17. **What are the characteristics of hypertension associated with thyrotoxicosis?**

    Thyrotoxicosis is classically associated with systolic hypertension, decreased diastolic blood pressure, and wide pulse pressure. Systolic hypertension is due to increased cardiac output and augmented myocardial contractility. Decreased diastolic blood pressure is due to peripheral vasodilatation, which occurs as a result of direct effect of thyroid hormones on vasculature and increased nitric oxide production. Peripheral vasodilatation is an adaptive response to enhanced thermogenesis to dissipate heat.

18. **What are the unusual cardiac manifestations of thyrotoxicosis?**

    The unusual cardiac manifestations of thyrotoxicosis, particularly seen in Graves' disease, are mitral valve prolapse, sick sinus syndrome, pulmonary hypertension, rate-related cardiomyopathy, and pleuro-pericardial friction rub (Means–Lerman scratch). Most of these are reversible with adequate and intensive treatment in early stages of the disease.

19. **What are the causes of weight gain in a patient with thyrotoxicosis?**

    Weight loss is the usual feature of thyrotoxicosis, seen in 85% of patients, but weight gain may be seen in 2% of patients. Young individuals with thyrotoxicosis, patients with mild thyrotoxicosis, those receiving glucocorticoids for coexisting thyroid-associated orbitopathy, and patients with congestive cardiac failure may present with weight gain.

20. **What are the alterations in body composition in a patient with thyrotoxicosis?**

    The effect of thyroid hormone excess on body composition includes reduction in lean body mass, fat mass, and bone mineral density. Weight loss in patients with thyrotoxicosis is predominantly due to a decrease in lean body mass, followed by decrease in fat mass. With attainment of euthyroid state, there is restoration of body composition to normal.

21. **What are the abnormalities in glucose–insulin homeostasis in thyrotoxicosis?**

    Patients with thyrotoxicosis may have glucose intolerance, which is attributed to increased intestinal absorption of glucose, enhanced hepatic gluconeogenesis, rapid clearance of insulin, and possibly insulin resistance at receptor level. Hepatic glucose output is increased due to elevated levels of counter-regulatory hormones like glucagon and catecholamines and high levels of lactate (Cori's cycle) due to increased anaerobic glycolysis. On the contrary, patients with Graves' disease may present with hypoglycemia which usually occurs after treatment with methimazole, as it acts as a hapten and induces anti-insulin antibodies. Rarely, treatment-naive patients may have hypoglycemia of autoimmune etiology.

22. **What are the causes of hepatic dysfunction in thyrotoxicosis?**

    Mild hepatic dysfunction is not uncommon in thyrotoxicosis and is seen in 20–30% of patients. The hepatic damage is due to relative hypoxia and commonly manifests as transaminitis. However, severe thyrotoxicosis may lead to advanced hepatic dysfunction due to centrilobular hepatic necrosis ("watershed zone" of liver), and can present as hyperbilirubinemia and transaminitis. Other causes of hepatic dysfunction in patients with thyrotoxicosis are concurrent autoimmune hepatitis, congestive hepatomegaly, and rarely use of antithyroid drugs or pulse methylprednisolone therapy for treatment of thyroid-associated orbitopathy. Propylthiouracil and methylprednisolone result in hepatocellular dysfunction, while carbimazole and methimazole leads to cholestatic jaundice.

23. **Why do patients with hyperthyroidism have gynecomastia?**

    Gynecomastia is present in one-third of patients with hyperthyroidism and is more commonly observed in elderly individuals. This occurs due to the direct stimulatory effect of T_4 on aromatase resulting in increased estradiol levels. In addition, increase in sex hormone-binding globulin (SHBG) due to excess T_4 results in elevated levels of total testosterone and estradiol; but free 17β-estradiol levels are higher than testosterone because of its lesser affinity to bind with SHBG as compared to testosterone, thereby shifting the free testosterone/estradiol ratio in favor of estradiol, leading to gynecomastia.

24. **What are the menstrual abnormalities in thyrotoxicosis?**

Menstrual irregularities are present in 20–60% of women with thyrotoxicosis and manifests as oligomenorrhea, hypomenorrhea, polymenorrhea, or rarely amenorrhea. Despite these menstrual disturbances, majority of women have ovulatory cycles. The mechanisms implicated for menstrual abnormalities are increased sex hormone-binding globulin, decreased free estradiol, impaired LH surge, secondary polycystic ovarian disease, and catabolic state associated with thyrotoxicosis. In addition, 5–6% of women with thyrotoxicosis have infertility, and there is an increased risk of fetal loss due to luteal phase defects and catabolic state.

25. **What are the testicular dysfunctions in thyrotoxicosis?**

Men with thyrotoxicosis can present with decreased libido, erectile dysfunction, gynecomastia, and infertility. These manifestations are due to normal/decreased free testosterone in the presence of increased free estradiol levels. Increase in SHBG due to excess T_4 results in normal/decreased free testosterone. In addition, free estrogen levels are increased because of increased aromatase activity and lesser affinity of estrogen for SHBG, thereby counteracting the effects of testosterone at nuclear receptors. Basal gonadotropin levels are normal or increased, and LH response to GnRH is exaggerated, while testosterone response to hCG is attenuated. Further, the sperm count may be normal or slightly reduced, but motility is consistently decreased (oligoasthenospermia) leading to infertility. These abnormalities are reversible with achievement of euthyroid state.

26. **What are the unusual manifestations of thyrotoxicosis?**

The unusual manifestations of thyrotoxicosis are enlisted in the table given below.

Unusual manifestations	**Remarks**
Apathetic hyperthyroidism	Elderly subjects (age-related neuropathy)
Sinus bradycardia	Use of β-blockers, sick sinus syndrome
Pyrexia of unknown origin	Subacute thyroiditis, Graves' disease
Weight gain	Young patient, mild thyrotoxicosis
Isolated thyroid-associated orbitopathy	May precede hyperthyroidism
Isolated thyroid-associated dermopathy	May precede hyperthyroidism/orbitopathy
Periodic paralysis	Hypokalemia or hyperkalemia
Rhabdomyolysis	Severe thyrotoxicosis
Fracture	Fibrous dysplasia (McCune Albright syndrome) Osteoporosis
Hypercalcemia	Severe bone resorption
Hypoglycemia	Autoimmune, use of methimazole
Gynecomastia	Altered T/E_2 ratio
Hyperpigmentation	Increased cortisol turnover
Lymphadenopathy, thymic hyperplasia, and hepatosplenomegaly	Lymphoreticular hyperplasia due to autoimmunity

27. **What are the causes of thyrotoxicosis?**

The common causes of thyrotoxicosis are Graves' disease, toxic multinodular goiter (MNG), toxic adenoma, subacute thyroiditis, and drugs like amiodarone and iodine-containing contrast agents. Rare causes of thyrotoxicosis are gestational thyrotoxicosis, human chorionic gonadotropin (hCG) secreting tumors, struma ovarii, thyrotropinoma, resistance to thyroid hormone, and McCune–Albright syndrome. Differentiating features among the three common causes of thyrotoxicosis are summarized in the table given below.

Features	Subacute thyroiditis	Graves' disease	Toxic MNG
Duration of illness	Days to weeks Usually timed by the patient	Weeks to months	Months to years
Age and sex	No age or gender predilection	20–40 years F/M = 10:1	Middle aged/elderly F/M = 4–10:1
Symptoms	Very severe	Severe	Mild–moderate
Neck pain	Present	Absent	Absent
Goiter	Small, asymmetrical	Diffuse, soft	Nodular, firm
Orbitopathy/dermopathy	Absent	Present	Absent
Thyroid function test	TSH ↓↓ T_4 ↑↑ T_3 normal/↑	TSH ↓ T_4 ↑ T_3 ↑↑	TSH ↓ T_4 ↑ T_3 ↑↑
$T_3 : T_4$ ratio (ng/dl: μg/dl)	<15	>20	>20
TSH receptor-stimulating antibodies	Absent	Present	Absent
Ultrasonography	Mildly enlarged thyroid gland with very low echogenicity	Diffusely enlarged gland with slightly reduced echogenicity	Multinodular goiter, with variable echogenicity
Color Doppler	Decreased vascularity, may be slightly increased during recovery phase	Increased vascularity	Variable
Radioiodine uptake/ technetium scan	Low uptake	High uptake	Variable depending on functional status of nodules

28. **What is the classical triad of Graves' disease?**

Diffuse toxic goiter, infiltrative orbitopathy, and infiltrative dermopathy constitute the classical triad of Graves' disease. Diffuse toxic goiter is the most common clinical manifestation; however, goiter may not be present in 4% of patients. Goiter is usually diffuse and soft due to increased vascularity in patients with Graves' disease, as against firm goiter in Hashimoto's thyroiditis. Infiltrative orbitopathy is clinically observed in 20–25%; however, on imaging it is present in 90–95% of patients. Infiltrative dermopathy is a rare manifestation, seen only in 3–5% of patients, and is invariably associated with orbitopathy.

29. **What are the causes of nodular goiter in Graves' disease?**

Graves' disease is usually associated with soft and diffuse goiter. However, a nodular goiter may be present in patients with long-standing Graves' disease, particularly who are on intermittent medical therapy. This occurs due to fluctuations in serum TSH levels associated with intermittent therapy. In addition, Graves' disease superimposed on Hashimoto's thyroiditis or MNG can also be associated with nodular thyroid disease.

30. **How to grade a goiter?**

There are various classifications available for the grading of goiter. However, there is marked heterogeneity and lack of clarity in description of goiter. The classification which is practiced at our institute is mentioned below.

Grade 0—No palpable thyroid gland[a]
Grade I—Thyroid gland is palpable and/or visible only in extended neck
Grade II—Thyroid gland is palpable and/or visible in neutral position
Grade III—Thyroid gland is visible from a distance
Grade IV—Monstrous goiter

[a]Normal thyroid gland is barely palpable

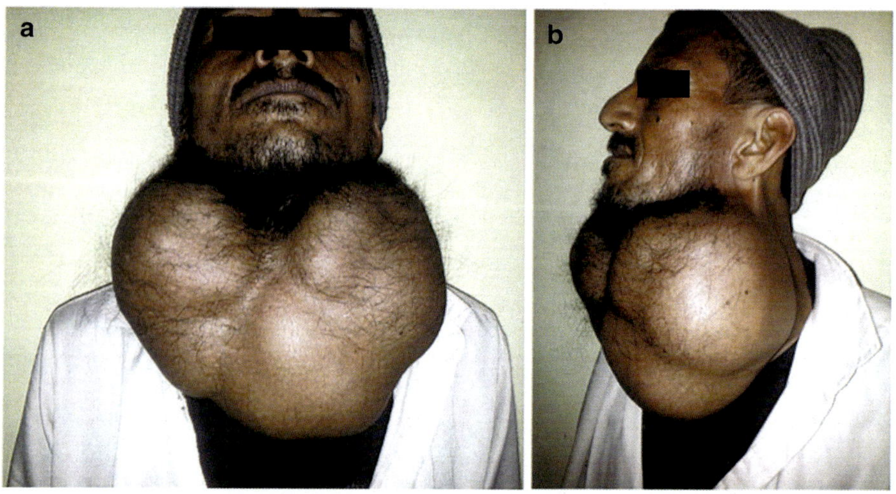

Fig. 10.2 (**a**, **b**) Monstrous euthyroid multinodular goiter in a patient from an iodine-sufficient area

31. **What are the causes of diffuse toxic goiter apart from Graves' disease?**

The most common cause of diffuse toxic goiter is Graves' disease. However, other causes include hereditary non-autoimmune hyperthyroidism (TSH receptor activating mutations, TRAbs negative), thyrotropinoma, and selective central thyroid hormone resistance.

32. **How to clinically suspect subacute thyroiditis?**

Short duration of symptoms, presence of fever and neck pain in a patient with thyrotoxicosis should raise a suspicion of subacute thyroiditis. However, the diagnosis is commonly missed because of monosymptomatic presentations (e.g., rapid weight loss or pyrexia of unknown origin), absence of neck pain, and lack of goiter. Moreover, even if the diagnosis of thyrotoxicosis is considered, many of these patients are managed with antithyroid drugs due to low index of suspicion of subacute thyroiditis. Therefore, every patient with thyrotoxicosis who present with short duration of symptoms and/or lack of goiter should undergo technetium pertechnetate scan or Doppler ultrasound of neck. β-blockers and nonsteroidal anti-inflammatory drugs are the mainstay of therapy, although glucocorticoids may be required in cases with persistent pain, fever, or severe symptoms.

33. **What are the autoimmune disorders associated with Graves' disease?**

The autoimmune disorders associated with Graves' disease include myasthenia gravis, type 1 diabetes mellitus, pernicious anemia, celiac disease, vitiligo, autoimmune thrombocytopenia, autoimmune hepatitis, systemic lupus erythematosus, and autoimmune hypoglycemia.

34. **What are disorders associated with clinical and biochemical discordance in thyroid function tests?**

Thyrotoxicosis is usually associated with elevated T_3 and T_4 and suppressed TSH. However, in certain situations there may be clinical and biochemical discordance which are summarized in the table given below. Therefore, complete thyroid profile including serum T_3, T_4, and TSH should be done to accomplish the correct diagnosis in a patient with suspected thyrotoxicosis.

Biochemical profile	Clinical profile	Diagnosis
Low TSH Normal T_3/T_4	Euthyroid/thyrotoxicosis	Subclinical hyperthyroidism Anti-thyroid drug therapy Pregnancy Corticosteroid therapy
Low TSH Low–normal T_3/T_4	Hypothyroid/euthyroid	Central hypothyroidism Non-thyroidal illness Over treatment with anti-thyroid drugs

Normal TSH
High T3/T4
	Euthyroid	TBG excess
		  Oral contraceptive pills
		  Acute hepatitis
		  Acute intermittent porphyria
		  Familial
		Presence of anti-T_4 antibody

Normal/high TSH *High T3/T4*	Thyrotoxic	TSH-secreting tumor
	Euthyroid/hypothyroid	Resistance to thyroid hormone Intermittent levothyroxine treatment

35. **What are the causes of relative "T_4 toxicosis"?**

The causes of relative "T_4 toxicosis" include hyperthyroidism in elderly, amiodarone-induced thyrotoxicosis, iodine-induced hyperthyroidism, hyperthyroidism with concurrent non-thyroidal illness (sick euthyroid syndrome), and exogenous T_4 therapy.

36. **What are the causes of relative "T_3 toxicosis"?**

Hyperthyroidism of any etiology (Graves' disease, toxic multinodular goiter, toxic adenoma) is associated with relative "T_3 toxicosis." In addition, patients receiving antithyroid drugs may also have relatively higher T_3 levels than T_4. This is because of inhibition of oxidation and organification by the drugs resulting in inability of the gland to utilize intra-thyroidal iodine, thereby leading to relatively higher secretion of T_3 (iodide economy). However, exogenous liothyronine therapy and hyperthyroidism associated with concurrent iodine deficiency will manifest as T_3 toxicosis with normal serum T_4.

37. **Why do patients with hyperthyroidism have relative T_3 toxicosis?**

In physiological states, circulating T_4 is exclusively produced from thyroid gland, while 80% of circulating T_3 is contributed by peripheral deiodination of T_4 to T_3 and only 20% by thyroid gland. Hyperthyroidism is characterized by a relatively greater increase in T_3 as compared to T_4. This relative T_3 toxicosis is due to increased intra-thyroidal as well as extra-thyroidal conversion of T_4 to T_3 because of activation of type 1 deiodinase (D1) by excess T_4. On the contrary, thyroiditis is characterized by release of preformed hormones; hence, it mimics the secretory profile of normal thyroid gland and has predominant T_4 secretion.

38. **What is the importance of estimating serum TSH in patients with thyrotoxicosis at diagnosis?**

Elevated serum free T_4 and/or free T_3 with suppressed TSH is the characteristic biochemical abnormality of thyrotoxicosis. Isolated measurement of free T_3 and T_4 may miss the diagnosis of subclinical hyperthyroidism, thyrotropinoma, and resistance to thyroid hormone. Therefore, in patients with suspected thyrotoxicosis, complete thyroid profile including free T_3, free T_4, and TSH should be measured.

39. **Why is the recovery of TSH delayed in patients with hyperthyroidism on treatment?**

In patients with hyperthyroidism on treatment, TSH may remain suppressed for a longer duration despite normalization of circulating T_3 and T_4. The delayed recovery of TSH may be a consequence of prolonged inhibitory effect of circulating T_3 and T_4 on thyrotropes. In addition, intrapituitary cytokines (TNF-α and IL-6 released by pituicytes) may exert a suppressive effect on thyrotropes by accelerating intrapituitary conversion of T_4 to T_3, resulting in delayed recovery of TSH particularly in patients with Graves' disease. The clinical implication of this biochemical observation is that the dose adjustment of antithyroid drugs should be based on serum T_3/T_4 levels rather than TSH in patients with hyperthyroidism.

40. **What are the indications for measuring TSH receptor antibodies?**

TSH receptor-stimulating antibodies are a specific marker of Graves' disease and are present in 80–95% of patients, whereas anti-TPO antibody and anti-Tg antibody are non-specific markers of autoimmune thyroid disease and are present in 80% and 70%, respectively. However, the routine estimation of TSH receptor antibodies is not advised. Specific indications for estimation of TSH receptor antibody include pregnant women with Graves' disease, isolated thyroid-associated orbitopathy/ dermopathy and to predict remission in Graves' disease during therapy.

41. **What are the indications for thyroid scintigraphy?**

In clinical practice thyroid scintigraphy is most commonly used to differentiate between subacute thyroiditis and Graves' disease. In addition, patients with congenital hypothyroidism, functioning thyroid nodule, suspected ectopic thyroid, thyroid carcinoma, and midline neck swelling (thyroglossal cyst) also require thyroid scintigraphy.

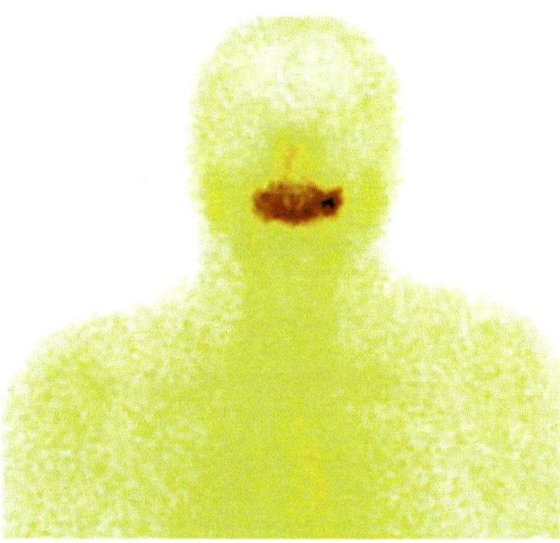

Fig. 10.3 ^{99m}Tc pertechnetate thyroid scan with negligible tracer uptake in the region of neck in a patient who presented with thyrotoxicosis. The scan is consistent with a diagnosis of subacute thyroiditis

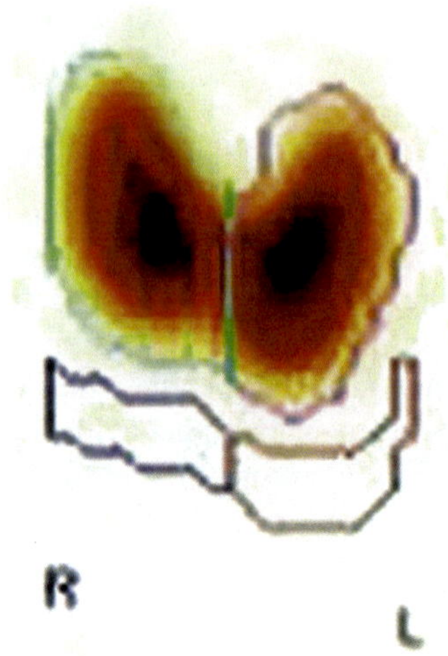

Fig. 10.4 ^{99m}Tc pertechnetate thyroid scan showing enlarged thyroid gland with homogenously increased tracer uptake in both the lobes with uptake at 20 min 53.6% (Normal <4%) suggestive of Graves' disease

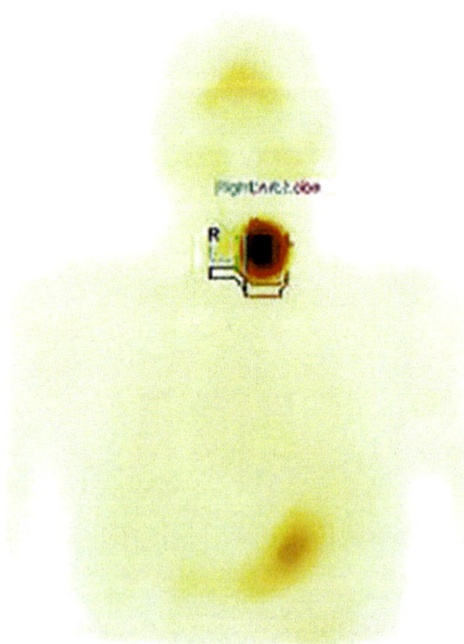

Fig. 10.5 ^{99m}Tc pertechnetate thyroid scan showing increased uptake in a nodule with reduced uptake in the rest of thyroid gland suggestive of toxic adenoma

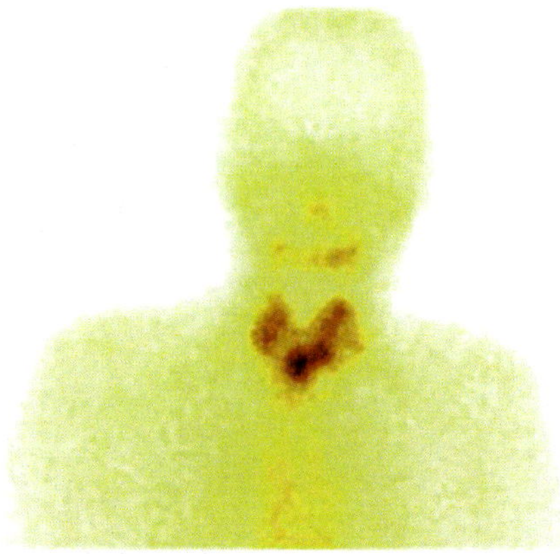

Fig. 10.6 ^{99m} Tc pertechnetate thyroid scan showing enlarged gland with increased uptake in multiple nodules and normal/ reduced uptake in the rest of thyroid gland suggestive of toxic multinodular goiter

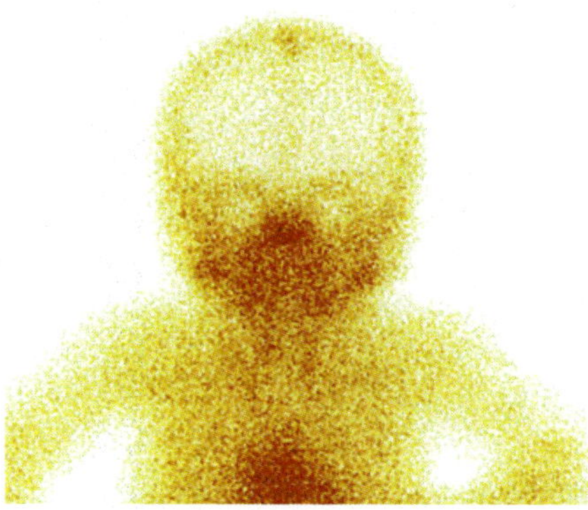

Fig. 10.7 ^{99m}Tc pertechnetate thyroid scan showing no uptake in the region of neck in a child with congenital hypothyroidism suggestive of thyroid aplasia

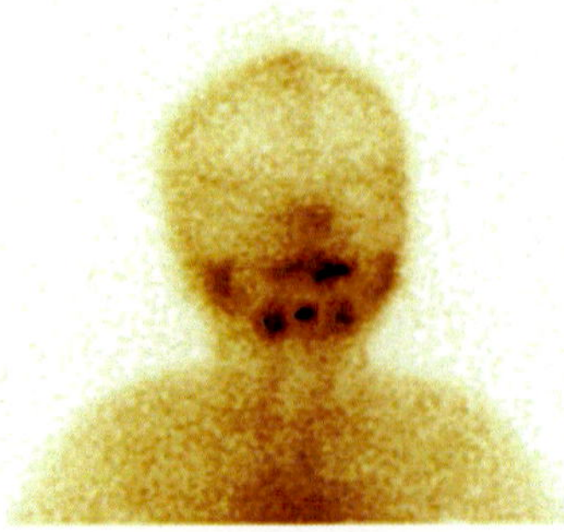

Fig. 10.8 ^{99m}Tc pertechnetate thyroid scan showing tracer uptake in the region of floor of mouth without any uptake in the neck suggestive of lingual thyroid

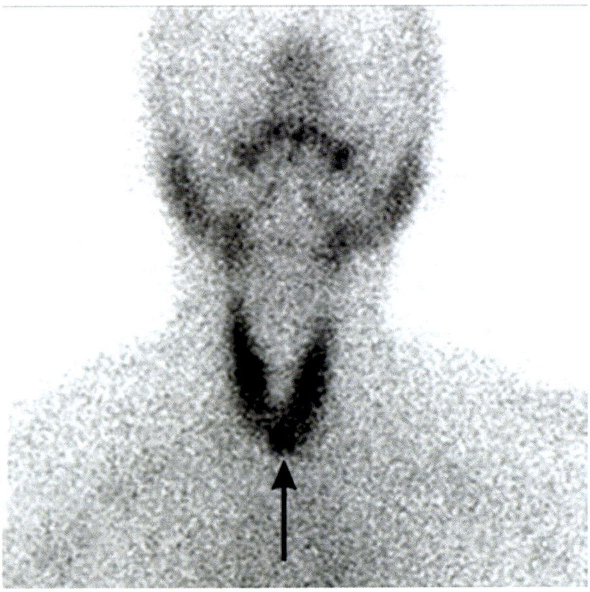

Fig. 10.9 ^{99m}Tc pertechnetate thyroid scan showing normal thyroid tissue and a thyroglossal cyst (arrow)

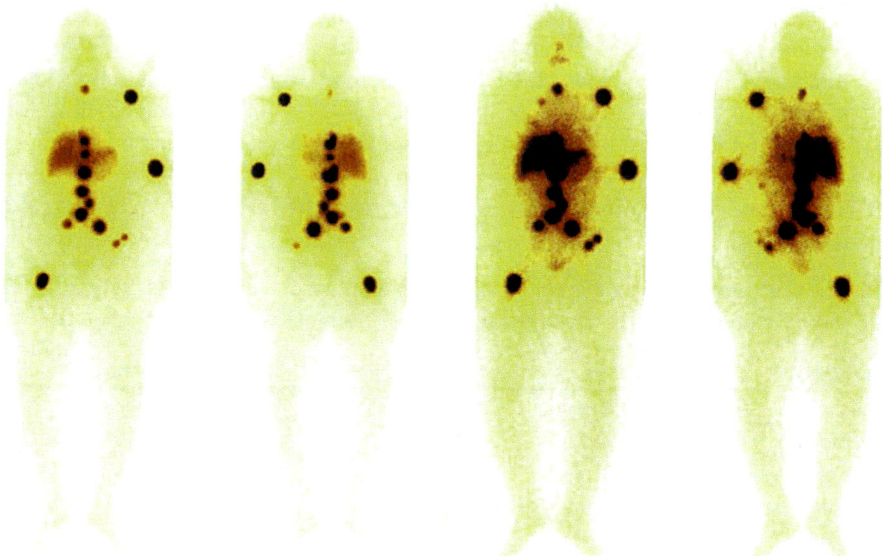

Fig. 10.10 ^{131}I scan showing skeletal metastasis in a patient with papillary thyroid carcinoma

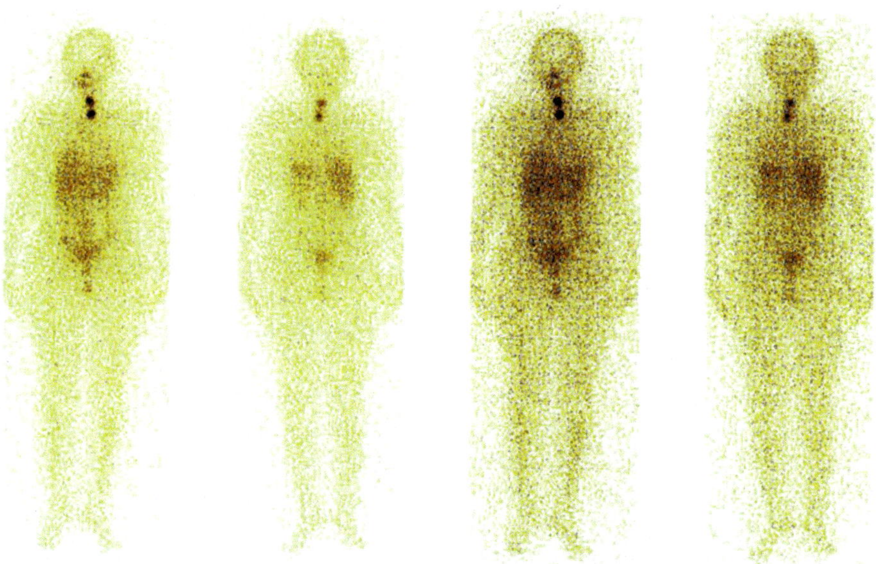

Fig. 10.11 ^{131}I scan showing cervical lymph node metastasis in a patient with papillary thyroid carcinoma

42. **What are the available isotopes of iodine?**

Natural iodine exists as ^{127}I and is the stable form of iodine. The available isotopes are ^{123}I, ^{124}I, ^{125}I, and ^{131}I, which are obtained from uranium fission. ^{125}I has the longest half-life of 60 days; therefore, it is used for hormone labeling for radioimmunoassay. ^{124}I has a half-life of 4.2 days and is used for PET scan.

43. **What are the radionuclides available for the assessment of thyroid disorders?**

The radionuclides available for the assessment of thyroid disorders include ^{123}I, ^{131}I, and ^{99m}Tc pertechnetate. Their properties are summarized in the table given below.

Parameters	**^{123}I**	**^{131}I**	**^{99m}Tc pertechnetate**
Source	Uranium	Uranium	Uranium/molybdenum
Half-life	13.2 h	8 days	6 h
Type of radiation	ϒ rays	β and ϒ rays	ϒ rays
Radiation exposure	Low	High	Lowest
Uptake via	NIS	NIS	NIS
Organification	Yes	Yes	No
Image quality	Excellent	Good	Very good
Route of administration	Oral	Oral	Intravenous
Background activity	Low	Low	High
Availability	Limited	Easily available	Easily available
Cost	Expensive	Inexpensive	Inexpensive

44. **Which is an ideal radionuclide for the assessment of thyroid disorders?**

^{123}I is an ideal radionuclide for the assessment of thyroid disorders. It is trapped via NIS and is organified within the thyroid gland. Its short half-life, minimum stunning effect, lesser radiation exposure, and pure ϒ emittance makes it a preferable radionuclide as compared to ^{131}I. Moreover, the images obtained after the procedure are distinct as it is organified within the gland and has minimal back ground activity. However, cost and limited availability precludes its routine clinical use. ^{99m}Tc pertechnetate is a pure ϒ emitter, has the shortest half-life, and has minimal procedural time (20 min), and its easy availability along with low cost makes it a suitable alternative in clinical practice. However, it is not involved in the process of organification; therefore, it is quickly washed out and the images obtained are less distinct.

45. **What are the advantages and disadvantages of ^{99m}Tc thyroid scintigraphy?**

Besides its easy availability, low cost, and early acquisition of images, ^{99m}Tc pertechnetate can also be used in patients who are on antithyroid drugs without discontinuation of therapy. This is because ^{99m}Tc is only trapped but not organified within the thyroid gland and antithyroid drugs interfere with organification, but not with trapping. However, antithyroid drugs should be omitted for at least 5–7 days prior to iodine scan, as ^{123}I and ^{131}I are organified within the thyroid gland. ^{99m}Tc is not useful in the diagnosis of dyshormonogenesis as technetium is not organified in the gland and has limited usefulness in cases of retrosternal goiter due to increased background activity.

46. **What are the disorders associated with discordant findings on ^{99m}Tc pertechnetate and ^{131}I scan?**

Although both ^{99m}Tc and ^{131}I are functional scans, at times the results of these modalities may be discordant. The most important cause of discordance between these modalities is thyroid dyshormonogenesis. In addition, patients with multinodular goiter and rarely, metastatic thyroid carcinoma may also show discordant results.

47. **What is the unique dual role of ^{131}I?**

^{131}I emits both ϒ and β rays. The ϒ rays are helpful in diagnostic imaging, while β rays are cytotoxic and useful in radio-ablation. Radioablative effect is mediated through free radical generation, decreased vascularity, and karyorrhexis.

48. **What are the precautions to be taken before subjecting a patient to thyroid scintigraphy?**

Patient should be enquired about drug intake, last menstrual period, and lactational status before thyroid scintigraphy. Those with history of exposure to iodine-containing contrast or amiodarone intake should wait for at least 3 months prior to scan. Thyroid scan should be deferred for 2–4 weeks in patients who are receiving expectorants containing potassium iodide. Exogenous administration of thyroid hormone or antithyroid drugs reduce radioiodine uptake and hence should be stopped at least for 4 weeks and 5–7 days, respectively, prior to scanning. β-blockers can be continued as they do not interfere with sodium–iodide symporter-mediated uptake. The patient need not be fasting, but heavy meal should be avoided. Pregnancy and lactation are absolute contraindications for ^{131}I scan; however, if essential, ^{99m}Tc scan may be performed.

49. **What are sodium-iodide symporter inhibitors?**

Sodium-iodide symporter (NIS) is essential for the transport of iodine from extracellular fluid to thyroid follicular cells. Fluoride, thiocyanate, perchlorate, and nitrate when present in excess can competitively inhibit NIS, thereby interfering with the transport of iodine into follicular cells, resulting in goiter.

50. **A 30-year-old male presented with rapid weight loss and tremor of 4 weeks duration. On evaluation, he had tachycardia, tremor, and grade I diffuse goiter. He had elevated T_3 and T_4 and suppressed TSH. How should he be investigated further?**

The close differential diagnoses with this clinical and biochemical profile are subacute thyroiditis and diffuse toxic goiter due to Graves' disease. The best investigation to differentiate these two disorders is a thyroid uptake study. Thyroid uptake will be low or suppressed in thyroiditis, while it will be high in Graves' disease. In such scenario, thyroid scan is not indicated as it does not provide any additional information over thyroid uptake study.

51. **What are the treatment modalities available for hyperthyroidism?**

    Available treatment modalities include antithyroid drugs (ATD), ^{131}I radio-ablation, and thyroid surgery. Treatment should be individualized based on age, etiology, size of goiter, concurrent comorbidities, patient's preference, and special situations like pregnancy.

52. **What are the available antithyroid drugs?**

    The available antithyroid drugs are carbimazole, methimazole, and propylthiouracil (PTU). Their properties are summarized in the table given below.

Parameters	Carbimazole	Methimazole	Propylthiouracil
Oral bioavailability	93%	93%	65–75%
Protein binding	Nil	Nil	75%
Serum half-life	6–8 h	6–8 h	1–2 h
Intra-thyroidal half-life	17–20 h	17–20 h	12 h
Equivalent dose	5 mg	3 mg	50 mg
T_4 to T_3 conversion	No effect	No effect	Inhibits
Metabolism in thyrotoxicosis	Increased	Increased	Normal
Effects on radio-ablation	Nil	Nil	Induces radio-resistance
Transplacental passage	High	High	Low
Secretion in breast milk	High	High	Low
Adverse events	Cholestasis	Cholestasis	Hepatitis

53. **Which is the preferred antithyroid drug?**

    Carbimazole and methimazole are the preferred antithyroid drugs in management of Graves' disease. Carbimazole is a prodrug which is converted to methimazole in liver. They are preferred over PTU because of once daily dosing, earlier achievement of euthyroid state, and lesser side effects. The rationale of once daily dosing despite a serum half-life of only 6–8 h is that both carbimazole and methimazole are actively concentrated in thyroid follicular cells (thyroid : plasma concentration—16:1) and have a longer intra-thyroidal half-life of 17–20 h. The higher potency and higher intra-thyroidal half-life of these drugs as compared to PTU aid in the achievement of early euthyroidism (6 weeks vs. 12 weeks). Further, side effects like agranulocytosis and hepatic failure are more common with the use of PTU.

54. **When is propylthiouracil preferred?**

    Propylthiouracil (PTU) is hepatotoxic and may result in fulminant hepatic failure; therefore, it is not recommended in routine clinical practice. However, it is preferred during first trimester of pregnancy due to its low transplacental passage because of its increased binding with serum albumin; thereby decreasing the risk of thionamide embryopathy. However, the recent literature does not support this observation. In addition, propylthiouracil is also preferred in patients with thyroid storm, as it inhibits peripheral T_4 to T_3 conversion.

55. **How to initiate and titrate antithyroid drugs in Graves' disease?**

The initiating dose of carbimazole is 30–40 mg per day in patients with Graves' disease who have serum T_4 levels >20 μg/dl and 20 mg per day in those with T_4 levels <20 μg/dl. Dose higher than 30–40 mg does not have any additional advantage, even in patients with severe thyrotoxicosis. The use of high doses of carbimazole (>20 mg) in patients with serum T_4<20 μg/dl leads to rapid development of hypothyroidism. Carbimazole is usually given once a day; however, it may be given twice daily in those with severe toxicosis, as the drug is rapidly washed out by the hyperfunctioning thyroid gland. Patients commonly achieve clinical and biochemical euthyroidism (normalization of both T_4 and T_3) within 6–12 weeks of therapy, and thereafter, dose should be reduced by 5 mg every 2–3 months with serial monitoring of serum T_4 and T_3 levels, followed by a maintenance dose of 5–10 mg till 18–24 months. The rationale of continuing low-dose antithyroid drugs for a prolonged duration despite normalization of T_3, T_4, and/or TSH is to prevent relapse by exploiting the immunomodulatory effects of the drug. These effects are mediated through a decrease in MHC class II antigen expression and reduction of intra-thyroidal inflammatory cytokines. In routine clinical practice, non-iodized salt is commonly advised during the management of hyperthyroidism; however, there is paucity of literature regarding its effectiveness.

56. **How to monitor a patient with Graves' disease on antithyroid drugs?**

Patients of Graves's disease on drugs should be monitored with serum T_3 and T_4 at intervals of 4–6 weeks, till serum T_4 is normalized. Serum T_3 may not return to normal for a longer period, despite normalization of T_4 as thyroid gland preferentially secretes T_3 due to intra-thyroidal iodine deficiency induced by antithyroid drugs. In this scenario, the dose of antithyroid drugs should not be decreased; rather, it may require increment. Once serum T_3 and T_4 are normalized, the dose of antithyroid drugs has to be decreased and TSH should also be monitored, along with T_3 and T_4, at a frequency of every 2–3 months. TSH takes a much longer time (>6–12 months) to recover. Once TSH is normalized, patients should be continued on maintenance doses of antithyroid drugs till 18–24 months and TSH should be monitored at a frequency of 3–6 months.

57. **A 40-year-old male, known case of Graves' disease on carbimazole 20 mg for 3 months, presented with serum T_3 2.5 ng/ml, T_4 6.5 μg/dl, and TSH 0.01 μIU/ml. What to do next?**

Serum T_4 is the earliest biochemical parameter to normalize on antithyroid drug treatment, followed by T_3 and finally TSH. If serum T_3 does not normalize despite normal or low T4, the doses of antithyroid drugs should not be decreased, rather may require increment in dose. Therefore, the aim of antithyroid drug therapy is to normalize both T_3 and T_4 levels and tapering of antithyroid drugs should be attempted thereafter.

58. **A 30-year-old female was diagnosed to have Graves' disease and was started on carbimazole 30 mg/day. After 6 months of treatment, she presented with features of hypothyroidism and her T_3 was 0.8 ng/ml, T_4 4 μg/dl, and TSH 20 μIU/ml. What to do next?**

    The index patient developed hypothyroidism after 6 months of antithyroid drug therapy. The most common cause of hypothyroidism in such a scenario is the failure to taper antithyroid drugs during follow-up. The possible management options are reduction in dose of carbimazole, addition of levothyroxine to carbimazole therapy (block–replacement therapy), and discontinuation of carbimazole with initiation of levothyroxine. The most appropriate strategy in this patient is to reduce the dose of carbimazole to 10 mg/day and repeat thyroid function test after 4–6 weeks, as this patient has received antithyroid drug therapy for only 6 months. The rationale for this approach is to continue antithyroid drug as an immunomodulator for 18–24 months to prolong the remission. The addition of levothyroxine to high-dose carbimazole has been tried as a modality to improve remission rate in patient with Graves' disease, as both carbimazole and levothyroxine have immunomodulatory action. But this regimen does not offer any additional advantage over low-dose carbimazole therapy alone. Discontinuation of carbimazole and initiation of levothyroxine is very tempting in this scenario; but the probability of resurgence of disease is very high as the patient has received antithyroid drugs for only 6 months.

59. **What are the causes of increase in size of goiter in a patient with Graves' while on treatment with antithyroid drugs?**

    Approximately one-third of patients of Graves' disease have a decrease in size of goiter with the use of antithyroid drugs. However, goiter may increase in size even on antithyroid drugs in certain situations which include development of hypothyroidism on treatment, worsening of Graves' disease, and rarely, evolution of thyroid malignancy. Further, intermittent therapy with antithyroid drugs and inadvertent treatment of thyrotropinoma as Graves' disease with antithyroid drugs may also result in an increase in size of goiter.

60. **When to stop antithyroid drug therapy in patients with Graves' disease?**

    Decision to discontinue antithyroid drugs may be taken after 18–24 months of therapy with normalization of T_3, T_4, and TSH while on maintenance dose of 5–10 mg of carbimazole along with disappearance of TRAbs. If TSH is not normalized and/or TRAbs titers are still measurable, then continuation of antithyroid drugs beyond 24 months may not be rewarding. Therefore, options in these patients include radio-ablation or surgery. However, recent data suggests that continuation of low-dose antithyroid drugs for 5–10 years is safe and may prevent relapses.

61. **How to define remission in Graves' disease?**

Remission in Graves' disease is defined as maintenance of euthyroid state for at least 1 year after discontinuation of antithyroid drugs. This definition is not applicable in those who are treated with ablative measures. Treatment with antithyroid drugs for 18–24 months yields remission in approximately 50% of patients. A period of 1 year is chosen for defining remission because majority of the relapses occur within the first 3–6 months of discontinuation of therapy and relapses are uncommon after 1 year.

62. **How does antithyroid drug therapy induce remission in Graves' disease?**

Although Graves' disease is an autoimmune disorder, hyperthyroidism per se leads to alterations in function of T_{reg} and B cells, resulting in increased generation of TRAbs. Therefore, achievement of euthyroidism by any treatment modality paves the way toward remission by decreasing the production of TRAbs. Antithyroid drugs inhibit thyroid peroxidase-mediated oxidation, organification, and coupling, thereby reducing thyroid hormone production. Further, antithyroid drugs also exert immunomodulatory effects on thyroid follicular cells and targets the pathogenic mechanisms implicated in Graves' disease. Therefore, prolonged immunosuppression for 18–24 months results in long-term remission in patients with Graves' disease.

63. **What are the predictors of remission in Graves' disease?**

The predictors of remission of Graves' disease are female gender, young age, small goiter, T_3 toxicosis, decrease in size of goiter during treatment, normalization of TSH, and declining levels of TRAbs on antithyroid drugs.

64. **Who are the patients of Graves' disease unlikely to achieve remission on antithyroid drugs?**

Patients with older age, large goiter (grade III and above), and severe thyrotoxicosis (T_3>9 ng/ml) are unlikely to achieve remission with antithyroid drug treatment. In addition, shorter duration of treatment (<18 months), inability to taper antithyroid drugs to maintenance doses (5–10 mg carbimazole) over 18–24 months, lack of normalization of TSH, development of nodularity, or persistence of TRAbs during treatment diminish the possibility of achieving remission. Further, males and chronic smokers are less likely to achieve remission.

65. **What are the strategies to prevent relapse in Graves' disease?**

The strategies that have been exploited to prevent relapse in patients with Graves' disease include prolonged duration of antithyroid drug therapy, high-dose antithyroid drugs, and block–replacement therapy. Treatment with antithyroid drugs for 18–24 months has been shown to be effective in preventing relapse in 50% of patients. Duration of therapy beyond 24 months does not influence the outcome. The use of high-dose antithyroid drugs (carbimazole >40 mg/day) or block–replacement therapy does not improve remission rate.

66. **A 40-year-old female was diagnosed to have Graves' disease and was started with 40 mg of carbimazole daily. After 3 months of therapy, her serum T_3 is 3.6 ng/ml, T_4 18 μg/dl, and TSH 0.001 μIU/ml. How to proceed further?**

Majority of patients with Graves' disease will achieve euthyroidism at this dose over a period of 3 months. In case of failure to respond, compliance to therapy must be ensured and use of iodine-containing drugs (e.g., cough expectorants) must be excluded. Patients who are severely thyrotoxic may require carbimazole in divided doses due to increased intra-thyroidal drug turnover and enhanced peripheral metabolism. If these measures are ensured and patient is still toxic, a further increase in dose of antithyroid drugs may not be useful. Therefore, these patients should be considered for ablative treatment. Although the term "drug failure" is not defined for antithyroid drugs, it should be considered if there is failure to achieve euthyroidism over a period of 12 weeks even after administering 30–40 mg of carbimazole per day.

67. **What is block–replacement therapy?**

Block–replacement therapy (BRT) comprises the use of high-dose antithyroid drugs (30 mg of carbimazole) with levothyroxine (100–150 μg). BRT was used in patients with Graves' disease to achieve a higher rate of remission by exploiting the immunomodulatory potential of antithyroid drugs and concurrent use of levothyroxine to prevent hypothyroidism. Further, levothyroxine decreases expression of thyroid antigens (TSH receptor) by inhibiting TSH and has immunomodulatory effects. However, BRT has not been shown to be superior in achieving higher remission rates, as compared to low-dose antithyroid drug therapy.

68. **What are the indications for block–replacement therapy?**

BRT may be beneficial in patients with thyroid-associated orbitopathy, as shown in a recent study where low-dose carbimazole (5 mg) and levothyroxine (100 μg) were shown to stabilize TSH and maintain euthyroid state without worsening of orbitopathy for a period of 5 years. Use of BRT in Graves' disease during pregnancy is not recommended as transplacental passage of antithyroid drugs is disproportionately higher than levothyroxine and fetal thyroid gland is extremely sensitive to antithyroid drugs, thereby increasing the risk of fetal hypothyroidism. However, pregnant women with Graves' disease who have undergone ablative therapies (radio-ablation or surgery) and are still TRAb positive should be treated with BRT if signs of fetal hyperthyroidism are present. In this scenario, antithyroid drugs help to control fetal thyrotoxicosis and levothyroxine restores euthyroidism in the mother.

69. **Is routine monitoring for neutropenia or hepatic dysfunction indicated in patients on antithyroid drugs?**

Complete blood count and liver function tests are recommended in all patients prior to initiation of antithyroid drug therapy. However, there is no recommendation for monitoring these parameters during therapy, as neutropenia and hepatic dysfunction are idiosyncratic adverse events and can occur at any time during treatment. Mild neutropenia (1,000–1,500/mm^3) is a feature of active Graves' disease per se and is not a contraindication for initiation of antithyroid drugs. However, appearance of sore throat and/or fever while on treatment should raise the possibility of drug-induced agranulocytosis (neutrophil count <500/mm^3). Transaminitis and hyperbilirubinemia can occur in severe thyrotoxicosis, but is not a contraindication to antithyroid drug therapy; rather, it may abate on treatment. Evolution of hepatic dysfunction on treatment suggests drug-induced liver damage and the offending drug should be omitted. Switching from carbimazole to propylthiouracil or vice versa is not recommended in patients with agranulocytosis because of cross-reactivity between these drugs, while in patients with hepatic dysfunction switchover has been tried as these drugs produce different types of hepatic injury, but it is not favored in clinical practice. Therefore, in these situations, patient should be initiated/continued with β-blockers and planned for radio-ablation/surgery.

70. **What are the indications of β-blockers in thyrotoxicosis?**

Current guidelines recommend the use of β-blockers as an adjunct therapy in all patients with thyrotoxicosis, as they ameliorate adrenergic symptoms rapidly. However, β-blockers are particularly useful in patients with atrial fibrillation with rapid ventricular rate, rate-related heart failure, thyrotoxic periodic paralysis, and thyroid storm. They are also effective in thyrotoxicosis-associated hypercalcemia, as T_4 increases bone resorption through β-adrenergic receptors. In addition, β-blockers are also indicated in those awaiting diagnostic evaluation and during the interim period post radio-ablation. β-blockers should be continued till serum T_3 and T_4 levels are normalized, except in patients with atrial fibrillation and thyrotoxic periodic paralysis where continued use of β-blockers is recommended till ablative treatment is ascertained. In patients with subacute thyroiditis, β-blockers are the prime modality of treatment. β-blockers should be used with caution during pregnancy as they may increase the risk of fetal/neonatal bradycardia, hypoglycemia, and intrauterine growth retardation.

71. **Which is the preferred β-blocker in the management of thyrotoxicosis?**

Nonselective β-blocker like propranolol is preferred as it inhibits peripheral conversion of T_4 to T_3 by inhibiting deiodinase type 1 and also alleviates anxiety by reducing central adrenergic drive. But, selective β-blockers like metoprolol or atenolol are also shown to be equally effective and may be an alternative to propranolol in patients with bronchial asthma. Esmolol, a short-acting β-blocker with rapid effect, is preferred in patients with thyroid storm. β-blockers are usually contraindicated in patients with heart failure; however, in those with rate-related heart failure, selective β1-blockers can be used with caution.

72. **What are the uses of inorganic iodide?**

Inorganic iodide is used in the management of thyroid storm and for preoperative preparation of patients with hyperthyroidism. Use of iodide reduces the vascularity of gland and makes it firm, thereby reducing blood loss during surgery. This is due to the direct effect of iodide on thyroid gland as well as its ability to prevent the effect of rising TSH (due to inhibitory effect of iodide on release of thyroid hormones) on thyroid gland. In addition, it is also used for shielding thyroid gland during nuclear scintigraphy performed for evaluation of extra-thyroidal disorders (e.g., ^{131}I MIBG scan for pheochromocytoma) and during nuclear disasters involving radioiodine.

73. **How to manage nuclear disasters involving radioiodine?**

Iodide is the best available option to protect thyroid gland during nuclear disasters, as it competes with radioiodine for NIS and does not allow the trapping of radioiodine. Theoretically, levothyroxine in high doses may also be used to protect the gland as it inhibits TSH and downregulates NIS, thereby preventing the uptake of radioiodine.

74. **When is ^{131}I radio-ablation preferred over other treatment modalities in the management of hyperthyroidism?**

^{131}I radio-ablation therapy is safe, effective, and inexpensive. It is the treatment of choice in patients with toxic adenoma. It is also preferred in patients with Graves' disease who are elderly and have large goiter (grade III) or comorbidities like cardiac failure or past history of thyrotoxic periodic paralysis. In addition, those who are intolerant to antithyroid drugs or have persistence/relapse of disease despite optimal medical treatment or have contraindications to antithyroid drugs may also be considered for radio-ablation. Further, patients with toxic multinodular goiter who are elderly, refuse surgery, or have comorbidities may also be subjected to radio-ablation. In patients who remain toxic despite ^{131}I, radio-ablation may require a repeat dose, which can be contemplated after 6 months of initial dose.

75. **What are the prerequisites before subjecting a patient of hyperthyroidism to ^{131}I radio-ablation?**

Pregnancy is an absolute contraindication for the use of ^{131}I therapy and urine pregnancy test is mandatory prior to radio-ablative therapy. Patients who are severely thyrotoxic (serum T_4>20 μg/dl) should be rendered euthyroid/mildly toxic before contemplating radio-ablative therapy. Mildly thyrotoxic patients respond better to radio-ablation than euthyroid subjects as the gland is more avid in patients who are toxic. Iodine-containing preparations should be discontinued for 2–4 weeks; however, an interval of 3–6 months may be required following use of amiodarone or radiocontrast. Antithyroid drugs should be discontinued for 5–7 days prior to ^{131}I therapy. This results in increased avidity of thyroid gland for ^{131}I and facilitates incorporation of ^{131}I in the process of oxidation and organification, leading to follicular cell destruction. Prior use of PTU, but not carbimazole/methimazole, makes the gland more radio-resistant because PTU acts as a free radical scavenger and free radicals are involved in follicular cell damage following ^{131}I therapy. Lithium, diuretics, pioglitazone, and retinoic acid have been tried to enhance the avidity of radioiodine, but they have not been found to be effective. β-blockers should be added/continued in the interim period after radio-ablation. Concurrent treatment with glucocorticoids is advised in those with clinically active thyroid-associated orbitopathy to prevent worsening after radioiodine ablation. Post-ablation, patient should avoid household and physical contact for a period of 1 week. Pregnancy should be avoided for at least 6 months after radio-ablation.

76. **How to follow up a patient after radio-ablation?**

After radio-ablation, thyroid hormones gradually decline over several weeks. Post-radio-ablation, there is a risk of exacerbation of symptoms due to radiation thyroiditis and increased TRAbs levels, and only 50–75% of patients are able to achieve euthyroidism in 6–8 weeks; therefore, β-blockers should be continued in the interim period. Antithyroid drugs should be reinitiated after 1 week of radio-ablation in patients with severe thyrotoxicosis and cardiac disease or those who are elderly, after performing a repeat thyroid function test. Thyroid function test should be monitored at 4–6 weekly intervals. Based on clinical profile and thyroid function tests, a decision can be taken regarding the use of levothyroxine or antithyroid drugs. However, ^{131}I can be readministered after 6 months of initial therapy, in patients who still remain toxic.

77. **How does ^{131}I act as an ablative agent?**

Orally administered ^{131}I is quickly absorbed and concentrated in the thyroid gland. After uptake, it is incorporated into the process of oxidation and organification, thereby retaining ^{131}I in the thyroid follicular cells. ^{131}I emits β rays, which results in increased free radical generation, reduced vascularity, and nuclear damage consequently resulting in thyroid follicular cell necrosis.

78. **When should ^{131}I radio-ablation be avoided in patients with hyperthyroidism?**

^{131}I radio-ablation is absolutely contraindicated in children <5 years of age and during pregnancy and lactation. Inadvertent exposure of ^{131}I during the first 10 weeks of gestation may not cause fetal hypothyroidism as thyroid gland develops after 10 weeks; but it may exert mutagenic effects on the developing embryo. However, if administered after 10 weeks of gestation, it is concentrated by the developing thyroid gland and causes fetal goiter and/or hypothyroidism. Data for the safety of ^{131}I during the first trimester of pregnancy are lacking; therefore, if administered inadvertently, the pros and cons should be discussed with the patient and family, regarding termination of pregnancy. Use of ^{131}I in a patient with clinically active orbitopathy can lead to worsening of eye disease. However, ^{131}I radio-ablation may be given along with steroids in these patients.

79. **What are adverse effects associated with ^{131}I radio-ablation?**

The adverse effects associated with ^{131}I radio-ablation (RAI) are radiation thyroiditis, permanent hypothyroidism, and exacerbation of thyroid-associated orbitopathy. After 1–2 weeks of RAI, there is a risk of radiation thyroiditis and patients present with a tender goiter and worsening of toxic symptoms. There is also an increased risk of cardiovascular events and probably mortality, not due to RAI per se but due to long-standing hyperthyroidism or subsequent untreated/ unrecognized subclinical hypothyroidism. Worsening of orbitopathy is attributed to the release of thyroid autoantigens and TRAbs from the gland after RAI. Although there is a concern for gonadal dysfunction after RAI, it has been shown that the therapeutic doses used in Graves' disease are safe, while the higher doses used in thyroid malignancy may be associated with transient gonadal dysfunction. Data regarding development of thyroidal or non-thyroidal malignancies like breast, stomach, and kidney after RAI is reassuring in adults. However, there is a risk of both thyroidal and non-thyroidal malignancies in children <5 years; hence radioablative therapy should be avoided in them.

80. **A 25-year-old female presented with weight loss, palpitation, and tremor of 8 months duration. On evaluation she had features of thyrotoxicosis, grade II goiter, and no orbitopathy. Her serum T_3 was 3.6 ng/ml, T_4 20 µg/dl, and TSH 0.01 µIU/ml. How to proceed further?**

Available therapeutic options for this patient are antithyroid drugs and radioablation. Antithyroid drugs may be preferred as the first-line therapy because of her age and small goiter, and there is a probability of achieving remission in 50% of patients after optimal duration of treatment without causing hypothyroidism. However, if she does not achieve remission after adequate duration of treatment or if there is a relapse, radio-ablative therapy is the treatment of choice. Alternatively, this patient can be offered radio-ablative treatment as a first-line therapy, but this will result in permanent hypothyroidism in majority of patients (80% over 1 year) and will require life-long replacement with levothyroxine. Although, it is easier to treat and monitor hypothyroidism than hyperthyroidism, the symptoms of hypothyroidism and quality of life (QOL) may not improve in all despite optimal thyroxine replacement and normalization of TSH.

81. **A 48-year-old male presented with palpitation and tremors. On evaluation he had features of thyrotoxicosis, grade III goiter, and no orbitopathy. His serum T_3 was 9.5 ng/ml, T_4 26 μg/dl, and TSH 0.001 μIU/ml. How to proceed further?**

Considering the age, size of the goiter, and severity of toxicosis, the probability of achieving remission with antithyroid drug therapy is low; therefore, such patients should not be treated with antithyroid drugs as a primary modality. This patient can be offered radio-ablative treatment or surgery after achieving euthyroid state with antithyroid drugs and β-blockers. As the patient preferred radio-ablative therapy over surgery, he was subjected to the same.

82. **A 20-year-old male presented with symptoms of thyrotoxicosis. On evaluation, he had grade I goiter and orbitopathy, with a clinical activity score of 4/7 and his serum T_3 was 3.9 ng/ml, T_4 22 μg/dl, and TSH 0.07 μIU/ml. What is the preferred treatment for hyperthyroidism?**

Antithyroid drugs should be preferred as first-line therapy in this patient. As he is young and has a small goiter, the probability of achieving remission is high with antithyroid drugs. In addition, the presence of clinically active orbitopathy favors the use of antithyroid drugs, as radio-ablation may worsen orbitopathy. Therefore, this patient was treated with antithyroid drugs, β-blockers, and pulse methylprednisolone therapy.

83. **Has thyroid surgery lost its place to antithyroid drugs and ^{131}I radio-ablation?**

No. Thyroid surgery is still the preferred modality in patients with large goiter (>80 g), compressive symptoms, retrosternal extension, and concurrent presence of thyroid cancer, or hyperparathyroidism. In addition, surgery is an alternative option for the treatment of Graves' disease in children <5 years of age and in pregnant women who are intolerant to antithyroid drugs. Further, occasional patients with severe thyroid-associated orbitopathy may be offered thyroid surgery to reduce the cumulative burden of thyroid autoantigens and TRAbs. Patients who fail to respond to multiple doses of RAI or those who are poorly compliant to medical therapy and refuse RAI can also be offered thyroid surgery.

84. **What is the recommended surgery for hyperthyroidism?**

Near-total or total thyroidectomy is the preferred surgery for the management of hyperthyroidism. Near-total thyroidectomy involves almost complete removal of the gland except 2 g as residual tissue, while subtotal thyroidectomy involves excision of 5/6th of the gland. The cure rate with near-total/total thyroidectomy is nearly 100% as compared to subtotal thyroidectomy, which is associated with persistent/recurrent disease in 8% of patients at 5 years with similar rate of complications.

85. **A 34-year-old woman with a known case of Graves' disease for the past 2 years presented with protrusion of both eyes of 8 months duration. She is on 40 mg of carbimazole and 120 mg of propranolol per day since diagnosis. On examination she had grade IV diffuse goiter and clinically inactive, moderate to severe TAO. Her T_3 was 3.4 ng/ml (0.8–1.8), T_4 26.4 μg/dl (4.8–12.6), and TSH 0.005 μU/ml (0.45–4.2). What to do next?**

The index patient has Graves' disease with grade IV goiter and inactive moderate to severe TAO. Despite being on maximal doses of carbimazole for 2 years, she did not attain euthyroidism. The available options for the index patient include further increase in dose of carbimazole, thyroid surgery, or radio-ablation. Increment in doses of carbimazole beyond 40 mg per day is usually not helpful. Radio-ablation may not be an ideal option in patients with grade IV goiter as the success rate in this scenario is low. Therefore, the best option in this patient is thyroidectomy. Although the index patient continues to be thyrotoxic, the risk of developing thyroid storm during surgery is possibly low as she is on carbimazole and β-blockers for a long duration. The risk of thyroid storm can further be reduced by preoperative use of inorganic iodide. After adequate preparation, she was subjected to near-total thyroidectomy which was uneventful. Post-operatively, anti-thyroid drugs were stopped and β-blockers continued. If she continues to remain toxic, radio-ablative treatment may be offered for the residual thyroid tissue.

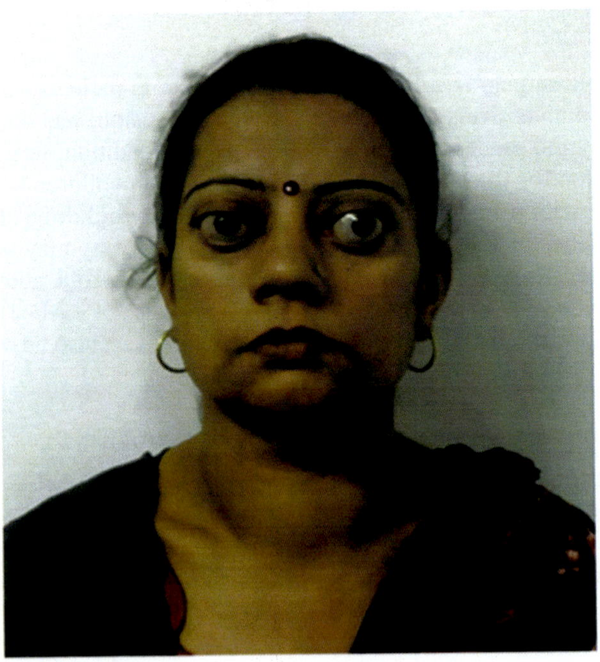

Fig. 10.12 Patient of Graves' disease with grade IV goiter and inactive TAO

86. **What is subclinical hyperthyroidism?**

Normal serum free T_4 and free T_3 levels in the presence of low serum TSH concentration (<0.5 μIU/ml) irrespective of presence or absence of symptoms is defined as subclinical hyperthyroidism. Suppressed TSH in the presence of normal free T_4 and free T_3 is because of the log-linear relationship between circulating free T_4 and TSH. The most common cause of subclinical hyperthyroidism is toxic multinodular goiter, followed by toxic adenoma, and Graves' disease.

87. **When to treat subclinical hyperthyroidism?**

Subclinical hyperthyroidism is associated with an increased cardiovascular risk, particularly atrial fibrillation, decreased bone mineral density, and possibly dementia. The risk increases with advancing age and declining TSH. However, overall mortality does not seem to be increased; hence, treatment decision needs to be individualized. All patients with TSH <0.1 μIU/mL and age >65 years need treatment. Those with TSH <0.1 μIU/mL and age <65 years with symptoms of thyrotoxicosis and presence of heart disease or cardiac risk factors or osteoporosis should be treated. In patients with TSH between 0.1 and 0.5 μIU/mL and age >65 years or TSH between 0.1 and 0.5 μIU/mL and age <65 years with comorbidities, treatment should be considered. In addition, treatment for subclinical hyperthyroidism may benefit women with infertility.

88. **How to treat subclinical hyperthyroidism?**

If treatment is indicated, subclinical hyperthyroidism associated with toxic adenoma or toxic MNG should be treated with radioactive iodine. Patients with Graves' disease with subclinical hyperthyroidism should be treated with low-dose antithyroid drugs as there is a higher probability of achieving remission. β-blockers are advised in those with predominant adrenergic symptoms. Patients should be periodically monitored with T_3, T_4, and TSH. However, the optimal duration of antithyroid drug therapy in these patients is not well defined.

89. **What is thyroid storm?**

Thyroid storm is a clinical disorder characterized by exaggerated symptoms of thyrotoxicosis with multiorgan dysfunction. It is a life-threatening condition with a mortality rate of 20–30% and requires urgent medical attention. Thyroid storm is commonly precipitated by infections, trauma, and surgical or medical emergencies and is common in those who are noncompliant to treatment than in treatment-naïve individuals. Although hyperthyroidism of any etiology may be complicated by thyroid storm, Graves' disease is the most common underlying disorder. Hyperpyrexia, tachycardia disproportionate to the degree of pyrexia, arrhythmias, and encephalopathy are the clinical clues to suggest the presence of thyroid storm. Despite severe manifestations of thyrotoxicosis, serum T_3 and T_4 levels may not be very high. The Burch–Wartofsky scoring for thyroid storm is useful for both diagnosis and prognosis. A score of ≥45 is suggestive of thyroid storm, a score of 25–44 supports the diagnosis, and a score <25 makes thyroid storm unlikely.

90. **Does circulating serum T_3/T_4 level predict the severity of thyroid storm?**

No. The circulating levels of T_3/T_4 are notably not higher as compared to uncomplicated thyrotoxicosis. Further, the level of T_3 may be normal/ mildly elevated in patients with thyroid storm due to concurrent sick euthyroid syndrome. Severe symptoms of thyrotoxicosis even without high levels of thyroid hormones can be attributed to increased adrenergic sensitivity, augmented peripheral response to circulating T_4, and increased levels of free T_3 and T_4 due to decreased binding with TBG during critical illness. Therefore, any patient with severe manifestations of thyrotoxicosis should be managed as thyroid storm.

91. **How to treat thyroid storm?**

Supportive measures are important in the management of thyroid storm. These include correction of dehydration by intravenous fluids containing dextrose, treatment of underlying infection with appropriate antibiotics, and use of antipyretics. Acetaminophen is preferred and aspirin is to be avoided as it interferes with protein binding, leading to elevated free T_3/T_4 levels. The specific treatment includes β-blockers (propranolol in doses of 40–80 mg every 6 h) along with either propylthiouracil in doses of 200 mg every 4 h or methimazole 20 mg orally every 4–6 h. Use of glucocorticoids preferably dexamethasone (4 mg every 6 h) not only provides adrenal support but also inhibits peripheral T_4 to T_3 neogenesis. After 2 h of initiation of antithyroid drugs, inorganic iodide should be administered, as it inhibits thyroid hormone release (Lugol's solution 10 drops twice daily or colossal iodine 40–50 ml twice a day [5 ml of colossal iodine/1 drop of Lugol's iodine contain 8mg of iodine]). Thionamides should be administered before iodine as prior administration of iodine may act as a fuel for the hyperfunctioning thyroid gland. In situations where oral administration of thionamides is not possible, per rectal administration is an alternative and is equally effective. Iodine treatment should be stopped within 5–7 days as the gland escapes from the inhibitory effect of iodine on thyroid hormone release (iodide escape). Patients usually recover within 5–7 days and require continuation of thionamides and β-blockers, while glucocorticoids and iodine are withdrawn.

92. **What are the clinical pointers to suggest malignancy in a thyroid nodule?**

Extremes of ages (<20 years and >65 years), male sex, family history of thyroid carcinoma, history of childhood radiation exposure, rapid increase in the size of nodule, fixation of nodule to surrounding structures, recurrent laryngeal nerve palsy, or concurrent cervical lymphadenopathy should raise a suspicion of malignancy. Neither the size nor the multiplicity of nodule predicts the risk of malignancy. Raised TSH is more likely to be associated with malignancy than a suppressed TSH.

93. **Which is the preferred imaging modality for evaluation of a thyroid nodule?**

Ultrasonography (USG) is the preferred modality to evaluate a thyroid nodule. Other modalities like CT and MRI are unable to distinguish between benign and malignant thyroid nodules; therefore, even incidentally detected thyroid nodules by these imaging modalities require further characterization by USG. However, incidentally detected thyroid nodules on ^{18}F-FDG-PET are likely to be malignant in one-third of patients and further evaluation should be actively pursued.

94. **What are the ultrasound characteristics of suspicious malignant thyroid nodule?**

Ultrasound characteristics of a suspicious malignant nodule are hypoechogenicity, solid nodule, increased intranodular vascularity, irregular infiltrative margins, microcalcifications, absent halo, and shape taller than width. Among these features, solid consistency has a highest sensitivity (86%), while microcalcifications and shape taller than width has a specificity of 90%.

95. **What is the differential diagnosis of a midline neck swelling?**

The differential diagnoses of a midline neck swelling include disorders of thyroid gland like thyroglossal cyst, thyroid nodule (benign or malignant), or thyroid abscess and non-thyroidal disorders like pretracheal lymphadenopathy, epidermal cyst, sebaceous cyst, branchial cyst, dermoid cyst, cystic hygroma, lymphangioma, and lipoma.

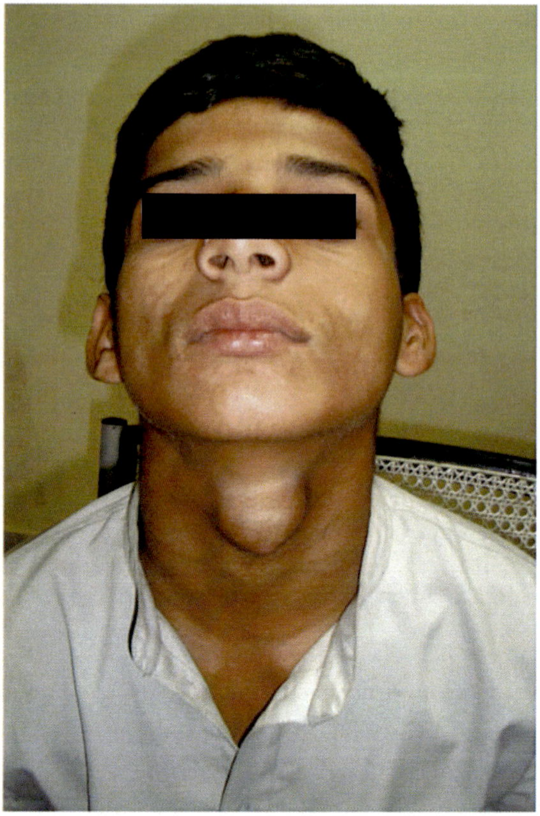

Fig. 10.13 Midline neck swelling due to thyroglossal cyst

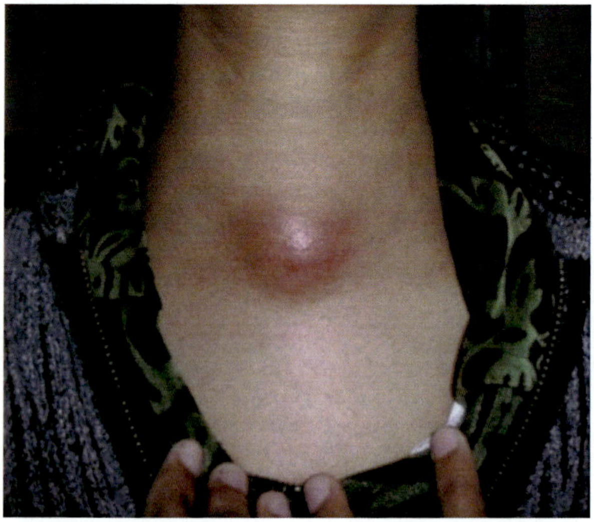

Fig. 10.14 Midline neck swelling due to pretracheal tubercular lymphadenopathy

Suggested Reading

1. Bahn RS, Burch HB, Cooper DS, Garber JR, Greenlee MC, Klein I, Laurberg P, et al. Hyperthyroidism and other causes of thyrotoxicosis: management guidelines of the American Thyroid Association and American Association of Clinical Endocrinologists. Thyroid. 2011;21(6):593–646.
2. Braverman LE, David C. Werner & Ingbar's the thyroid, a fundamental and clinical text. 10th ed. Philadelphia: Wolters Kluwer Health/Lippincott Williams & Wilkins; 2012.
3. Jameson LJ, DeGroot LJ. Endocrinology: adult and pediatric. Philadelphia: Elsevier Health Sciences; 2010.
4. Longo D, Fauci A, Kasper D, Hauser S, Jameson J, Joseph Loscalzo J. Harrison's principles of internal medicine. 18th ed. New York: McGraw Hill Professional; 2012.
5. Melmed S, Polonsky KS, Reed Larsen P, Kronenberg HM. Williams textbook of endocrinology: expert consult. London: Elsevier Health Sciences; 2011.

Extra-thyroidal Manifestations of Autoimmune Thyroid Disease

11

11.1 Case Vignette

A 60-year-old man presented with history of weight loss, palpitations, and tremor for the last 6 months. He also had protrusion of both eyes, which was gradually progressive. For the last 2 weeks, he developed retrobulbar pain and redness of both eyes. There was no history of diplopia or visual loss. He denied history of smoking. On examination, his pulse rate was 128/min, regular, BP 140/60 mmHg, and had diffuse, soft, grade I goiter. He had proptosis (24 mm) of both eyes with marked chemosis and swelling of eyelids with a clinical activity score of 6/7 and severity score moderate to severe. Ocular movements were restricted in all the quadrants bilaterally. He had normal visual acuity and color vision, and there was no papilledema. Pupillary reflexes were normal. He had no evidence of dermopathy or acropachy. On investigation, serum T_3 was 3.4 ng/ml (0.8–1.8), T_4 20.4 μg/dl (4.8–12.6), and TSH 0.001 μIU/ml (0.45–4.2), and TPO antibodies were 200 IU/ml (<35). CT orbit revealed enlargement of extraocular muscles (size >5 mm) with sparing of tendons and increased volume of retro-orbital tissue without any evidence of apical crowding. He was diagnosed to have Graves' disease with active and moderate to severe thyroid-associated orbitopathy. He was advised artificial teardrops, sunglasses with side cover and elevation of head end of bed while sleeping. He was initiated on carbimazole 30 mg once a day and propranolol 40 mg thrice daily along with pulse methylprednisolone therapy. A week later, he had improvement in clinical activity score (4/7) and symptoms of toxicosis. Liver function tests were monitored periodically and were within normal limits. Repeat thyroid function test at 4 weeks revealed serum T_3 2.2 ng/ml, T_4 14.6 μg/dl (4.8–12.6), and TSH 0.001 μIU/ml (0.45–4.2). He was continued with 30 mg carbimazole and propranolol. A cumulative dose of 4.5 g methylprednisolone was administered over a period of 12 weeks. Subsequently at 3 months, he had resolution of clinical symptoms and normalization of T_3 and T_4; however, TSH remained suppressed. Dose of carbimazole was decreased to 20 mg per day, and β-blockers were discontinued. His clinical activity score (CAS) improved further (2/7); proptosis remained static, and there was no

A. Bhansali, Y. Gogate, *Clinical Rounds in Endocrinology: Volume I - Adult Endocrinology*, DOI 10.1007/978-81-322-2398-6_11

deterioration in vision during follow-up. He was continued on carbimazole for 2 years with close monitoring of thyroid function tests. Later, he was subjected to decompressive eye surgery for severe proptosis after 6 months of consistently inactive disease. On follow-up, he is doing fine.

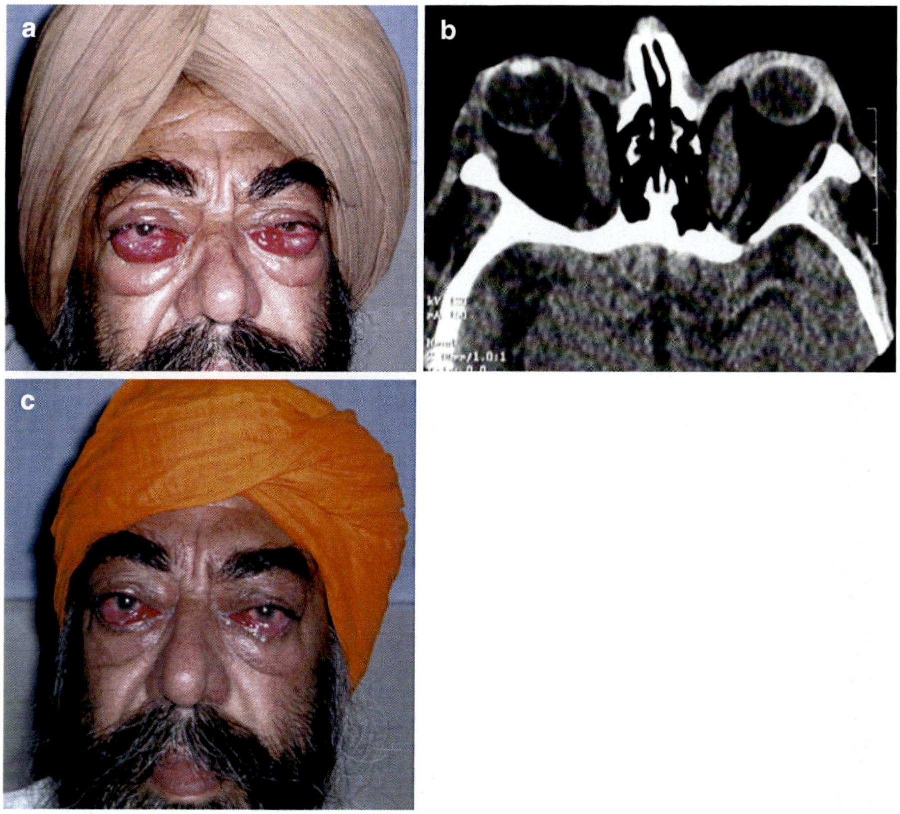

Fig. 11.1 (**a**) Clinically active, moderate–severe TAO in a patient with Graves' disease. (**b**) CT scan of the orbit showing thickening of extraocular muscles (medial rectus) and sparing of tendons with bilateral proptosis. (**c**) Improvement in clinical activity score and proptosis following pulse methylprednisolone therapy

11.2 Stepwise Analysis

Long duration of symptoms of thyrotoxicosis, presence of diffuse goiter and orbitopathy are consistent with the diagnosis of Graves' disease. Further, he had CAS of 6/7 which indicates the presence of active (CAS $\geq$3/7) thyroid-associated orbitopathy. Disease was moderate to severe as proptosis was >20 mm, and there was severe soft tissue involvement. He had marked restriction of eyeball movements (frozen globe) without any cranial nerve involvement. Orbital CT was done to exclude the presence of orbital apex syndrome as he had severe TAO. Imaging features were consistent with the diagnosis of TAO (extraocular muscle belly thickening with tendon sparing) without any evidence of dysthyroid optic neuropathy. Thyroid function test confirmed the diagnosis of thyrotoxicosis, and he was started on carbimazole and propranolol. Presence of active eye disease suggests ongoing inflammation and merits glucocorticoid treatment. Surgery is indicated only in patients with dysthyroid optic neuropathy, corneal breakdown, and globe subluxation who do not respond to glucocorticoids within 1–2 weeks. He was started on methylprednisolone therapy. The reduction in CAS from 6/7 to 4/7 within a week's time suggests significant response to therapy and predicts favorable outcome. Further, absence of smoking in the index case appears to be complimentary for the long-term outcome. It is important to monitor liver function test as pulse methylprednisolone therapy can rarely induce fatal hepatic failure. Further, thyroid function test was closely monitored in the index case as hypothyroidism may lead to worsening of TAO. He was continued on antithyroid drugs for 2 years. Rehabilitative surgeries are undertaken once the eye disease is consistently inactive for 6 months; therefore, the patient was subjected to decompressive eye surgery after 6 months of persistently inactive eye disease.

11.3 Clinical Rounds

1. **What are the extra-thyroidal manifestations of autoimmune thyroid diseases?**

   The extra-thyroidal manifestations of autoimmune thyroid disease include thyroid-associated orbitopathy, infiltrative dermopathy, and thyroid acropachy.

2. **What is thyroid-associated orbitopathy?**

   Thyroid-associated orbitopathy (TAO) is an autoimmune disorder characterized by immuno-inflammation of the extraocular muscles and retro-orbital tissue, and invariably occurs in the presence of autoimmune thyroid disease, irrespective of presence of hyper-, hypo-, or euthyroidism. Autoimmune thyroid disease is the prerequisite for the development of TAO as evidenced by consistent presence of antithyroid antibodies (TRAbs, TPO, or anti-Tg antibodies) in these patients and absence of TAO in patients with thyroid aplasia and toxic multinodular goiter. Ninety percent of patients with TAO have hyperthyroidism, while 6–10% are euthyroid, and 3–4% have hypothyroidism. Hyperthyroid or euthyroid patients with TAO commonly have Graves' disease, while those with hypothyroidism have Hashimoto's thyroiditis or rarely Graves' disease with blocking antibodies. TAO associated with hyperthyroidism is usually moderate to severe, bilateral, and symmetrical, while TAO with hypothyroidism is milder and tends to be asymmetrical.

3. **Is there any difference between Graves' orbitopathy and thyroid-associated orbitopathy?**

   Yes. The term thyroid-associated orbitopathy denotes orbitopathy associated with autoimmune thyroid disease, either Graves' or Hashimoto's thyroiditis, while Graves' orbitopathy is a specific term for orbitopathy associated with Graves' disease.

4. **Is Graves' ophthalmopathy and Graves' orbitopathy synonymous?**

   No. Although the terms Graves' ophthalmopathy and Graves' orbitopathy are used interchangeably, they are not synonymous. The ocular manifestation in patients with thyroid disorder is due to involvement of retro-orbital tissue and ocular muscles. Therefore, the term "Graves' ophthalmopathy" is a misnomer as it does not address orbital involvement in the disease process. Hence, the appropriate term should be Graves' orbitopathy.

5. **Why is the onset of TAO not always synchronous with development of hyperthyroidism?**

   Onset of TAO can precede, follow, or may occur concurrently with hyperthyroidism in patients with Graves' disease. Therefore, TAO and hyperthyroidism were considered as different diseases in the past. However, patients with euthyroid TAO often have subtle thyroid function abnormalities, and there is a qualitative correlation between the presence of TRAbs and the occurrence of TAO and thyrotoxicosis. Hence, it has been reconciled that both TAO and hyperthyroidism are spectrum of same autoimmune thyroid disease. Differential responsiveness of orbital fibroblast to circulating TRAbs as compared to thyroid follicular cells, variability in TSH receptor density and affinity in the target tissue, and co-expression of IGF1 receptor along with TSH receptor in the orbital fibroblast may explain the discordance between the onset of TAO and hyperthyroidism in patients with Graves' disease.

6. **What are the extra-thyroidal effects of TSH?**

   TSH regulates growth and development of thyroid gland and stimulates thyroid hormone synthesis by upregulation of expression of sodium iodide symporter, activation of thyroid peroxidase and augmentation of thyroglobulin proteolysis. In addition to its thyrotrophic effects, TSH has various extra-thyroidal actions. It acts as a lipolytic hormone by activating hormone-sensitive lipase. TSH receptors are present on osteoblasts and osteoclasts, and TSH has been shown to inhibit bone remodeling. TSH receptors are also expressed in ovary and testes, and it may play a role in the development of multicystic ovaries and macroorchidism in primary hypothyroidism. In addition, the presence of TSH receptors on orbital fibroblasts, extraocular muscles, adipocytes, and dermal fibroblasts explains its role in the pathogenesis of TAO and dermopathy.

7. **What are the risk factors for the development of Graves' orbitopathy?**

   Risk factors for Graves' orbitopathy include old age, male sex, severe thyrotoxicosis at presentation, large goiter, persistent elevation of TRAbs, smoking, and use of radioiodine. In addition, use of drugs like pioglitazone may worsen TAO due to orbital adipocyte proliferation.

8. **What are the characteristic features of Graves' orbitopathy?**

   Clinically evident orbitopathy is seen in nearly one-third of patients with Graves' disease, although imaging may show evidence of orbitopathy in almost all. However, sight-threatening orbitopathy occurs in only 3–5% of patients. Graves' disease is highly prevalent in women with a female to male ratio of 10:1, while the ratio of female to male for Graves' orbitopathy (GO) is narrowed to 2:1. It is usually bilateral, but may be asymmetrical in 10–15% and is rarely unilateral. Further, GO may precede, accompany, or follow hyperthyroidism. The most common muscles involved in GO are inferior rectus and medial rectus and are characterized by involvement of muscle belly with sparing of tendons.

9. **What is the natural history of Graves' orbitopathy?**

   Natural history of Graves' orbitopathy in a treatment-naive patient is characterized by an initial active phase of 6–12 months, followed by a plateau for 1–3 months and eventually an inactive phase lasting 1–2 years. The clinical activity of disease progressively declines over time; however, parameters of severity like exophthalmos, diplopia, and lid retraction may not remit completely. Further, once disease remits it is unlikely to relapse.

10. **What is clinically active TAO?**

    Pain on eye movement, spontaneous retro-orbital pain, conjunctival and eyelid injection, and swelling of eyelid, conjunctiva, and caruncle are the parameters used for the assessment of clinical activity of TAO. A score of $\geq$3/7 is considered to be clinically active and requires immunosuppressive therapy.

11. **How to assess severity score in a patient with TAO?**

    Lid retraction, soft tissue involvement, proptosis diplopia, corneal exposure, and optic nerve dysfunction are the parameters used for assessment of severity of TAO. Mild TAO is defined as presence of lid retraction <2 mm, mild soft tissue involvement, exophthalmos <3 mm above normal for race and gender or transient diplopia. The presence of any one of the following defines moderate–severe TAO; lid retraction >2 mm, moderate/ severe soft tissue involvement, exophthalmos >3 mm above the reference range, and inconstant or constant diplopia. The presence of corneal breakdown and optic nerve dysfunction indicates sight-threatening TAO.

12. **What is the difference between clinical activity score and severity score?**

    The objective parameters for the assessment of TAO include clinical activity score (CAS) and severity score (SS). Clinical activity score represents acute inflammation in the orbit with extension into anterior region of eye. Clinical activity is the result of cytokine-mediated injury to retro-ocular and ocular tissues, and venous outflow obstruction. Severity score represents anatomical/ functional aberrations and is due to retro-orbital fibroblast and adipocyte proliferation and thickening of extraocular muscles along with glycosaminoglycan deposition in a closed retro-orbital space and thereby compressing neighboring tissues including optic nerve. Patients with clinically active disease (CAS $\geq$3/7) requires immunosuppressive therapy, while those with moderate–severe TAO and CAS <2/7 require orbital decompression/reconstructive surgery as immunosuppression is not effective. If disease is active and severe, immunosuppressive therapy should be started first, and surgery should be contemplated later if indicated, and as with improvement in clinical activity, severity score may also improve.

13. **What are the endocrine causes of proptosis?**

    TAO is the most common endocrine cause of proptosis, and the other causes include Cushing's syndrome, acromegaly, morbid obesity, and primary hyperparathyroidism.

14. **What are the non-endocrine causes of proptosis?**

    The non-endocrine causes of proptosis include cavernous sinus thrombosis, carotid–cavernous fistula, orbital myositis, orbital tumors and granulomatous infiltration of orbit. In addition, systemic disorders like chronic obstructive airway disease, chronic liver disease, and chronic kidney disease can also be associated with proptosis.

15. **Why is there proptosis in Graves' disease?**

    Proptosis is defined as forward protrusion of eyeball. It is a measure of position of cornea in relation to lateral margin of orbit. The degree of protrusion of eyeball depends on age, sex, ethnicity, extent of myopia, and method used to measure it. Normally it does not exceed 17 mm in Asian adults, and >20 mm is considered as moderate–severe proptosis. In TAO, proptosis is due to proliferation of retro-orbital fibroblasts and adipocytes along with deposition of glycosaminoglycans (GAG) in the retrobulbar space and extraocular muscles. In addition ocular muscle tone, that normally retracts the globe, is lost in TAO due to deposition of GAG in extraocular muscles leading to proptosis.

16. **What is "frozen globe"?**

    "Frozen globe" is a clinical entity in which there is restriction of movements of eyeball in all quadrants. It commonly occurs due to ocular cranial nerve involvement. However, in patients with Graves' disease, "frozen globe" can occur due to involvement of extraocular muscles per se without any cranial nerve palsy.

17. **What are the causes of ptosis in patients with Graves' disease?**

    Ptosis is uncommon in patients with Graves' disease, and if present, the patient should be evaluated for myasthenia gravis. Other causes include superior orbital fissure syndrome, orbital apex syndrome, and rarely mechanical failure of levator palpebrae superioris due to long-standing severe proptosis. Ptosis can occur either due to involvement of the Muller's muscle or levator palpebrae superioris, innervated by sympathetic nerve fibers and 3rd cranial nerve, respectively. Ptosis is usually mild with sympathetic nerve involvement, whereas it is severe with oculomotor nerve palsy.

18. **What is superior orbital fissure syndrome?**

    Superior orbital fissure is a passage for oculomotor, trochlear, and abducens nerves, ophthalmic branch of trigeminal nerve, inferior and superior ophthalmic veins, and sympathetic fibers. Superior orbital fissure syndrome (SOFS) is characterized by ptosis, proptosis, ophthalmoplegia, fixed and dilated pupil, and sensory loss involving upper eyelid and forehead. The close differential diagnosis of SOFS is orbital apex syndrome. It shares all the features of SOFS, and in addition, there is visual loss due to optic nerve involvement as optic nerve passes through optic canal which lies in close proximity to superior orbital fissure.

19. **What are the causes of vision loss in patients with thyroid-associated orbitopathy?**

    Causes of vision loss in patients with thyroid-associated orbitopathy are exposure keratitis with severe corneal involvement and dysthyroid optic neuropathy either due to optic nerve compression or stretching of optic nerve.

20. **What is dysthyroid optic neuropathy?**

    Dysthyroid optic neuropathy (DON) is characterized by reduced visual acuity, loss of color vision, visual field defects, papilledema, relative afferent pupillary defect, and apical crowding on imaging. Optic neuropathy is caused by compression of optic nerve due to crowding of retro-orbital tissue and thickened extraocular muscles at the apex (orbital apex syndrome) and/or stretching of optic nerve either due to severe proptosis or subluxation of the globe. This is an important cause of visual loss in patients with GO and is an urgent indication to initiate pulse methylprednisolone therapy (1 g intravenous for 3 consecutive days). If there is no improvement in optic nerve function after 1–2 weeks of glucocorticoid therapy, orbital decompression is recommended. Orbital radiotherapy is not recommended as a monotherapy in the management of DON; however, it may be used as an adjunct to glucocorticoids.

21. **How does smoking exacerbate thyroid-associated orbitopathy?**

    Smoking is associated with increased incidence of TAO, severe eye disease, poor response to therapy, and risk of worsening of TAO post-radio-ablation. Smoking exacerbates TAO by causing local hypoxia and increased free radical generation resulting in fibroblast proliferation and increased deposition of glycosaminoglycans. In addition, increased production of interleukin-1 in smokers has been shown to induce orbital adipogenesis and may worsen orbitopathy. Therefore, complete cessation of smoking is recommended in all patients with Graves' disease.

22. **What are the indications of orbital imaging in a patient with thyroid-associated orbitopathy?**

    Patients with unilateral or asymmetrical proptosis, clinically suspected DON, euthyroid/ hypothyroid orbitopathy, and TAO associated with ptosis should undergo orbital imaging. In addition, patients who are planned for rehabilitative surgery need imaging for anatomical details of the orbit. Lastly, in the presence of atypical clinical features, imaging must be done to exclude alternative diagnosis, e.g., orbital tumors, orbital myositis, orbital mycosis, or granulomatous infiltrative disease of the eye.

23. **What are the imaging characteristics of thyroid-associated orbitopathy?**

    Imaging modalities available for detection of thyroid-associated orbitopathy (TAO) are A/B mode ultrasonography, CT scan, and MRI. MR imaging is the best available modality for the detection of TAO. Imaging features of TAO include proptosis, thickening of extraocular muscles (>5 mm) with sparing of tendons (Coca-Cola bottle sign), increased retro-orbital fat, intracranial fat prolapse, and apical crowding. Inferior and medial recti are the most common muscles to be affected, although any ocular muscle can be involved. Tendon sparing is due to decreased expression of TSH receptors over the tendons as compared to belly of the muscle. Intracranial fat prolapse is a surrogate evidence of raised retro-orbital tension.

24. **What are the indications for glucocorticoids in the management of thyroid-associated orbitopathy?**

    The indications for glucocorticoids in the management of thyroid-associated orbitopathy are clinically active disease and dysthyroid optic neuropathy.

25. **How to treat clinically active thyroid-associated orbitopathy?**

    Clinically active TAO is defined as CAS ≥3/7 and mandates immunosuppressive therapy. Glucocorticoids are the drug of choice and intravenous therapy is preferred over oral therapy. The effect of intravenous therapy is dramatic and sustained with higher response rate (77% vs. 51%), better tolerance, and reduced risk of Cushing's syndrome. The preferred regimen is pulse therapy with intravenous methylprednisolone, administered over a period of 12 weeks with a dose schedule of 500 mg weekly for 6 weeks followed by 250 mg weekly over the next 6 weeks with a cumulative dose of 4.5 g. Rarely, fulminant hepatitis may occur with pulse methylprednisolone therapy; therefore, liver function tests should be monitored. Alternatively, oral prednisolone may be administered at a dose of 1 mg/kg/day for 4–6 weeks and tapered over the next 4–6 weeks. If there is no response to steroids after 3 months of therapy, other treatment options like rituximab, azathioprine, cyclosporine, etanercept, somatostatin analogues, and immunoglobulin may be considered. However, data with the use of these drugs is scanty and not encouraging. Orbital radiotherapy is another option available for the management of TAO.

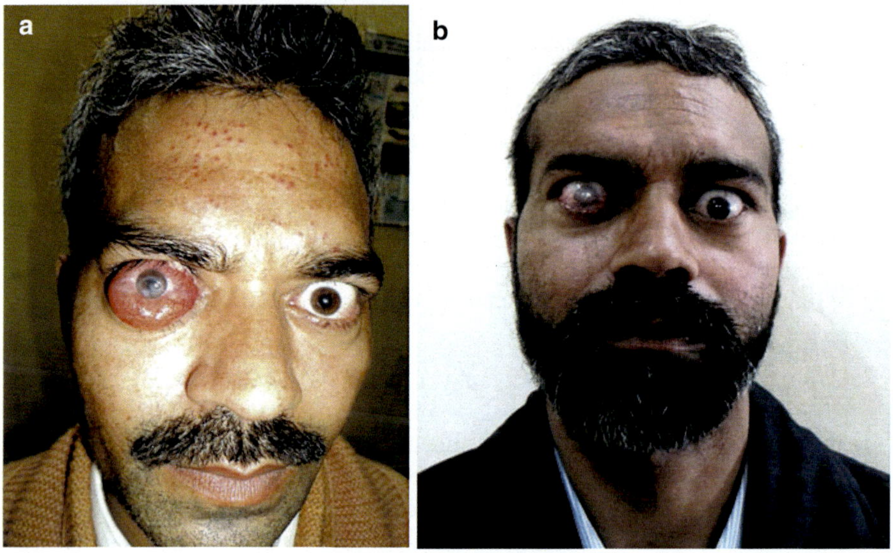

Fig. 11.2 (**a**) Unilateral active disease (CAS 7/7) with keratitis in a patient with TAO. Note the proptosis in other eye with CAS 0/7. (**b**) Posttreatment image of the same patient showing marked reduction in CAS of the right eye to 1/7 along with corneal opacity

26. **How to treat mild TAO with CAS 2/7?**

Thyroid-associated orbitopathy with mild severity is treated with artificial tears, dark protective glasses with side cover and use of prism, if diplopia is present. In addition, elevation of head end of the bed at nighttime improves disease activity by reducing venous congestion. As the disease is clinically inactive (CAS <3/7), there is no indication for immunosuppressive therapy, because the risks outweigh the benefits. In addition, the disease is self-limiting as evidenced by the fact that majority of patients with active disease experience spontaneous remission. Use of selenium may be beneficial in patients with mild TAO and CAS ≤3/7, as it results in modest improvement in clinical activity score as well as in severity score because of its anti-inflammatory and antioxidant effect.

27. **How to treat clinically inactive but moderate–severe thyroid-associated orbitopathy?**

Clinical activity and severity of TAO do not always go together despite similar pathophysiology, as seen in clinical practice. Therefore, it is prudent to assess CAS and SS in all patients of TAO for therapeutic decision. Patients with clinically inactive disease (CAS <3/7) do not benefit from immunosuppressive therapy, rather may have adverse consequences. However, the presence of moderate–severe disease requires decompressive/reconstructive surgery. In addition, thyroid function should be monitored periodically, and hypothyroidism must be avoided.

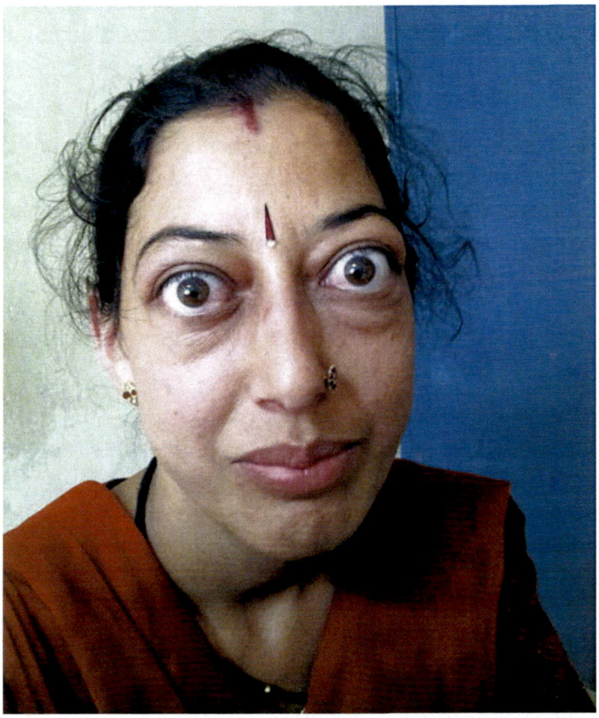

Fig. 11.3 Patient of Graves' disease with CAS 0/7 and moderate–severe TAO

28. **What are the indications for orbital radiotherapy in the management of TAO?**

Orbital radiotherapy is indicated in patients with clinically active TAO who are either intolerant or have contraindications for the use of glucocorticoids. In addition, it can also be used as an adjunct to glucocorticoids in those with active disease. It is most effective in patients with recent-onset active disease who have diplopia or restricted mobility. However, orbital radiotherapy is contraindicated in patients <35 years of age and in those with diabetic and hypertensive retinopathy. Orbital radiation as monotherapy is contraindicated in patients with DON.

29. **How effective is orbital radiotherapy in the management of TAO?**

External beam radiation suppresses intraorbital T-lymphocytes, thereby decreasing immuno-inflammation in the orbit. The recommended dose is 10–20 Gy in each orbit, focused on retro-orbital tissues, and delivered in ten fractions over a period of 2 weeks. A short course of prednisolone (10–20 mg/d for a week) along with radiotherapy is administered to avoid transient worsening of eye disease. External beam radiation therapy (EBRT) has been shown to be as effective as oral prednisolone (1 mg/kg/day) in the management of clinically active TAO as monotherapy; however, the response is slow in onset with a delayed peak effect. The combined use of radiotherapy and glucocorticoids may be indicated in those with higher CAS (6–7/7) as both therapies are complimentary, and response rate increases by approximately 10% as compared to glucocorticoids alone.

30. **What are the predictors of response in TAO?**

Patients with recent-onset disease respond better than those with long-standing TAO as extraocular muscle fibrosis occurs in patients with prolonged duration of disease. Further, a good clinical response within a week of initiating glucocorticoids usually predicts a favorable outcome. However, smokers and those with persistently elevated TRAb levels are poor responders.

31. **What are the limitations of glucocorticoid therapy in thyroid-associated orbitopathy?**

Intravenous methylprednisolone for thyroid-associated orbitopathy (TAO) is associated with a failure of response in approximately 20%, relapse in 10–20%, and progression of dysthyroid optic neuropathy in 5% of patients. Rarely, fulminant hepatic failure may occur with the use of pulse methylprednisolone therapy. Moreover, use of steroids may not preclude the need for reconstructive surgery later.

32. **What is the role of rituximab in thyroid-associated orbitopathy?**

Rituximab is a chimeric mouse–human monoclonal antibody against CD20, a human B-cell-specific antigen. CD20 is expressed by pre- and mature B lymphocyte but not by stem cells or plasma cells. Although, Graves' disease is a T-cell-mediated autoimmune disease, rituximab is effective in TAO, despite its activity against B cell. This is because B cells are involved in antigen presentation, cytokine production, and suppression of T_{reg} cells, thus contributing to orbitopathy. The available literature favors the use of rituximab in clinically active TAO; however, the data is derived mostly from case reports or case series and few non-randomized trials. The dose used is 1,000 mg intravenously on days 1 and 15. There is an improvement in clinical activity score as well as thyroid function. However, TRAb levels do not decrease as plasma cells which secrete immunoglobulins (TRAbs) do not express CD20 antigen. It has been mainly used in refractory TAO, but rituximab may be an attractive treatment option even in glucocorticoid-naïve patients. Adverse events associated with rituximab include infusion related flu-like symptoms and transient (<6 months) immune suppression.

33. **What are indications for orbital decompression?**

    Orbital decompression is indicated in dysthyroid optic neuropathy, corneal breakdown, or globe subluxation not responding to methylprednisolone for 1–2 weeks. In addition, those with active disease but are intolerant/nonresponsive to glucocorticoids can also be considered for orbital decompression. Patients with inactive disease may also require orbital decompression for disfiguring exophthalmos for cosmetic reasons.

34. **What are the surgical options available in the management of inactive TAO?**

    Rehabilitative surgery in the management of TAO includes orbital decompression, squint correction, and eyelid surgery (lid lengthening, blepharoplasty, and browplasty). If more than one procedure is required, then orbital decompression should be performed first, followed by squint surgery and lastly eyelid surgery. Before any surgical procedure is undertaken, the disease should be consistently inactive for at least 6 months.

35. **Why is there a worsening of TAO after radioiodine ablation?**

    New onset or worsening of TAO has been reported in 15–30% of patients after radio-ablation and usually occurs within 6 months of therapy. This is commonly observed in smokers and those who develop hypothyroidism after radio-ablation. Release of thyroid autoantigens and TRAbs along with elevated TSH after radio-ablation activates intraorbital T-lymphocytes, which results in worsening of TAO. Therefore, periodic monitoring of thyroid function is essential to detect development of hypothyroidism and consequent worsening of eye disease. Concurrent administration of glucocorticoids (0.5 mg/kg/day prednisolone for 4–8 weeks) in patients with active TAO prevents the risk of worsening of orbitopathy.

36. **What is infiltrative dermopathy?**

    Infiltrative dermopathy is an extra-thyroidal manifestation of autoimmune thyroid disorder, seen in approximately 5% of patients with Graves' disease and rarely in patients with Hashimoto's thyroiditis. Infiltrative dermopathy is invariably associated with thyroid-associated orbitopathy. The lesions are classically present over the shin (pretibial myxedema); however, it may also be present on the dorsum of hands, sacrum, or face. Several clinical variants have been described; diffuse nonpitting edematous form is the most common, and other variants include nodular or plaque-like lesions and rarely elephantiasis. Histologically, there is involvement of dermis (reticular zone) with fragmentation of collagen due to glycosaminoglycan deposition and infiltration with lymphocytes. Treatment includes topical and sometimes intralesional steroids.

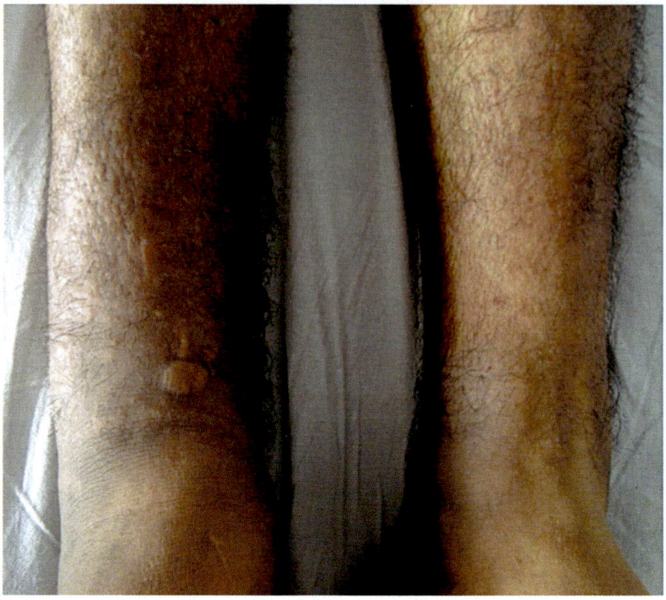

Fig. 11.4 Nodular and plaque-like lesions and diffuse nonpitting edema suggestive of infiltrative dermopathy in a patient with Graves' disease

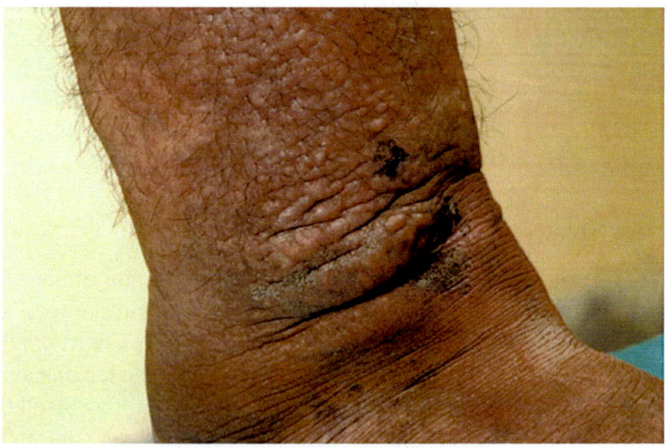

Fig. 11.5 Nodular lesions and diffuse nonpitting edema suggestive of infiltrative dermopathy in a patient with Graves' disease

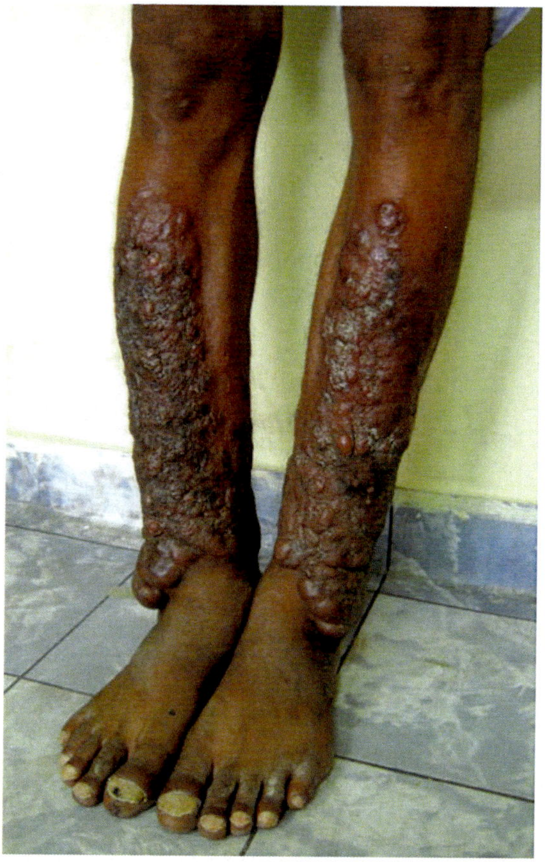

Fig. 11.6 Severe, nodular, and plaque-like lesions on both shins in a patient with Graves' disease

37. **What is thyroid acropachy?**

Thyroid acropachy is defined as acral changes in patients with Graves' disease. It is a manifestation of severe thyrotoxicosis and is characterized by digital soft tissue swelling, clubbing, and subperiosteal bone formation. It is painless, lacks warmth, and does not involve joints, and these features differentiate it from hypertrophic pulmonary osteoarthropathy. Thyroid acropachy is usually associated with orbitopathy and dermopathy. Thyroid acropachy is due to localized proliferation of digital soft tissue as a result of relative hypoxia, opening up of arteriovenous connections, and increased platelet-derived growth factor. In addition, autoimmune activation of periosteal fibroblasts has also been suggested.

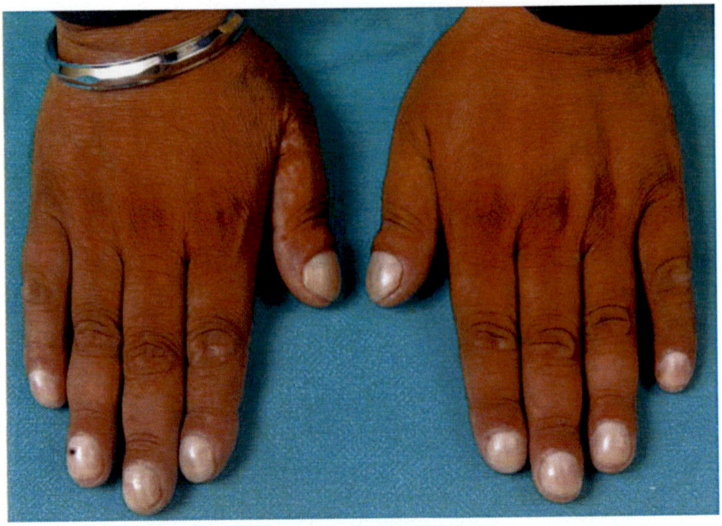

Fig. 11.7 Acropachy in a patient with Graves' disease. Note the presence of vitiligo.

38. **What is onycholysis?**

Onycholysis, also called as Plummer's nail is the separation of the nail from the nail bed and is seen as deposition of dirt underneath the nail bed. This can occur in patients with thyrotoxicosis of any etiology, while the term acropachy is specific for Graves' disease.

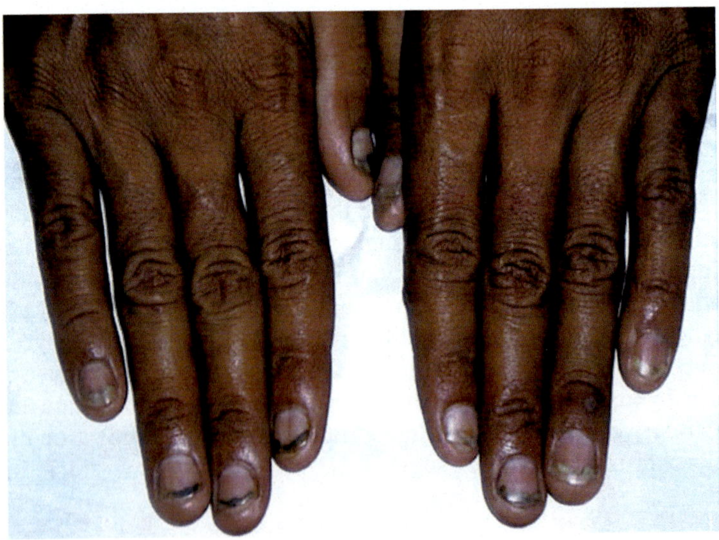

Fig. 11.8 Onycholysis in a patient with Graves' disease

39. **What is thyrotoxic periodic paralysis?**

Thyrotoxic periodic paralysis (TPP) is a recurrent, episodic, acute-onset flaccid, para-/quadriparesis due to hypokalemia in patients with thyrotoxicosis. TPP is rare with a prevalence of 0.1–2% among patients with thyrotoxicosis and is predominantly seen in men of Asian origin. It usually occurs in patients with Graves' disease, though it has been reported with thyrotoxicosis of other etiologies. Precipitating factors include carbohydrate-rich meals and rest following strenuous exercise. TPP can masquerade acute inflammatory demyelinating polyneuropathy or spinal shock. Presence of goiter, clinical features of toxicosis, or orbitopathy in a patient with acute-onset paraparesis or quadriparesis should raise a suspicion of TPP. It is due to an acquired channel defect associated with enhanced Na^+/K^+- ATPase pump activity leading to increased intracellular shift of potassium causing hypokalemic paralysis. The increased activity of Na^+/K^+- ATPase is due to excess T_4, augmented adrenergic sensitivity, and hyperinsulinemia due to thyrotoxicosis. In addition, inactivating mutations of Kir2.6 channels has also been implicated. Treatment of TPP includes supplementation with potassium, β-blockers, and thionamides followed by radio-ablation to prevent recurrence.

40. **What are the differences between thyrotoxic periodic paralysis and familial periodic paralysis?**

Parameters	Thyrotoxic periodic paralysis	Familial periodic paralysis
Age of onset	20–40 years	<25 years
Gender (M:F)	17–70:1	1:1
Inheritance	Sporadic	Autosomal dominant
Ethnicity	Asians	Caucasians
Thyrotoxicosis	Present	Absent
Pathogenesis	↑ Na^+/K^+- ATPase channel activity ↓ Kir2.6 channel activity	Voltage-sensitive calcium (90%) and sodium (10%) channels
Treatment	Thyroid ablation, β-blockers K^+ supplementation	K^+ supplementation, spironolactone

Suggested Reading

1. Bartalena L, Baldeschi L, Dickinson A, et al. Consensus statement of the European Group on Graves' orbitopathy (EUGOGO) on management of GO. Eur J Endocrinol. 2008;158:273–85.
2. Braverman LE, David C. Werner & Ingbar's the thyroid, a fundamental and clinical text. 10th ed. Philadelphia: Wolters Kluwer Health/Lippincott Williams & Wilkins; 2012.

3. Garber JR, Cobin RH, Gharib H, Hennessey JV, Klein I, Mechanick JI, Pessah-Pollack R, Singer PA, Woeber KA. Clinical practice guidelines for hypothyroidism in adults: cosponsored by the American Association of Clinical Endocrinologists and the American Thyroid Association. Endocr Pract. 2012;18(6):988–1028.
4. Jameson LJ, DeGroot LJ. Endocrinology: adult and pediatric. Philadelphia: Elsevier Health Sciences; 2010.
5. Melmed S, Polonsky KS, Reed Larsen P, Kronenberg HM. Williams textbook of endocrinology: expert consult. London: Elsevier Health Sciences; 2011.

12 Thyroid Disorders During Pregnancy

12.1 Case Vignette

A 27-year-old woman presented with primary infertility. She had regular menstrual cycles and had no galactorrhea. On evaluation, she was found to have features of thyrotoxicosis and bilateral proptosis. She had grade III diffuse goiter and clinically inactive, and moderate to severe thyroid associated orbitopathy. Her serum T_3 was 2.4 ng/ml (0.8–1.8), T_4 15.6 μg/dl (4.8–12.6), and TSH 0.01 μIU/ml (0.45–4.2). She was started on carbimazole 30 mg per day, and she achieved euthyroidism within 3 months of therapy, and the dose was reduced to 15 mg per day. She conceived after 11 months of therapy without any assisted reproductive techniques. During her first trimester, she had worsening of symptoms and her serum T_3 was 2.8 ng/ml, T_4 18.3 μg/dl, and TSH 0.001 μIU/ml. The dose of carbimazole was increased to 30 mg per day. At 4 months of gestation, she attained euthyroidism and the dose of carbimazole was decreased to 15 mg per day which was continued thereafter with regular monitoring of thyroid function tests. She delivered a term baby with a birth weight of 2.45 kg with normal APGAR score. The child was active and was accepting feed normally. Thyroid function of newborn was done on 5th day, which showed a serum T_3 1.2 ng/ml, T_4 10.3 μg/dl, and TSH 2.6 μIU/ml. The baby was discharged. At 3 weeks of life, the baby was brought to the hospital with lower respiratory tract infection, and he had weight loss of 0.6 kg despite normal feeding. Examination revealed a pulse rate of 170/min, sunken eyes, and no goiter. Repeat thyroid function test showed serum T_3 3.5 ng/ml, T_4 23.7 μg/dl, and TSH 0.005 μIU/ml. He was started on methimazole at a dose of 0.5 mg/kg/day and propranolol at a dose of 2 mg/kg/day, and the child progressively improved with a weight gain of 2 kg over the next 2 weeks. Thyroid function test at 6 weeks showed serum T_3 0.9 ng/ml, T_4 7.2 μg/dl, and TSH 1.4 μIU/ml, and the dose of methimazole was tapered to 0.25 mg/kg per day. Six weeks postpartum, mother had exacerbation of symptoms of toxicosis, with a heart rate of 120/min, tremors, and grade III goiter. TAO remained static during pregnancy and postpartum period. Her serum T_3 was 1.8 ng/ml, T_4 16.5 μg/dl, and TSH 0.05 μIU/ml; the dose of carbimazole was increased to 20 mg/day and

A. Bhansali, Y. Gogate, *Clinical Rounds in Endocrinology: Volume I - Adult Endocrinology*, DOI 10.1007/978-81-322-2398-6_12

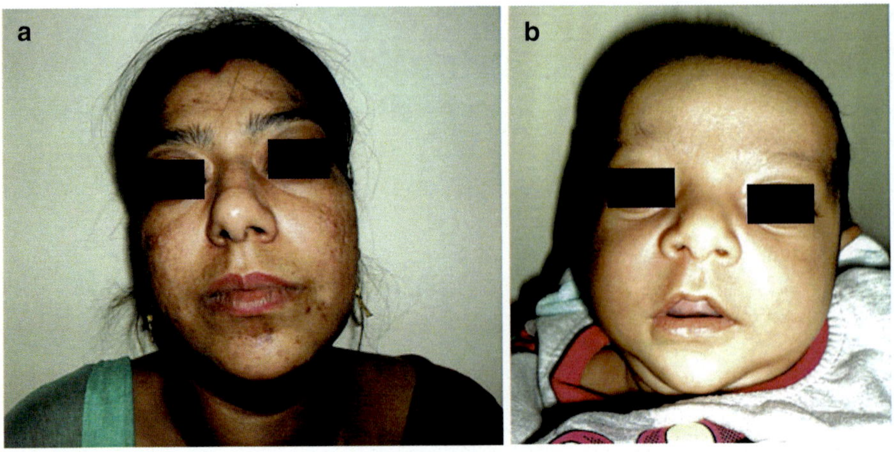

Fig. 12.1 (**a**) A 27-year-old lady with diffuse goiter and bilateral proptosis suggestive of Graves' disease. (**b**) A 6-week-old infant born to the mother with Graves' disease, who developed neonatal thyrotoxicosis

β-blocker was added. After 3 months of follow-up, the mother is clinically and biochemically euthyroid and is planned for thyroidectomy in view of large goiter. The baby is growing well and his thyroid function is normal without antithyroid drugs at 3 months.

12.2 Stepwise Analysis

The index patient had infertility despite regular menstrual cycles. Majority of women with Graves' disease have regular ovulatory cycles (around 80%), and infertility is present in only 5–10% of patients. After achievement of euthyroidism with the use of antithyroid drugs, the index patient conceived and pregnancy could be sustained. She had worsening of thyrotoxicosis during the first trimester with an increase in requirement of carbimazole. This is due to rising levels of hCG, which stimulates the thyroid gland due to "specificity spillover." After the first trimester, there was a decline in the requirement of antithyroid drugs due to increase in thyroxine-binding globulin and quiescence of Graves' disease due to suppression of autoimmunity by rising estradiol and progesterone. At 7 months of gestation, her thyroid function test (TFT) was T_3 2.3 ng/ml, T_4 17.9 μg/dl, and TSH 0.01 μIU/ml. She was continued on the same dose of carbimazole (15 mg per day) as these serum T_4 levels correspond to the normal range for pregnancy (one and a half times upper limit of normal). The higher reference range of serum total T_3 and T_4 in pregnancy is due to estrogen-mediated rise in thyroid-binding globulin. Ideally serum TRAb level should be estimated between 22 and 26 weeks of gestation in a patient with active Graves' disease to predict the risk of fetal and neonatal thyrotoxicosis and a close monitoring for fetal thyrotoxicosis, in case TRAbs are positive. Unfortunately, these measures could not be contemplated in our patient. She delivered a term baby with a low birth weight. However, thyroid function test of the newborn done on the 5th day was apparently normal. Ideally, TFT should be done on the first day of life in a neonate born to a mother with active Graves' disease, to recognize the disease at the earliest as neonatal TSH surge may not occur because of fetal thyrotoxicosis. Despite transplacental passage of TRAbs, neonatal thyrotoxicosis may not be present at birth. This may be due to the effect of maternal antithyroid drugs which readily cross placenta and prevents neonatal hyperthyroidism. Symptoms of neonatal thyrotoxicosis usually appear after 5–7 days, when antithyroid drugs are completely metabolized in the newborn. In some neonates, the onset of neonatal thyrotoxicosis may be further delayed if TSH blocking antibodies as well as stimulating antibodies are coexisting and blocking antibodies dominate over stimulating antibodies. After a diagnosis of hyperthyroidism was made in the index neonate, antithyroid drugs and β-blockers were initiated. There was resolution of thyrotoxicosis and antithyroid drugs were discontinued at 3 months. Neonatal thyrotoxicosis due to maternal Graves' disease is almost always transient and abates within 3–12 weeks with disappearance of TRAbs. In fact, if neonatal thyrotoxicosis does not ameliorate within 3–6 months, alternate diagnosis like McCune–Albright syndrome and TSH receptor-activating mutation should be considered. Patients with Graves' disease often have exacerbation of symptoms in the postpartum period due to withdrawal of estrogen and progesterone, as was seen in the index case at 6 weeks postpartum. In addition, patients with Graves' disease are predisposed for the development of postpartum thyroiditis, usually between 8 and 24 weeks postpartum, and present with symptoms of new-onset/worsening thyrotoxicosis.

12.3 Clinical Rounds

12.3.1 Pregnancy and Hypothyroidism

1. **What are the hormones of physiological importance to fetal thyroid axis that cross placenta?**

   Hormones that cross placenta are TRH (smallest peptide, three amino acids) and T_4. Maternal TRH plays an important role in the growth and development of fetal hypothalamo–pituitary–thyroid (HPT) axis, and T_4 is necessary for fetal neural growth and development, particularly during the first trimester, as the fetal HPT axis starts functioning after 12 weeks of intrauterine life. The deiodinase type 3 is expressed in placenta and modulates availability of free T_4; thereby preventing overexposure of thyroid hormones to the fetus.

2. **What are the molecules of clinical importance to thyroid gland that cross the placenta?**

   Iodine is the most important molecule which freely crosses placenta as syncytiotrophoblasts express sodium iodide symporter (NIS). Iodine helps in fetal thyroid growth and development and is a precursor for thyroid hormone biosynthesis. In addition, iodine per se plays a role in neural growth and development. Apart from iodine, TSH receptor antibody (TRAb) which includes thyroid stimulating immunoglobulin (TSI) and TSH-binding inhibitory immunoglobulin (TBII) can also cross placenta. Antithyroid drugs like carbimazole, methimazole, and propylthiouracil can cross placenta and may result in fetal goiter and hypothyroidism and can rarely cause "thionomide embryopathy." In addition, levothyroxine also crosses placenta.

3. **Why is iodine requirement increased during pregnancy?**

   During pregnancy, demand for iodine is increased by approximately 50%. This is due to increased maternal thyroid hormone synthesis, enhanced urinary iodine excretion, and utilization of iodine by the fetus. Production of T_3 and T_4 increases by 50% during pregnancy in response to rising hCG and increasing TBG, to maintain circulating free T_4 levels. Enhanced urinary iodine excretion is due to increased glomerular filtration rate during pregnancy resulting in hyperfiltration of iodine. Iodine is required by the fetus not only for thyroid hormone synthesis but also for neurocognitive development. Hence, recommended daily allowance of iodine is increased from 150 to 250 μg during pregnancy.

4. **Should all pregnant women be screened for thyroid dysfunction?**

   Ideally all pregnant women should be screened for thyroid dysfunction during the first trimester. Current data favors universal screening in view of increased risk of fetal loss in patients with untreated subclinical hypothyroidism and improvement in pregnancy outcome with levothyroxine therapy. Although fetal neurocognitive development may be impaired in patients with untreated subclinical hypothyroidism, there is insufficient data to show improvement in these parameters with treatment. Therefore, universal screening is debatable. However, high-risk individuals must be screened for thyroid dysfunction preferably preconceptionally or else during the first trimester, and these risk factors include: age >30 years, presence of goiter, TPO positivity, bad obstetric history, morbid obesity (BMI >40 kg/m^2), personal or family history of autoimmune thyroid disease or autoimmune disorders, presence of iodine deficiency, prior thyroid surgery, and use of amiodarone or lithium.

5. **What is the best screening test for evaluation of thyroid dysfunction during pregnancy?**

   Measurement of serum TSH is the best screening test for evaluation of thyroid dysfunction during pregnancy. However, levels of TSH should be interpreted according to trimester-specific range. If serum TSH is out of reference range for pregnancy, then estimation of free T_4/total T_4 should be performed. Serum T_3 is not indicated during pregnancy unless TSH is suppressed and free T_4 is normal.

6. **Why is serum TSH low in pregnant women as compared to nonpregnant women?**

   During pregnancy, placental human chorionic gonadotropin (hCG), a glycoprotein hormone that shares homology with TSH, directly stimulates the thyroid gland due to "specificity spillover." This results in an increased production of T_4, thereby inhibiting endogenous TSH. The clinical significance of this alteration is that median TSH is low in all trimesters as compared to nonpregnant women and especially so in the first trimester due to peak hCG levels. Hence, reference range for TSH during first trimester is 0.1–2.5 μIU/ml, second trimester 0.2–3.0 μIU/ml, and third trimester 0.3–3.0 μIU/ml.

7. **How to define subclinical and overt hypothyroidism during pregnancy?**

   The reference range for TSH during the first trimester is 0.1–2.5 μIU/ml, second trimester 0.2–3.0 μIU/ml, and third trimester 0.3–3.0 μIU/ml. Those with TSH values above the trimester-specific reference range with normal free T_4 are diagnosed to have subclinical hypothyroidism. Those with TSH value above the reference range but <10 μIU/ml with a low free T_4 or TSH >10 μIU/ml irrespective of free T_4 level are considered to have overt hypothyroidism during pregnancy.

8. **What to estimate during pregnancy, free T_4 or total T_4?**

   During pregnancy, total T_4 is increased as thyroxine-binding globulin (TBG) starts rising by 6–8 weeks and remains elevated throughout the pregnancy because of estrogen-mediated increased production and decreased clearance due to sialylation. Therefore, estimation of free T_4 is preferred during pregnancy. Free T_4 should be estimated by equilibrium dialysis as other available methods lack precision. However, non-availability and difficult assay technique precludes the routine use of equilibrium dialysis. An alternative to free T_4 estimation is to multiply the normal reference range of total T_4 for non-pregnant population by one and a half time.

9. **What are the risks associated with subclinical hypothyroidism during pregnancy?**

   Maternal risks associated with subclinical hypothyroidism are miscarriage, preterm delivery, and stillbirths, whereas fetal risks include low birth weight and possibly impaired neurocognitive development.

10. **Is treatment recommended for all women with subclinical hypothyroidism during pregnancy?**

    Yes. Treatment of subclinical hypothyroidism during pregnancy is associated with favorable maternal outcome. However, the effect of maternal subclinical hypothyroidism on fetal neurocognitive development is not so clear. Theoretically there is an increased risk of cognitive dysfunction in these newborns but data regarding improvement in cognitive outcome with levothyroxine in children born to mothers with subclinical hypothyroidism is not robust. However, ethically it is not appropriate to withhold a treatment having virtually no adverse effects.

11. **Is treatment with levothyroxine advised in euthyroid TPO-positive pregnant women?**

Pregnant women who have normal thyroid function but are TPO positive have an increased risk of recurrent miscarriages due to autoimmunity. The data regarding pregnancy outcome with the use of low dose levothyroxine in such subset of patients is variable. Available guidelines also do not support the use of levothyroxine in these patients. However, TSH should be monitored more frequently, and if increased beyond the upper limit of trimester-specific cutoff, levothyroxine should be initiated. Although therapy with selenium reduces TPO titers, it is not recommended.

12. **Should medical termination of pregnancy be considered in a patient with hypothyroidism detected during pregnancy?**

No. Maternal T_4 is essential for neural growth and development during first trimester, as fetal hypothalamo–pituitary–thyroid axis is functional only after 10–12 weeks of intrauterine life. Deficiency of maternal T_4 theoretically signals a poor neurological outcome, but the available literature in women with subclinical as well as overt hypothyroidism do not consistently support this risk. Hence, in women with subclinical or overt hypothyroidism detected any time during pregnancy, medical termination is not recommended. However, in pregnant women having severe T_4 deficiency with a history of previous child with mental/physical handicap/congenital malformation, especially from an iodine deficient area, the decision regarding medical termination of pregnancy can be taken after a detailed discussion with both parents.

13. **What are the causes of bad obstetric history in hypothyroidism?**

Optimal T_4 levels are necessary for a successful pregnancy outcome. Hypothyroidism, whether subclinical or overt, is associated with recurrent miscarriages due to impaired folliculogenesis, luteal phase defect, and senescent ova fertilization as a result of aberrant gonadotropin secretion. Further, the presence of secondary polycystic ovarian disease, hyperprolactinemia, impaired LH surge, and altered estrogen metabolism also contributes to ovarian dysfunction. Other causes of poor pregnancy outcome in hypothyroidism include gestational hypertension and placental abruption. TPO positivity with normal thyroid function has also been demonstrated to cause fetal loss which may be related to autoimmunity and is a surrogate marker of graft-versus-host disease. Concurrent presence of other autoimmune disease like anti-phospholipid antibody syndrome and celiac disease may further contribute to bad obstetric history.

14. **What should be the TSH target in a hypothyroid woman planning pregnancy?**

The recommended TSH level in a nonpregnant individual with hypothyroidism is 0.4–4.1 μIU/ml. However, when a woman is planning pregnancy, TSH should be targeted <2.5 μIU/ml as TSH even in the upper normal range (2.5–4.1 μIU/ml) is considered as relative hypothyroidism for a pregnant female during first trimester.

15. **A 26-year-old lady, who is a known hypothyroid for 5 years, on levothyroxine 50 μg per day presented at 12 weeks of gestation with a TSH of 13 μIU/ml. How to optimize the therapy?**

    Patients receiving therapy for overt/subclinical hypothyroidism prior to conception should be advised to increase the dose of levothyroxine by 30–50% at 4–6 weeks of gestation. However, failure to increase the dose during this period may result in elevated TSH. In women who are on levothyroxine therapy during pregnancy and have elevated TSH, a suggested dose adjustment schedule is as follows: TSH between 5–10 μIU/ml, increment of levothyroxine by 25–50 μg/day; TSH 10–20 μIU/ml, increment by 50–75 μg/day; and TSH >20 μIU/ml, increment by 75–100 μg/day. In the index case the dose of levothyroxine was increased to 125 μg/day, and she was advised to take iron and calcium supplements 6–8 h after intake of levothyroxine as they interfere with the absorption of levothyroxine. Her repeat TSH after 4 weeks was 1.2 μIU/ml.

12.3.2 Pregnancy and Hyperthyroidism

16. **Is suppressed TSH abnormal during pregnancy?**

    Human chorionic gonadotropin (hCG) is a glycoprotein hormone which shares homology with TSH and directly stimulates thyroid gland due to "specificity spillover". During pregnancy, placental hCG starts rising by the 3rd week, peaks by 12th week, and progressively declines thereafter. This results in an increased production of T_4, leading to suppression of endogenous TSH. The clinical significance of this alteration is that the median TSH is low in all trimesters. Hence, the reference range for TSH during first trimester is 0.1–2.5 μIU/ml, second trimester 0.2–3.0 μIU/ml, and third trimester 0.3–3.0 μIU/ml. TSH value less than the trimester-specific lower reference range is said to be suppressed, and possibility of thyrotoxicosis should be considered. However, the suppressed TSH value does not always suggest thyrotoxicosis as small percentage of normal pregnant women and women with multiple pregnancies may have TSH <0.01 μIU/ml.

17. **How to interpret a suppressed TSH value in pregnancy?**

    TSH value less than the trimester-specific lower reference range is considered to be suppressed. A suppressed TSH value should be accompanied with estimation of free T_4. Normal free T_4 with a suppressed TSH is suggestive of subclinical hyperthyroidism. In a subset of patients who have suppressed TSH and normal free T_4 with clinical signs of toxicosis, estimation of total T_3 may be useful as occasionally, Graves' disease may only have T_3 toxicosis. Suppressed TSH with elevated free T_4 suggests gestational thyrotoxicosis, molar pregnancy or Graves' disease.

18. **Does subclinical hyperthyroidism require treatment during pregnancy?**

Subclinical hyperthyroidism during pregnancy does not require treatment as it is not associated with adverse maternal or fetal outcome because serum free T_4 levels are within the normal range. Moreover, incidence of pregnancy-associated hypertension has been shown to be lower in those with subclinical hyperthyroidism. Further, treatment may be detrimental as it may result in fetal hypothyroidism because antithyroid drugs readily cross the placenta.

19. **How to suspect thyrotoxicosis during pregnancy?**

Failure to gain weight, heat intolerance, excessive sweating, and tachycardia disproportionate to duration of gestation are the clues which suggest thyrotoxicosis during pregnancy.

20. **How to differentiate between gestational thyrotoxicosis and Graves' disease?**

Gestational thyrotoxicosis is a transient, self-limiting, non-autoimmune hyperthyroidism which usually manifests between 10 to 16 weeks of gestation. High levels of placental hCG cross-react with the TSH receptors on the thyroid gland and lead to increased serum T_3 and T_4 during the first trimester and manifest as gestational thyrotoxicosis. If gestational thyrotoxicosis is associated with severe nausea, vomiting, weight loss, and ketonemia/ketonuria, it is called as gestational thyrotoxicosis with hyperemesis gravidarum. Gestational thyrotoxicosis should be differentiated from Graves' disease as the management is primarily symptomatic in the former due to the self-limiting nature of illness, whereas patients with Graves' disease require antithyroid drugs. Though it is difficult to differentiate between the two disorders based on clinical features or thyroid function tests, a prior history of thyroid disease, presence of goiter, infiltrative orbitopathy, and TRAbs positivity favor the diagnosis of Graves' disease.

21. **Why is molar pregnancy associated with hyperthyroidism?**

Molar pregnancy is characterized by excessive production of hCG by the trophoblastic tissue and is associated with hyperthyroidism in 7% of affected pregnancies. hCG has a weak TSH-like activity, and it has been shown that for every 10,000 mU/ ml increase in serum hCG, fT_4 increases by 0.1 ng/ dl and, therefore, extreme elevations of serum hCG results in hyperthyroidism. Patients present with classical symptoms of thyrotoxicosis and, rarely, with thyroid storm. The definitive treatment of hyperthyroidism associated with molar pregnancy is evacuation; however, many patients require β-blockers and antithyroid drugs for control of thyrotoxicosis prior to evacuation.

22. **What is the natural history of Graves' disease during pregnancy?**

Women with Graves' disease experience exacerbation of symptoms during the first trimester, and there is a gradual improvement during the second and third trimester. The initial aggravation is related to hCG-mediated increased thyroid hormone production, while the increase in TBG and suppression of autoimmunity by rising estradiol, progesterone, and cortisol levels leads to reduction in severity of disease in second and third trimester. This is evidenced by reduction in TRAb titer and decrease in requirement of antithyroid drugs during the second and third trimester. Further, 20–30% of patients may not require antithyroid drugs in the last trimester. However, soon after delivery there may be aggravation of disease due to sudden decline in placental steroids and reactivation of autoimmunity. This is evidenced by the fact that patients with Graves' disease who are in remission preconceptionally have a higher rate of relapse during post-partum period, as compared to non-pregnant women (84 vs 56%).

23. **When to estimate TRAbs during pregnancy?**

Indications for estimation of TRAbs during pregnancy include active Graves' disease, history of radio-ablative therapy or surgery for Graves' disease prior to pregnancy, history of a previous neonate with Graves' disease, and elevated TRAbs prior to pregnancy. Estimation of TRAbs during pregnancy is performed between 22 to 26 weeks of gestation as transplacental passage of TRAbs peaks during the second trimester and fetal TSH receptors becomes responsive to TRAbs by this time.

24. **How to suspect fetal thyrotoxicosis?**

Fetal thyrotoxicosis manifests as persistent tachycardia (>170 bpm lasting >10 min), intrauterine growth retardation, goiter, congestive cardiac failure, hydrops fetalis, and accelerated bone maturation. If remained undiagnosed, it may result in still birth.

25. **What are the causes of goiter in a fetus?**

Goiter in a fetus commonly results from the use of antithyroid drugs or iodine-containing preparations by the mother. In addition, maternal Graves' disease with transplacental passage of TRAbs or fetal thyroid dyshormonogenesis can also cause fetal goiter. Rarely, TSH receptor-activating mutations may result in fetal goiter.

26. **How to plan a pregnancy in a patient with Graves' disease?**

Patients of Graves' disease should be rendered euthyroid prior to conception. Women who are euthyroid on maintenance doses of antithyroid drugs (5–15 mg carbimazole) can safely proceed for pregnancy. A patient with Graves' disease who is drug-naïve or toxic on antithyroid drugs or euthyroid on higher doses of antithyroid drugs (>15 mg carbimazole) should be considered for ablative therapy prior to conception. This is because of difficulties in controlling hyperthyroidism during pregnancy, risk of fetal thyroid dysfunction due to transplacental passage of antithyroid drugs, and the possibility of resurgence of disease in postpartum period. After radio-ablation, conception should be avoided for the next 6 months for optimizing levothyroxine therapy. Surgery may be preferred over radio-ablation as the level of TRAbs may increase and remain so for up to 1 year post radio-ablation, while after surgery the levels decline faster.

27. **How to treat Graves' disease during pregnancy?**

Hyperthyroidism can be associated with preterm delivery, preeclampsia, fetal/neonatal thyrotoxicosis, and increased perinatal and maternal mortality; hence treatment is indicated. The treatment of choice for Graves' disease during pregnancy is antithyroid drugs. Propylthiouracil (PTU) is indicated in the first trimester and carbimazole/methimazole in second and third trimesters. PTU has a theoretical advantage of lower transplacental transfer due to its high protein binding; however, recent evidence suggests that both methimazole and PTU cross the placenta readily. Therefore, switching over to propylthiouracil in the first trimester may not be associated with lesser risk of thionamide embryopathy. Moreover, PTU is associated with a risk of severe hepatotoxicity; hence in the present clinical scenario, carbimazole/methimazole seems to be an appropriate choice throughout the pregnancy. β-Blockers should be stopped during the first trimester and may be used with caution later as it may be associated with intrauterine growth retardation, fetal bradycardia, poor lung development, and neonatal hypoglycemia. Radioactive iodine is absolutely contraindicated during pregnancy. Iodized salt should be continued in pregnant women even with Graves' disease as it is required for fetal thyroid and neural growth and development.

28. **How to monitor a patient of Graves' disease during pregnancy?**

Free T_4/total T_4 and TSH should be monitored at 4–6-week interval during pregnancy. Free T_4 should be maintained at or just above trimester-specific upper limit of normal, or if total T_4 is opted, then it should be kept one and a half times upper limit of normal. Serum T_3 is not useful for monitoring, as attempts to normalize serum T_3 during pregnancy result in overtreatment with antithyroid drugs and fetal hypothyroidism. TSH may remain suppressed throughout the pregnancy; however, if it increases, dose of antithyroid drugs should be reduced to maintain TSH in trimester-specific ranges. In addition, estimation of TRAbs is useful during pregnancy to predict the risk of fetal and neonatal thyrotoxicosis.

29. **What is "thionamide embryopathy"?**

"Thionamide embryopathy" is associated with defects like choanal atresia, esophageal atresia, omphalocele, omphalomesenteric duct anomalies, and aplasia cutis due to exposure to thionamides (propylthiouracil, carbimazole, methimazole) in the first trimester. Theoretically, propylthiouracil has lesser risk of congenital malformations due to its increased protein binding and lower transplacental transfer. However, recent data do not support this notion.

30. **What are the indications for thyroid surgery in Graves' disease during pregnancy?**

Patients of Graves's disease who are intolerant to anti-thyroid drugs or experience serious drug-related adverse events, require high doses of anti-thyroid drugs (over 30 mg/d methimazole or 450 mg/d PTU) or non-compliant to therapy should be offered surgery in the second trimester.

12.3.3 Thyroid Dysfunction in the Newborn

31. **What is the normal thyroid function profile in a neonate?**

    Immediately after birth of a term baby, there is a neonatal TSH surge, which can be as high as 80 μIU/ml. This elevation of TSH is physiological and occurs in response to exposure to cold environment after birth. The elevated TSH increases free T_4 within 24 h, to induce nonshivering thermogenesis. Thereafter, there is a gradual decline in TSH and free T_4 levels, and by second week free T_4 normalizes and TSH levels falls to <10 μIU/ml.

32. **What are the thyroid dysfunction in newborn of a mother with subclinical hypothyroidism?**

    Maternal subclinical hypothyroidism is usually not associated with fetal thyroid dysfunction; hence neonatal thyroid function test is likely to be normal. However, if the cause of maternal subclinical hypothyroidism is iodine deficiency, the neonate may develop subclinical or overt hypothyroidism. Further, if the mother is harboring TSH receptor-blocking antibodies, the neonate is at risk for developing hypothyroidism. This has been reported only in a handful of cases.

33. **How to suspect hypothyroidism in a neonate?**

    Unexplained post-maturity, macrosomia, open posterior fontanel, poor feeding, hypothermia, prolonged physiological jaundice, umbilical hernia, constipation, macroglossia, and hoarse cry are the clues to suspect hypothyroidism in a neonate. Serum TSH and T_4 should be estimated immediately and an abnormal thyroid function test (low T_4 and elevated TSH) mandates urgent therapy. Technetium scintigraphy helps in defining the etiology and hence should be performed in all newborn with congenital hypothyroidism; however, therapy should not be delayed awaiting scan. Estimation of bone age (X-ray knee) is complementary in establishing the diagnosis and monitoring of therapy. As most newborns with hypothyroidism are asymptomatic, universal thyroid screening is an important tool to identify neonatal hypothyroidism at the earliest to prevent neurocognitive dysfunction.

34. **What are the endocrine causes of prolonged physiological jaundice?**

    The endocrine disorders associated with prolonged physiological jaundice (>2 weeks in term and >3 weeks in preterm baby) include congenital hypothyroidism and isolated growth hormone deficiency. Glucuronyl transferase is a key enzyme involved in bilirubin metabolism, and its activity is regulated by thyroxine and growth hormone. Therefore, infants with deficiency of these hormones manifest as prolonged physiological jaundice.

35. **What are the endocrine causes of post-maturity?**

Post-maturity is defined as prolongation of gestation beyond 42 weeks. The endocrine causes include congenital hypothyroidism, placental sulfatase deficiency, and congenital adrenal hypoplasia. Initiation of labor depends upon fetal movements and optimal levels of estrogen, prostaglandins, and oxytocin. Congenital hypothyroidism is associated with decreased fetal movement, and the latter two disorders are accompanied with decreased production of fetal estrogen.

36. **What are the causes of congenital hypothyroidism?**

The most common cause of congenital hypothyroidism is thyroid dysgenesis (65%) which includes ectopia, aplasia, hypoplasia, and hemi-agenesis. Other causes include thyroid dyshormonogenesis (10%) and severe iodine deficiency. All these disorders result in permanent hypothyroidism. Use of antithyroid drugs or iodine-containing preparation by the mother, TSH receptor-blocking immunoglobulins, and DUOX-2 gene mutation are important causes of transient neonatal hypothyroidism. In addition, multiple pituitary hormone deficiency due to pituitary transcription factor defects may also present as neonatal hypothyroidism.

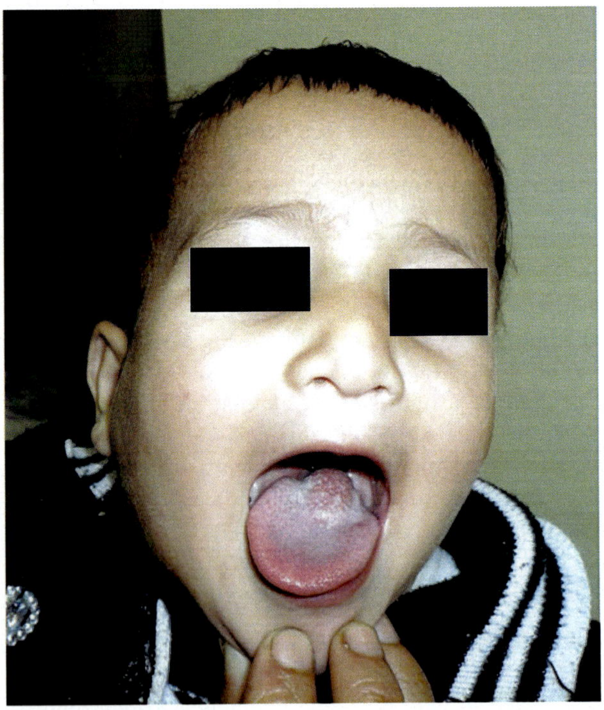

Fig. 12.2 A child with lingual thyroid

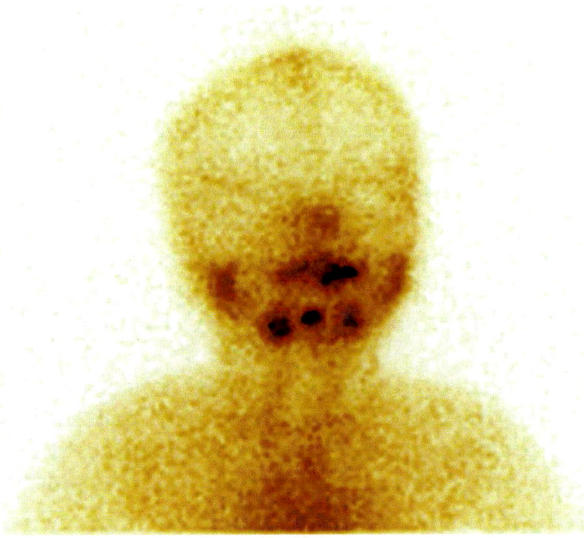

Fig. 12.3 ^{99m}Tc pertechnetate thyroid scan showing tracer uptake in the region of base of tongue without any uptake in the neck suggestive of lingual thyroid

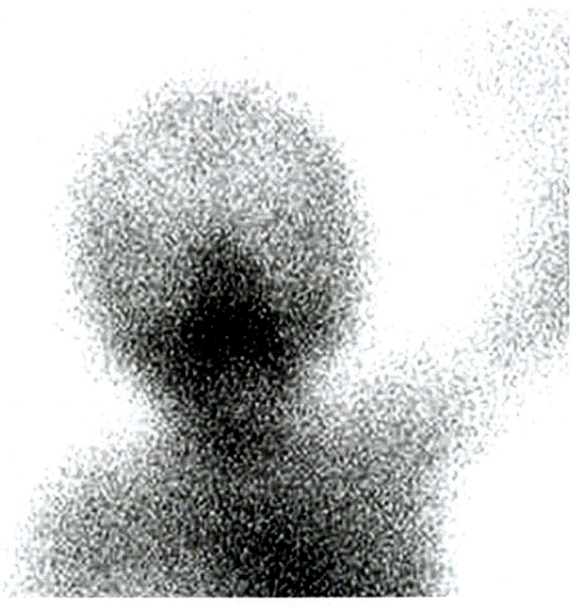

Fig. 12.4 ^{99m}Tc pertechnetate thyroid scan showing no tracer uptake in region of neck suggestive of thyroid agenesis in a child with congenital hypothyroidism

37. **Why is it important to establish the etiological diagnosis of congenital hypothyroidism?**

Investigation required to establish the etiological diagnosis of congenital hypothyroidism includes ^{99m}Tc pertechnetate scan, USG thyroid, serum thyroglobulin, and, if indicated, MRI of the sella. ^{99m}Tc pertechnetate scan, is a useful modality to identify the presence and location of thyroid gland. If there is no uptake found on ^{99m}Tc scan, measurement of serum thyroglobulin is indicated and undetectable levels confirm a diagnosis of thyroid aplasia. Absent or ectopic gland suggests permanent hypothyroidism and the need for lifelong levothyroxine replacement. Further, localization of ectopic thyroid gland may prevent inadvertent removal of thyroid gland. Eutopic thyroid gland in the presence of hypothyroidism signifies dyshormonogenesis or transient hypothyroidism. USG is useful for detection of goiter associated with dyshormonogenesis, where ^{99m}Tc pertechnetate scan, shows increased uptake. MR imaging should be performed in those with suspected secondary hypothyroidism.

38. **When to do thyroid scintigraphy in a neonate with hypothyroidism?**

^{99m}Tc scintigraphy should be performed in all neonates with hypothyroidism, ideally at diagnosis, before initiating treatment; however, therapy should not be delayed awaiting scan. Thyroid scintigraphy can even be performed within 3–4 days of initiation of therapy, provided serum TSH is high (>30 μIU/ml). If thyroid scintigraphy was not performed at diagnosis, it is prudent to continue levothyroxine till 3 years of age as neuronal growth and development are nearly complete by this age. Thereafter, thyroid scan can be performed after discontinuation of levothyroxine for 1 month.

39. **How to treat congenital hypothyroidism?**

Need for immediate initiation of levothyroxine therapy, requirement of higher doses of levothyroxine, need for rapid achievement of euthyroidism, and monitoring of therapy by serum T_4 rather than TSH are distinctive features in the management of congenital hypothyroidism. Initiation of treatment even on clinical suspicion (awaiting biochemical confirmation) and rapid achievement of euthyroidism is important to improve neurocognitive outcome. Higher doses of levothyroxine (10–15 μg/kg/day) are required as compared to adults because of greater body surface area of infants. Serum T_4 and TSH should be monitored on treatment.

40. **What are the thyroid dysfunction in the newborn of a mother with subclinical hyperthyroidism?**

Maternal subclinical hyperthyroidism is usually not associated with adverse pregnancy outcome, and neonatal thyroid function is expected to be normal. However, if the etiology of subclinical hyperthyroidism is Graves' disease, the neonate is at risk for thyrotoxicosis due to transplacental transfer of TRAbs.

41. **What are the characteristics of neonatal thyrotoxicosis?**

Neonatal thyrotoxicosis is characterized by low birth weight, poor feeding, failure to thrive, diarrhea, prominent eyes, microcephaly, tachycardia, and heart failure. Thyroid profile is consistent with severe thyrotoxicosis with markedly elevated T_3, T_4, and suppressed TSH. The most common cause of neonatal thyrotoxicosis is transplacental passage of TRAbs and usually remits spontaneously within 3–12 weeks as half-life of TRAbs is 2 weeks. However, persistence of disease beyond 6 months raises the possibility of rare causes like McCune–Albright syndrome and TSH receptor-activating mutations.

42. **How to treat neonatal thyrotoxicosis?**

Neonatal thyrotoxicosis should be managed as thyroid storm as mortality is high (30%) in untreated neonates. Treatment includes antithyroid drugs (methimazole 0.25 mg to 1 mg/kg/day in two to three divided doses), propranolol 2 mg/kg/day, and iodides if required. Propylthiouracil is contraindicated as neonates are at a higher risk of hepatotoxicity. Glucocorticoids should be instituted to tide over the crisis. Antithyroid drugs are required only for short duration as TRAb-mediated neonatal thyrotoxicosis remits by itself within 2–3 months. However those with McCune–Albright syndrome and TSH receptor-activating mutations require definitive therapy later, after attaining euthyroidism with antithyroid drugs.

43. **How to monitor a patient of subclinical hypothyroidism during lactation?**

A patient who is on levothyroxine replacement therapy during pregnancy for subclinical hypothyroidism usually needs a reduction in doses by 20–30% soon after delivery. The treatment needs to be continued throughout lactation (~6 months) for postpartum well-being of the mother. Stoppage of levothyroxine immediately in postpartum period may lead to exacerbation of autoimmune thyroid disease and may also predispose for postpartum thyroiditis. The risk of developing hypothyroidism in an infant born to a mother with subclinical hypothyroidism is very low; however, thyroid function tests are indicated in these newborns.

44. **How to monitor a patient of Graves' disease during lactation?**

Patients of Graves' disease who are either in remission or on maintenance doses of carbimazole (10–15 mg per day) may experience exacerbation of symptoms in the postpartum period. Therefore, a periodic thyroid function monitoring is required. The dose of carbimazole which is considered safe during lactation is <15 mg. If it exceeds more than 15 mg, then the drug concentration secreted in the breast milk is sufficient to interfere with the development and maturation of HPT axis of the newborn. Caution should be exercised to feed the baby 4 h after intake of carbimazole. However, if the mother requires higher doses of carbimazole, periodic monitoring of thyroid function test of mother as well as newborn is required.

Suggested Reading

1. Alex S-G, Marcos A, Erik A. Guidelines of the American Thyroid Association for the Diagnosis and Management of Thyroid Disease During Pregnancy and Postpartum. Thyroid. 2011;21(10):1081–125.
2. Braverman LE, Cooper D. Werner & Ingbar's the thyroid: a fundamental and clinical text. 10th ed. Philadelphia: Wolters Kluwer Health/Lippincott Williams & Wilkins; 2012.
3. De Groot L, Abalovich M, Alexander EK. Management of thyroid dysfunction during pregnancy and postpartum. An endocrine society clinical practice guideline. J Clin Endocrinol Metab. 2012;97:2543–65.
4. Jameson JL, De Groot LJ. Endocrinology: adult and pediatric. Philadelphia: Elsevier Health Sciences; 2010.
5. Melmed S, Polonsky KS, Larsen PR, Kronenberg HM. Williams textbook of endocrinology: expert consult. London: Elsevier Health Sciences; 2011.

Disorders of Mineral Homeostasis 13

13.1 Case Vignette

A 55-year-old male presented with epigastric pain for the past 6 weeks. It was intermittent, moderate in severity, and associated with nausea and vomiting. He also had anorexia, constipation, and weight loss of 15 kg in the last 6 months. He underwent pyelolithotomy 2 months back for renal stone disease. There was no history of gallstone disease, bone pains, or fragility fracture. He was nonalcoholic and nonsmoker. On examination, he was dehydrated with a blood pressure 90/72 mmHg, pulse rate 126/min, and central venous pressure 2 cm H_2O. Abdominal examination revealed a 10×8 cm mass in the epigastrium extending to right hypochondrium. Ultrasonography of the abdomen showed a bulky pancreas with multiple collections in the peripancreatic region. On investigations, hemoglobin was 12.4 g/dl, total leukocyte count 12,300/cumm^3, serum sodium 129 mEq/L, potassium 5 mEq/L, creatinine 2.6 mg/dl, corrected calcium 15.1 mg/dl, ionized calcium 1.75 mmol/L, phosphorus 3 mg/dl, and alkaline phosphatase 240 IU/L. His serum lipase was 77 U/L, amylase 24 U/L, and liver function tests were normal. Serum iPTH was 8.1 pg/ml (9–65), 25(OH)D 10 ng/ml, and 1,25$(OH)_2$D 62.2 pg/ml (19.6–54.3). Based on clinical and biochemical profile, a diagnosis of PTH-independent hypercalcemia and pancreatitis was considered. There was no history of intake of lithium, thiazides, vitamin A, or D. Angiotensin-converting enzyme levels were normal and workup for multiple myeloma was noncontributory. Contrast-enhanced CT of chest and abdomen revealed hilar lymphadenopathy and bulky pancreas with multiple collections in the lesser sac. ^{18}F-FDG-PET showed avid uptake in the mediastinal lymph nodes. Transbronchial lymph node biopsy was suggestive of sarcoidosis. The patient was managed with intravenous saline, diuretics, zoledronic acid 5 mg, and prednisolone 1 mg/kg/day. There was a rapid normalization of serum calcium levels within 3–4 days, and prednisolone was gradually tapered over a period of 6 months with sustained normalization of serum calcium during follow-up. Later, he was subjected to cystogastrostomy for pancreatic pseudocyst.

A. Bhansali, Y. Gogate, *Clinical Rounds in Endocrinology: Volume I - Adult Endocrinology*, DOI 10.1007/978-81-322-2398-6_13

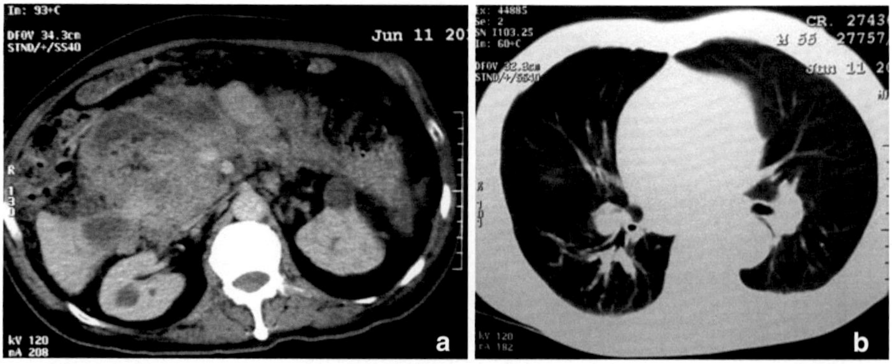

Fig. 13.1 (**a**) CECT abdomen showing bulky pancreas with necrosis and peripancreatic fat stranding suggestive of pancreatitis. (**b**) CT chest in the same patient showing bilateral hilar adenopathy

13.2 Stepwise Analysis

The presence of anorexia, constipation, and significant weight loss for the past 6 months in the index patient mandates evaluation for chronic infectious disease, inflammatory disorders, and malignancy. Patient had epigastric pain and an abdominal lump; therefore, a possibility of gastrointestinal malignancy was considered initially. However, ultrasonography revealed bulky pancreas and peripancreatic collections. Presence of renal stone disease along with pancreatitis raised the suspicion of primary hyperparathyroidism. But, the biochemistry revealed hypercalcemia with low iPTH, suggestive of PTH-independent hypercalcemia. The differential diagnosis of PTH-independent hypercalcemia includes malignancy (lung, breast, kidney, lymphoma, and multiple myeloma), chronic granulomatous disorders (tuberculosis and sarcoidosis), and drugs (lithium, thiazide, calcium containing antacids, and vitamin D). The possibility of malignancy-associated hypercalcemia was high in the index patient as he had history of significant weight loss, short duration of symptoms, and severe hypercalcemia (serum calcium >14 mg/dl). To establish the etiology of hypercalcemia, CT chest and abdomen, serum and urine protein electrophoresis, ACE levels, 25(OH)D and 1,25$(OH)_2$D levels were performed. CT chest showed bilateral hilar adenopathy and a parenchymal nodule which suggested the diagnosis of sarcoidosis. ^{18}F-FDG-PET showed avid uptake only in the mediastinal lymph nodes thereby excluding possibility of disseminated disease. The diagnosis of sarcoidosis was further substantiated by high serum 1,25(OH)2D levels and was confirmed on histopathology. Serum ACE levels were normal in our patient as elevated ACE levels are seen only in 60% of patients with active disease. The significant weight loss in our patient can be attributed to anorexia and nausea associated with hypercalcemia and possibly due to IL-6 and IFN-ϒ secreted from noncaseating granulomas in sarcoidosis. Pancreatitis in the index patient may be due to severe hypercalcemia and possibly because of involvement of the pancreas by sarcoid granulomas. However, the cause and effect relationship between hypercalcemia and pancreatitis is not well established. Hypercalcemia occurs in 4–11% of patients with sarcoidosis and 10% of patients may have nephrolithiasis, as was seen in our patient. Severe hypercalcemia is uncommon in sarcoidosis; however, in our patient it could be attributed to marked intravascular volume depletion due to recurrent vomiting, pancreatitis, and nephrogenic diabetes insipidus. Volume repletion followed by saline diuresis is the initial management strategy in hypercalcemia. Bisphosphonates are useful in hypercalcemia of any etiology and the reduction in serum calcium with intravenous bisphosphonates is apparent by 48–72 h. Zoledronic acid can be safely administered in patients with an eGFR of >60 ml/min; however, in those with eGFR 30–60 ml/min, the standard dose can be given, but at a slower rate. Zoledronic acid is best avoided in those with eGFR <30 ml/min and dialysis should be preferred in this scenario. Glucocorticoids are the definitive treatment for hypercalcemia associated with sarcoidosis. They inhibit macrophage 1α-hydroxylase and decrease the production of PTHrP, IFNϒ, and bone-resorbing cytokines. In addition, they also inhibit intestinal calcium absorption and cause hypercalciuria. Vitamin D supplementation should be avoided in patients with chronic granulomatous disorders because they are at an increased risk of developing hypercalcemia due to upregulated 1α-hydroxylase activity in the macrophages.

13.3 Clinical Rounds

1. **How to define hypercalcemia?**

   Serum calcium level above the reference range is considered as hypercalcemia. The reference range for serum calcium is based on the data derived from healthy subjects and is dependent on age, vitamin D status, and analytical method. Increasing age and postmenopausal status is associated with modest rise in serum calcium. Older biochemical methods underestimate serum calcium, while the newer auto-analyzer system accurately measures it.

2. **What are the precautions to be taken while sampling and interpreting calcium value?**

   Application of tourniquet while sampling, hydration status, serum albumin, and analytical method influence serum calcium level. Serum calcium can be measured at any time of day irrespective of fasting state and posture (sitting/supine). Use of tourniquet falsely elevates serum calcium due to local increase in protein binding and acidosis leading to release of tissue calcium. Dehydration results in hemoconcentration and false elevation of total serum calcium. Serum albumin also influence total serum calcium; therefore, calcium should be corrected for albumin. Older biochemical methods (Clark and Collip) tend to underestimate serum calcium; hence, newer methods (auto-analyzer) are preferred. After considering these factors, an elevated serum calcium value requires reconfirmation especially if it is mildly elevated.

3. **Why does serum calcium need to be corrected for albumin?**

   Almost 99% of total body calcium is present in the bone and only 1% is present in the extracellular fluid. Half of the circulating calcium is bound to albumin and the rest is free. Therefore, alterations in serum albumin levels significantly influence the total serum calcium. As a result, serum calcium needs to be adjusted in relation to albumin based on the following formula:

Corrected calcium (mg/dl) = 0.8 × (4.0 − serum albumin [g/dl]) + measured total Ca [mg/dl].

This correction is important to avoid underestimation or overestimation of serum calcium depending upon the low or high serum albumin, respectively. If available, it is preferable to measure serum ionized calcium.

4. **What are the causes of pseudo-hypercalcemia?**

   Pseudo-hypercalcemia is characterized by increased total serum calcium with normal ionized calcium. This is seen in patients with severe dehydration and paraproteinemia (e.g., multiple myeloma) and is due to increased protein binding.

5. **What is the next biochemical investigation required after confirmation of hypercalcemia?**

   After confirmation of hypercalcemia, serum parathyroid hormone (PTH) should be estimated along with phosphate and creatinine. These investigations help in the differential diagnosis of hypercalcemia. An elevated PTH level above the reference range in the setting of hypercalcemia suggests PTH-dependent hypercalcemia. However, 10–20% of patients with PTH-dependent hypercalcemia may have serum PTH levels within the reference range. Those with PTH value <20 pg/ml are considered to have PTH-independent hypercalcemia.

6. **Why to measure serum phosphate after overnight fast?**

   A healthy individual can have a variation in serum phosphate levels by as much as 50% during the day. Therefore, certain precautions are required while estimating serum phosphate. Serum phosphate should be measured in fasting state as postprandial rise in insulin, particularly after carbohydrate-rich meal, promotes intracellular shift of phosphate and falsely lowers it. In addition, the circadian variation in phosphate levels, being higher in morning than evening, necessitates morning sampling for phosphate. Therefore, the sample for phosphate should be taken in the morning after an overnight fast. Further, it should be ensured that the blood sample should not be hemolyzed as it can falsely elevate the phosphate level.

7. **What are the precautions to be taken during sampling for PTH?**

   PTH is a heat-labile peptide; therefore, the sample should be collected in a prechilled EDTA tube with immediate cold centrifugation and stored at −20 °C. The sample should be processed within 72 h of venipuncture. However, the sample should be stored at −80 °C if PTH is to be estimated later but not exceeding 2 months (DiaSorin Liaison) or 2 years (Roche Elecsys).

8. **What is "intact PTH" assay?**

   PTH is an 84 amino acid peptide with amino- and carboxy-terminal regions. The amino-terminal region imparts biological activity to PTH, while carboxy terminal region is biologically inactive. Normally, intact PTH (1–84) and inactive carboxy-terminal PTH fragments are secreted from the parathyroid gland, while amino-terminal fragments (1–34) are not secreted. Difficulties in the estimation of serum PTH include very low concentrations of intact PTH and presence of very high concentration of biologically inactive carboxy-terminal fragments. Therefore, a two-site assay called "intact PTH" assay, which requires the presence of both amino-terminal and carboxy-terminal sequences in the same molecule, is preferred as it measures only the biologically active form of circulating PTH, i.e., intact PTH (1–84).

9. **What are the causes of PTH-dependent hypercalcemia?**

The causes of PTH-dependent hypercalcemia include primary hyperparathyroidism (adenoma/hyperplasia/carcinoma), tertiary hyperparathyroidism, familial hypocalciuric hypercalcemia, anti-CaSR antibody-mediated hyperparathyroidism, and lithium therapy. Use of thiazide diuretics per se does not cause hypercalcemia, but may unmask hypercalcemia of any etiology including primary hyperparathyroidism.

10. **What are the causes of low PTH in a patient with parathyroid adenoma?**

Serum PTH >20 pg/ml suggests PTH-dependent hypercalcemia. However, patients with PTH-dependent hypercalcemia can rarely have low or undetectable serum PTH even in the presence of histologically proven parathyroid adenoma. This can be attributed to improper sampling and transportation, "hook effect" with sandwich immunoassays (e.g., immunoradiometric assay, IRMA), and secretion of bioactive but non-immunoreactive PTH fragments by the tumor. Rarely PTH-related peptide (PTHrP) can be secreted from parathyroid tumor and biochemically mimics PTH-independent hypercalcemia.

11. **What are the causes of normal/high serum phosphate in primary hyperparathyroidism?**

Primary hyperparathyroidism is commonly associated with hypercalcemia and hypophosphatemia. The causes of normal/high serum phosphate in the presence of PHPT include hemolyzed sample, asymptomatic hyperparathyroidism, and coexisting renal insufficiency. Rarely, MEN1 syndrome with PHPT and acromegaly can also be associated with normal serum phosphate due to the opposing effects of GH and PTH on renal tubular phosphate reabsorption. In children with PHPT, age-specific range should be considered for the interpretation of serum phosphate levels.

12. **How does lithium cause hypercalcemia?**

Chronic lithium administration interferes with the action of calcium-sensing receptor in the parathyroid gland and results in higher set point for suppression of PTH, thereby leading to uninhibited PTH secretion. Occasionally, this may result in development of parathyroid hyperplasia and rarely parathyroid adenoma. Hypercalcemia associated with lithium therapy is usually mild and resolves after discontinuation of therapy in majority. However, patients who develop parathyroid hyperplasia or adenoma may have persistent hypercalcemia even after discontinuation of lithium.

13. **What is familial hypocalciuric hypercalcemia?**

    Familial hypocalciuric hypercalcemia (FHH) is an autosomal dominant disorder characterized by hypercalcemia, hypocalciuria, and normal or mildly elevated PTH. It is due to inactivating mutation of calcium-sensing receptor (CaSR) at both thick ascending limb of loop of Henle and parathyroid gland. In normal physiology, activation of CaSR result in excretion of calcium at renal tubular level and inhibits secretion of PTH from parathyroid gland. Patients with FHH are mostly asymptomatic and are detected incidentally. Hypercalcemia is usually mild and is present since birth. Therefore, any child with hypercalcemia should be evaluated for FHH. A urinary calcium/creatinine clearance ratio <0.01 suggests FHH. Chondrocalcinosis, premature vascular calcification, pancreatitis, and gallstone disease may rarely be seen in patients with FHH. Majority of patients do not require any treatment and inadvertent parathyroid surgery has not yielded any benefit. Rarely, biochemical profile mimicking FHH is seen in adults harboring autoimmune disorders and is due to the presence of anti-CaSR antibodies.

14. **What are the causes of parathyroid-independent hypercalcemia?**

    The most common cause of PTH-independent hypercalcemia is malignancy-related hypercalcemia, either due to solid tumors (e.g., carcinoma lung, carcinoma breast) or hematological malignancies (e.g., multiple myeloma, lymphoma). Other common causes of PTH-independent hypercalcemia include chronic granulomatous disorders (e.g., sarcoidosis, tuberculosis), vitamin D/A intoxication and milk-alkali syndrome. In addition, hyperthyroidism, immobilization and adrenal insufficiency may also result in PTH-independent hypercalcemia.

15. **What are the investigations required in a patient with PTH-independent hypercalcemia?**

    25-hydroxyvitamin D, 1,25-dihydroxyvitamin D, serum ACE level, and serum and urine protein electrophoresis, are the first-line biochemical investigations required in a patient with PTH-independent hypercalcemia. CECT chest and abdomen, mammography, ^{99m}Tc MDP bone scan and ^{18}F-FDG-PET are also helpful in establishing the etiology. Serum parathyroid hormone-related protein (PTHrP) may be estimated when the source of hypercalcemia remains obscure despite all investigations.

16. **What is humoral hypercalcemia of malignancy?**

    Humoral hypercalcemia of malignancy (HHM) is a paraneoplastic manifestation of solid tumors without osseous metastasis and is mediated by circulating PTHrP. HHM contributes to 80% of malignancy-related hypercalcemia and the remaining 20% of malignancy-related hypercalcemia is due to osteolytic metastasis. Most common tumors associated with HHM are squamous cell cancer (lung, esophagus, head and neck, cervix), renal cell carcinoma, and breast carcinoma. PTHrP acts on PTH/PTHrP receptor leading to hypercalcemia and hypophosphatemia. Osteolytic metastasis-associated hypercalcemia is mediated by cytokines, chemokines, and local PTHrP leading to increased bone resorption and is seen in patients with multiple myeloma, lymphoma, and breast carcinoma. Rarely, ectopic production of PTH or calcitriol may also contribute to malignancy-related hypercalcemia. The differences between HHM and osteolytic metastasis-related hypercalcemia are summarized in the table below.

Parameters	HHM	Osteolytic metastasis
Prevalence	80%	20%
Mechanism	Circulating PTHrP	Cytokines, chemokines, and local PTHrP
Serum calcium	Elevated	Elevated
Serum phosphate	Low	Normal
Serum PTH	Low	Low
Malignancy	Squamous cell cancer	Lymphoma, multiple myeloma

17. **What are the differences between PTH- and PTHrP-mediated hypercalcemia?**

The differences between PTH and PTHrP in physiology and PTH- and PTHrP-mediated hypercalcemia are summarized in the table given below.

Parameters	PTH	PTHrP
Structure	84 amino acids	139–173 amino acids
Expression	Post-natal life	Fetal life
Receptor	PTH/PTHrP	PTH/PTHrP
Effect on 1α-hydroxylase	Stimulates	No action
Effect on urinary calcium reabsorption	Increase	Increase
Actions	Endocrine	Autocrine, paracrine, and endocrine
Physiological role	Bone remodeling	Fetal chondro-osteogenesis Placental calcium transport

Parameters	PTH-mediated hypercalcemia	PTHrP-mediated hypercalcemia
Disorder	Hyperparathyroidism	HHM
Presentation	Insidious	Rapid
Serum calcium	Mild to moderate hypercalcemia	Severe hypercalcemia
Serum phosphate	Low	Low
Alkaline phosphatase	Elevated	Normal
Bone turnover		
Formation	Stimulates	No effect
Resorption	Stimulates	Stimulates

18. **Why are granulomatous diseases associated with hypercalcemia?**

Granulomatous diseases like tuberculosis, sarcoidosis, fungal infections, and Wegener's granulomatosis are associated with hypercalcemia. It is due to increased 1α-hydroxylase activity, decreased degradation of 1,25-OHD_3, and secretion of PTHrP and bone-resorbing cytokines like IL-6 from granulomatous lesions. Increased 1α-hydroxylase activity and decreased degradation of 1,25-OHD_3 in the macrophage are mediated by interferon-ϒ secreted from granulomas. Hypercalcemia in these disorders may be accompanied with hyperphosphatemia. These patients are exquisitely sensitive to cholecalciferol supplementation or UV radiation and may develop hypercalcemia due to unregulated 1α-hydroxylase activity in granulomas. Treatment includes glucocorticoids (prednisolone 0.5–1 mg/kg/day) and specific therapy for the underlying disease. Glucocorticoids inhibit 1α-hydroxylase activity and decrease the secretion of cytokines from the granulomatous lesions.

19. **What are the regulators of renal 1α-hydroxylase activity?**

The enzyme 1α-hydroxylase is expressed in proximal convoluted tubule and converts 25 (OH)D to active form 1,25$(OH)_2$D (calcitriol). Renal 1α-hydroxylase activity is stimulated by PTH, hypophosphatemia, hypocalcemia, GH, estrogen, and prolactin, while it is inhibited by FGF23, 1,25(OH)2D, hypercalcemia, hyperphosphatemia, and drugs like glucocorticoids and ketoconazole. Measurable levels of 1,25(OH)2D even in anephric patients suggest the presence of extrarenal source of 1α-hydroxylase activity as seen in macrophages and lymphocytes.

20. **Why is there no vitamin D toxicity with sun exposure?**

Vitamin D is synthesized in the epidermis (stratum malpighian). The precursor 7-dehydrocholesterol (provitamin D) is converted to previtamin D under the influence of UVB rays at a frequency of 290–320 nm, and further previtamin D is isomerized by body heat to vitamin D_3. However, the capacity of cutaneous biosynthesis of provitamin D to previtamin D is limited (15%), and in case of prolonged sun exposure, previtamin D is metabolized to inactive compounds like lumisterol and tachysterol. Therefore, prolonged sun exposure never results in vitamin D toxicity.

21. **Can there be milk–alkali syndrome without milk?**

Yes. Milk–alkali syndrome is a triad of hypercalcemia, metabolic alkalosis, and renal failure. In the past, milk and alkali was used as a treatment for acid peptic disease and their excessive consumption was associated with "milk–alkali syndrome." In the present clinical context, the most common cause of milk–alkali syndrome is excessive administration of calcium as calcium carbonate, usually for the treatment of hypoparathyroidism or osteoporosis.

22. **Why do patients with milk–alkali syndrome have hypercalcemia?**

Milk–alkali syndrome is a triad of PTH-independent hypercalcemia, metabolic alkalosis, and renal insufficiency. It occurs due to intake of large amount of calcium (4–60 g/day) as calcium carbonate, but not as acetate or citrate. Hypercalcemia in milk–alkali syndrome is due to increased supplemental calcium intake, enhanced intestinal absorption of calcium, reduced reposition of calcium into bone, and decreased renal excretion of calcium.

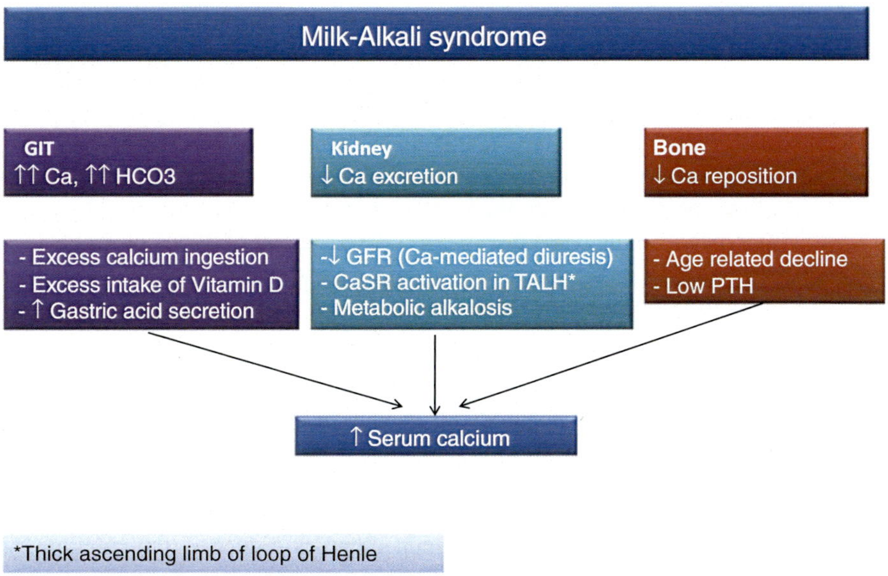

Fig. 13.2 Pathophysiology of milk–alkali syndrome

- Enhanced intestinal absorption of calcium is due to concurrent vitamin D ingestion and increased gastric acid secretion by calcium-mediated CaSR activation in the gastric mucosa.
- Bone reposition of calcium is reduced due to low PTH and limited capacity of skeleton to uptake calcium.
- Decreased renal excretion of calcium is due to reduction in GFR which is consequent to diuresis and natriuresis induced by hypercalcemia.

Metabolic alkalosis is due to increased intestinal bicarbonate absorption (calcium carbonate is converted into bicarbonate in the presence of gastric acid) and augmented bicarbonate reabsorption from the proximal tubule due to decreased GFR. Metabolic alkalosis results in increased renal tubular reabsorption of calcium, thereby perpetuating hypercalcemia. The treatment is discontinuation of the offending agent, saline diuresis, and dialysis. Bisphosphonate should be avoided as they themselves are nephrotoxic.

23. **What is hypercalcemic crisis?**

Hypercalcemic crisis is characterized by severe hypercalcemia (>14 mg/dl) with signs and symptoms related to multiorgan dysfunction, predominantly neurological. The presenting manifestations include altered sensorium, severe dehydration, nausea, vomiting, renal failure, and cardiac arrhythmias. The most common cause of hypercalcemic crisis is malignancy-related hypercalcemia.

24. **Why all patients with severe hypercalcemia do not present with hypercalcemic crisis?**

Severity of symptoms of hypercalcemia does not exclusively depend on absolute level of serum calcium, but also on the rapidity of rise in serum calcium. Hypercalcemic crisis is rare in patients with PHPT despite having severe hypercalcemia because the disease is insidious in onset and allows the homeostatic mechanisms to operate thereby preventing the development of hypercalcemic crisis. However, patients with malignancy-related hypercalcemia usually present with hypercalcemic crisis due to rapid development of hypercalcemia.

25. **How to treat hypercalcemic crisis?**

The first and foremost treatment for hypercalcemic crisis is volume repletion. Patients with hypercalcemic crisis are severely dehydrated due to polyuria caused by hypercalcemia-induced nephrogenic diabetes insipidus. Rehydration with isotonic saline (2–4 l over 24 h) is preferred as it not only restores intravascular volume, but also facilitates calcium excretion. Once optimal fluid repletion has been achieved, loop diuretics may be administered to enhance urinary calcium excretion. Saline administration and loop diuretics reduce serum calcium by 1–3 mg/dl within 24 h; however, the effect is not sustained and mandates additional treatment. Bisphosphonates are useful in hypercalcemia of any etiology. Zoledronic acid is the most potent bisphosphonate and normalizes serum calcium in 60–90% of patients within 4–7 days and if required may be repeated after 7 days. In those with impaired renal function, ibandronate is a safer alternative and can be used if eGFR >30 ml/min. Salmon calcitonin (2–8 IU/kg) administered s.c./i.m./i.v. twice daily rapidly reduces serum calcium by 1–2 mg/dl. However, its therapeutic potential is limited due to tachyphylaxis within 3–5 days. Calcitonin nasal spray is not effective in the treatment of hypercalcemia. Glucocorticoids are useful, particularly in patients with hypercalcemia related to vitamin D intoxication and granulomatous disorders. Hemodialysis is the preferred modality of treatment in the presence of renal failure or refractory hypercalcemia. The underlying cause of hypercalcemia needs to be addressed to prevent recurrence.

26. **What is hypocalcemia?**

Hypocalcemia is defined as serum calcium level below the reference range. Estimation of ionized calcium is preferred for the diagnosis of hypocalcemia; however, if it is not available, albumin-corrected total calcium should be used.

27. **Can tetany occur in the presence of hypercalcemia?**

Multiple blood transfusions is associated with elevated total serum calcium, but reduced ionized calcium. Elevated total serum calcium is due to binding of calcium with EDTA present in the transfused blood, resulting in low ionized calcium, and may manifest clinically as tetany.

28. **What are the causes of chronic hypocalcemia?**

The pivotal mechanisms involved in chronic hypocalcemia include impaired intestinal absorption of calcium, suppressed bone resorption, and increased renal loss of calcium and are the consequence of impaired secretion/action of PTH and/or calcitriol. The common causes of chronic hypocalcemia are chronic kidney disease, vitamin D deficiency or resistance, hypoparathyroidism, and pseudohypoparathyroidism. Estimation of serum phosphate, creatinine, PTH, and 25(OH)D is crucial in establishing the etiological diagnosis of chronic hypocalcemia. High serum phosphate in the presence of chronic hypocalcemia suggests the diagnosis of chronic kidney disease, hypoparathyroidism, and pseudohypoparathyroidism. Low serum PTH in the presence of high phosphate and low calcium is consistent with hypoparathyroidism, while high serum PTH with high phosphate, low calcium, and normal serum creatinine establishes the diagnosis of pseudohypoparathyroidism. Low serum phosphate in the presence of normocalcemia/hypocalcemia suggests vitamin D deficiency/resistance.

29. **A 13-year-old boy presented with tonic–clonic seizures. On evaluation, EEG was abnormal, but had a normal neuroimaging. He was started on phenytoin in optimal doses; however, he reported a week later with worsening of seizures. How to proceed further?**

Phenytoin is commonly used as a first-line drug in the management of seizure disorder. However, it can worsen seizure in a patient having hypocalcemia or in a patient with hyperosmolar nonketotic diabetic coma. Phenytoin worsens hypocalcemia by decreasing calcium absorption from the intestine (decreased calcium-binding protein in jejunal epithelium), by increasing the metabolism of 25(OH)D to inactive metabolites and by inhibiting PTH- and calcitriol-mediated bone resorption. Therefore, every child who presents with seizure should be evaluated for hypocalcemia. In the index patient, corrected serum calcium was 5.2 mg/dl, phosphate 7.5 mg/dl, magnesium 2.4 mg/dl, PTH 2.4 pg/ml, and 25(OH)D 20 ng/ml. He also had bilateral immature senile cataract. There was no history of radiation exposure or any neck surgery in the past. He did not have features of any autoimmune disorders or mucocutaneous candidiasis. Therefore, a diagnosis of idiopathic hypoparathyroidism was considered. He was treated with calcium, calcitriol, and sodium valproate. On follow-up, the child is seizure-free without any antiepileptic drugs and is doing well.

30. **What are the causes of hypoparathyroidism?**

The most common cause of hypoparathyroidism is inadvertent injury to parathyroid glands during thyroid surgery. The causes of hypoparathyroidism are summarized in the table given below.

Congenital	Acquired
Polyglandular endocrinopathy type 1 (AIRE gene mutation)	Post-surgical
Polyglandular endocrinopathy type 2	Neck irradiation
Infiltrative diseases Hemochromatosis Wilson's disease	Anti-CaSR antibodies
Parathyroid transcription factor defects DiGeorge syndrome (TBX1 gene mutation) Hypoparathyroidism, deafness, and renal dysplasia syndrome (GATA3 gene mutation)	
PTH gene mutations	
Activating CaSR gene mutations	

31. **How to predict the duration of hypoparathyroidism?**

Enamel hypoplasia, cataract, and basal ganglia calcification in a patient with hypoparathyroidism suggest the presence of long-standing untreated disease with onset during childhood.

32. **What are the manifestations of hypoparathyroidism?**

The manifestations of hypoparathyroidism may be due to hypocalcemia, hyperphosphatemia, and low PTH. The symptoms related to hypocalcemia include neuromuscular irritability, tetany, refractory seizures, pseudotumor cerebri, and rarely heart failure. Hyperphosphatemia leads to metastatic calcification and may present as cataract and basal ganglia calcification. Low serum PTH results in decreased bone remodeling and manifests as increased BMD with low bone turnover markers. Presence of premature cataract, refractory seizures, and dystonia are the clinical clues for the diagnosis of hypoparathyroidism. In addition, patients with mucocutaneous candidiasis and concurrent autoimmune endocrine disorders particularly adrenal insufficiency during childhood should be evaluated for hypoparathyroidism. In patients with childhood-onset adrenal insufficiency, treatment with hydrocortisone may unmask underlying hypoparathyroidism.

33. **What are the differences in soft tissue calcification of hypoparathyroidism and hyperparathyroidism?**

The fundamental basis of soft tissue calcification in patients with a disorder of mineral homeostasis is elevated calcium phosphate solubility product (>55 mg^2/dl^2). In patients with hypoparathyroidism, soft tissue calcification occurs in basal ganglia, cerebellum, cerebrum (gray and white matter junction), and lens, while renal pelvicalcyceal calcification can occur during treatment. In patients with secondary hyperparathyroidism due to CKD, who also have similar or higher solubility product compared to patients with hypoparathyroidism, the sites of calcification are different and include medium- to small-sized arteries (metacarpal and metatarsal arteries), skin (calcinosis cutis), and soft tissues like heart and lung. The variation in sites of metastatic calcification in these two disorders is attributed to the difference in circulating PTH levels. In pseudohypoparathyroidism, calcium profile exactly mimics secondary hyperparathyroidism due to CKD, but the sites of calcification are similar to hypoparathyroidism suggesting that not only the level of PTH but its action is also important in determining the sites of calcification. In patients with primary hyperparathyroidism, the sites of calcification include renal parenchyma and pelvicalyceal system, small vessels, pancreas, pericardium, and rarely endometrium. Therefore, the determinant of ectopic calcification in disorders of calcium phosphorus homeostasis is not only the solubility product, but also the circulating level of PTH and its action. The sites of ectopic calcification in disorders of mineral homeostasis are summarized in the table given below.

Disorder	Sites of calcification
Primary hyperparathyroidism	Renal pelvicalyceal system, small vessels, pancreas, periarticular tissues, pericardium, endometrium
Secondary hyperparathyroidism (CKD-related)	Medium–small vessels, skin, soft tissue like heart and lung
Hypoparathyroidism	Basal ganglia, cerebellum, cerebrum, lens
Pseudohypoparathyroidism	Basal ganglia, cerebellum, cerebrum, lens

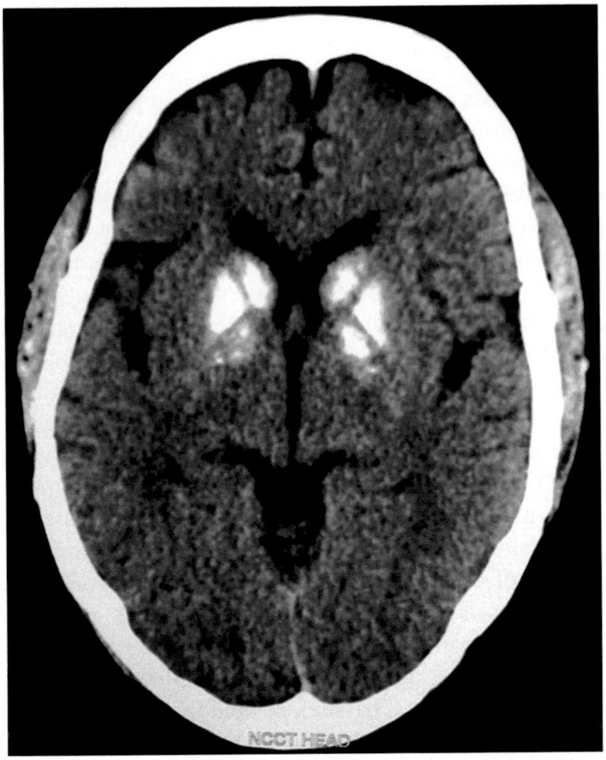

Fig. 13.3 CT head showing bilateral basal ganglia calcification in a patient with hypoparathyroidism

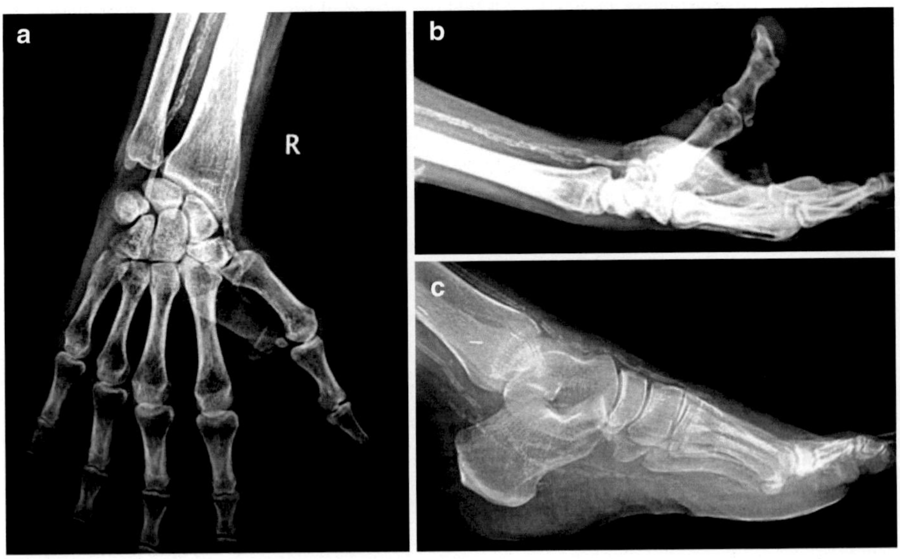

Fig. 13.4 (**a**–**c**) Plain radiograph of the hand (**a**), distal forearm (**b**), and foot (**c**) demonstrating arterial calcification in a patient with secondary hyperparathyroidism due to chronic kidney disease

34. **What are the causes of interosseous membrane calcification?**

Calcification of interosseous membrane is pathognomonic of fluorosis. However, it is also seen in patients with osteogenesis imperfecta type V and rarely in patients with hypoparathyroidism.

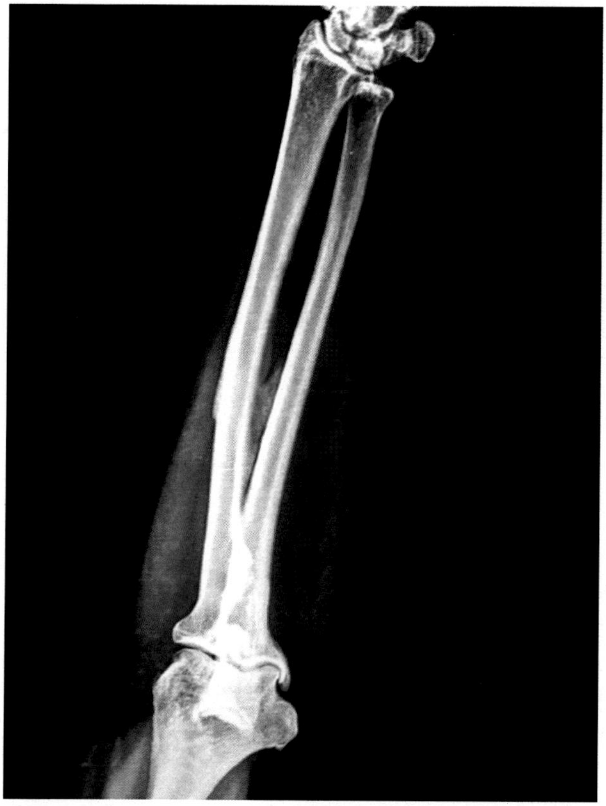

Fig. 13.5 X-ray of forearm showing interosseous membrane calcification in a patient with fluorosis

35. **What are the drugs that can be detrimental in patients with hypoparathyroidism?**

Certain drugs, if used inadvertently, may have undesirable consequences in patients with hypoparathyroidism. Metoclopramide, a D_2 receptor antagonist, may result in worsening or appearance of dystonia in those with basal ganglia calcification. Antiepileptic drugs particularly phenytoin and phenobarbitone can aggravate hypocalcemia and may induce seizure. Loop diuretics should also be avoided as they result in hypercalciuria and may exacerbate hypocalcemia.

36. **What is reversible hypoparathyroidism?**

The crucial defect in the pathogenesis of reversible hypoparathyroidism is transient suppression of PTH secretion. This is seen in patients with hypo- or hypermagnesemia and critical illness. Patients with chronic alcohol intake, malnutrition, malabsorption, renal tubular disorders, uncontrolled diabetes, and those on total parenteral nutrition or loop diuretics are predisposed for hypomagnesemia, whereas use of magnesium salts as cathartics, antacids, or tocolytics may cause hypermagnesemia. Dysmagnesemia is associated with decreased PTH secretion due to activation of CaSR and interferes with PTH action; this is reversible with normalization of serum magnesium. In patients with critical illness, interleukins increase the expression of CaSR on parathyroid gland and reduces PTH secretion which improves after recovery of underlying illness.

37. **What is the ideal treatment of hypoparathyroidism?**

Ideally, PTH replacement should be the treatment of choice in patients with hypoparathyroidism. PTH therapy normalizes serum calcium and phosphorus, effectively reduces hypercalciuria, and increases bone remodeling. However, in clinical practice, this is impractical because of daily injections and higher cost. Further, to sustain normocalcemia PTH has to be administered twice daily. Therefore, calcium and calcitriol supplementation remain the mainstay of treatment in patients with hypoparathyroidism. However, this therapy does not reduce hypercalciuria and has no effect on bone remodeling.

38. **How to treat hypoparathyroidism?**

Calcium is supplemented at doses of 1–9 g/d and calcitriol 0.25–2 μg per day in divided doses. Calcitriol is preferred over alfacalcidol (1α-(OH)D) because of its shorter duration of action that enables rapid reversal in the event of iatrogenic hypercalcemia. Treatment with calcium and calcitriol commonly results in worsening of hypercalciuria and formation of renal stones. Addition of thiazides may reduce the risk of renal stone by reducing calcium excretion and helps to normalize serum calcium. Despite the use of calcitriol in high doses, hyperphosphatemia usually does not worsen as chronic calcitriol therapy is associated with phosphaturia. In those who are vitamin D deficient, replacement with cholecalciferol may decrease the requirement of calcitriol and calcium, as 25(OH)D and its metabolites also have direct effects on intestinal calcium absorption. Calcilytic agents may be useful in those who have a defect in CaSR. Phosphate binder like calcium carbonate is advised in patients with severe hyperphosphatemia to normalize the solubility product; however, data supporting the use of sevelamer and lanthanum are not available.

39. **How to monitor a patient of hypoparathyroidism on treatment?**

Aims of treatment in a patient with hypoparathyroidism are resolution of symptoms and prevention of long-term complications. Biochemical targets include maintenance of serum calcium in the low–normal range, serum phosphate in the high–normal range, calcium phosphate solubility product <55 mg^2/dl^2, and urinary calcium <300 mg/day. Maintenance of serum calcium in the low–normal range is advised, as efforts to raise serum calcium to normal range might exacerbate hypercalciuria due to lack of PTH. If 24-h urinary calcium excretion exceeds 250 mg, addition of thiazides and low salt intake should be considered. Therefore, serum calcium, phosphate, creatinine, and urinary calcium should be measured weekly at initiation of treatment to titrate the doses and once in 3 months later on. Serum PTH monitoring is not required.

40. **What is the fate of orally ingested calcium in a healthy individual?**

Calcium homeostasis in a healthy individual who ingests 1g of calcium per day is shown in figure 13.6. Of this 1,000 mg of calcium, 300 mg is absorbed from the duodenum and jejunum, but 100 mg is secreted back into the intestine with net absorption of 200 mg. Therefore, 800 mg of ingested calcium is excreted in feces. Two-hundred milligram of absorbed calcium enters into circulation and there is a constant exchange between blood pool and bone calcium pool to maintain the normal serum calcium. The influx of calcium to bone and the efflux of calcium from bone are almost similar (200–500 mg) in young adults, whereas influx is less than efflux in elderly. Further, kidney plays an important role in the regulation of calcium homeostasis. Approximately, 9,000 mg of calcium is filtered every day and 8,800 mg of this is effectively reabsorbed with a net excretion of 200 mg in urine per day irrespective of calcium intake. Therefore, the net calcium balance is nil in a healthy individual with an adequate intake of calcium. However, inadequate intake of dietary/supplemental calcium will induce bone resorption to maintain blood calcium pool as there is sustained renal loss of calcium, and this eventually will diminish bone calcium reserve.

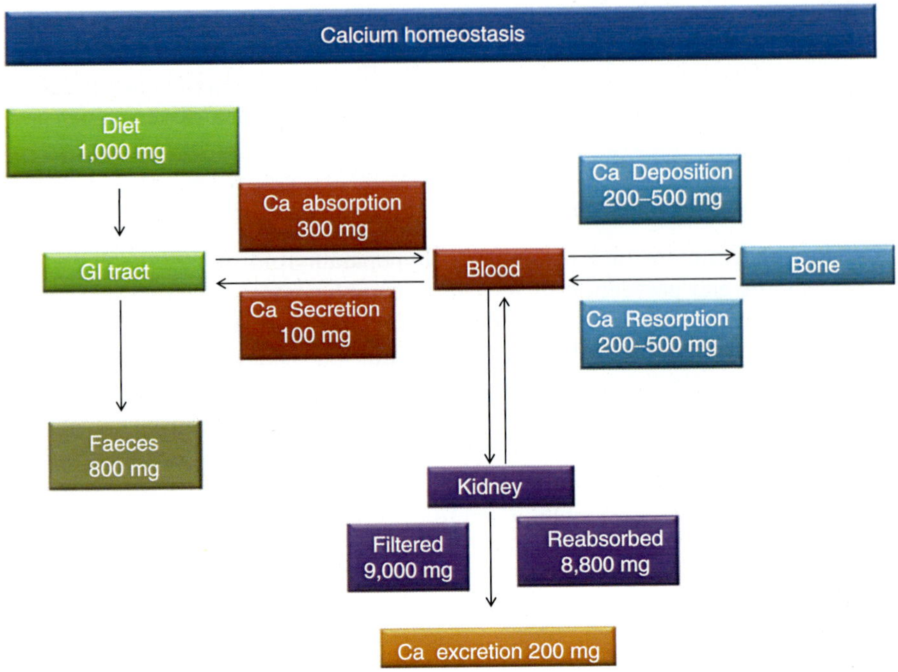

Fig. 13.6 Calcium homeostasis in a healthy adult

41. **Why is there increase in calcium requirement with advancing age?**

With advancing age, there is an increase in calcium requirement to 1.2–1.5 g/day. This increase in demand for calcium is attributed to age-related decline in 1α-hydroxylase activity and decreased absorption of calcium as a result of reduced sensitivity to 1,25(OH)2D and low gastric acid output with aging. Moreover, many elderly people receive proton pump inhibitors which further reduce calcium absorption.

42. **Why does calcium supplementation lead to increased cardiovascular risk?**

A recent study showed that calcium supplementation is associated with increased cardiovascular risk. Acute rise in serum calcium levels after oral calcium administration is associated with increased procoagulant activity, release of proinflammatory cytokines, elevated FGF23 levels, and vascular calcification and thereby contributes to increased cardiovascular risk. In addition, calcium supplementation suppresses endogenous 1,25(OH)2D, and this decrease in 1,25(OH)2D, induces the renin–angiotensin–aldosterone system (RAAS) activity and further increases the cardiovascular risk. Therefore, to meet the recommended daily allowance (RDA), calcium intake from natural source like dairy products should be encouraged as it is associated with regulated and steady serum calcium levels.

43. **What is FGF23?**

FGF23 is a 251 amino acid peptide predominantly secreted by osteocytes. It is a major phosphotonin (possibly a misnomer as it is a phosphaturic hormone) involved in phosphate homeostasis. It acts in association with its co-receptor α-Klotho and inhibits the translocation of intracellular sodium phosphorus co-transporter (NaPi-2a and 2c) to the cell membrane in proximal convoluted tubule, resulting in phosphaturia. In addition, it also inhibits renal 1 α-hydroxylase activity, thereby decreasing intestinal phosphate reabsorption.

44. **What is Klotho?**

Klotho is named after Greek Goddess "Clotho" who spins the thread of human life. Klotho is a gene that encodes a protein which is present in three forms: transmembrane klotho, secreted klotho, and soluble klotho. The shedding of extracellular domain of transmembrane klotho into circulation forms soluble klotho. Transmembrane form is expressed in multiple tissues, especially in kidney, and acts as a co-receptor for FGF23 and results in phosphaturia and suppresses renal 1α-hydroxylase and PTH. In addition, it has an antiaging and anti-IGF1 effects. Secreted as well as soluble klotho may act alone or in concert with FGF23 and has antioxidant, anti-apoptotic, and anti-*wnt* signaling effects.

45. **How does FGF 23 and PTH cross-talk?**

Both FGF23 and PTH exert phosphaturic effect by inhibiting NaPi co-transporter activity at proximal convoluted tubule (PCT). However, FGF23 requires the presence of PTH for its phosphaturic effect. This is evidenced in patients with hypoparathyroidism, where high levels of FGF23 fail to exert its phosphaturic effect due to lack of PTH. In addition, normalization of serum phosphate after total parathyroidectomy, even in the presence of high FGF23 in patients with difficult-to-treat tumor-induced osteomalacia, further supports the fact that PTH acts as a second messenger for FGF23.

46. **What is the role of FGF23 in chronic kidney disease?**

Patients with chronic kidney disease (CKD) have high serum FGF23 levels. Increase in FGF23 precedes any alterations in calcium, phosphorus, or calcitriol levels. Elevated FGF23 is attributed to acquired Klotho deficiency due to renal oxidative stress. The rise in FGF23 leads to reduction in 1α-hydroxylase activity, consequently resulting in hypocalcemia.

47. **Why is there vascular calcification in CKD?**

The common denominator of soft tissue calcification in patients with CKD is elevated calcium phosphate solubility product (>55 mg^2/dl^2). In addition, Klotho deficiency has been incriminated in the pathogenesis of vascular calcification. Klotho prevents vascular calcification possibly by enhancing phosphaturia, by inhibiting the phosphate uptake by vascular smooth muscle cells, and by preserving renal function. Further, FGF23 has also been shown to be associated with increased incidence of vascular calcification; however, the cause and effect relationship is not established.

48. **What is tumoral calcinosis?**

Tumoral calcinosis is a rare autosomal recessive metabolic disorder characterized by periarticular and surrounding soft tissue calcification. Hip joint is most commonly involved followed by elbow and shoulder. Patients commonly present with painless boggy swelling with or without a discharging sinus. The biochemical hallmarks are hyperphosphatemia, normo- or hypercalcemia, normal PTH, and elevated 1,25(OH)2D. X-ray reveals densely calcified "cauliflower"-like lesion in periarticular soft tissues. Tumoral calcinois is due to defective synthesis of FGF23 (inactivating mutations of FGF23 gene/ineffective glycosylation) or resistance to action of FGF23 (absence of Klotho). This results in increased translocation of sodium phosphorus co-transporter (NaPi-2a and 2c) and enhanced 1α-hydroxylase activity in PCT, thereby leading to hyperphosphatemia. Repeated microvascular trauma at joints in the presence of increased solubility product (calcium x phosphate >55 mg^2/dl^2) results in metastatic calcification. The treatment strategies are directed to reduce serum phosphate and include restriction of dietary phosphate and use of phosphate binders (sevelamer, lanthanum, calcium acetate) and acetazolamide. Bisphosphonates have been used with limited success. Surgery may be required in cases with painful joints and/or limited mobility.

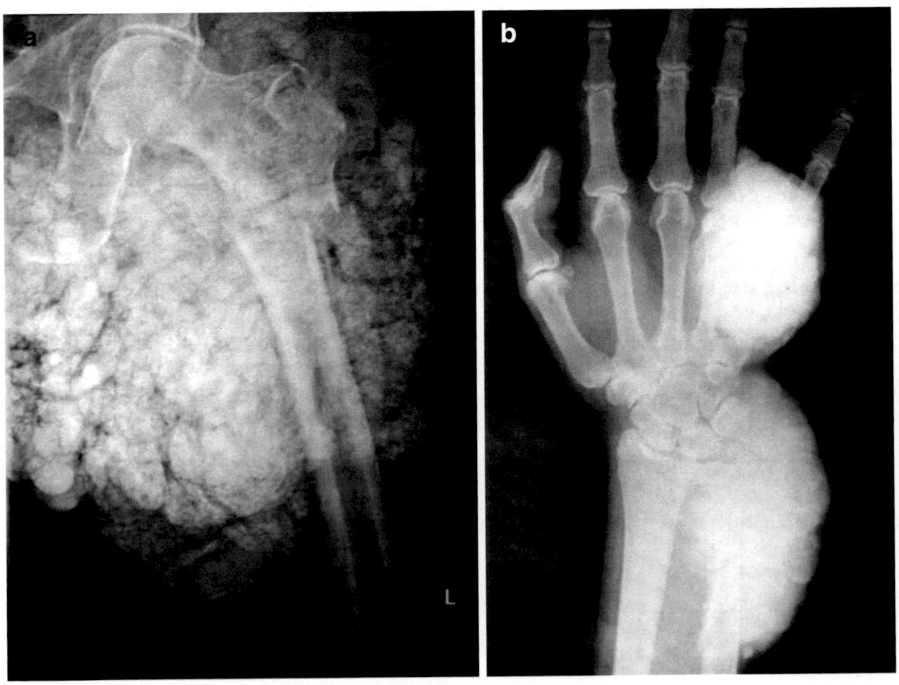

Fig. 13.7 (**a**, **b**) Plain radiograph of the hip (**a**) and hand (**b**) showing large calcified lesions involving upper thigh, distal forearm, and palm suggestive of tumoral calcinosis

49. **What is hypophosphatemic osteomalacia?**

Hypophosphatemic osteomalacia is a clinico-biochemical entity characterized by rickets/osteomalacia and hypophosphatemia. Increased renal excretion of phosphate is the key abnormality in the development of hypophosphatemic osteomalacia. The renal phosphate wasting may be FGF23 or non-FGF23 mediated. The common causes of FGF23-mediated hypophosphatemic rickets/osteomalacia are X-linked/autosomal dominant/autosomal recessive hypophosphatemic osteomalacia, tumor-induced osteomalacia, fibrous dysplasia, and linear sebaceous nevus syndrome. Serum calcium, alkaline phosphatase, and PTH levels are usually normal in patients with FGF23-mediated hypophosphatemic osteomalacia. Non-FGF23-mediated hypophosphatemic osteomalacia includes primary hyperparathyroidism, hereditary hypophosphatemic rickets with hypercalciuria, and Fanconi's syndrome.

50. **What is tumor-induced osteomalacia?**

Tumor-induced osteomalacia, also called as oncogenic osteomalacia, is a paraneoplastic syndrome due to secretion of phosphatonins (e.g., FGF23) from mesenchymal tumors and results in severe hypophosphatemia and low 1,25(OH)2D. These tumors arise from bone or soft tissue and may be located anywhere in the body but are commonly located in extremities and paranasal sinuses. They are typically very small in size and are difficult to localize. Histologically, they are grouped as "phosphaturic mesenchymal tumors—mixed connective tissue variant (PMT-MCT)" and include hemangiopericytomas (most common), hemangioma, sarcoma, ossifying fibroma, and rarely osteoblastoma. Majority of these tumors are benign (90%).

51. **When to suspect tumor-induced osteomalacia?**

Any patient with osteomalacia having normocalcemia, severe hypophosphatemia, normal or mildly elevated alkaline phosphatase, and normal PTH and 25(OH) D levels, should be evaluated for hypophosphatemic osteomalacia. Other clinical clues to suspect hypophosphatemic osteomalacia are failure to respond to cholecalciferol/calcitriol given for the treatment of osteomalacia or worsening of hypophosphatemia after rPTH therapy initiated inadvertently for the management of osteoporosis with fracture. High levels of FGF23 and inappropriately low–normal 1,25(OH)D in relation to serum phosphate confirm the diagnosis of hypophosphatemic osteomalacia. Absence of family history and onset of disease in adulthood are strong pointers towards tumor-induced osteomalacia (TIO). Functional scan followed by anatomical imaging is recommended for the localization of source of FGF23 excess.

52. **What are the phosphotonins implicated in TIO?**

FGF23 is the clinically most relevant phosphatonin and majority of patients with TIO have elevated levels of FGF23. However, other phosphatonin have also been implicated in the pathogenesis of TIO and include secreted frizzled-like protein 4, matrix extracellular phosphoglycoproteins, and FGF7, which have been demonstrated only in tumor tissue but not in serum.

53. **How to explain the biochemical abnormalities in TIO?**

The hallmark biochemical abnormality in TIO is severe hypophosphatemia, which occurs as a result of renal phosphate wasting due to secretion of FGF23 from mesenchymal tumors. FGF23 exerts its phosphaturic effect in concert with PTH. Serum calcium and PTH are usually in normal range, while 1,25(OH) D_3 is low or inappropriately normal due to direct suppressive effect of FGF23 on renal 1α-hydroxylase. Serum alkaline phosphatase is normal even in the presence of osteomalacia because of normal PTH levels.

54. **How to localize the tumor in TIO?**

In endocrine disorders, biochemical confirmation of the disease is followed by structural localization. However, in TIO functional localization precedes structural imaging, as these tumors are too small and are frequently missed by anatomical imaging. Most preferred modality for tumor localization is octreotide-based scintigraphy (e.g., DOTANOC, DOTATATE) followed by CT or MRI to assess the anatomical details. However, only 50–70% of these tumors can be localized by octreotide-based scintigraphy. Selective venous sampling is indicated when the lesion is suspicious or multiple.

55. **Which is the preferred functional imaging for the localization of tumor in patients with TIO?**

Octreotide-based scintigraphy (e.g., 68Ga-DOTATATE PET-CT) is more sensitive and specific than ^{18}F-FDG-PET scan for the localization of tumor in TIO. The decreased sensitivity of ^{18}F-FDG-PET is due to low proliferative indices of these tumors and lower specificity is because of FDG uptake by metabolically active fracture sites. Further, whole body functional scan should be performed for localization as these tumors are frequently present in extremities particularly hands and feet. In routine clinical practice, extremities are usually not scanned and tumors in these locations may therefore be missed. The following images illustrate the importance of functional scan in localizing the tumor in a patient with TIO.

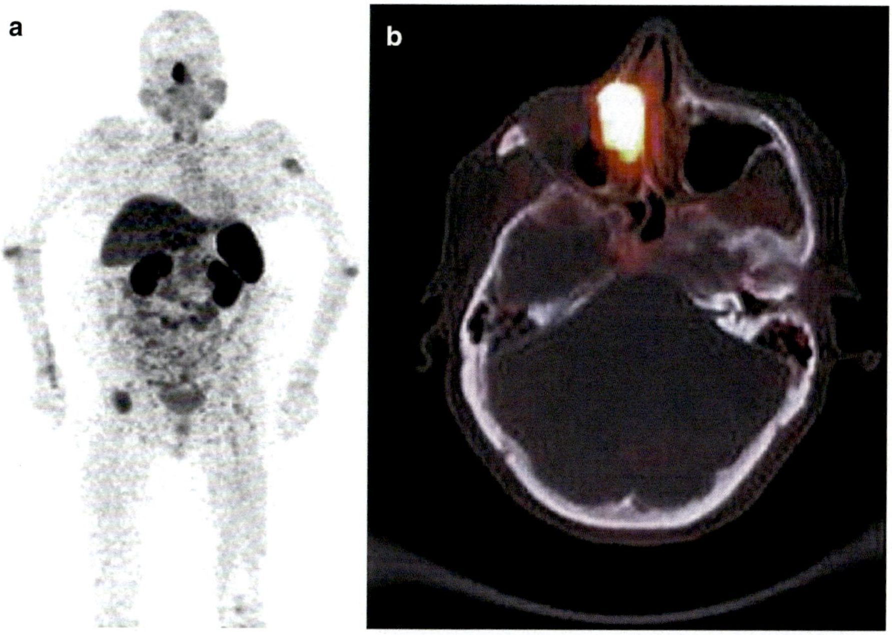

Fig. 13.8 (**a**) ^{68}Ga-DOTATATE PET scan showing somatostatin receptor expressing soft tissue lesion in the right nasal cavity. (**b**) ^{68}Ga-DOTATATE PET/CT fusion image showing intense tracer uptake (SUV max-22) in a soft tissue thickening in the right nasal cavity

56. **What are the treatment modalities for TIO?**

Complete surgical excision of a well-localized tumor with wide margins is curative. If the tumor is inaccessible, radiofrequency ablation and lutetium-based therapies are other alternatives. In situations where the tumor is not localized, phosphate supplementation (15–60 mg/kg/d) along with calcitriol (15–60 ng/kg/d) is useful in the management of osteomalacia. Calcitriol helps in maintaining serum phosphate level by stimulating intestinal phosphate absorption and inhibiting renal phosphate wasting, which occurs as a result of phosphate therapy-induced rise in PTH. Further, calcitriol may prevent the development of secondary/tertiary hyperparathyroidism associated with phosphate therapy. Calcimimetic agents like cinacalcet have been tried with limited success. Recently, a case report showed resolution of hypophosphatemia after total parathyroidectomy, and this opens new vistas in the management of TIO. Anti-FGF23 antibodies have been found to be effective in mouse models of hypophosphatemic osteomalacia and may be a promising alternative in the future.

57. **What is the importance of measurement of calcium profile in patients with McCune–Albright syndrome?**

McCune–Albright syndrome is due to post-zygotic somatic mutation associated with constitutive action of Gsα subunit manifesting as fibrous dysplasia (monostotic/polyostotic), cafe-au-lait macules, and endocrinopathies. The common endocrine disorders include gonadotropin-independent precocious puberty, toxic nodular goiter, acrogigantism, and hypophosphatemic rickets/osteomalacia. Hyperphosphatemia in a patient with McCune–Albright syndrome should prompt evaluation for hypersomatotropism, while hypophosphatemia suggests the possibility of fibrous dysplasia-associated hypophosphatemic rickets/osteomalacia, renal tubular defects (due to Gsα mutation), or rarely primary hyperparathyroidism.

58. **Is universal screening for vitamin D deficiency recommended prior to vitamin D replacement?**

Ideally, screening for vitamin D deficiency should be done prior to vitamin D replacement. However, vitamin D deficiency is rampant and is an independent risk factor for fracture; therefore, in routine clinical practice, it should be supplemented without screening. Supplementation with oral vitamin D should be preferred over parenteral preparations, as the risk of vitamin D toxicity is negligible with oral preparations. However, estimation of 25(OH)D is indicated in patients with osteoporosis, rickets/osteomalacia, chronic kidney disease, hypercalcemia, and hyperparathyroidism and patients on statin therapy who complain of myalgia.

59. **What are the indications of calcitriol therapy?**

Calcitriol $\{1,25(OH)_2D_3\}$ is synthesized from $25(OH)D_3$ by the enzyme 1α-hydroxylase, which is present in proximal convoluted tubule of kidney. The prime regulators of 1α-hydroxylase activity are PTH and FGF23. Therefore, disorders associated with impaired 1α-hydroxylase activity or deficient secretion/action of PTH or increased FGF23 requires calcitriol therapy. These include chronic kidney disease, hypoparathyroidism, pseudohypoparathyroidism, hypophosphatemic osteomalacia, and renal tubular acidosis. Further, patients with primary hyperparathyroidism who develop hungry bone syndrome or hypoparathyroidism postoperatively also require treatment with calcitriol. In addition, vitamin D-dependent rickets, type 1 (inactivating mutations of 1α-hydroxylase) and type 2 (vitamin D receptor defects), are indications for calcitriol therapy. Elderly subjects (>70 years) may also require calcitriol supplementation for their bone health, as there is a decline in 1α-hydroxylase activity with advancing age due to progressive decline in eGFR. However, the benefit in prevention of osteoporotic fracture in this population is not proven.

Suggested Reading

1. Larry JL, De Groot LJ. Endocrinology: adult and pediatric. Philadelphia.: Elsevier Health Sciences; 2010.
2. Longo D, Anthony F, Dennis K, Stephen H, Jameson J, Joseph L. Harrison's principles of internal medicine. 8th ed. New York: EB. McGraw Hill Professional; 2012.
3. Melmed S, Polonsky KS, Larsen PR, Kronenberg HM. Williams textbook of endocrinology: expert consult. London: Elsevier Health Sciences; 2011.

Hyperparathyroidism

14

14.1 Case Vignette

A 35-year-old lady presented with pain and swelling in left knee for the last 10 months. On evaluation, she was found to have a lytic lesion in the upper part of left tibia and underwent bone curettage with implantation of fibular graft. Histopathology revealed giant cell tumor, for which localized radiation therapy was advised, and she received external beam radiotherapy (30 Gy in 10 fractions over 2 weeks). Subsequently, a bone scan was performed which showed multiple lytic lesions, and she was referred to endocrinology for opinion. On evaluation, she was found to have corrected serum calcium 15.1 mg/dl (8.6–10.2), phosphate 2.4 mg/dl (2.7–4.2), alkaline phosphatase (ALP) 943 IU/ml (40–129), iPTH 1,687 pg/ml (15–65), 25(OH)D 13.2 ng/ml (11–43), and serum creatinine 1.1 mg/dl (0.5–1.2). Her serum prolactin was 18 ng/ml (5–25). 24-h urinary calcium was 174 mg with urinary creatinine of 640 mg. Ultrasonography (USG) of abdomen revealed bilateral nephrolithiasis. She did not have gallstone disease or pancreatitis. Her T-score was −3.8 at lumbar spine and −4.7 at femoral neck. USG of neck and ^{99m}Tc-sestamibi scan localized right inferior parathyroid adenoma (RIPA). Preoperatively, hypercalcemia was managed with saline diuresis and intravenous zoledronic acid (5 mg), after which serum calcium decreased to 9.7 mg/dl. She underwent successful resection of RIPA through unilateral neck exploration. Weight of the excised adenoma was 1.9 g, and histopathology was consistent with parathyroid adenoma. 24 h after surgery, she developed symptomatic hypocalcemia with serum calcium 6.7 mg/dl, phosphate 1.3 mg/dl, alkaline phosphatase 1,100 IU/ml, and iPTH 104.6 pg/ml. She was managed with intravenous calcium infusion, calcitriol, and cholecalciferol with frequent monitoring of serum calcium and phosphate. Her symptoms improved with increase in serum calcium to 8.0 mg/dl and phosphate to 2.2 mg/dl. She was discharged on oral calcium, calcitriol, and cholecalciferol. At 6 weeks of follow-up, she is asymptomatic and has serum calcium 8.2 mg/dl, phosphate 3.0 mg/dl, and ALP 800 IU/ml. She was continued on 2 g elemental calcium and 1.5 μg calcitriol per day along with 60,000 IU cholecalciferol once per month and was advised serial monitoring of calcium profile.

A. Bhansali, Y. Gogate, *Clinical Rounds in Endocrinology: Volume I - Adult Endocrinology*, DOI 10.1007/978-81-322-2398-6_14

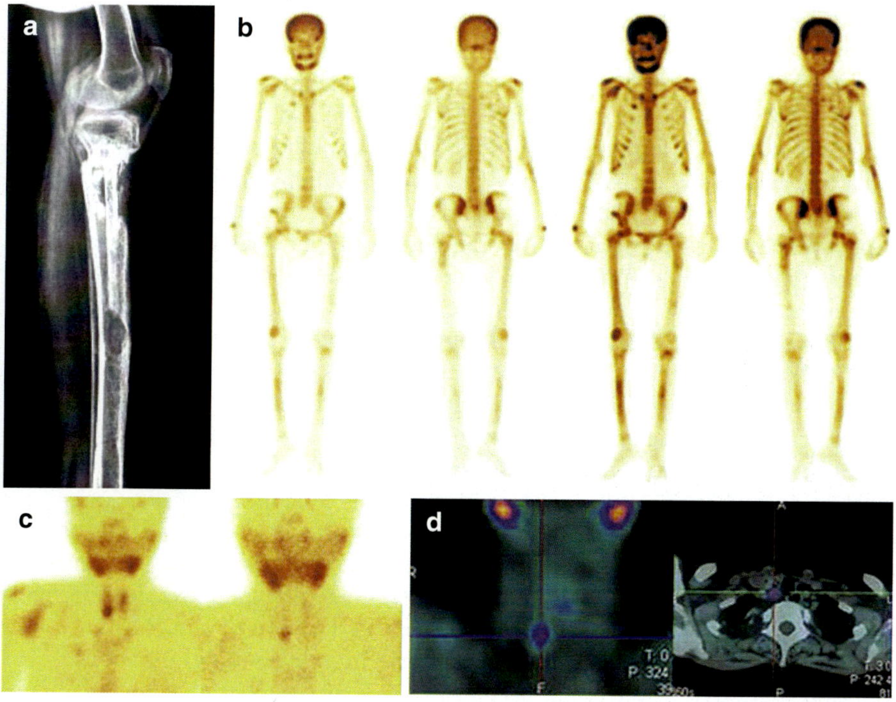

Fig. 14.1 (**a**) Lateral radiograph of the leg showing cystic lytic lesions in the tibia with bone graft in situ. (**b**) ^{99m}Tc MDP scintigraphy shows diffusely increased tracer uptake in the mandible, skull bones, bilateral femora, and tibia suggestive of metabolic bone disease. (**c**) ^{99m}Tc MIBI parathyroid scintigraphy showing focal tracer uptake in lower pole of right lobe of the thyroid gland in early image and retention of tracer in delayed image suggestive of right inferior parathyroid adenoma. (**d**) SPECT–CT fusion images showing localization of tracer to a well-defined lesion inferior and posterior to lower pole of right lobe of the thyroid gland suggestive of right inferior parathyroid adenoma

14.2 Stepwise Analysis

Our patient, a 35-year-old lady, presented with a lytic lesion in the upper part of tibia. The differential diagnosis for a lytic lesion at this site includes osteoclastoma, osteitis fibrosa cystica, fibrous dysplasia, simple/aneurysmal bone cyst, and osteosarcoma. Imaging and histopathology may help in the diagnosis of these disorders, but not conclusively in all cases. In the index case, histopathology revealed a giant cell tumor, and she was managed accordingly. Bone scan was performed to exclude the possibility of malignant giant cell tumor, which revealed multiple lytic lesions. The closest differential diagnosis of osteoclastoma (giant cell tumor) is osteitis fibrosa cystica; however, the two disorders cannot be differentiated either by imaging or histopathology. Nevertheless, estimation of serum calcium clinches the diagnosis. Hypercalcemia and multiple lytic lesions favor the diagnosis of osteitis fibrosa cystica due to primary hyperparathyroidism, while single lytic lesion with eucalcemia supports the diagnosis of osteoclastoma. Hypercalcemia, hypophosphatemia, raised alkaline phosphatase, normal eGFR, high iPTH, bilateral nephrolithiasis, osteoporosis, and multiple lytic lesions suggestive of osteitis fibrosa cystica substantiate the diagnosis of primary hyperparathyroidism (PHPT) in the index patient. Multiple endocrine neoplasia should be considered in all patients of PHPT with young age at onset. However, PHPT is likely to be sporadic in our case, as her serum prolactin was normal, and had no family history of PHPT. As majority of patients (85%) with sporadic PHPT have a single adenoma, preoperative localization provides an opportunity for limited neck exploration. Preoperative imaging consistently localized right inferior parathyroid adenoma in the index patient. Preoperatively severe hypercalcemia, if present (serum calcium >14 mg/dl), should be managed in view of high risk of arrhythmia. Prior use of zoledronic acid not only reduces serum calcium but also decreases the risk of postoperative hungry bone syndrome. Subsequently, she underwent unilateral neck exploration and successful parathyroidectomy as evidenced by the decline in serum PTH >50% from baseline, though it was performed on day 1 postoperatively. She developed symptomatic hypocalcemia with biochemical evidence of hungry bone syndrome (hypocalcemia, worsening of hypophosphatemia, and rising ALP) on day 1 postoperatively. Advanced duration of symptoms, severe bone disease (high ALP, multiple lytic lesions), high serum calcium, high iPTH, and large parathyroid adenoma predict the risk of postoperative hungry bone syndrome (HBS), and our patient had all these risk factors. HBS should be aggressively managed to prevent life-threatening consequences of hypocalcemia and hypophosphatemia. Initially, she was managed with calcium infusion, calcitriol, and cholecalciferol, and after resolution of symptoms of hypocalcemia, she was continued on oral calcium, calcitriol, and cholecalciferol. Biochemical abnormalities of HBS usually improve over several weeks; however, improvement in bone mineral density may take longer time (9–12 months) despite optimal therapy. After resolution of HBS, inadvertent therapy with calcitriol and high-dose calcium can result in milk–alkali syndrome. Therefore, periodic monitoring of calcium profile is required, and therapy should be optimized accordingly. After parathyroidectomy, intervention should also be planned for nephrolithiasis to prevent deterioration in renal function. In view of her severe bone disease, she requires long-term regular follow-up for optimal bone health.

14.3 Clinical Rounds

1. **What is primary hyperparathyroidism**?

   Primary hyperparathyroidism (PHPT) is a metabolic bone disease characterized by hypercalcemia, hypophosphatemia, and inappropriately elevated PTH due to autonomous production of parathormone by a parathyroid adenoma, hyperplasia or rarely, carcinoma.

2. **What is the classical pentad of primary hyperparathyroidism**?

   The classical clinical pentad of PHPT comprises of mnemonic "**stones** (renal stone disease), **bones** (osteitis fibrosa cystica, fracture), abdominal **groans** (gallstone disease, pancreatitis, acid peptic disease), psychiatric **moans** (mood disorders), and fatigue **overtones** (myalgia, myopathy)."

3. **What are the unusual presentations of primary hyperparathyroidism**?

   The unusual presentations of PHPT include rickets, distal renal tubular disorders, facial asymmetry, proptosis, anemia, and recurrent pancreatitis.

4. **How does primary hyperparathyroidism cause rickets**?

   PHPT can manifest as rickets in children and adolescents. This is attributed to high levels of PTH which results in renal phosphate wasting and increased bone turnover, which prevents optimal mineralization of matrix. In addition, poor oral intake because of hypercalcemia-induced anorexia and increased demand of calcium during puberty further worsens mineralization.

5. **What are the causes of PHPT**?

   A single parathyroid adenoma accounts for approximately 80–85% of patients with PHPT, and double adenomas are found in 4–5%. Multiple gland hyperplasia contributes to approximately 10% of patients with PHPT, while parathyroid carcinoma is rare (<1%).

6. **Is there any correlation between clinical phenotype and histology of parathyroid adenoma in patients with PHPT**?

   Parathyroid gland predominantly comprises of chief cells in addition to oxyphil cells and clear cells. The chief cells are rich in glycogen and fat globules, are equipped with calcium-sensing receptor (CaSR) and G protein-coupled receptor (GPCR), and exclusively contribute to circulating PTH, while oxyphil cells are rich in mitochondria, are devoid of CaSR/GPCR, and minimally secrete PTH. Most parathyroid adenomas or hyperplasia arise from chief cells. Rarely (3%) adenomas can arise from oxyphil cells which are usually larger than chief cell adenomas and have modestly elevated PTH. Clear cell adenomas are rare with anecdotal case reports.

7. **Why is PHPT a disease of postmenopausal women**?

   Postmenopausal state is characterized by estrogen deficiency. Estrogen inhibits the action of PTH by interfering with post-receptor signaling (cAMP-dependent protein kinase) and antagonizes cytokine-mediated bone resorption. Hence, estrogen deficiency in postmenopausal state leads to unopposed PTH action, thereby unmasking PHPT. In addition, estrogen deficiency may have a role in parathyroid tumorigenesis. Calcitriol has antiproliferative effects on parathyroid cells, and estrogen deficiency results in decreased 1α-hydroxylase activity, thereby promoting parathyroid cell growth and proliferation. Further, estrogen deficiency is associated with upregulation of estrogen receptors in parathyroid cells and may potentiate the generation of local IGF1 resulting in parathyroid cell proliferation.

8. **What are the mechanisms implicated in parathyroid tumorigenesis**?

The exact pathogenesis of parathyroid tumorigenesis is still elusive, but it seems to be multifactorial in origin, except in familial syndromes where exact mutation can be detected. Sporadic PHPT accounts for 95% of patients and harbors single or double adenoma, while the rest are contributed by familial syndromes and usually have parathyroid hyperplasia. However, parathyroid hyperplasia can rarely be sporadic. The predisposing factors for PHPT are previous neck irradiation, low calcium intake, and lithium exposure. The putative genes involved in sporadic PHPT include cyclinD1/PRAD1, menin, vitamin D receptor, and possibly gain-of-function mutation of phosphate-sensing receptors. The familial syndromes associated with PHPT include MEN1 (menin), MEN2A (RET proto-oncogene), MEN4 (CDKN1B), hyperparathyroidism–jaw tumor syndrome (HRPT2), and familial isolated hyperparathyroidism (menin, HRPT2, CaSR).

9. **Why is inferior parathyroid gland more likely to be ectopic**?

Parathyroid glands are endodermal in origin and develop from the pharyngeal pouch. Superior parathyroid glands originate from the fourth pharyngeal pouch, while inferior parathyroid glands from third pharyngeal pouch. Superior parathyroid glands descend along with thyroid gland to their eutopic location in the neck, whereas inferior parathyroid glands descend along with thymus and have to migrate a longer distance to reach their final destination in the neck. Because inferior parathyroid glands have to travel a longer distance as compared to superior parathyroid glands, they are more likely to be ectopic in location. The most common site of ectopic parathyroid gland is intrathyroidal, followed by thymus, mediastinum, retro-esophageal groove, and pericardium.

10. **Why is there a differential effect of parathyroid hormone on cortical and cancellous bone**?

The skeletal tissue is composed of cortical and cancellous bone in varying proportions. Distal forearm predominantly have cortical bone, and spine has cancellous bone, while the hip comprises of cortical and cancellous bone in equal proportions. PTH has an anabolic effect on cancellous bone and resorptive effect on cortical bone in patients with mild PHPT, but it has deleterious effects both on cortical and cancellous bone in patients with severe PHPT. The osteoanabolic effect of PTH on cancellous bone in patients with mild PHPT is related to modest elevation of PTH, which promotes osteoblast and osteocyte survival and stimulates *Wnt*-signaling pathway. In addition, higher metabolic activity of cancellous bone with increased bone turnover results in increased BMD in patients with mild PHPT. Despite its osteoanabolic effect on cancellous bone in mild PHPT, PTH exerts its catabolic effects on cortical bone through RANKL-OPG-RANK pathway resulting in decreased BMD (10–20%) at cortical sites. The mechanism of dual action of mildly elevated PTH remains elusive; differential expression of PTH receptors on cancellous and cortical bone or alterations in post-receptor signaling pathway may explain this dual effect of PTH. However, patients with severe PHPT have decreased BMD at both cortical and cancellous sites, although cortical bone is more severely affected. This effect is primarily due to stimulation of RANKL-OPG-RANK pathway by high circulating levels of PTH at both sites. Therefore, in clinical practice it is not uncommon to find vertebral fractures in addition to forearm/hip fractures in patients with severe PHPT.

11. **What is the distribution of cortical and cancellous bone at different sites in an adult**?

    The adult human skeleton is composed of 80% cortical bone and 20% cancellous bone. The ratio of cortical to cancellous bone is different in different bones, and even within the same bone, it is different at different sites. The vertebra is composed of cortical and cancellous bone in a ratio of 25:75. This ratio is 50:50 in the femoral head and 95:5 in distal radius.

12. **What are the skeletal manifestations of PHPT**?

    Osteitis fibrosa cystica (OFC) is the protean skeletal manifestation of hyperparathyroidism of any etiology, characterized by increased osteoclast activity resulting in bone resorption (cystica) followed by fibrosis. Radiological features of OFC include subperiosteal phalangeal bone resorption, acrosteal resorption of terminal phalanx, brown tumors (trabecular portion of long bones, pelvis, rib, jaw, and rarely in vertebrae), "salt and pepper" appearance of skull and bone cysts. Excess PTH also leads to osteopenia and increased risk of fractures. Dental abnormalities in PHPT include thinning of lamina dura and early loss of teeth.

13. **What is brown tumor**?

    In clinical practice, the terms brown tumor and OFC are used interchangeably, but the two are not synonymous. Brown tumor is a severe form of OFC. It commonly occurs in the trabecular portion of long bones, pelvis, ribs, and mandible

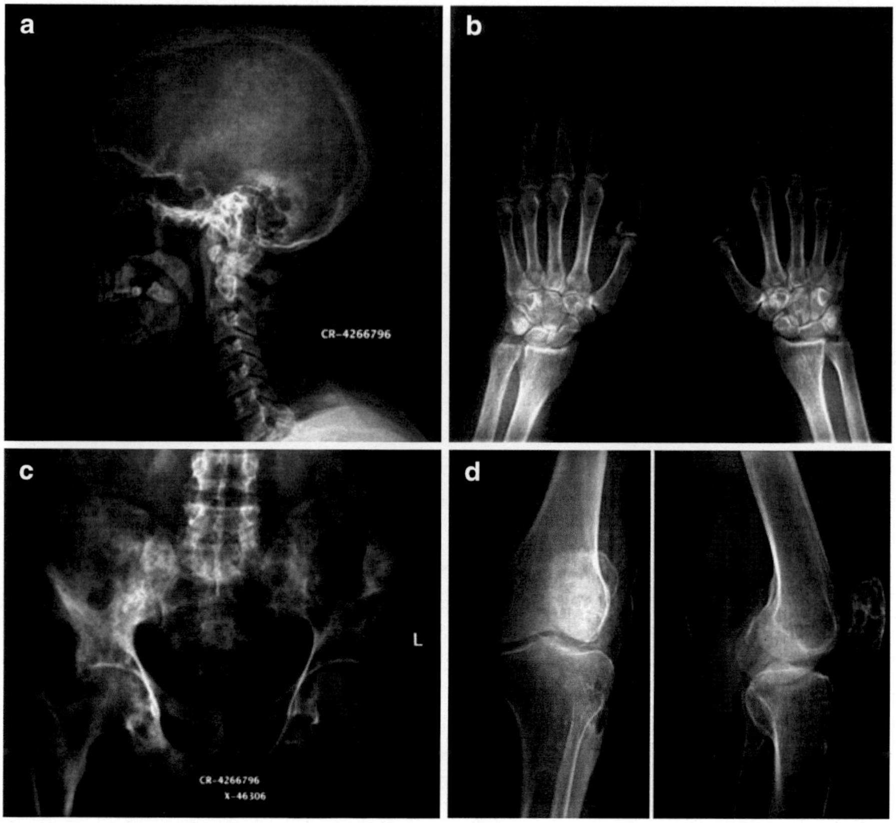

Fig. 14.2 (**a**) Plain radiograph of skull lateral view showing osteopenia with multiple lytic lesions, "salt and pepper" appearance. (**b**) Plain radiograph of both hands showing subperiosteal resorption involving proximal phalanges. (**c**) Plain radiograph of pelvis showing diffuse osteopenia with lytic lesions in iliac blades and pubic bones. (**d**) Plain radiograph of knee AP and lateral views showing lytic lesions in the patella and tibial metaphysis

and is visualized as a lytic lesion on X-ray. The name brown tumor is actually a misnomer, as it is not a tumor but represents hemorrhage into a cystic lesion, and the brown color is a result of hemosiderin deposition. Brown tumor associated with PHPT usually heals after curative parathyroidectomy, but rarely may require surgery if it persists >6 months after curative surgery.

14. **How to differentiate between osteoclastoma and brown tumor**?

Brown tumor is a manifestation of hyperparathyroidism and is not a tumor. They are usually multiple and present in long as well as in flat bones. However, osteoclastoma (giant cell tumor) is a neoplasm of bone and manifest as a solitary lytic lesion in long bone. Brown tumor and osteoclastoma are indistinguishable on imaging and histology; however, calcium profile can differentiate between the two disorders. Treatment for brown tumor is parathyroidectomy, while osteoclastoma requires local excision.

15. **What is the differential diagnosis of a bony swelling in a patient with PHPT?**

The causes of bony swelling in a patient with PHPT include brown tumor, bone cysts, mono-/polyostotic fibrous dysplasia (McCune–Albright syndrome), and ossifying fibroma (hyperparathyroidism–jaw tumor syndrome).

16. **What is epulis?**

Epulis is a swelling situated on gingiva or alveolar mucosa. In the context of PHPT, epulis is a bony swelling arising from maxilla or mandible.

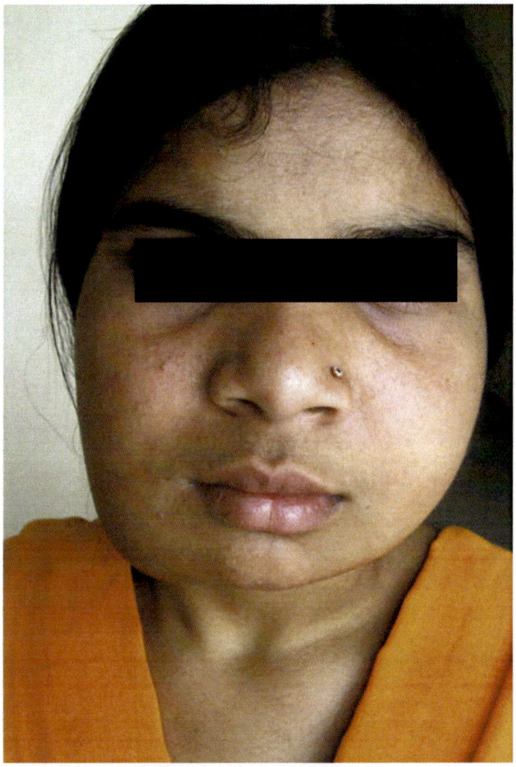

Fig. 14.3 Right-sided jaw swelling (epulis) due to brown tumor in a patient with primary hyperparathyroidism

17. **What are the oral manifestations of PHPT?**

Patients with PHPT may have jaw swelling (epulis) as presenting manifestation due to OFC, ossifying fibroma, or fibrous dysplasia. These may also present as intraoral bony swellings. In addition, dental caries, enamel hypoplasia, loss of lamina dura, and early loss of teeth may occur in these patients.

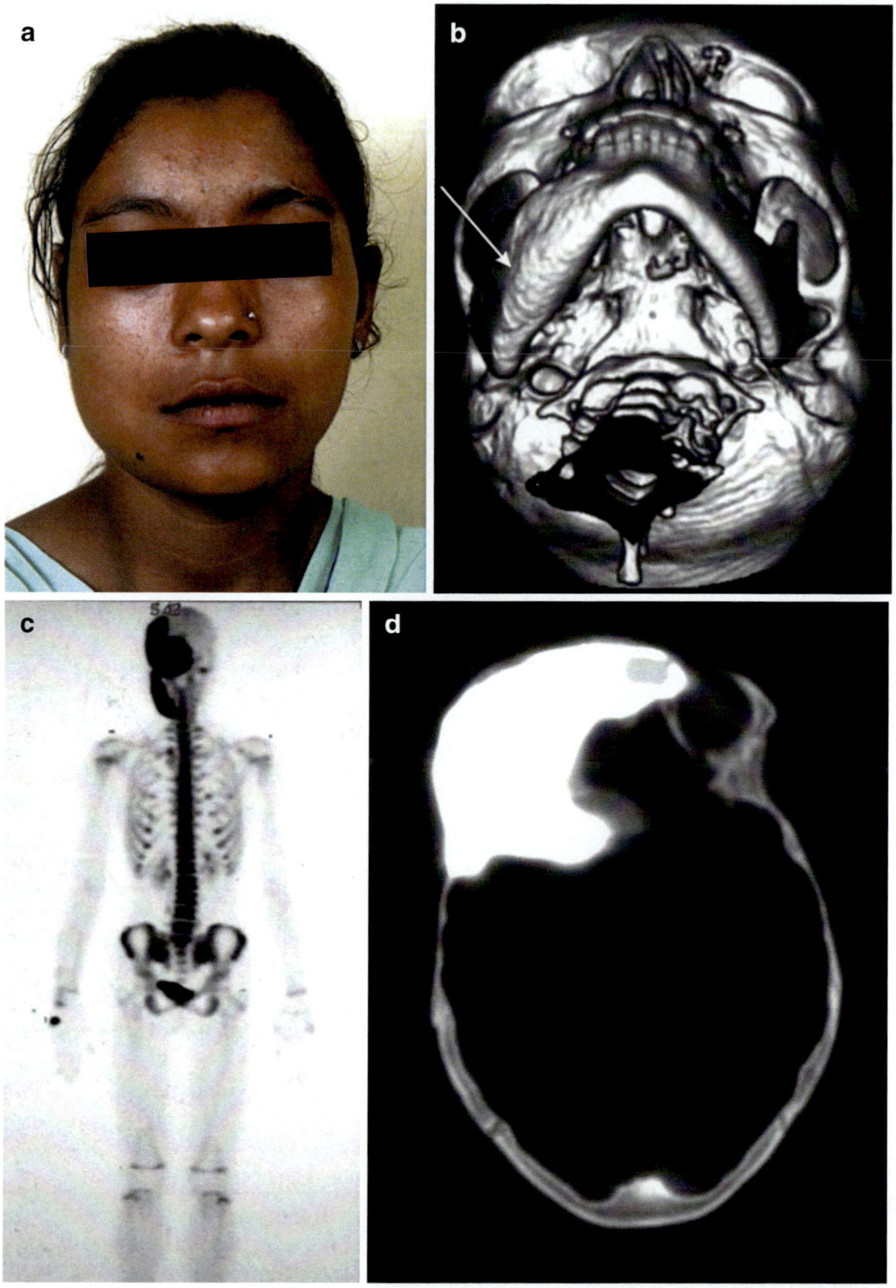

Fig. 14.4 (**a**) Right-sided jaw swelling due to fibrous dysplasia in a patient with McCune–Albright syndrome. (**b**) 3D CT volume-rendered image showing expansile lesion of mandible in the same patient. ^{18}F-FDG-PET scan (**c**) showing increased tracer uptake in right frontal and temporal bone and in right side of mandible. PET–CT fusion image (**d**) showing increased tracer uptake in right frontal and temporal bone in the same patient

18. **What is the difference between brown tumor and bone cyst?**

Brown tumor and bone cyst are skeletal manifestations of primary hyperparathyroidism. Brown tumors are located in the trabecular portion of the jaw, ribs, and long bones and may be single or multiple. These are composed of multinucleated giant cells, fibroblasts, and red blood cells, whereas bone cysts tend to occur in the shaft of the metacarpals, ribs, and pelvis and contain a brownish serous fluid. Brown tumors usually heal after curative parathyroidectomy, while bone cysts may additionally require bone grafting.

19. **A 22-year-old lady presented with a painful swelling over the left shin for the past 2 years. X-ray revealed an expansile lytic lesion and fine-needle aspiration cytology showed giant cell tumor. How to proceed further?**

The differential diagnosis of a bony swelling in this patient includes brown tumor, giant cell tumor (osteoclastoma), aneurysmal bone cyst (ABC), simple bone cyst (SBC), fibrous dysplasia, and chondroblastoma. The closest differential diagnosis of giant cell tumor (GCT) is brown tumor, and the two cannot be easily differentiated either by imaging or histology. Therefore, a calcium profile must be done in all patients to establish the etiological diagnosis. In the index patient, calcium profile revealed hypercalcemia, hypophosphatemia, and inappropriately elevated PTH, and the diagnosis of brown tumor due to PHPT was confirmed. The differences between common lytic bony lesions are summarized in the table given below.

Parameters	Brown tumor	GCT	FD	SBC	ABC
Site	Upper tibia, pelvis, mandible, ribs, vertebra	Knee, distal radius	Femur, tibia, skull, jaw, ribs	Proximal humerus and femur	Any bone, common in spine
Location	Diaphysis	Epiphysis	Metaphysis/diaphysis (intramedullary)	Metaphysis (intramedullary)	Metaphysis (intramedullary)
Lesions	Single/multiple	Single	Single/multiple	Single	Single
Age (years)	20–40, >50	20–40	10–20	0–20	10–20
X-ray	Well-defined expansile lytic lesion	Well-defined expansile lytic lesion with metaphyseal extension	Large elongated, well-defined expansile lesion with "ground-glass" appearance	Well-defined expansile lytic lesion, centrally placed, may be multiloculated	Well-defined expansile lytic lesion, eccentric, may be multiloculated

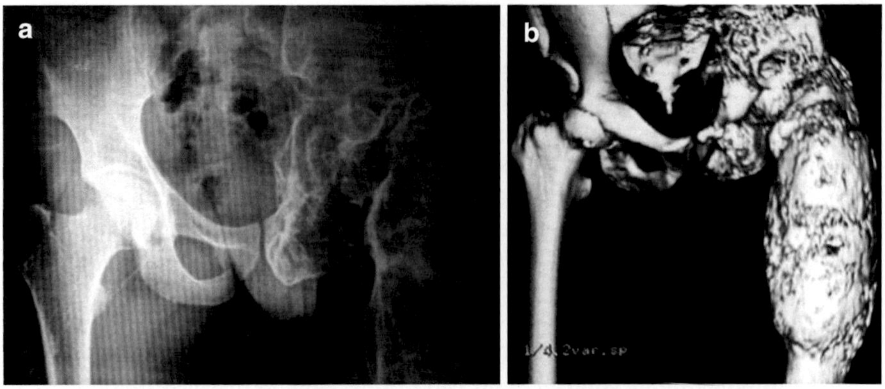

Fig. 14.5 Plain radiograph pelvis (**a**) and volume-rendered CT scan (**b**) showing multiple expansile lytic lesions in left ischium, pubis, acetabulum, and proximal femur suggestive of polyostotic fibrous dysplasia

20. **What are the renal manifestations of PHPT**?

    The renal manifestations of PHPT include hypercalciuria, nephrolithiasis, nephrocalcinosis, renal tubular dysfunction, and renal insufficiency. In addition, distal renal tubular acidosis and hypermagnesuria may also occur. Hypercalciuria is the result of increased filtered calcium overwhelming the reabsorptive capacity of PTH and leading to renal stone disease. Renal tubular dysfunction manifests as polyuria because of the decreased concentrating ability of tubules. Renal insufficiency is usually due to obstructive uropathy, but may also occur even in the absence of renal stone disease, possibly due to the direct effect of elevated PTH or calcium on renal function.

21. **What are the characteristics of renal stone disease in PHPT**?

    Renal stone disease is present in 4–20% of patients with PHPT. However, a higher prevalence (60–80%) has been reported from developing countries, which possibly may be related to delayed presentation and severe disease. Presence of recurrent renal stone disease, bilateral stone disease, nephrocalcinosis, nephrolithiasis with nephrocalcinosis, and lack of family history of renal stone disease points towards the diagnosis of PHPT. The most common type of stone in patients with PHPT is calcium oxalate, contrary to expectation of calcium phosphate stones. Renal stone disease is an important cause of renal insufficiency, and progression of renal dysfunction may occur even after curative parathyroidectomy, if the renal stone disease is not adequately intervened.

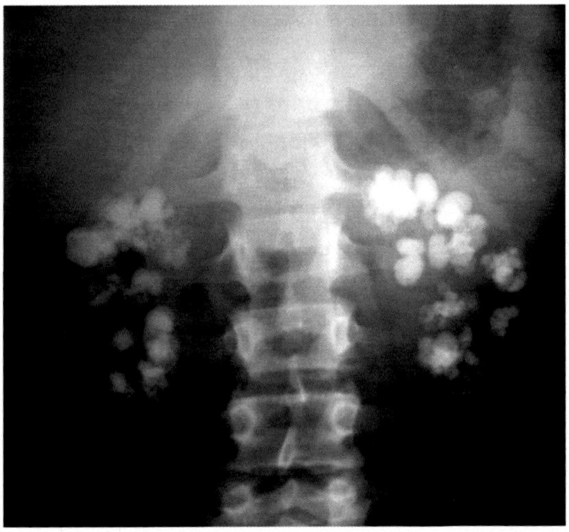

Fig. 14.6 Plain radiograph showing bilateral medullary nephrocalcinosis in a patient with PHPT

22. **What are the differences between nephrocalcinosis and nephrolithiasis**?

    The deposition of calcium into pelvi-calyceal system of kidney is called as nephrolithiasis, while the deposition of calcium into renal parenchymal tissue is termed nephrocalcinosis, which may occur in cortical zone or medullary zone. The most common cause of cortical calcification is ischemic injury to the kidney (dystrophic calcification), while medullary calcification occurs in primary hyperparathyroidism, renal tubular acidosis, hyperoxaluria, medullary sponge kidney, and drugs like acetazolamide and amphotericin B. Primary hyperparathyroidism and hyperoxaluria can be associated with both nephrolithiasis and nephrocalcinosis.

23. **What are the causes of concurrent renal stone and gallstone disease**?

    Primary hyperparathyroidism is characteristically associated with both renal stone and gallstone disease. However, they may occur synchronously or metachronously. The other disorders associated with calculi in both these organs include acromegaly, Cushing's syndrome, and chronic alcoholism.

24. **What are the cardiovascular manifestations of PHPT**?

    PHPT is associated with increased prevalence of hypertension, left ventricular hypertrophy, endothelial dysfunction, increased carotid intima–media thickness, vascular calcification, and increased cardiovascular mortality. These effects are mediated through elevated PTH and hypercalcemia. Further, excess PTH is implicated in insulin resistance and has been shown to stimulate aldosterone biosynthesis. Curative parathyroidectomy results in improved cardiovascular outcome in patients with severe hyperparathyroidism, while hypertension may not resolve in all.

25. **What are hematological manifestations of PHPT?**

The hematological manifestations of PHPT are anemia and thrombocytopenia. These hematological abnormalities are possibly due to marrow fibrosis mediated by PTH and cytokines. Curative parathyroidectomy leads to improvement in anemia and thrombocytopenia.

26. **What is parathyroid crisis?**

Hypercalcemic crisis caused by excess PTH is called parathyroid crisis. Patients commonly present with altered sensorium and serum calcium >14 mg/dl and highly elevated PTH levels (>20 fold). Parathyroid crisis is rare in patients with PHPT because of the insidious nature of disease, which allows tissues to adapt to hypercalcemic milieu over a period of time. The mechanism for the development of parathyroid crisis is not known, but may be related to life-threatening intercurrent illness, volume depletion, or infarction/hemorrhage in a parathyroid adenoma.

27. **What is asymptomatic primary hyperparathyroidism?**

Incidentally detected hypercalcemia with elevated PTH is called as asymptomatic primary hyperparathyroidism. In the western world, 80% of patients with PHPT are asymptomatic, while in developing countries only minority of patients (5–10%) are incidentally diagnosed. Some patients with asymptomatic PHPT, when carefully questioned, have nonspecific symptoms, such as fatigue, weakness, anorexia, depression, and mild cognitive or neuromuscular dysfunction.

28. **What is the natural history of asymptomatic PHPT?**

In a study, 63% of untreated subjects with asymptomatic PHPT when followed up for up to 15 years did not develop any indication for surgery. In another prospective study of 8 years, one-third of patients with asymptomatic PHPT developed worsening of hypercalcemia and decrease in bone mineral density (at cortical sites) especially in those who were younger and had a longer duration of follow-up. Therefore, patients with asymptomatic PHPT who do not have indications for surgery at diagnosis should be monitored annually with serum calcium, creatinine (estimated glomerular filtration rate), and bone mineral density estimation at the spine, hip, and distal radius.

29. **What is normocalcemic primary hyperparathyroidism?**

Normocalcemic primary hyperparathyroidism is a biochemical entity characterized by normal total and ionized serum calcium and consistently elevated PTH levels, after exclusion of secondary causes of hyperparathyroidism. It is considered as a *forme fruste* of PHPT. In a study, 19% of patients with normocalcemic PHPT, who had low BMD at presentation, developed overt hypercalcemia over a period of 3 years. The possible mechanisms of normocalcemic PHPT include target tissue resistance to PTH or rise in PTH which precedes the development of hypercalcemia during evolution of PHPT.

30. **What are the secondary causes of normocalcemic primary hyperparathyroidism?**

Patients with primary hyperparathyroidism may have normocalcemia with elevated PTH due to presence of concurrent disorders which mask hypercalcemia. The secondary causes of normocalcemic PHPT include vitamin D deficiency, reduced eGFR, hypoalbuminemia, use of loop diuretics, idiopathic hypercalciuria, gastrointestinal disorders associated with calcium malabsorption (celiac disease, chronic pancreatitis, and bariatric surgery), and prior bisphosphonate therapy.

31. **How to differentiate between PHPT with concurrent vitamin D deficiency from secondary hyperparathyroidism due to vitamin D deficiency?**

PHPT is characterized by high normal to elevated serum calcium, low phosphate, and inappropriately elevated PTH (>20 pg/ml) and can present with fragility fracture, recurrent renal stone disease, gallstone disease, and pancreatitis or may be asymptomatic. It is invariably due to autonomous secretion of PTH either from an adenoma or hyperplasia. Secondary hyperparathyroidism due to vitamin D deficiency is characterized by low to low-normal calcium, hypophosphatemia, and markedly elevated PTH and alkaline phosphatase and presents with features of rickets/osteomalacia and pseudofractures. The differentiation between PHPT with concurrent vitamin D deficiency and secondary hyperparathyroidism due to vitamin D deficiency poses a diagnostic dilemma in clinical practice. However, the presence of renal stone disease, pancreatitis, fractures, high-normal serum calcium, and marked hypophosphatemia suggests the diagnosis of PHPT even in the presence of vitamin D deficiency. Low-normal serum calcium, low serum phosphate, very high ALP, presence of pseudofractures, and features of rickets/osteomalacia suggest a diagnosis of secondary hyperparathyroidism due to vitamin D deficiency. Parathyroid imaging may be helpful in differentiating the two, but even localization of a single adenoma does not exclude the diagnosis of secondary hyperparathyroidism. The correction of vitamin D deficiency may lead to development of overt hypercalcemia in patients of PHPT with concurrent vitamin D deficiency, whereas decrease/normalization of PTH without development of hypercalcemia occurs in patients with secondary hyperparathyroidism due to vitamin D deficiency.

32. **What are familial causes of PTH-dependent hypercalcemia?**

The familial causes of PTH-dependent hypercalcemia are multiple endocrine neoplasia (MEN1, MEN2a, and MEN4), familial hypocalciuric hypercalcemia, neonatal severe hyperparathyroidism, hyperparathyroidism–jaw tumor syndrome, and familial isolated hyperparathyroidism. The familial causes contribute to only 5% of PTH-dependent hypercalcemia, and majority of these patients have parathyroid hyperplasia.

33. **What are the characteristics of PHPT in MEN1?**

Multiple endocrine neoplasia type 1 is an autosomal dominant disorder with loss-of-function mutation of MENIN gene located on chromosome 11q13. The most common endocrine manifestation of MEN1 is PHPT and is present in 90% of patients. On the contrary, only 1–18% of patients with "sporadic" PHPT have MEN1-related PHPT. The differences between PHPT in MEN 1 and sporadic PHPT are summarized in the table.

Parameters	MEN1-related PHPT	Sporadic PHPT
Age of onset	20–25 years	>50 years
Male/female	1:1	1:3
Phenotypic markers	Facial angiofibromas (85%) Collagenomas (70%) Lipomas (30%)	Absent
Hypercalcemia	Mild	Mild to severe
Imaging	Usually normal	Single adenoma (85%)
Pathology	Hyperplasia	Adenoma
Carcinoma	Almost never	<1%
Surgery	$3^{1/2}$ gland excision	Adenoma excision
Outcome	High risk for hypoparathyroidism and recurrent/persistent disease	Usually curative, low risk for hypoparathyroidism

34. **How to manage PHPT in patients with MEN1?**

PHPT in MEN1 may occur as early as 8 years of age, but surgery is recommended only if the patient is symptomatic. Bilateral neck exploration is the preferred approach as almost all patients have multiglandular involvement and $3^{1/2}$ gland excision is recommended. Asymptomatic patients with PHPT should be kept under regular surveillance. The reasons for deferring the surgery in asymptomatic patients despite earlier recognition of their disease include presence of mild hyperparathyroidism, very low probability of malignant transformation, and higher risk of developing hypoparathyroidism or recurrence of disease after surgery.

35. **What is hyperparathyroidism–jaw tumor syndrome?**

Hyperparathyroidism–jaw tumor syndrome (HPT–JT) is an autosomal dominant disorder characterized by fibro-osseous tumors of mandible and/or maxilla with primary hyperparathyroidism. Ossifying fibromas of the jaw are present in 25–50% of patients with HPT–JT. These tumors are benign, unrelated to PHPT, and are devoid of giant cells on histology. Approximately 95% of patients with HPT-JT have PHPT. HPT-JT-related PHPT is characterized by multiglandular involvement with cystic adenomas, and is malignant in 10–15% of patients. HPT–JT may also be accompanied with Wilms' tumor, uterine tumors, and multiple renal cysts. HPT–JT has been mapped to HPRT2 gene (CDC73), which produces a protein "parafibromin" that negatively regulates cell growth and proliferation. Inactivating mutations of parafibromin promotes cell proliferation via *Wnt*-signaling pathway and cyclin D1 gene expression.

36. **What are the features suggestive of parathyroid carcinoma?**

Presence of a palpable neck mass, recurrent laryngeal nerve involvement, cervical lymphadenopathy, serum calcium >14 mg/dl, and serum PTH >1,000 pg/ml in a patient with PHPT suggest the possibility of parathyroid carcinoma. In addition, patients with HPT–JT should also be evaluated for parathyroid carcinoma. Further, presence of surrounding tissue invasion and distant metastasis favors a diagnosis of parathyroid carcinoma.

37. **Is there a need for preoperative localization in patients with PHPT?**

Preoperative localization is recommended in patients with PHPT who are planned for minimally invasive parathyroidectomy (MIP) and in those with recurrent/persistent PHPT. Preoperative localization is not advisable in patients with PHPT <30 years of age or in familial PHPT, as they are likely to have multiglandular disease and require bilateral neck exploration. In patients with "sporadic PHPT," after preoperative localization of a single adenoma by USG or sestamibi (MIBI) or both in concordance, MIP is curative in 84% of patients.

38. **What are the available modalities for preoperative localization in PHPT?**

The available modalities for parathyroid imaging include ultrasound, CT, MRI, technetium 99m-sestamibi planar scintigraphy, ^{99m}Tc-sestamibi single-photon emission computed tomography, and ^{99m}Tc-sestamibi SPECT combined with computed tomography. Ultrasound, CT, and MRI yield information about structural abnormalities of the gland, while ^{99m}Tc-sestamibi is a functional scan.

39. **What is the utility of ultrasonography for preoperative localization in patients with PHPT?**

Ultrasonography is a useful modality for preoperative localization in patients with PHPT. It is easily available, inexpensive, and is devoid of ionizing radiation. Normal parathyroid glands are not identified by USG because of their small size ($5 \times 3 \times 1$ mm) and isoechogenicity to thyroid gland. Parathyroid adenoma are usually larger in size and are hypoechoic to the surrounding thyroid tissue and USG has a sensitivity of 72–85% and positive predictive value of 60–92% in localizing a solitary adenoma. However, the sensitivity of USG for detection of double adenoma and hyperplasia is only 35% and 16%, respectively. The lower sensitivity in multiglandular disease may be due to smaller size of these abnormal glands and isoechogenicity to thyroid tissue.

40. **What is the utility of CT and MRI in preoperative localization in patients with PHPT**?

CT and MRI offer an advantage to visualize the entire neck and mediastinum in a single imaging. However, these imaging modalities have a sensitivity of only 46–87% in localizing abnormal parathyroid gland/s in patients with PHPT. Because of their lower sensitivity, use of these modalities is not routinely recommended. Nevertheless, these modalities are particularly useful in patients with recurrent/persistent disease and in those with ectopic parathyroid gland identified on scintigraphy to delineate the anatomical details.

41. **What is the principle of ^{99m}Tc-sestamibi scintigraphy**?

^{99m}Tc-sestamibi is taken up by many tissues in body but is concentrated in only those tissues which are rich in mitochondria including thyroid, parathyroid, myocardium, and salivary glands. The radiotracer is retained for a longer duration by the mitochondria-rich oxyphil cells in the abnormal parathyroid gland than in normal parathyroid and thyroid tissue. This differential uptake helps in localizing the abnormal parathyroid gland. ^{99m}Tc-sestamibi planar scintigraphy and ^{99m}Tc-sestamibi SPECT scintigraphy are functional scans and yield 2D images and 3D images, respectively. The sensitivity of sestamibi SPECT in localizing a solitary adenoma is 68–95%, while for hyperplasia and double adenoma, 44% and 30%, respectively. ^{99m}Tc-sestamibi SPECT–CT (Hybrid SPECT–CT) displays both structural and functional abnormalities of the parathyroid gland with a sensitivity of 88–93% for solitary adenoma. Further, this imaging modality is particularly useful in localization of ectopic parathyroid gland and in those with distorted neck anatomy.

42. **What are the advantages and disadvantages with ultrasound and ^{99m}Tc-sestamibi for preoperative localization in PHPT**?

The advantages and disadvantages of both these modalities are listed in the table given below.

Modality	Advantages	Disadvantages
Ultrasonography	Structural scan Highly sensitive (72–85%) in experienced hands for solitary adenoma Inexpensive and noninvasive Reproducible No radiation exposure	Operator dependent Decreased accuracy in smaller adenoma (<1 cm), ectopic gland, and obese individuals Falsely positive in the presence of coexisting thyroid nodule and lymph nodes
^{99m}Tc-sestamibi	Functional scan Sensitivity to localize single adenoma-68–95% If combined with SPECT-CT sensitivity for single adenoma –88–93%	Not easily available Expensive False positivity with thyroid nodule, Hurthle cell adenoma, lymph nodes

43. **What is the sensitivity of ^{99m}Tc-sestamibi and ultrasonography in localizing abnormal parathyroid gland**?

The sensitivity of ^{99m}Tc-sestamibi and ultrasonography in localizing abnormal parathyroid gland is listed in the table given below. If both these modalities are combined together, sensitivity increases to 95%, but the concordance rate is only 64% for localization of a single adenoma.

Abnormality	^{99m}Tc-sestamibi	USG
Single adenoma	68–95%	72–85%
Double adenoma	30%	35%
Hyperplasia	44%	16%

44. **What are the causes of discordant findings between ultrasonography and ^{99m}Tc-sestamibi scintigraphy during preoperative localization**?

The causes of discordant findings between ultrasonography and ^{99m}Tc-sestamibi scintigraphy during preoperative localization are listed below.

USG +, MIBI –	USG –, MIBI +
Double adenoma	Ectopic gland
Use of calcium channel blockers	Small adenoma (<1 cm)
Adenoma with paucity of oxyphil cell	Multiglandular hyperplasia
	Inexperienced operator

45. **What is the advantage of 4D-CT for preoperative localization**?

4D-CT employs four phases and include pre-contrast, immediate (30s), early-delayed (60s), and late-delayed (90s) phases. The differential uptake of contrast during the immediate vascular phase (30s) allows distinction of parathyroid adenoma from normal thyroid/lymph node. Parathyroid adenoma, being highly vascular, shows early and maximum uptake of contrast as compared to surrounding normal tissues. 4D-CT is useful to localize abnormal parathyroid in patients with sporadic PHPT planned for MIP with an accuracy of 96.5% and in those with recurrent and persistent disease. In addition, 4D-CT may localize adenoma even in those with negative USG and MIBI scan.

46. **A 25-year-old woman presented with recurrent renal stone disease. On evaluation, she had PTH-dependent hypercalcemia without localization on USG and MIBI. How to proceed further**?

Preoperative localization is not recommended in younger patients (<30 years) as they are likely to have multiglandular disease. In such a scenario, the patient should be evaluated for familial causes of hyperparathyroidism. The presence of concurrent hyperprolactinemia suggests a diagnosis of MEN1 syndrome which can be further confirmed on genetic analysis. Other rare causes of PTH-dependent hypercalcemia like familial hypocalciuric hypercalcemia, anti-CaSR antibody, and lithium therapy should also be excluded. After exclusion of these causes, patient should be subjected to four-gland exploration.

47. **A 40-year-old lady presented with fragility fracture of right neck of femur. On evaluation, she had hypercalcemia and inappropriately elevated PTH. USG neck and MIBI scintigraphy were noncontributory. What to do next**?

    The most common cause of PTH-dependent hypercalcemia is PHPT, and in 85% of patients it is due to a solitary parathyroid adenoma. However, USG and MIBI may be negative in 5–10% of patients with PHPT, particularly in those with parathyroid hyperplasia, double adenoma, ectopic parathyroid adenoma, or small eutopic adenoma (<1 cm). In such a situation, other modalities like ^{99m}Tc-sestamibi-SPECT-CT/4D-CT may localize a solitary adenoma with a sensitivity of 85–93%. If localized, patient can be subjected to minimally invasive surgery. If adenoma is not localized on either of these modalities, patient should be subjected to bilateral neck exploration. In this patient SPECT–CT scintigraphy localized a mediastinal lesion, and patient was subjected to surgery. Histopathology was consistent with parathyroid adenoma.

48. **A 45-year-old male presented with recurrent pancreatitis. On evaluation he had PTH-dependent hypercalcemia. USG neck localized an adenoma in the right inferior gland while MIBI in the left superior gland. How to proceed further**?

    The combined use of USG and MIBI scintigraphy for the localization of an abnormal gland is common in clinical practice and has a sensitivity of 95% in localizing a solitary adenoma, with a concordance of 64%. However, the available literature does not recommend dual scanning for localization in a patient with suspected sporadic PHPT. The discordance between USG and MIBI scintigraphy in localizing a solitary adenoma is nearly 28% and is due to presence of multiglandular disease (double adenoma/hyperplasia), ectopic adenoma, oxyphil cell adenoma, and concurrent thyroid nodule. In such a scenario the evidence to proceed further with imaging modalities like ^{99m}Tc-sestamibi-SPECT-CT/4D-CT are sparse, and hence the patient should be subjected to bilateral neck exploration.

49. **What are the indications for surgery in asymptomatic PHPT**?

    The indications for surgery in asymptomatic PHPT are serum calcium >1 mg/dl above upper limit of normal, T-score ≤−2.5 (any site) or presence of vertebral fracture, eGFR <60 ml/min, 24 h urine calcium >400 mg/day with an increased risk for calcium-containing stones, presence of nephrolithiasis/nephrocalcinosis, and age <50 years.

50. **What are the indications for surgery in symptomatic PHPT**?

Ideally all patients with symptomatic PHPT should be subjected to surgery. These include renal stone disease/nephrocalcinosis, classic neuromuscular disease, fracture or OFC, and symptomatic hypercalcemia.

51. **Should vitamin D be replaced in patients with PHPT who have coexisting vitamin D deficiency**?

There is a theoretical risk of hypercalcemia and hypercalciuria with vitamin D repletion in patients of PHPT with concurrent vitamin D deficiency. But, the available evidence does not support this risk in patients of PHPT with mild hypercalcemia (within 1 mg/dl above reference range). Rather, vitamin D supplementation may be associated with significant reduction in serum PTH and probably reduce the risk of postoperative hungry bone syndrome. However, in patients with severe hypercalcemia (>12 mg/dl), vitamin D supplementation should be avoided.

52. **What are the benefits of bisphosphonate therapy in patients with PHPT**?

Bisphosphonates are potent osteoclast inhibitors and prevent bone resorption. They are useful in patients of PHPT with severe hypercalcemia, in those with severe bone disease (as they are at higher risk of hungry bone syndrome postoperatively), and in those who opt for medical treatment. However, their preoperative use may be associated with a risk of postoperative recalcitrant hypocalcemia and possibly an unfavorable effect on bone remodeling after curative parathyroidectomy.

53. **What are the different surgical approaches in a patient with PHPT**?

The available surgical options include bilateral neck exploration (BNE), unilateral neck exploration (UNE), and minimally invasive parathyroidectomy (MIP). BNE is the gold standard procedure which does not require preoperative localization as it involves exploration of all four glands. In addition, it provides an opportunity to visualize thyroid gland. The procedure is safe and highly effective with a cure rate of 95% in experienced hands. UNE involves an incision towards the side of localized abnormal gland (Kocher incision) and provides an opportunity to explore ipsilateral "normal" superior or inferior parathyroid gland. Advantages of UNE are smaller incision, shorter hospital stay, and reduced morbidity. MIP involves targeted excision of a preoperatively localized abnormal gland through a mini-incision.

54. **What is minimally invasive parathyroidectomy**?

Minimally invasive parathyroidectomy (MIP) is a surgically refined procedure which focuses on reducing the size of the incision (2.5–3 cm) and minimizing surgical dissection. The concept of MIP stems from the fact that 85% of patients with "sporadic PHPT" have a solitary adenoma which is potentially identifiable and resectable with a mini-incision, thereby avoiding bilateral neck exploration in majority. Preoperative localization of a single abnormal gland is mandatory before proceeding for MIP in a patient with biochemically confirmed PHPT. MIP encompasses a number of different techniques, including open minimally invasive parathyroidectomy, minimally invasive radio-guided parathyroidectomy, video-assisted parathyroidectomy, and purely endoscopic parathyroidectomy. Advantages of MIP include shorter operative time, less postoperative hypocalcemia, shorter hospital stay, and better cosmetic outcome. Contraindications for MIP include coexisting thyroid disease, multiglandular parathyroid disease, PHPT in young (<30 years), non-localization of an abnormal gland, and parathyroid malignancy.

55. **What is turbo PTH assay**?

Turbo PTH assay is a method which allows rapid estimation of serum PTH and is used intraoperatively to confirm successful excision of abnormal parathyroid gland(s). It provides faster results as compared to conventional assays, because of shorter incubation time (7 min vs. 1–2 h) required during processing of sample. This is achieved by increasing the incubation temperature from 20 °C to 45 °C and shaking speed from 180 to 400 rpm. Further, the analytic range of the turbo PTH assay is almost comparable to the conventional assay.

56. **What is Miami criterion**?

Miami criterion is used for defining the success of parathyroidectomy. It includes >50% reduction in serum PTH levels 10 min after excision of suspected abnormal gland as compared to the highest pre-incision or pre-excision serum PTH level. The accuracy of intraoperative PTH (IOPTH) in predicting cure in solitary adenoma is 97%, while 58% in those with multiglandular disease. The IOPTH measurement for confirmation of curative parathyroidectomy is feasible due to the short half-life of PTH (3–5 min) and availability of turbo PTH assay. Measurable levels of PTH even after curative surgery suggest that rest of parathyroid glands are not completely suppressed by hypercalcemia.

57. **What are the biochemical alterations after parathyroid surgery**?

After successful removal of abnormal parathyroid gland, PTH levels decline intraoperatively by >50% and return to the reference range within 30 h; however, the secretory response to hypocalcemia may take several weeks to recover. Decrease in serum calcium occurs by 12 h and reaches a nadir by 24–36 h postoperatively. After curative parathyroidectomy serum phosphate may normalize or decline, depending upon the severity of preexisting bone disease. Decrease in serum phosphate along with increase in alkaline phosphatase suggests hungry bone syndrome, whereas increase in serum phosphate above reference range signals hypoparathyroidism, which may be due to inadvertent injury/

ischemia to neighboring parathyroid glands. Bone turnover markers may take longer time (~1 year) to recover and correlate with increase in BMD.

58. **What is the effect of curative parathyroidectomy on BMD?**

After curative parathyroidectomy, there is a significant increase in BMD at spine and hip, sites which are rich in trabecular bone. BMD increases by ~5–10% in first year and continues to increase by 12–15% over ten years. However, there is minimal or no change in BMD at distal radius, which is composed predominantly of cortical bone.

59. **What are the causes of hypocalcemia after parathyroidectomy?**

Hypocalcemia after parathyroidectomy occurs due to hungry bone syndrome, transient hypoparathyroidism, hypomagnesemia, and permanent hypoparathyroidism. Hungry bone syndrome is the most common cause of post-operative hypocalcemia in patients with symptomatic PHPT. Transient hypoparathyroidism is due to suppression of normal parathyroid gland by high levels of calcium, which recovers slowly over a week's time. However, inadvertent injury/ischemia or accidental removal of normal parathyroid glands during surgery may cause transient, but sometimes permanent hypoparathyroidism. In addition, prior bisphosphonate therapy and severe vitamin D deficiency can also manifest as hypocalcemia after curative parathyroidectomy.

60. **What is hungry bone syndrome?**

Hungry bone syndrome (HBS) is characterized by "increased appetite of bone" for calcium and phosphorus, due to sudden decrease in osteoclastic activity with continued osteoblast activity driving the influx of calcium and phosphorus into bone. Biochemically, it is characterized by hypocalcemia, hypophosphatemia, hypomagnesemia, raised alkaline phosphatase and hypocalciuria. The prerequisite for development of HBS is measurable levels of PTH which is required for bone remodeling, as HBS does not occur in patients who develop hypoparathyroidism.

61. **What are the causes of hungry bone syndrome?**

The most common cause of hungry bone syndrome (HBS) is parathyroidectomy for hyperparathyroidism (primary/secondary/tertiary). It may also occur in patients with rickets/osteomalacia who are replaced with vitamin D alone without calcium. The other causes include patients with untreated severe hyperthyroidism following thyroid surgery, correction of metabolic acidosis in patients with renal tubular acidosis, and after administration of antiresorptive therapy in patients with osteoblast metastasis (e.g., carcinoma prostate). Rarely, patients with Cushing's syndrome may also develop HBS after curative surgery, particularly in those who have severe bone disease, vitamin D deficiency, and are on ketoconazole therapy.

62. **What are the predictors of hungry bone syndrome in patients with primary hyperparathyroidism**?

    Predictors of HBS in patients with primary hyperparathyroidism include old age (>60 years), postmenopausal status, vitamin D deficiency, severe bone disease (osteitis fibrosa cystica, high ALP), high preoperative serum calcium and PTH, and large parathyroid adenoma (>5 cm). Preoperative use of bisphosphonates has been shown to reduce the occurrence of HBS.

63. **How to prevent hungry bone syndrome following curative parathyroidectomy**?

    There is a dearth of literature regarding the preventive strategies for HBS following curative parathyroidectomy. Prior use of bisphosphonate reduces the risk of HBS by causing osteoclast apoptosis, thereby preventing the crosstalk between osteoblast and osteoclasts. This leads to suppression of bone remodeling, which is the driving force for entry of calcium into bone. In patients with severe bone disease, prior use of bisphosphonate may not prevent HBS possibly due to ongoing intense bone remodeling. In addition, preoperative vitamin D replacement in vitamin D-deficient individuals with mild hypercalcemia may also favorably influence the outcome.

64. **How to differentiate between hypocalcemia due to hungry bone syndrome and prior bisphosphonate therapy in a patient with primary hyperparathyroidism postoperatively**?

    Hypocalcemia after curative surgery may be due to hungry bone syndrome, hypoparathyroidism or prior bisphoshponate therapy. Low serum phosphate is characteristic of HBS; however, it may also occur with the prior use of bisphosphonate. Rising serum alkaline phosphatase (ALP) favors hypocalcemia due to HBS, while normal/decreasing levels of ALP suggest prior bisphosphonate therapy as the cause of hypocalcemia.

65. **How to treat hungry bone syndrome**?

    Frequent, regular monitoring of serum calcium, preferably ionized calcium during immediate postoperative period, is advised. With the development of symptomatic hypocalcemia, signs of latent tetany or serum calcium <8.4 mg/dl, calcium supplementation should be initiated. Oral calcium (elemental calcium 2–4 g) in divided doses, preferably between meals is administered, to minimize phosphate binding. Oral calcitriol (1–2 μg) should also be administered along with calcium. Calcitriol is required as PTH-mediated 1α-hydroxylation is reduced following parathyroidectomy, and its rapid onset and offset of action provide flexibility in adjusting the dose to prevent inadvertent hypercalcemia.

In addition, patients with concurrent vitamin D deficiency, cholecalciferol should be supplemented to provide optimal substrate for 1α-hydroxylation. Phosphorus supplementation is generally not required; moreover, phosphorus can reduce intestinal calcium absorption. Intravenous calcium should be administered cautiously if patients develop seizures, cardiac arrhythmias, laryngeal spasm, or ionized calcium <0.9 mmol/l, which can be life-threatening. Overzealous administration of i.v. calcium can result in pancreatitis.

66. **What are the indicators of resolution of hungry bone syndrome**?

The indicators of resolution of HBS include normalization of serum calcium, phosphorous, ALP and bone turnover markers, healing of osteitis fibrosa cystica, and significant gain in BMD. Complete recovery after HBS usually occurs over a period of ~9–12 months.

67. **How to follow a patient with PHPT postoperatively**?

Postoperatively, serum calcium, phosphorus, and alkaline phosphatase should be carefully monitored in patients with PHPT. In case of persistent hypocalcemia, hungry bone syndrome should be differentiated from permanent hypoparathyroidism. Hypocalcemia/normocalcemia suggests curative parathyroidectomy, while lack of normalization of serum calcium suggests either failed surgery or multiglandular disease. Patients with hypocalcemia due to transient hypoparathyroidism require calcium and calcitriol supplementation for 3–6 months as there is a delay in recovery of calcium–PTH axis. Mild hypocalcemia is preferred in these patients as it acts as a modest stimulus to allow the recovery of the calcium–PTH axis. Serum PTH should be estimated in the immediate postoperative period and in case of persistent hypocalcemia/hypercalcemia. Bone mineral density must also be monitored.

68. **What are the causes of worsening of bone diseases after curative parathyroidectomy**?

Recurrence of PHPT, persistent vitamin D deficiency, and progressive renal failure due to untreated nephrolithiasis and/or nephrocalcinosis may lead to worsening of bone disease even after curative parathyroidectomy. In addition, chronic pancreatitis due to PHPT may result in worsening of bone disease due to calcium and vitamin D malabsorption.

69. **What are the medical options available to treat patients with PHPT**?

A patient with PHPT should be advised adequate hydration, and to avoid the use of thiazide diuretic and prolonged immobilization. In addition, dietary calcium should not be restricted. The medical options for the management of PHPT are enlisted in the table given below.

Modality of treatment	Mechanism of action	Effect on calcium	Effect on BMD
Estrogen, selective estrogen receptor modulator (raloxifene)	Promotes osteoclast apoptosis Antagonizes the action of PTH at receptor level Inhibits cytokine (IL-1, IL-6, and TNF-α)-mediated osteoclast resorption	Modest decline (0.5–1 mg/dl)	Improvement in spine and hip BMD
Bisphosphonates	Potent inhibitors of osteoclastogenesis and prevents bone resorption	Transient reduction in serum calcium	Improvement in spine and hip BMD
Cinacalcet	Calcimimetic	Normalizes serum calcium	No effect
Non-calcemic vitamin D analogues (24 oxo-calcitriol)	Directly suppresses PTH	Modest	No effect

70. **What is the role of cinacalcet in the management of hyperparathyroidism**?

Calcium-sensing receptor (CaSR) is present on chief cells of parathyroid gland and thick ascending limb of loop of Henle. Binding of calcium with CaSR in parathyroid gland inhibits PTH secretion, and at kidney, it increases calcium excretion. Cinacalcet is a calcimimetic agent that activates CaSR and inhibits PTH secretion. Cinacalcet leads to normalization of serum calcium in 70–100% of patients with asymptomatic PHPT, while serum calcium is normalized only in 28–68% of patients with symptomatic (severe) PHPT. However, reduction in serum PTH is modest (30–50%) despite normalization of serum calcium in majority of patients. This discordance may be explained by the activation of CaSR at kidney, and possibly at bone, resulting in hypercalciuria and increased calcium influx into bone, respectively. There is increase in serum phosphate, although it remains in a low-normal range. Surprisingly, there is no significant improvement in BMD, even with prolonged use of cinacalcet. In addition, cinacalcet has also been used in patients with parathyroid carcinoma and in those with secondary hyperparathyroidism due to chronic kidney disease on maintenance dialysis.

71. **What are the complications of parathyroid surgery**?

The complications of parathyroid surgery with bilateral neck exploration include recurrent laryngeal nerve injury (<1%) and transient (10%) or permanent hypoparathyroidism (<1%). In addition, failed surgery in 1–6% of patients results in persistent hyperparathyroidism. However, complications are much less with minimally invasive parathyroidectomy.

72. **What is curative parathyroidectomy?**

Curative parathyroidectomy may be defined as persistent normalization of serum calcium, phosphate, and PTH with restoration of calcium–PTH axis after surgery. Bone turnover markers, and bone mineral density may take a longer time to normalize and should not be considered as indicators of curative parathyroidectomy.

73. **What is persistent or recurrent PHPT?**

Persistent PHPT is defined as hypercalcemia that either persists or recurs within 6 months of parathyroid surgery. Reappearance of hypercalcemia after 6 months of curative parathyroid surgery is termed as recurrent PHPT. The causes of persistent/recurrent PHPT include failure to localize abnormal parathyroid gland intraoperatively, incomplete excision of adenoma, multiglandular disease (familial syndromes), ectopic parathyroid adenoma, and rarely parathyroid carcinoma.

74. **What is the role of preoperative imaging in patients with recurrent/persistent PHPT?**

Preoperative localization is mandatory prior to any surgical intervention in patients with recurrent/persistent PHPT. USG neck and ^{99m}Tc-sestamibi-SPECT scintigraphy are recommended as the initial imaging modalities. If the results of these imaging are concordant, accuracy of this combined approach is 90%, and no further investigation is required for localization. However, if the results of USG and MIBI are negative, discordant, or inconclusive, further imaging is needed. CT and MRI are helpful in localizing ectopic lesion in the mediastinum with a sensitivity of 46–87%. Hybrid SPECT–CT and 4D-CT are helpful particularly in patients with negative USG and MIBI scan, with a sensitivity of 88% and 82%, respectively. At times, invasive tests are to be performed, when there is failure to localize with noninvasive tests. USG-guided FNAC of suspected lesion with assessment of tissue PTH level has a sensitivity of 87% and specificity of 74% in the diagnosis of parathyroid lesion. Selective arteriography and venous sampling for PTH is an invasive and expensive test which requires considerable experience, and is associated with a risk of vascular injury; however, it localizes abnormal glands in 75% of patients, which were not identified by any of the noninvasive methods.

75. **How to treat patients with recurrent/persistent PHPT?**

Indications for surgery are essentially the same as in surgically naive patients with PHPT. All symptomatic patients should be subjected to surgery. Those who have well-localized adenoma with concordance on USG and MIBI can be offered MIP. Those with non-localization or discordant results on USG and MIBI should undergo further imaging (Hybrid SPECT–CT, MRI, 4D-CT), and failure to localize warrants bilateral neck exploration. Surgical cure rate is

85–90% in patients with recurrent/persistent disease as compared to 95–97% in surgically naive patients. Patients with recurrent/persistent hyperparathyroidism who are asymptomatic or who have mild disease should be kept under regular surveillance and if required, may be managed medically. This is because of difficulties associated with redo surgery due to distorted neck anatomy, higher risk of recurrent laryngeal nerve injury, and hypocalcemia.

76. **What are the causes of hypercalcemia in a patient with renal failure**?

Hypocalcemia is common in patients with renal failure and can be due to decreased renal 1α-hydroxylase activity, vitamin D deficiency, hyperphosphatemia, PTH resistance, and poor oral intake. Nevertheless, hypercalcemia can occur in patients with renal failure, and the causes include overzealous treatment with calcium and calcitriol, tertiary hyperparathyroidism, adynamic bone disease, and milk–alkali syndrome.

77. **Why does secondary hyperparathyroidism develop in chronic kidney disease**?

Chronic kidney disease (CKD) is characterized by progressive loss of renal mass resulting in decreased glomerular filtration rate. This leads to hyperphosphatemia and reduced renal 1α-hydroxylase activity and consequently hypocalcemia. All these metabolic abnormalities act as strong stimuli for PTH secretion and parathyroid gland proliferation, resulting in secondary hyperparathyroidism. In addition, skeletal PTH resistance (due to PTH receptor downregulation), bioinactive PTH fragments (acting as PTH antagonists), and uremic toxins aggravate secondary hyperparathyroidism. Further, intrinsic abnormalities within parathyroid gland, particularly alterations in set point or expression of CaSR also contribute to secondary hyperparathyroidism. There is an emerging role of FGF23 in the development of secondary hyperparathyroidism as CKD is associated with FGF23 resistance, due to reduced Klotho expression.

78. **What is tertiary hyperparathyroidism**?

Tertiary hyperparathyroidism is characterized by autonomous hypersecretion of PTH leading to hypercalcemia and is invariably a sequel of long-standing undiagnosed/untreated secondary hyperparathyroidism. Parathyroid hyperplasia involving all four glands is a consistent feature in these patients; however, 20% of these patients may additionally have a single or double adenoma.

79. **What are the causes of tertiary hyperparathyroidism**?

The stimuli for parathyroid cell growth and proliferation includes chronic hypocalcemia, hyperphosphatemia, low 1,25(OH)2D, and alteration in the set point of calcium-sensing receptor. These stimuli lead to secondary hyperparathyroidism and if persistent may result in tertiary hyperparathyroidism. The causes of tertiary hyperparathyroidism are chronic kidney disease (CKD), vitamin D deficiency, and phosphate supplementation without calcitriol in patients with hypophosphatemic osteomalacia and rarely patients with pseudohypoparathyroidism type 1b. It is postulated that an acquired altered set point at high threshold for calcium-sensing receptor (CaSR) results in monoclonal/polyclonal expansion of parathyroid cells, leading to either hyperplasia or adenoma.

80. **How to differentiate between secondary versus tertiary hyperparathyroidism associated with chronic kidney disease?**

Secondary hyperparathyroidism is an adaptive response to hypocalcemia, hyperphosphatemia, and reduced $1,25(OH)_2D$, in chronic kidney disease (CKD). Biochemically it is characterized by low to normal serum calcium, high phosphate, and very high levels of PTH. PTH excess clinically manifests as pruritus, anemia, high turnover bone disease, and myopathy. Periosteal bone resorption, salt and pepper appearance of skull bone, and brown tumors are radiological features of PTH excess irrespective of etiology of hyperparathyroidism, while rugger-jersey spine (alternate bands of sclerosis and lucency) is specific to secondary hyperparathyroidism due to CKD. Tertiary hyperparathyroidism associated with CKD is a consequence of long-standing untreated/inadequately treated secondary hyperparathyroidism resulting in autonomous secretion of PTH. Development of hypercalcemia in a patient with CKD signals the onset of tertiary hyperparathyroidism. Normal to high levels of serum calcium, normal to low phosphate (due to metastatic calcification), and elevated PTH are the biochemical hallmarks. Patients can develop fracture, renal stone disease, pancreatitis, and soft tissue and vascular calcifications. Radiological features are similar to secondary hyperparathyroidism.

81. **How to differentiate primary hyperparathyroidism from tertiary hyperparathyroidism?**

PHPT is primarily a disorder of parathyroid gland, while tertiary hyperparathyroidism is a consequence of long-standing untreated secondary hyperparathyroidism. Although etiopathologically they are different, biochemically both present as PTH-dependent hypercalcemia. Hypercalcemia, hypophosphatemia, normal serum creatinine, inappropriately elevated PTH, and localization of an adenoma on imaging suggest PHPT, while normal to mild hypercalcemia in the presence of high serum creatinine, normal to high phosphorus, elevated PTH, and failure to localize the source on imaging suggests tertiary hyperparathyroidism. However, distinction between PHPT with renal failure and tertiary hyperparathyroidism due to chronic kidney disease is a challenge in clinical practice. History of recurrent renal stone disease, fragility fracture, pancreatitis, gallstone disease, short duration of renal disease, and obstructive uropathy on USG suggests PHPT. Presence of long-standing renal disease, small kidneys on USG, anemia, and hypertension suggests the diagnosis of chronic kidney disease and favors tertiary hyperparathyroidism, rather than PHPT. Patients with PHPT with a localized single adenoma will be cured with adenomectomy, while patients with tertiary hyperparathyroidism usually require three and a half gland excision, even in the presence of a localized adenoma on imaging. This underscores the importance of differentiating these two akin conditions.

82. **Why to treat secondary hyperparathyroidism associated with CKD**?

PTH excess is associated with anemia (PTH-induced myelofibrosis), pruritus (accumulation of inactive carboxy-terminal PTH fragments), high turnover bone disease, dysglycemia (PTH-mediated insulin resistance), cardiac dysfunction (PTH-mediated myocardial fibrosis), and hypertension (PTH-mediated vascular injury, endothelial dysfunction, and hyperaldosteronism). Therefore, treatment of secondary hyperparathyroidism is of paramount importance and may improve outcome.

83. **How to treat secondary/tertiary hyperparathyroidism associated with CKD**?

Management of secondary/tertiary hyperparathyroidism associated with CKD includes dietary restriction of phosphate, use of phosphate binders (sevelamer, lanthanum, or calcium acetate), calcitriol supplementation, and correction of acidemia. Serum PTH levels should be targeted between 35 and 70 pg/ml in those with stage 3 CKD (eGFR 30–59 ml/min), between 70 and 110 pg/ml in stage 4 CKD (eGFR 15–29 ml/min), and between 150 and 300 pg/ml in stage 5 CKD (eGFR <15 ml/min). With worsening eGFR, higher levels of PTH are required to prevent the development of adynamic bone disease. Serum calcium and phosphorus should be maintained in the reference range, and calcium phosphorus product should be maintained <55. If these measures fail to achieve the defined targets of PTH, calcimimetics (cinacalcet) or parathyroidectomy should be considered.

84. **What are the indications of parathyroidectomy in CKD**?

Indications for parathyroidectomy in patients with CKD include persistently high iPTH >800 pg/ml, sustained hypercalcemia (>11 mg/dl) and hyperphosphatemia despite optimal medical management. In addition, calciphylaxis with iPTH >500 pg/ml, presence of fragility fracture, and refectory pruritus also mandate parathyroidectomy. Excision of three to three and a half parathyroid glands is preferred as opposed to total parathyroidectomy, to avoid the risk of recalcitrant hypocalcemia.

85. **What is CKD–MBD**?

CKD–MBD denotes chronic kidney disease–mineral and bone disorder. It refers to abnormalities of mineral metabolism, metabolic bone disease, and/or metastatic calcification in a patient with chronic kidney disease. The metabolic bone disease associated with CKD is also known as renal osteodystrophy. Abnormalities in mineral homeostasis include alterations in the metabolism of calcium, phosphorus, PTH, $1,25(OH)_2D$, and FGF23. These mineral derangements lead to metabolic bone disease which manifests as alterations in bone histology (OFC, osteomalacia, and adynamic bone disease), bone strength, and impaired linear growth. Further, vascular and soft tissue calcification may also ensue from altered mineral homeostasis.

86. **What is renal osteodystrophy**?

Renal osteodystrophy (ROD) refers to the metabolic bone disease associated with CKD. It is a constellation of osteitis fibrosa cystica, osteomalacia, and adynamic bone disease, with varying combinations, as a consequence of chronic kidney disease. Decreased renal 1α-hydroxylase activity, PTH resistance, increased FGF23, concurrent vitamin D deficiency, altered calcium phosphate solubility product, and poor oral calcium intake result in renal osteodystrophy. Renal osteodystrophy may be associated with a high, normal, or low bone turnover. The high turnover state is due to elevated PTH and manifests as osteitis fibrosa cystica, while adynamic bone disease is a low bone turnover state due to inappropriately suppressed PTH. However, osteomalacia is associated with normal bone turnover. Periodic surveillance of calcium, phosphate, alkaline phosphatase, intact PTH, and 25(OH)D should be done in patients with CKD stage 3 and beyond. Skeletal survey is indicated in asymptomatic patients when iPTH is at extremes (<50 or >800 pg/ml). Treatment of high turnover bone disease/osteomalacia includes phosphorus restriction, phosphate binders, calcium supplementation, and calcitriol, but caution is advised as overzealous treatment may result in adynamic bone disease.

87. **What is adynamic bone disease**?

Adynamic bone disease is characterized by suppressed bone remodeling due to low PTH (<50 pg/ml), which is usually a result of overzealous treatment with calcitriol and calcium-containing phosphate binders and is commonly seen in patients on dialysis. Treatment with aluminum-containing antacids (as phosphate binders) was an important cause for adynamic bone disease in the past. Patients with adynamic bone disease commonly present with bone pain, fragility fracture, and metastatic calcification. Biochemical abnormalities include hypercalcemia with low iPTH. Hypercalcemia is a result of reduced influx of calcium from circulation into bone due to decreased bone remodeling, consequent to low PTH. Treatment includes discontinuation of calcitriol and calcium-contacting phosphate binders with restriction of oral calcium to 2 g/day. In refractory cases, treatment with recombinant PTH may be useful. Bisphosphonates are contraindicated as bone remodeling is already suppressed.

Suggested Reading

1. Jameson JL, De Groot LJ. Endocrinology: adult and pediatric. Philadelphia: Elsevier Health Sciences; 2010.
2. Longo D, Fauci A, Kasper D, Hauser S, Jameson J, Loscalzo J. Harrison's principles of internal medicine. 18th ed. New York: McGraw Hill Professional; 2012.
3. Melmed S, Polonsky KS, Larsen PR, Kronenberg HM. Williams textbook of endocrinology: expert consult. London: Elsevier Health Sciences; 2011.

Osteoporosis

15

15.1 Clinical Rounds

1. **What is osteoporosis?**

   Osteoporosis is a diffuse skeletal disease characterized by decreased bone mass and deterioration of bone microarchitecture, resulting in enhanced bone fragility and a consequent increase in fracture risk.

2. **What are the lacunae of this definition?**

   The definition of osteoporosis includes low bone mass. However, in clinical practice bone mass is not measured, as it requires bone biopsy; rather, bone mineral density (BMD), is used to define osteoporosis. Deterioration of bone microarchitecture is not specific to osteoporosis and it occurs in almost all metabolic bone disorders. The enhanced bone fragility and increased fracture risk are consequences of osteoporosis and do not add to the definition. Hence, Albright's description of osteoporosis as "too little bone in the bone" seems most appropriate.

3. **What are the fallacies in defining osteoporosis based on bone mineral density?**

   Organic component constitutes around 30–40% of bone mass, while inorganic component comprises the rest. Bone mineral density (BMD) measurement only estimates the inorganic component and does not represent the total bone mass and true strength of bone. Therefore, even individuals with normal BMD can also have fragility fractures. The T-score based definition of osteoporosis was derived from the bone mineral density data obtained from Caucasian women. However, race/ethnicity based normative BMD data for definition of osteoporosis is not available. Further, the definition of osteoporosis based on bone mineral density (T-score <–2.5) is only applicable to postmenopausal women and men >50 years of age. BMD measurement at one or two sites does not necessarily represent the overall decrease in bone mineral density.

A. Bhansali, Y. Gogate, *Clinical Rounds in Endocrinology: Volume I - Adult Endocrinology*, DOI 10.1007/978-81-322-2398-6_15

4. **Why is bone mass and bone mineral density used interchangeably?**

In physics, density and mass are different. However, in routine clinical practice, the terms bone mass and bone mineral density are used interchangeably. In children because of growing bones, bone mass increases, while bone mineral density may decrease, due to lag in mineralization of laid-down matrix. However, in adults, bone length remains stable; therefore, bone mass and bone mineral density remain proportionate to each other. Thus, for all practical purposes, bone mineral density reflects bone mass in adults.

5. **Why bone mineral density is considered a surrogate marker of the fracture risk?**

Bone mineral density represents 75–85% of total bone strength and correlates well with the weight-bearing capacity of the skeleton. The relationship between fracture risk and decline in bone mineral density is linear. Therefore, BMD is used in clinical practice to predict the fracture risk.

6. **What are the causes of increased fracture risk despite high bone mineral density?**

Low bone mineral density (BMD) is associated with increased risk of fracture. However, certain disorders are associated with high BMD and an increased fracture risk and these include fluorosis, osteopetrosis, Paget's disease (sclerotic form), osteoblastic skeletal metastasis, prolonged bisphosphonate therapy, and T2DM. These disorders are associated with impaired bone remodeling thereby increasing the fracture risk.

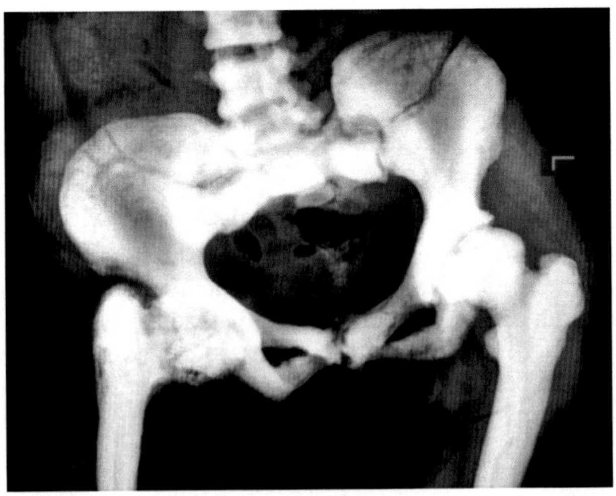

Fig. 15.1 X-ray of pelvis with both hip joints showing diffuse osteosclerosis with fracture of right neck of femur in a patient with osteopetrosis. Note the obliteration of medullary cavity of femur which is classical of osteopetrosis

7. **What is the difference between bone mineral content and bone mineral density?**

Bone mineral content represents the mineral mass expressed as grams, whereas bone mineral density corresponds to bone mineral mass within a defined area or volume, expressed as gm/cm^3 (volumetric BMD as measured with quantitative CT) or gm/cm^2 (areal BMD as measured by DXA).

8. **What are the constituents of bone?**

The bone is made up of cells and the matrix. The cellular components include osteoblasts, osteoclasts, and osteocytes. The matrix is composed of inorganic and organic components. The inorganic components comprises of calcium hydroxyapatite, phosphorus, and magnesium. The organic component consists of collagen, predominantly type 1, and non-collagenous proteins like bone sialoprotein, osteopontin, osteonectin, and osteocalcin.

9. **What are osteocytes?**

Osteocytes are terminally differentiated osteoblasts and account for 90% of all cells of bone and are scattered throughout the matrix. Osteocytes act as mechanostat and sense mechanical stress to the bone. It also secretes sclerostin which is an inhibitor of *Wnt* signaling pathway, thereby suppressing bone formation. In addition, it secretes FGF23 which is the key regulator of phosphate homeostasis.

10. **What is bone remodeling?**

Bone remodeling is a well-coordinated and sequential process of bone formation and resorption due to crosstalk between osteoblast and osteoclast. The steps involved in bone remodeling are quiescence, activation, resorption, reversal, and formation in a basic multicellular unit. Bone remodeling is stimulated by mechanical factors and hormones. Osteocytes act as mechanostat and initiate bone remodeling, while hormones which increase bone remodeling include PTH, $1,25(OH)_2D$, and possibly FGF23. Bone remodeling cycle takes about 90–120 days to result in new bone formation. Bone remodeling is required for repair of microfractures, maintenance of nutrition and blood supply, regulation of calcium homeostasis, and removal of nonfunctional cellular components.

11. **What is the difference between bone modeling and remodeling?**

Bone modeling occurs during childhood and peripubertal period and helps in attainment of peak bone mass. This process involves formation of new bone without preceding bone resorption. Bone remodeling is a sequential process involving resorption and formation of bone and begins after peripubertal period. Remodeling maintains bone strength by repairing microfractures and preserves resilience.

12. **What are the hormonal regulators of bone health?**

Skeletal tissue is composed of both cortical and cancellous (trabecular) bone in varying proportions. Vertebra is composed of cortical to cancellous bone in a ratio of 25:75, while in femoral head this ratio is 50:50 and 95:5 in distal radius. Primary regulators of cortical bone health are PTH and $1{,}25(OH)_2D$. Cancellous bone is metabolically more active and is mainly influenced by gonadal steroids and PTH. GH, IGF1, thyroxine, cortisol, and FGF23 play a permissive role in the maintenance of bone health.

13. **What is receptor activator of nuclear factor kappa β (RANK) and receptor activator of nuclear factor kappa β ligand (RANKL)?**

RANKL is a member of tumor necrosis factor (TNF) family and is a product of osteoblasts. It binds with RANK, a receptor expressed on osteoclast, and initiates the process of osteoclastogenesis. RANKL–RANK pathway is activated by cytokines (TNF-α, IL-1, IL-6), PTH, PTHrP, $1{,}25(OH)_2D$, and glucocorticoids, while it is inhibited by estrogen/testosterone, TGF-β, and possibly GH-IGF1.

14. **What is osteoprotegerin?**

Osteoprotegerin is a decoy receptor produced by osteoblasts. It binds with RANKL and prevents the interaction of RANKL with RANK, thereby resulting in suppression of osteoclast activation. PTH, $1{,}25(OH)_2D$, prostaglandinE_2, and glucocorticoids reduce production of osteoprotegerin, whereas estrogen and GH stimulate it.

15. **What is the importance of *Wnt*/β-catenin signaling pathway in bone physiology?**

Wnt/β-catenin signaling pathway is the prime regulator of osteoblast differentiation. Activation of *Wnt* pathway results in conversion of pre-osteoblasts into osteoblasts and leads to bone formation, while inhibitors of *Wnt* pathway such as sclerostin and Dickoff1 prevent bone formation. *Wnt*/β-catenin signaling pathway is now being targeted in the management of osteoporosis.

16. **What drives the influx of calcium into the bone?**

The factors which drive the entry of calcium into bone are not well elucidated. However, the most important factor is ongoing bone modeling/remodeling. Further, optimum levels of circulating calcium, phosphate, $1{,}25(OH)_2D$, and PTH, and IGF1 are required for influx of calcium and phosphate into bone. In addition, appropriately laid-down matrix and suppression of inhibitors of mineralization are prerequisite for bone mineralization.

17. **What is fragility fracture?**

A fracture that occurs as a result of minimal trauma or a fall from standing height or less of an individual is called as fragility fracture. The usual sites of fragility fractures are vertebrae, hip, and distal radius. However, it can occur at any site, except the face and skull.

18. **What is the most common manifestation of osteoporosis?**

Majority of patients with osteoporosis are asymptomatic. However, the most common manifestation of osteoporosis is vertebral fracture in those >50 years and distal radius fracture in those <50 years. The vertebral fracture commonly occurs in thoracic vertebrae below T_6 or in lumbar vertebrae. These fractures are usually asymptomatic and require a high index of suspicion to diagnose and can be confirmed on X-ray lateral view of thoracolumbar spine.

19. **Why is there a loss of teeth in patients with osteoporosis?**

Maxilla and mandible are composed predominantly of trabecular bone, which is metabolically more active, and its microarchitecture and remodeling are dependent upon gonadal steroids. In postmenopausal women, due to estrogen deficiency, there is an accelerated maxillary/mandibular bone resorption, eventually resulting in loss of teeth. Treatment with estrogen or bisphosphonates prevents loss of teeth.

20. **What is the barometer of osteoporosis?**

Hip fracture is considered as the barometer of osteoporosis for multiple reasons. It is associated with highest morbidity and mortality among all the fragility fractures. Almost all patients with hip fracture need hospital care, making it easier to estimate. Therefore, it is a reliable tool to gauge the incidence/prevalence of osteoporosis across different populations.

21. **How to diagnose osteoporosis?**

Osteoporosis is quantified by using bone mineral density derived T-score value compared to young Caucasian females. The table depicts the criteria to define osteoporosis based on T-score value.

Categories	T-score
Normal	T-score ≥ -1 SD
Osteopenia	T-score < -1 SD and > -2.5 SD
Osteoporosis	T-score ≤ -2.5 SD
Severe osteoporosis	T-score ≤ -2.5 SD in the presence of one or more fragility fractures

22. **How to calculate T-score?**

T-score is used to define osteoporosis and it estimates the difference between measured BMD of the patient and ideal peak BMD achieved in a young adult. Ideally, it should be based on normative data for that particular ethnicity and gender. T-score is calculated as follows:
T-score = (measured BMD—young adult mean BMD)/young adult BMD standard deviation (SD)

23. **How to calculate z-score?**

Z-score measures the difference between patient's measured BMD and bone mineral density in age-matched peer. Ideally, it should be based on normative data for that particular ethnicity and gender. Z-score <–2SD indicates low BMD in children and adolescents. However, osteoporosis in children and adolescents is defined as presence of low BMD and history of fracture. Although, it is not used for diagnosis of osteoporosis in adults, it provides a clue for the presence of secondary causes of decreased BMD. Z-score is calculated as follows:
Z-score = (measured BMD—age-matched BMD)/age-matched BMD standard deviation (SD)

24. **What are the limitations of T-score-based classification of osteoporosis?**

The T-score classification system has several limitations. T-score data has been derived from young Caucasian females and hence is not applicable to other ethnic groups, men, and children. T-score has been derived from dual-energy X-ray absorptiometry (DXA), hence should not be used when BMD is measured by other modalities. T-score is based on bone mineral density, which is not the only factor that determines the fracture risk.

25. **What are the modalities to assess bone mineral density?**

Modality	Principle	Site	Advantages	Disadvantages
Dual-energy X-ray absorptiometry (DXA)	X-ray tube produces two photon beams of different energy and the difference in attenuation of these beams help to quantify BMD	Hip Spine Distal radius	Most widely used Precise and accurate Used in FRAX tool Useful in monitoring response to therapy	Not portable Expensive Radiation exposure False results at site of fracture Measures areal BMD Observer dependent
Peripheral dual-energy X-ray absorptiometry	Same as DXA	Forearm Calcaneum	Good predictor of fracture risk Portable Inexpensive	Not validated for defining osteoporosis Imprecise Radiation exposure
Quantitative ultrasonography	Measures the transmission of ultrasound through limb bones or the reflectance of ultrasound waves from the bone surface	Calcaneum	Inexpensive Portable No radiation exposure	Not validated for defining osteoporosis
Quantitative computed tomography	Three-dimensional X-ray absorptiometry	Hip Spine	Measures volumetric BMD Allows differentiation between cortical and cancellous bone Better predictor of vertebral fracture risk than DXA	Expensive Very high radiation Exposure Not validated for defining osteoporosis

26. **What are precautions before performing a DXA scan?**

Detailed history regarding previous fracture should be enquired before subjecting a patient to DXA scan, as is to be avoided at fracture site. Pregnancy must be excluded prior to DXA scan. Calcium supplements should be avoided at least 48 h prior and bisphosphonates on the day of procedure. Scan should be postponed at least for 2 weeks if radiocontrast has been used previously. Repeat scan should be performed by the same operator at the same site, in the same position, and using the same system.

27. **A 40-year-old male presented with low backache for the last 2 years. On evaluation, he was found to have vertebral fracture with a T-score −2.5 and Z-score −3.5 at neck of femur. Should he be treated with antiresorptive/ anabolic therapy?**

    In males <50 years, T-score should not be used to define osteoporosis. However, a Z-score <−2 suggests low bone mineral density and requires evaluation for secondary causes of decreased BMD. In the index patient, a detailed evaluation revealed history of decreased shaving frequency, reduced libido, and erectile dysfunction. His bilateral testicular volume was 4 ml with serum testosterone of 4 nmol/L and low LH and FSH suggestive of hypogonadotropic hypogonadism. He was started on testosterone replacement along with vitamin D and calcium. Therefore, osteoporosis in a young patient requires evaluation and treatment of underlying cause, rather than antiresorptive/anabolic therapy.

28. **What are the causes of drug-induced osteoporosis?**

    Drugs are the most common cause of secondary osteoporosis. Glucocorticoids (parenteral/oral/ topical/ inhaled preparations), warfarin, heparin, anticonvulsants, cyclosporine, lithium, aromatase inhibitors, GnRH agonists, and overzealous treatment with thyroxine are associated with osteoporosis.

29. **What are the endocrine causes of secondary osteoporosis?**

    Cushing's syndrome, hyperparathyroidism, thyrotoxicosis, and hypogonadism are associated with osteoporosis and should actively be sought in young patients with osteoporosis.

30. **Why is estrogen essential for bone health?**

    Estrogen helps in accrual of peak bone mass, and maintains BMD in both genders. It has predominant effect on osteoclast and effectively reduces bone resorption. This effect is mediated through increased production of osteoprotegerin, inhibition of PTH-mediated RANKL–RANK interaction, and reduction of cytokine-mediated bone resorption (TNF-α, IL-1, and IL-6). In addition, estrogen increases bone formation by reducing osteoblast apoptosis and inhibiting sclerostin. Besides this, estrogen also increases renal 1-α hydroxylase activity and promotes local IGF1 generation. Therefore, in estrogen deficiency states, bone resorption is enhanced as a large number of basic multicellular units are recruited with consequent disparity between bone resorption and bone formation.

31. **How does glucocorticoid cause osteoporosis?**

    Glucocorticoids predominantly affect cancellous bone. It increases bone resorption by inducing osteoclastogenesis, promotes osteoblast and osteocyte apoptosis. In addition, it preferentially diverts primitive mesenchymal stem cells (which are destined to differentiate into osteoblasts) to adipocytes, decreases osteoprotegerin, reduces local IGF1 generation, disrupts cross-linking of bone collagen, and inhibits *Wnt* signaling pathway. Glucocorticoids also results in alterations in mineral homeostasis by inhibiting intestinal absorption of calcium and promoting renal loss of calcium.

32. **What are the biochemical investigations required in a patient with osteoporosis?**

Minimum investigations in a patient with osteoporosis include calcium, phosphorus, alkaline phosphatase, 25(OH)D, and creatinine. Further investigations depend upon history and physical findings and include iPTH, complete blood count, erythrocyte sedimentation rate, serum protein electrophoresis, IgA tissue transglutaminase, and thyroid function test to rule out secondary causes of osteoporosis. Estimation of serum FSH, LH, estrogen/testosterone, and prolactin is indicated in those with osteoporosis at a younger age.

33. **What are the markers of bone formation?**

Bone formation markers are the product of osteoblasts and include bone specific alkaline phosphatase, osteocalcin, carboxy-terminal propeptide of type 1 procollagen (P1CP), and amino-terminal propeptide of type 1 procollagen (P1NP). In addition, osteonectin and osteopontin also reflect osteoblast activity.

34. **What are the markers of bone resorption?**

Bone resorption markers are the degradation products of bone proteins (either collagen or non-collagen) or are osteoclast-specific enzymes. The markers of bone collagen are hydroxyproline, hydroxylysine, pyridinoline, deoxypyridinoline, carboxy-terminal cross-linked telopeptide of type 1 collagen (CTX), and amino-terminal cross-linked telopeptide of type 1 collagen (NTX). Bone sialoprotein is the degradation product of non-collagen bone protein. Osteoclast-specific enzyme includes tartrate-resistant acid phosphatase (TRAP).

35. **What is the utility of bone turnover markers?**

Bone turnover markers is a noninvasive modality to detect the status of bone remodeling. They are useful to predict fracture risk independent of bone mineral density. They are also helpful in monitoring treatment response, as alteration in bone turnover markers occurs much earlier than improvement in bone mineral density. Further, estimation of bone turnover markers also helps to understand the mechanism of action of new therapies for osteoporosis. The near complete suppression of both bone formation and bone resorption markers suggests the diagnosis of severe suppression of bone turn over, as seen with prolonged bisphosphonate therapy and adynamic bone disease.

36. **Who should be screened for osteoporosis?**

Screening for osteoporosis by estimation of BMD is recommended in individuals who have a high risk for fragility fracture. The indications as recommended by the National Osteoporosis Foundation are summarized in the table given below.

Indications for BMD measurement
All women ≥65 years or men ≥70 years
Younger postmenopausal women, perimenopausal women, and men age 50–69 with clinical risk factors for fracture
Adults with fracture after the age >50 years
Disorders and/or drugs associated with osteoporosis (rheumatoid arthritis, glucocorticoids in a daily dose ≥5 mg prednisone or equivalent for ≥3 months)

37. **What is the need for fracture prediction tool?**

The occurrence of fragility fracture is not solely dependent on decreased bone mineral density, but is rather a culmination of multiple risk factors. The important risk factors include advanced age, female sex, low body weight, past/family history of fracture, visual impairment, neuromuscular dysfunction, smoking, alcohol, and use of glucocorticoids. Hence, there is a need to devise a comprehensive tool to precisely predict the fracture risk in an individual. Various fracture prediction tools available are FRAX score, Nguyen algorithm, and Garvan fracture calculator.

38. **What is FRAX score?**

FRAX is a web-based algorithm designed to calculate the 10-year probability of a major osteoporosis-related fracture (hip, forearm, humerus, or spine), or hip fractures alone. FRAX score is applicable for both men and women. The risk factors used for fracture prediction were derived from meta-analysis of multiple studies. These risk factors include body weight, previous history of fracture, history of hip fracture in parents, current smoking, use of glucocorticoids (≥5 mg/day of prednisolone equivalent for ≥ 3 months), rheumatoid arthritis, alcohol use (≥3 units/day), and secondary osteoporosis (type 1 diabetes, osteogenesis imperfecta, hypogonadism, chronic malnutrition, and chronic liver disease). The intervention threshold is based upon economic cost-effectiveness analysis (10-year probability of major osteoporotic fracture ≥20% and hip fracture ≥3%).

39. **What are the advantages of FRAX score?**

FRAX score is an inexpensive, convenient, easy to use, and comprehensive tool to predict an individual's fracture risk. In addition, FRAX score also takes into account the effect of race and ethnicity for the assessment of fracture risk. Furthermore, it can be used in a primary healthcare setting as fracture risk can be calculated without estimation of bone mineral density.

40. **What are the limitations of FRAX score?**

FRAX tool was devised to create a definite fracture prediction model, but it has its own inherent flaws. The limitations with FRAX score are that it does not consider independent risk factors like number of falls, visual impairment, neuromuscular dysfunction, vitamin D deficiency, and physical inactivity. In addition, fracture risk cannot be assessed in individuals aged <40 or >90 years. Although glucocorticoid exposure (≥5 mg/day of prednisolone equivalent for ≥3 months) is considered a risk factor, there is no further subcategorization for doses higher than this. (i.e., a person taking 7.5 mg or 30 mg of prednisolone for >3 months are presumed to have a similar risk of fracture). FRAX score is validated only in drug-naive patients and is not useful for monitoring the therapeutic response.

41. **Which is the preferred calcium preparation in a patient with osteoporosis?**

Commonly available preparations include calcium carbonate and calcium citrate. Their properties are enlisted in the table given below.

Characteristics	Calcium carbonate	Calcium citrate
Elemental calcium	40%	20%
Absorption	Fair	Good
Requirement of acidic pH	Yes, hence given with meals	No, can be given any time
GI side effects	Yes	Minimal
Milk–alkali syndrome	May occur	Very rare
Colloidal liquid form	No	Yes
Cost	Inexpensive	Expensive

42. **What are the drugs available for the management of osteoporosis?**

The available drugs for the management of osteoporosis are enlisted in the table below.

Drugs	Target	Route of administration
Anabolic drugs		
$rPTH_{1-34}$ or $rPTH_{1-84}$	Osteoblast, *Wnt*/β-catenin	s.c.
Calcilytics	CaSR	p.o.
Romosozumab (Anti-sclerostin antibody)	Sclerostin (*Wnt*/β-catenin)	s.c.
Abaloparatide (rPTHrP1-34 analogue)	Osteoblast, *Wnt*/β-catenin	s.c.
Antiresorptive drugs		
Estrogen, SERM	Estrogen receptor on osteoclasts	p.o.
Bisphosphonates	Osteoclast	p.o./i.v.
Denosumab (Antibody against RANKL)	RANKL	s.c.
Odanacatib (Cathepsin K inhibitor)	Cathepsin K (collagen-degrading enzyme secreted from osteoclast)	p.o.
Saracatinib (c-Src inhibitor)	c-Src kinase (osteoclast-activating enzyme)	p.o.

43. **How do bisphosphonates act?**

Bisphosphonates (BPs) are pyrophosphate derivatives that bind to calcium hydroxyapatite at active bone remodeling sites to exert their antiresorptive effects. This effect is mediated by inhibition of crystal dissolution and suppression of bone resorption by blocking osteoclast action. Bisphosphonates are classified into non-nitrogen-containing BPs and nitrogen-containing BPs as given in the table below. Non-nitrogen-containing BPs are metabolically incorporated into non-hydrolyzable ATP analogues within osteoclasts, resulting in osteoclast apoptosis. Nitrogen-containing BPs inhibit mevalonate pathway by blocking farnesyl diphosphate synthase (FDPS), a key regulatory enzyme catalyzing the production of isoprenoid lipids. Inhibition of FDPS blocks the synthesis of farnesyl pyrophosphate (FPP) and geranylgeranyl pyrophosphate (GGPP), which in turn prevents prenylation of small GTPases, thereby disrupting cytoskeletal arrangement and vesical transport resulting in osteoclast apoptosis. Nitrogen-containing BPs, particularly zoledronate has been shown to have anti-apoptotic effects on osteoblasts via connexin43 and protein kinase activity. The mechanism of action of nitrogen-containing BPs is illustrated in the figure given below.

Class	Drugs	Action	Potency
Non-nitrogen-containing BPs	Etidronate Clodronate	Form cytotoxic intracellular ATP analogues resulting in osteoclast apoptosis	Weak
Nitrogen-containing BPs (amino-BPs)	Pamidronate Alendronate Risedronate Ibandronate Zoledronate	Inhibit mevalonate pathway which causes cytoskeletal abnormalities resulting in osteoclast apoptosis	Potent

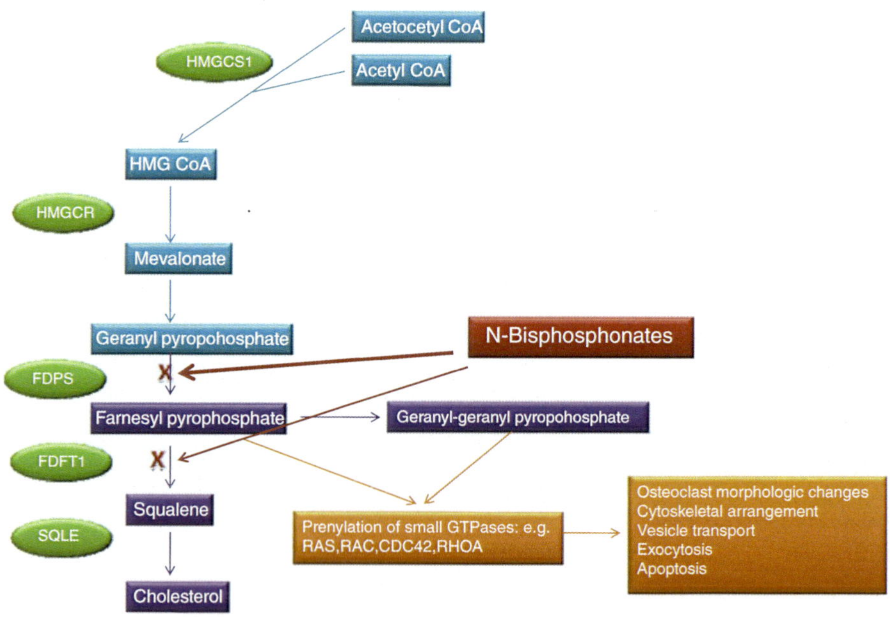

Fig. 15.2 Mechanism of action of bisphosphonates

44. **What are the precautions to be taken before administering bisphosphonates?**

Detailed history, examination, and appropriate investigations are necessary to rule out secondary causes of osteoporosis and also to establish a definite indication for bisphosphonate use. Vitamin D should be estimated and, if found deficient, should be supplemented. Renal function should be assessed and if eGFR is <30 ml/min, bisphosphonates should preferably be avoided. Oral cavity must be examined for periodontal diseases/caries and if present, should be treated before bisphosphonate therapy. Oral bisphosphonates should be avoided in those with upper gastrointestinal disease.

45. **Which is the preferred bisphosphonate for the management of osteoporosis?**

Zoledronate is the most potent bisphosphonate and is administered once in a year, making it convenient to patients in clinical practice. However, all newer generation bisphosphonates are equally effective in preventing both hip and spine fractures.

46. **What are the adverse events associated with bisphosphonate therapy?**

The adverse events associated with bisphosphonate use are listed in the table below.

Adverse effects	Remarks
Acute	
Flu-like syndrome	Accumulation of isopentenyl pyrophosphate that causes release of TNF-α
GI intolerance	Nausea, vomiting, diarrhea, esophagitis with oral bisphosphonates
Hypocalcemia	Concurrent vitamin D deficiency Severe bone disease
Hypophosphatemia	Occasional
Atrial fibrillation	More with zoledronate
Renal failure	Only with rapid infusion
Chronic	
Severe suppression of bone turnover related atypical fractures	Dose-dependent effect Impaired bone remodeling
Osteonecrosis of jaw	Dose-dependent effect Impaired bone remodeling More common in patients with malignancy and diabetes
Esophageal carcinoma	Rare, only with oral bisphosphonates

47. **How do bisphosphonates cause hypocalcemia and hypophosphatemia?**

Bisphosphonates inhibit osteoclasts, thereby suppressing bone resorption. This leads to reduced efflux of calcium from the bone, resulting in hypocalcemia. Serum PTH levels rise in response to hypocalcemia, leading to phosphaturia and consequently hypophosphatemia.

48. **What are the non-osteoporotic uses of bisphosphonates?**

Non-osteoporotic uses of bisphosphonates include hypercalcemia of any etiology, asymptomatic hyperparathyroidism, osteogenesis imperfecta, fibrous dysplasia, Paget's disease of bone, malignancy with osseous metastasis, and multiple myeloma.

49. **What is the effect of parathyroid hormone on bone?**

PTH is an important regulator of calcium homeostasis and bone remodeling and maintains bone mass and microarchitecture. It enhances the differentiation of pre-osteoblasts to mature osteoblast, increases the production of RANKL, and decreases osteoprotegerin leading to synchronized crosstalk between osteoblasts and osteoclasts. In addition, it increases bone mass by promoting the release of growth factors (e.g., IGF1, amphiregulin, and FGF2) and suppressing sclerostin, an inhibitor of the *Wnt* signaling pathway.

50. **What is the secretory pattern of PTH?**

In physiology, PTH is secreted in a pulsatile manner with a pulse frequency of 6–7 bursts per hour. The pulsatile secretion contributes to nearly 30% of circulating PTH, while 70% is by tonic (basal) secretion. Probably, the pulsatile secretion is helpful in maintaining bone mass (anabolic effect), while the basal secretion is responsible for bone remodeling (catabolic effect). In pathological states like primary hyperparathyroidism, pulse frequency remains unaltered, but pulse amplitude and tonic secretion are increased remarkably.

51. **Why is intermittent parathyroid hormone therapy beneficial in osteoporosis?**

Continuous exposure to high levels of PTH has an overwhelming effect on osteoblasts, leading to inappropriate production of RANKL, decreased osteoprotegerin, and excessive osteoclastogenesis, resulting in bone resorption. Intermittent exogenous administration of PTH mimics normal physiology and leads to decreased expression of sclerostin from osteocytes resulting in activation of *Wnt* pathway and consequently bone formation. In addition, intermittent PTH therapy also stimulates RUNX2 in osteoblasts, which is required for differentiation of pre-osteoblasts to osteoblasts. Factors determining the dual effects of PTH are not well elucidated.

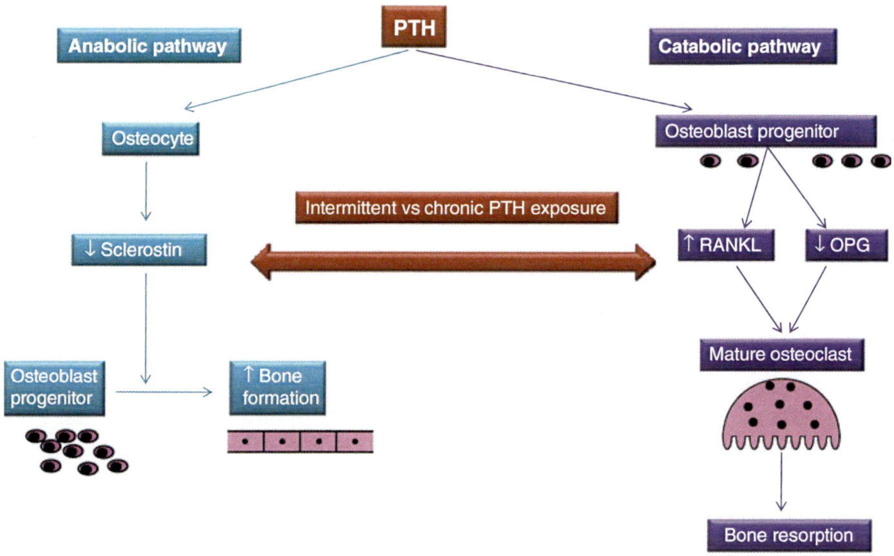

Fig. 15.3 Differential effects of PTH during continuous versus intermittent exposure

52. **What is the role of teriparatide in osteoporosis?**

    Recombinant PTH 1-34 (teriparatide) is a potent osteo-anabolic agent in the therapeutic armamentarium against osteoporosis. It is administered daily subcutaneously, preferably between 2000h and 2100h, to mimic the circadian rhythm. Teriparatide is administered at a dose of 20 μg per day for 18–24 months. It has also been shown to be effective when administered once weekly, at dose ranging from 28.2 to 56.5 μg in few studies. The adverse effects associated with teriparatide are transient hypercalcemia and allergic reactions. Discontinuation of treatment with teriparatide should be sequentially followed by use of bisphosphonates, to preserve the gain in BMD achieved with anabolic therapy.

53. **What are the differences between $rPTH_{1\text{-}34}$ and $rPTH_{1\text{-}84}$ in the treatment of osteoporosis?**

    $rPTH_{1\text{-}34}$ and $rPTH_{1\text{-}84}$ differ in many aspects including bioavailability, half-life, and side effects. The bioavailability of $rPTH_{1\text{-}34}$ and $rPTH_{1\text{-}84}$ is 95 and 55%, half-life is 75 and 150 min, and the dose recommended is 20 μg and 100 μg, respectively. In addition, the use of $rPTH_{1\text{-}84}$ is associated with higher levels of bone formation markers, as compared to $rPTH_{1\text{-}34}$. However, it does not translate into increased BMD. Recently, it has also been shown that there is a decrease in bone strength with the use of $rPTH_{1\text{-}84}$ as compared to $rPTH_{1\text{-}34}$, the significance of which requires further elucidation. Further, use of $rPTH_{1\text{-}84}$ is associated with hypercalcemia and hypercalciuria, which are rare with $rPTH_{1\text{-}34}$ possibly due to higher levels of PTH achieved for a longer duration with $rPTH_{1\text{-}84}$.

54. **What is anabolic window?**

Intermittent rPTH therapy is initially associated with overwhelming bone formation with minimal resorption, followed by activation of bone resorption (after 3 months); however, the bone formation still exceeds resorption. This period of increased bone formation, which usually lasts for 12–18 months after initiation of rPTH therapy, is called "anabolic window." During anabolic window, 30% of bone formation is due to bone modeling and the rest is by remodeling. It must be noted that in adults bone modeling is virtually absent otherwise, and the new bone formation exclusively depends upon bone remodeling. The differential effect of low-dose intermittent PTH (initially anabolic, later catabolic) is probably due to activation of *Wnt* signaling pathway during the initial period resulting in anabolic phase (direct effect as well as via inhibition of sclerostin), followed by inhibition of *Wnt* signaling pathway (via activation of Dickkopf-related protein) and activation of RANKL–RANK pathway on prolonged exposure, resulting in catabolic phase. This explains the rationale of use of rPTH for 18–24 months in the management of osteoporosis, as beyond this period bone formation as well as resorption markers decline, resulting in minimal/ no change in BMD.

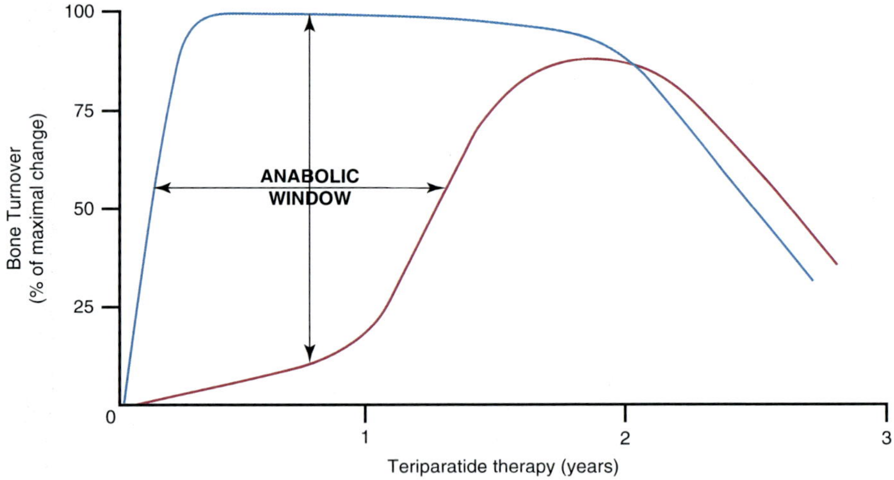

Fig. 15.4 Anabolic window during teriparatide therapy

55. **What is "expanded" anabolic window?**

Anabolic window can simply be defined as a period in which bone formation exceeds bone resorption. This concept is exploited in the management of osteoporosis by using teriparatide. This window period usually lasts for 12–18 months, as both bone formation and resorption decline after this period. Unfortunately, this anabolic window period cannot be extended further, possibly because of osteoblast senescence and/or PTH receptor downregulation due to prolonged use of teriparatide. However, the area under curve for this anabolic window can be "expanded" by the use of bisphosphonates along with teriparatide, thereby resulting in increased new bone formation due to suppression of bone resorption.

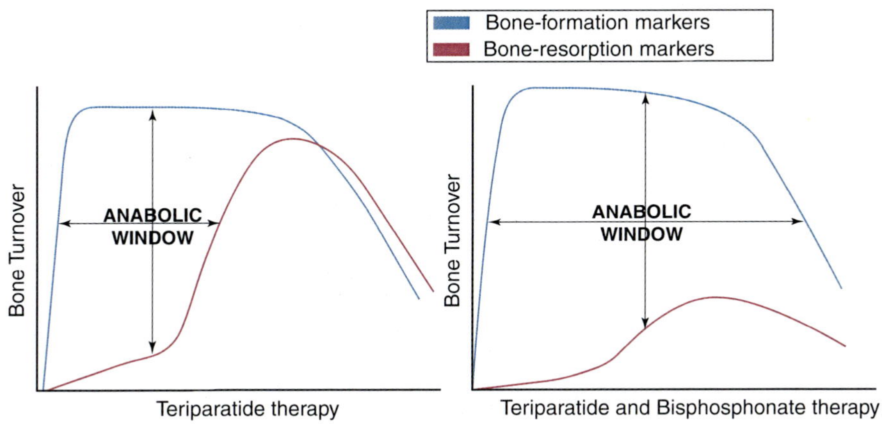

Fig. 15.5 "Expanded" anabolic window during combination therapy with teriparatide and bisphosphonate

56. **What is the role of combined use of bisphosphonate and teriparatide therapy?**

The combined use of bisphosphonate and teriparatide therapy seems attractive as they have complementary mechanism of actions in increasing BMD. The use of teriparatide is associated with an "anabolic window" and bisphosphonates lead to an "expanded anabolic window" by suppression of osteoclast activity. Some studies suggest a beneficial effect of combined therapy in patients with osteoporosis, while others do not support this notion. Therefore, the combined use of bisphosphonates and teriparatide is not routinely recommended.

57. **What are the differences between teriparatide and bisphosphonate in the management of osteoporosis?**

The differences between teriparatide and bisphosphonate in the management of osteoporosis are summarized in the table given below.

Parameters	Teriparatide	Bisphosphonates
Class	Anabolic	Antiresorptive
Lumbar BMD Femoral BMD	Increase by 9–13% Increase by 3–6%	Increase by 4.3–5.1% Increase by 3.1–3.5%
Effect on bone microarchitecture	Improves	Possibly no effect
Duration of therapy	18–24 months	5–7 years
Fracture outcome Vertebral Non-vertebral	65% reduction 53% reduction	70% reduction 25% reduction
Drug holiday	Not recommended	Recommended
Persistence of effects after discontinuation	No	Yes
Side effects	Hypercalcemia and hypercalciuria, rarely osteosarcoma	Atypical fractures Osteonecrosis of jaw Atrial fibrillation (zoledronate)

58. **What are the disorders in which recombinant PTH therapy is associated with worsening of bone disease?**

Recombinant PTH is an effective anabolic agent and is recommended in the management of osteoporosis. Its use is associated with significant increase in BMD and reduction in fracture risk. However, inadvertent use of rPTH can be detrimental especially in patients with hypophosphatemic osteomalacia and severe vitamin D deficiency, due to worsening of hypophosphatemia and consequent impaired bone mineralization.

59. **What are the indications of anti-osteoporotic therapy?**

NOF recommends pharmacotherapy for postmenopausal women and men >50 years if they have sustained a fragility fracture (irrespective of BMD/FRAX score), or T-score < −2.5. In addition, patients with osteopenia (T-score between −1 and −2.5) who have a 10-year probability of a hip fracture ≥ 3% or a 10-year probability of a major osteoporosis-related fracture ≥ 20% also merits therapy.

60. **A 72-year-old postmenopausal female was incidentally detected to have osteopenia (T-score −2.3) without any fragility fracture. However, her mother had history of hip fracture. Should she be treated?**

Patients with osteopenia have a higher risk of fracture as compared to those with normal BMD. Guidelines recommend estimation of 10 year probability of fracture risk in individuals with osteopenia. In the index case, FRAX score risk was 7.2% for hip fracture and 15% for major osteoporotic fracture; hence, she was started on bisphosphonates.

61. **A 65-year-old postmenopausal female was incidentally detected to have osteoporosis (T-score−2.7) without any fragility fracture. She had received yearly zoledronic acid for the past 3 years and did not have any fragility fracture. Should she be continued on treatment?**

The long-term use of bisphosphonates is associated with atypical fractures and osteonecrosis of jaw, due to severe suppression of bone turnover. In addition, bisphosphonates have a prolonged tissue half-life which exceeds more than 10 years. Further, use of bisphosphonates beyond 5 years is beneficial only in those with high risk of fracture. Hence, a patient with no new fragility fracture or low risk of fracture may be given a "drug holiday," after 3–5 years of their use. In the index case, as there was no history of fragility fracture, she was given a drug holiday. The patient who is given a drug holiday should be kept under regular surveillance for deterioration in bone mineral density and/or bone turnover markers every 1–2 years, if previously received alendronate and 2–3 years for zoledronic acid.

62. **How do antiresorptive agents cause severe suppression of bone turnover?**

The prolonged use of bisphosphonates may result in osteoclast apoptosis and complete cessation of crosstalk between osteoblasts and osteoclasts, leading to severe suppression of bone turnover (SSBT) and accumulation of microfractures, which clinically manifests as atypical fractures and osteonecrosis of jaw. The risk of SSBT is increased when bisphosphonates are used concurrently with estrogen or glucocorticoids. There is a theoretical risk of SSBT with denosumab, as it was demonstrated that osteoclasts were absent in bone biopsy specimens in 50% of patients who were treated with denosumab. On the contrary, newer class of antiresorptive drugs like odanacatib and saracatinib impair osteoclast function without exerting deleterious effect on osteoclast viability; hence, they are associated with minimal risk of SSBT.

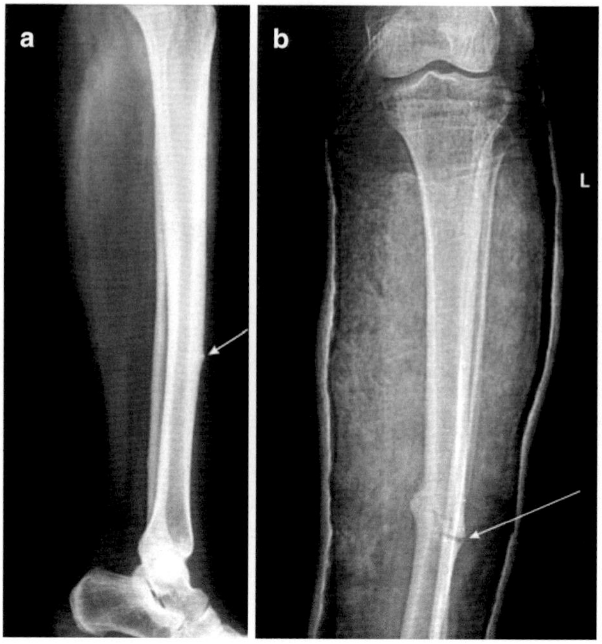

Fig. 15.6 (**a**, **b**) Plain radiograph of leg (**a**) showing anterior beaking of mid-diaphysis of the tibia (*arrow*) with subsequent development of fracture (**b**) on follow-up at the same site in a patient on bisphosphonate therapy

63. **When to suspect SSBT-related fracture?**

SSBT-related fracture should be suspected in a patient who is on long-term bisphosphonate therapy and complains of thigh or groin pain. This prodrome is present in 50% of patients before sustaining a fracture related to SSBT. The fracture sites are atypical as compared to osteoporotic fractures and include shaft of femur, pubic bone, and ischium; sites which are predominantly composed of cortical bone. The radiological hallmarks include thickened cortices and transverse orientation of fracture line. These fractures can be bilateral and may be preceded by beaking of cortex. Further, SSBT-related fractures have impaired healing and consequently lack callous formation. Histologically, decreased osteoblastic and osteoclastic surface with reduced/absent tetracycline labeling is classical of SSBT-related fracture. Treatment of SSBT-related fracture includes discontinuation of bisphosphonates and administration of teriparatide.

64. **What are the endocrine causes of delayed healing of fractures?**

Delayed healing of fracture despite adequate orthopedic management suggest the presence of underlying metabolic bone disease. This may be due to defective bone collagen (osteogenesis imperfecta) , impaired bone remodeling (primary hyperparathyroidism), and poor mineralization (osteomalacia).

65. **How to monitor a patient on pharmacotherapy for osteoporosis?**

Physical activity should be encouraged and compliance to treatment including adequate amount of calcium and vitamin D intake must be ensured. The clinical, biochemical, and radiological parameters to be monitored on follow-up are summarized in the table given below.

Parameters	**Remarks**
Clinical	
History	Fragility fracture
Height measurement annually	Height loss ≥ 2 cm, repeat X-ray spine
Radiological	
DXA	Every 1–2 yearly
Biochemical	
Bone turnover markers	Not routinely advised

DXA scan should be interpreted in context to change in baseline BMD. Stable or increase in bone mineral density should be considered as a beneficial response to treatment. A significant change in BMD should be greater than the least significant change (LSC) for that densitometer, which is usually 3–6% for hip BMD and 2–4% for spine BMD. During follow-up, increase in bone mineral content may be more foretelling of treatment response than change in BMD, as increase in bone mineral content occurs earlier than BMD.

66. **What should be done if there is no significant improvement in bone mineral density in a patient with osteoporosis on pharmacotherapy?**

The approach to a patient who has significant decrease in BMD on treatment for osteoporosis is described in the figure given below.

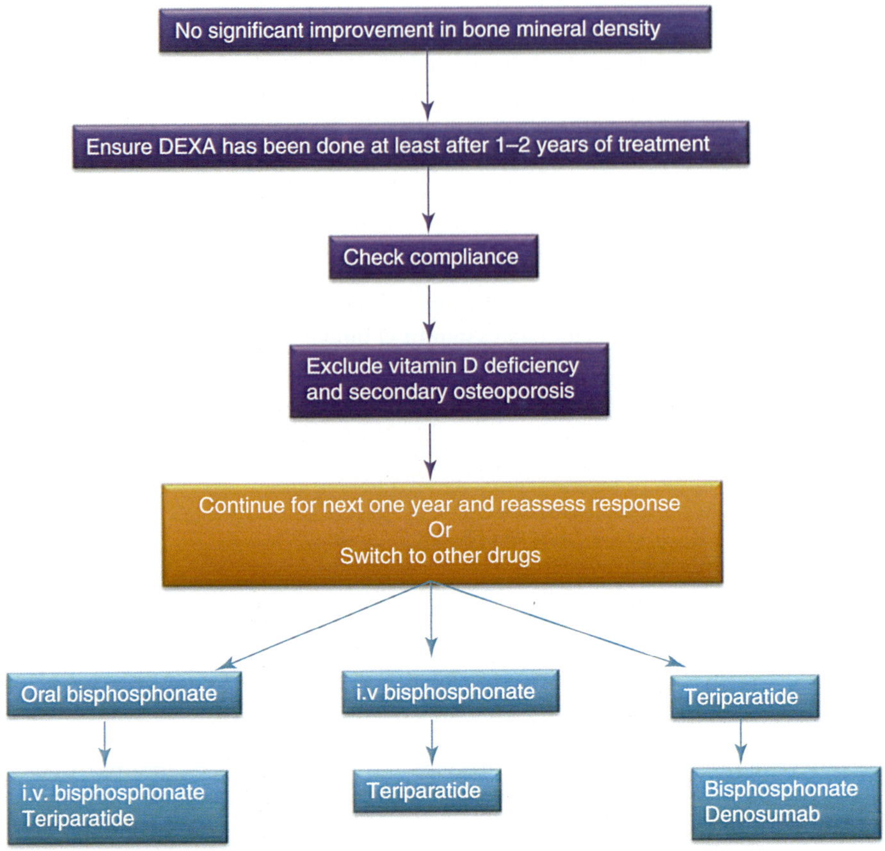

Fig. 15.7 Approach to a patient with worsening of BMD despite therapy

67. **What is the role of denosumab in the management of osteoporosis?**

Denosumab is a human monoclonal antibody that binds with RANKL, thereby preventing the interaction of RANKL with RANK, resulting in inhibition of osteoclastogenesis and osteoclast activation, and consequently reduced bone resorption. The dose recommended is 60 mg s.c. once in 6 months. It has been shown to increase BMD by 3–6.7% at lumbar spine and 1.9–3.6% at hip with relative risk reduction of hip and vertebral fracture by 40 and 68%, respectively. Hypocalcemia; dermatological manifestations like eczema, cellulitis, and erysipelas; and possibly increased risk of serious infections are the adverse events associated with denosumab. The unique features of denosumab as compared to bisphosphonates include subcutaneous administration at a frequency of 6 months, lack of gastrointestinal adverse events, safety in renal failure, and rapid reversibility of its action, because it is not accumulated into bone tissue. The quick reversibility of its effect can be a disadvantage if patient misses a dose. There are few reports of osteonecrosis of jaw and atypical fractures with the use of denosumab.

68. **What is the role of odanacatib in the management of osteoporosis?**

Cathepsin K is a lysosomal protease present in mature osteoclasts. It breaks down bone collagen, an event crucial for bone resorption. Odanacatib is a cathepsin K inhibitor and is an efficient antiresorptive agent. Unlike bisphosphonates and denosumab, odanacatib does not affect osteoclast survival; rather, it only inhibits osteoclast function. The advantages of odanacatib include oral route of administration and very low risk of SSBT-related atypical fracture. Nonspecific cathepsin inhibitors are associated with scleroderma-like skin thickening and rashes, which have not been reported with odanacatib, as cathepsin K is bone specific.

69. **What is anti-sclerostin antibody?**

The canonical *Wnt* signaling pathway is involved in new bone formation by binding of *Wnt* ligands to LRP5/6 and frizzled protein receptor on osteoblasts. Sclerostin, a protein secreted by osteocyte, binds with LRP5/6 on osteoblast and inhibits *Wnt* signaling pathway, thereby preventing new bone formation. Anti-sclerostin antibody (romosozumab) is an effective anabolic agent which promotes new bone formation by facilitating *Wnt* pathway. It is administered subcutaneously monthly or every 3 months and is associated with minimal adverse events, e.g., local site reactions.

70. **What is saracatinib?**

Saracatinib is a tyrosine Src kinase inhibitor and is an antiresorptive agent. Tyrosine Src kinase plays an important role in osteoclast activation and consequent bone resorption. Like odanacatib, it only impairs osteoclast function and does not lead to osteoclast apoptosis. Side effects include papular rash and loose stools. The drug is currently explored for osteosarcoma and in skeletal metastasis, rather than osteoporosis.

Suggested Reading

1. Compston J, Cooper A, Cooper C, Francis R, Kanis JA, Marsh D, McCloskey EV, Reid DM, Selby P, Wilkins M. Guidelines for the diagnosis and management of osteoporosis in postmenopausal women and men from the age of 50 years in the UK. Maturitas. 2009;62(2):105–8.
2. Jameson JL, De Groot LJ. Endocrinology: adult and pediatric. Philadelphia: Elsevier Health Sciences; 2010.
3. Longo D, Fauci A, Kasper D, Hauser S, Jameson J, Loscalzo J. Harrison's principles of internal medicine 18E EB. New York: McGraw Hill Professional; 2012.
4. Melmed S, Polonsky KS, Reed Larsen P, Kronenberg HM. Williams textbook of endocrinology: expert consult. London: Elsevier Health Sciences; 2011.
5. Rosen HN, Drezner MK. In: Post TW, editor. UpToDate. Waltham: UpToDate.

Type 1 Diabetes Mellitus

1

16.1 Clinical Rounds

1. **Why was nomenclature changed from insulin-dependent diabetes mellitus to type 1 diabetes mellitus?**

   The earlier classification of diabetes by the National Diabetes Data Group (NDDG, 1979) was based on pharmacotherapy and categorized diabetes into two major subgroups, namely, insulin-dependent diabetes mellitus (IDDM) and non-insulin-dependent diabetes mellitus (NIDDM). However, with advancing duration of diabetes, majority of patients with NIDDM also require insulin for good glycemic control making the classification redundant. Thereafter, ADA proposed a new classification of diabetes in 1997 based on its aetiopathogenesis; nomenclature of IDDM was renamed to type 1 diabetes (immuno-inflammatory destruction of β-cell leading to absolute insulin deficiency) and NIDDM to type 2 diabetes (non-immune-mediated decline in β-cell function leading to relative insulin deficiency with insulin resistance).

Year	**1979**	**1997**
Proposed by	NDDG	ADA
Subtypes of diabetes	IDDM NIDDM GDM MRDM Other types	Type 1 diabetes (T1DM) Type 2 diabetes (T2DM) Other specific types GDM
Prediabetes	IGT	IFG, IGT

IDDM insulin-dependent diabetes mellitus, *NIDDM* non-insulin-dependent diabetes mellitus, *MRDM malnutrition*-related diabetes mellitus, *GDM* gestational diabetes mellitus

2. **What is type 1.5 diabetes?**

   Type 1.5 diabetes is a synonym for latent autoimmune diabetes in adults (LADA) and is also known as slowly progressive T1DM or "smoldering" T1DM. These

A. Bhansali, Y. Gogate, *Clinical Rounds in Endocrinology: Volume I - Adult Endocrinology*, DOI 10.1007/978-81-322-2398-6_16

patients have clinical phenotype of T1DM but lack ketosis/ketoacidosis at presentation, despite evidence of islet autoimmunity. This occurs because of slow progression of immuno-inflammatory destruction of β-cells. Patients with LADA are usually <35 years of age, insulin independent for at least initial 6 months after the diagnosis, and have at least one of the autoantibodies (islet-cell autoantibody and autoantibodies to GAD-65, IA-2, insulin, and zinc transporter 8). They are predisposed for other autoimmune disorders and may have familial clustering of diabetes. Insulin is the treatment of choice in patients with LADA, and sulfonylureas should be avoided as they may augment the ongoing immuno-inflammatory destruction of β-cell by stimulating insulin secretion. The important differences between T1DM and LADA are summarized in the table below.

Parameters	T1DM	LADA
Age of onset	Childhood	Young adults
Presentation with DKA	Common	Unusual
Islet autoimmunity	Multiple autoantibodies	Single autoantibody Most common GAD65
Treatment	Insulin dependence since diagnosis	Insulin independence for at least initial 6 months

3. **What is type 1b diabetes?**

Type 1b diabetes, also called as fulminant type 1 diabetes, is commonly seen in Japanese population and is characterized by acute onset severe hyperglycemia, ketosis/ketoacidosis, near-normal glycated hemoglobin (suggest short duration of disease), predisposition in those with HLA-DR-DQ4, and negative islet autoimmunity (non-autoimmune disorder). It usually occurs in patients >20 years of age. Flu-like symptoms at onset are not uncommon. The following criteria have been proposed for the diagnosis of fulminant type 1 diabetes

- Ketosis or ketoacidosis within a week after onset of hyperglycemic symptoms
- Plasma glucose level ≥288 mg/dl and HbA1c<8.5% at first visit
- Fasting plasma C-peptide <0.3 ng/ml and glucagon-stimulated C-peptide <0.5 ng/ml at onset

Pancreatic histopathology demonstrates subclinical pancreatitis but not insulitis in these patients. Viral infections, particularly enterovirus and herpes virus in an HLA-predisposed individual have been implicated in the pathogenesis of fulminant type 1 diabetes. Treatment includes intravenous saline and insulin during ketoacidosis followed by basal-bolus insulin after recovery from ketoacidosis.

4. **Can a child with hyperglycemia at the age of 4 months have T1DM?**

No. T1DM does not occur prior to the age of 6 months as the immune system (T-regulatory cells) is immature to trigger an immune response till this age. In addition, the infants are exclusively breast-fed till the age of 6 months, which minimizes the exposure to environmental antigens. Therefore, occurrence of diabetes before the age of 6 months suggests the possibility of neonatal diabetes.

5. **What is neonatal diabetes?**

The onset of diabetes mellitus before 6 months of age is termed as neonatal diabetes (NDM). Clinically, there are three forms of NDM: transient NDM, permanent NDM, and syndromic NDM. Approximately 50% of neonatal diabetes is transient. These patients typically present within first few days to weeks of life, and the disease commonly remits by 12 weeks of age. However, 50% of these patients may have a relapse of disease during adolescence or young adulthood. Persistence of diabetes beyond 6 months of life suggests permanent NDM. The most common cause of permanent NDM includes activating mutations in KCNJ11 gene (encode Kir6.2), followed by ABCC8 gene (encode SUR1). Kir6.2 and SUR1 are two subunits of K_{ATP} channel in the pancreatic β-cell. In addition, mutations in insulin and glucokinase gene may also result in permanent NDM. Syndromic NDM is permanent and is associated with IPEX syndrome, Wolcott–Rallison syndrome, Wolfram syndrome, and syndromes associated with mutations in genes PDX/IPF1, PTF1A, GLIS3, NEUROD1, and HNF1B. Sulfonylureas are the drug of choice for NDM associated with KCNJ11 and ABCC8 gene mutations, while insulin is required for the management of other forms of NDM.

6. **What is Flatbush diabetes?**

Flatbush diabetes was described in African-American obese adults who presented with osmotic symptoms and diabetic ketosis/ketoacidosis similar to T1DM, but the subsequent course was akin to T2DM. This has been described in other ethnic groups and is now referred to as ketosis-prone diabetes (KPD). Patients with KPD differs from T1DM in that they are obese, have strong family history of T2DM, and lack evidence of islet autoimmunity. The mechanism of ketosis-prone diabetes remains elusive. However, glucotoxicity has been proposed as a possible mechanism for rapid decline in β-cell function, which improves after treatment with insulin.

7. **Do all patients with ketosis-prone diabetes maintain glycemic control on oral hypoglycemic drugs after an episode of diabetic ketoacidosis?**

No. About 50% of patients with ketosis-prone diabetes (KPD) can maintain glycemic control on oral hypoglycemic drugs. Initially, all patients with KPD should be treated with insulin. Basal and stimulated C-peptide level and markers of islet autoimmunity should be assessed after resolution of DKA. Based on the Aβ classification {the presence or absence of autoimmunity (A) and/or β-cell function (β)}, nature of long-term therapy can be determined in patients with KPD.

Category of KPD	Prevalence (%)
A−β+	50
A−β−	22
A+β−	17
A+β+	11

Those with lean phenotype, islet autoimmune positivity, and undetectable C-peptide (A+ β−) should be continued on insulin, and those with obese phenotype, negative islet autoimmunity, and preserved β-cell function(A−β+) are the best responders to OHAs. Nevertheless, majority (50%) of patients with KPD are A−β+, which suggests preserved β-cell function and subsequent insulin independence.

8. **What are the environmental factors that predispose to T1DM?**

   The environmental factors that predispose to type 1 diabetes include viral infections (congenital rubella, coxsackie virus, and mumps), dietary factors (bovine milk and gliadin), and toxins (nitrates). Coxsackie virus (enterovirus) inclusion bodies were demonstrated in the islets of patient with T1DM who died of DKA, suggesting the etiological role of Coxsackie virus in T1DM. Coxsackie virus specifically affects β-cells in genetically predisposed individuals, and consequently results in insulitis. Molecular mimicry has been proposed as the mechanism for virus-mediated insulitis due to structural similarity between 2C protein of coxsackie virus and β-cell GAD65 antigen. Other viruses that have been implicated in causation of T1DM include mumps, rubella, rotavirus, and cytomegalovirus. However, childhood vaccination against these viral infections does not predispose to T1DM. Bovine milk consists of beta-casein and ABBOS (17-Amino-Acid Bovine Serum Albumin Peptide) and these antigens have been implicated for islet autoimmunity. ABBOS has structural similarity with GAD65 (molecular mimicry) and beta-casein acts as a hapten. However, recent studies refute the association between cow's milk and T1DM. Breast feeding and supplementation with vitamin D and ω-3 fatty acids have been shown to be protective against T1DM.

9. **What are the non-HLA genes associated with type 1a diabetes?**

   The most important loci determining the risk of T1DM are within the major histocompatibility complex on chromosome 6p21, in particular HLA class II molecules (DR3-DQ2 or DR4-DQ8). But certain non-HLA genes associated with type 1a diabetes are autoimmune regulator gene (AIRE) on chromosome 21, gene encoding fork head box P3 (FOXP3) leading to IPEX syndrome, insulin gene, PTPN22 gene encoding a lymphoid-specific phosphatase, and cytotoxic T-lymphocyte-associated protein 4 gene (CTLA-4). Most of these genes are involved in T-cell lymphocyte function and signaling. AIRE and FOXP3 gene-mediated insulitis are the cause of monogenic type 1 diabetes.

10. **Why is there an increase in incidence of T1DM?**

The incidence of T1DM is increasing by 2–5% per year worldwide, especially in children <5 years of age. This may be partially attributed to increase in personal hygiene ("hygiene hypothesis") and rising incidence of obesity ("accelerator hypothesis"). According to hygiene hypothesis, improvement in living conditions in modern society result in lack of exposure to pathogens early in life, leading to inadequate maturation of immune system and thereby increased predisposition to autoimmune disorders, including T1DM. Accelerator hypothesis proposes that there is an enhanced immuno-inflammatory destruction of β-cells in response to increased insulin resistance associated with obesity.

11. **What are the HLA loci protective for T1DM?**

The HLA loci DRB1*1501, DQA1*0102, DQ6, and DRB1*1401 are protective for T1DM. However, the presence of these loci may not confer protection in all, as 3% of patients with T1DM have these haplotypes.

12. **Does obesity predispose to T1DM?**

Possibly yes. The adiposity increases the risk of developing type 1 diabetes because insulin resistance and adipocytokines (IL6 and TNFα) accelerate the immuno-inflammatory destruction of β-cells. Insulin resistance leads to increased β-cell antigen expression mediated through rising glucose and free fatty acids levels, thereby augmenting insulitis. In addition, adipocytokines released from adipocytes act as fuel to the fire in patients with obesity. Therefore, obese children who are genetically predisposed for type 1 diabetes have a faster destruction of β-cells. This combination of type 1 diabetes with insulin resistance is also called as "double diabetes."

13. **What are the animal models of T1DM?**

Animal models of T1DM can be spontaneous or induced. The spontaneous models include Nonobese diabetic (NOD) mouse, BioBreeding (BB) rat, and Long–Evans Tokushima Lean (LETL) rat, while the induced models include streptozotocin- or alloxan-induced diabetic Wistar rat. The NOD mouse and BB rat have HLA predisposition and spontaneously develop diabetes; therefore, they are ideal for studying the pathogenesis of T1DM. Both these models are characteristically associated with T-cell lymphopenia. LETL rat is also a spontaneous model of T1DM with histologic evidence of insulitis, but without T-cell lymphopenia. The Wistar rat is commonly used for induction of T1DM, and the agents employed are streptozotocin or alloxan. Both these agents cause selective destruction of β-cells because they enter β-cells through GLUT2. Streptozotocin is administered intraperitoneally at a dose of 50–100 mg/kg, and it causes cell damage by karryorrhexis, while alloxan leads to free radical-mediated β-cell damage.

14. **What is "pseudoatrophic" islet?**

Normal pancreas weighs about 100–150 g and consists of one million islets that contribute 2% of its weight. β-cells are uniformly distributed throughout the pancreas, while the α-cells are predominantly present in body and tail of the pancreas. In patients with T1DM, there is selective destruction of β-cells by the immuno-inflammatory cells, while α-cells remain intact. In patients with long-standing T1DM, β-cells and the infiltrates eventually disappear, leaving behind the clumps of islet containing α-cells, which are termed as "pseudo-atrophic" islet.

15. **What are the distinctive features of T1DM?**

The distinctive features of T1DM are young age of onset, absolute insulin deficiency, and presence of islet autoimmunity. T1DM has tri-modal presentation with the first peak at 3–6 years, second at peripubertal age, and finally at 35–40 years of age. Absolute insulin deficiency manifest as sarcopenia, ketosis/ keto-acidosis and the need for insulin for glycemic control since diagnosis.

16. **Do all patients with T1DM have ketosis/ketoacidosis at presentation?**

The most common presenting manifestation in patients with T1DM is osmotic symptoms in the form of polyuria, polydipsia, and weight loss despite increased appetite. Only 25–67% of children with type T1DM present with ketosis/ ketoacidosis. Destruction of 90% of β-cells is required to manifest as diabetic ketoacidosis (DKA). The absence of DKA at presentation in (17–30%) approximately 1/3rd to 2/3rd of patients is due to early detection of disease (presence of residual β-cell function) and variability in the rate of destruction of β-cells.

17. **What are the autoimmune disorders associated with T1DM?**

The common autoimmune disorders associated with T1DM are autoimmune thyroid disease (17–30%) and celiac disease (1–16%). Hence, screening with TSH, anti-TPO, and anti-tissue transglutaminase (IgA-tTG) should be done at diagnosis in all patients with T1DM. If the screening tests are negative, retesting should be done periodically at intervals of 1–2 years. Other associated autoimmune diseases are pernicious anemia (2.6%) and Addison's disease (0.5%).

18. **What is GAD65?**

Glutamic acid decarboxylase (GAD) is an enzyme that catalyzes the decarboxylation of glutamate to gamma-aminobutyric acid (GABA). GAD exists in two isoforms: GAD65, which is expressed in pancreas, and GAD67, in central nervous system. In the pancreas, GAD65 is selectively expressed in β-cells and mediates the synthesis of GABA which has been shown to inhibit insulin and glucagon release in a paracrine manner. However, the exact significance of GAD65/GABA in islet physiology is unclear.

19. **Are all patients with T1DM anti-GAD65 antibody positive?**

No. Age at onset of diabetes and duration of disease determines the presence or absence of a particular autoantibody in a patient with T1DM. The autoantibodies of importance in T1DM include anti-GAD65 antibody, islet-cell autoantibody (ICA), insulinoma-associated antigen 2 (IA-2) antibody, anti-insulin antibody (IAA), and anti-zinc transporter antibody (ZnT8). One or more of these autoantibodies are present in >95% of patients with newly diagnosed T1DM, and presence of two or more autoantibodies have a high predictive value for the diagnosis of T1DM. The characteristics of islet antibodies are summarized in the table given below.

	Age at diagnosis		**Duration of disease**	
Antibody	<15 years (%)	>15 years (%)	At diagnosis (%)	At 10 years (%)
ICA	80–85	60–80	85	10
Anti-GAD65	60	70–80	80	50
IA-2	70–80	40–60	80	50
IAA	30–65	20–35	–	–
ZnT8	–	–	60–80	–

In those with onset of T1DM in childhood, ICA and IA-2 are the most prevalent autoantibodies, while anti-GAD65 antibody is the most common antibody in adolescents and adults. The prevalence of autoantibody positivity progressively declines with advancing duration of disease. However, anti-GAD65 antibody is positive in 50% of patients even 10 years after the onset of disease.

20. **What is the role of C-peptide in the diagnosis of diabetes?**

C-peptide is a 31 amino-acid peptide that connects A and B chains of insulin in the proinsulin molecule. In clinical practice, it is not uncommon to encounter difficulties in categorizing the patients into T1DM or T2DM, especially in those with young onset of disease. In this scenario, assessment of endogenous β-cell reserve may help in differentiating the two. C-peptide is cosecreted with insulin and is a marker of β-cell function. The advantages of estimation of C-peptide over insulin include its longer half-life (30 min vs. 4 min), negligible hepatic extraction, and usefulness even in patients on exogenous insulin therapy. C-peptide should be measured only after optimizing blood glucose profile to avoid the effect of glucotoxicity on β-cells. Fasting C-peptide level ≥0.6 ng/ml and glucagon-stimulated C-peptide ≥0.96 ng/ml suggest optimal endogenous β-cell reserve.

21. **Can C-peptide measurement replace islet autoimmune markers for differentiating type 1 from type 2 diabetes?**

No. C-peptide is a marker of β-cell function and cannot replace islet autoimmune markers. However, estimation of C-peptide can be complementary in differentiating between T1DM and T2DM, along with autoantibodies. The limitations with C-peptide estimation include less validated cutoffs for defining β-cell reserve and poor diagnostic value in the presence of renal insufficiency. In addition, estimation of C-peptide has low discriminatory value in predicting the development of T1DM in high-risk individuals.

22. **A couple with T1DM plans to have a child and is worried about the risk of T1DM in the progeny. How to counsel?**

    Majority (>85%) of patients with T1DM lack family history of T1DM. The risk of developing T1DM in the offspring is 10%, if both parents have T1DM. However, in case of a single parent having T1DM, the risk to offspring is higher if father (4.6%) has T1DM as compared to mother (2%). The risk of developing T1DM in a sibling with a dizygotic twin is 6%, while the risk becomes 8-fold higher (50%) in monozygotic twins. In the present case scenario, parents can be counseled that the probability of not having T1DM in the offspring is 90%.

23. **What are the predictors for the development of T1DM in high-risk individuals?**

    The aim of prediction is to identify individuals who are at high-risk for development of T1DM among first-degree relatives of patients with T1DM, to prevent progression of immune-mediated destruction of β-cells. The predictors for development of T1DM in these high-risk individuals include presence of islet autoantibodies, HLA haplotype, and loss of first-phase insulin response (FPIR) to glucose during an intravenous glucose tolerance test. The usual strategy is to initially screen for anti-GAD65 antibody and either IAA or IA-2 antibody. IAA should be preferred in children <10 years of age. If both these autoantibodies are positive, the risk for developing T1DM is 70% at 10 years and 84% at 15 years. If only one autoantibody is positive, testing for other autoantibodies (ZnT8 and ICA) associated with T1DM is suggested. In individuals who have positivity for two auto-antibodies, HLA typing and intravenous glucose tolerance test should be performed. However, at present routine screening for T1DM is not recommended in high-risk individuals due to lack of familial clustering, variability in latent period for development of hyperglycemia, poor standardization of the available assays for autoantibodies and ineffective preventive strategies.

24. **What are the strategies to prevent T1DM?**

    Various strategies which have been tried for the prevention of T1DM are summarized in the table given below.

Prevention	Candidates	Measures
Primary	Family history of T1DM HLA predisposition	Docosahexaenoic acid Vitamin D Gluten-free diet

Prevention	Candidates	Measures
Secondary	Multiple autoantibody positivity	Parenteral and oral insulin Nicotinamide Cyclosporine Vitamin E
Tertiary	Recent-onset T1DM	Intensive insulin therapy Rituximab Azathioprine Anti-thymocyte globulin CD3 monoclonal antibody GAD65 with alum Mesenchymal stem cells

However, most of these intervention strategies have yielded futile results.

25. **What are the causes of anemia in patients with T1DM?**

    The presence of anemia in patients with T1DM should raise a suspicion of celiac disease, hypothyroidism, and pernicious anemia. In addition, diabetes-related complications like diabetic kidney disease, gastroparesis, and blind-loop syndrome can also contribute to anemia.

26. **What are the causes of diarrhea in patients with T1DM?**

    The causes of diarrhea in patients with T1DM include celiac disease, autonomic neuropathy, Graves' disease, Addison's disease, and rarely IPEX syndrome (immunodysregulation, polyendocrinopathy, enteropathy, X-linked).

27. **How did Diabetes Control and Complication Trial change the management of T1DM?**

    Diabetes Control and Complication Trial (DCCT) was a landmark study involving 1,441 patients with T1DM who were randomized to receive either intensive or conventional insulin therapy, and followed up for 6.5 years. DCCT demonstrated that intensive glycemic control using multiple subcutaneous injections or continuous subcutaneous insulin infusion (with an average HbA1c 7.2%) led to prevention as well as delayed the progression of microvascular complications, as compared to those who received conventional treatment (with an average HbA1c 9%). The follow-up of DCCT cohort, i.e., the Epidemiology of Diabetes Interventions and Complications (EDIC) study, demonstrated the beneficial effect of initial good glycemic control on future development of cardiovascular complications. Hence, intensive glycemic control with use of multiple subcutaneous injections/CSII should be initiated at diagnosis of T1DM to achieve target HbA1c and to prevent long-term micro- and macrovascular complications.

28. **What is metabolic memory?**

A period of early intensive glycemic control in patients with diabetes prevents the development of micro- and macrovascular complications in the long run, despite discontinuation of intensive therapy later on. The long-term beneficial effect of intensive glycemic control early in the course of disease is termed as good "metabolic memory" or "legacy effect." This was first demonstrated in the EDIC study and later in the follow-up cohort of UKPDS. The legacy effect is attributed to decreased oxidative stress, reduction in advanced glycated end products, and epigenetic changes (DNA methylation/histone acetylation) associated with reduction in gluco-lipotoxicity.

29. **What is "glucose hypothesis"?**

Glucose hypothesis states that chronic and persistent hyperglycemia results in micro- and macrovascular complications and intensive glycemic control prevents the onset/delay the progression of these complications. The convincing evidence for "glucose hypothesis" was provided by the DCCT in patients with T1DM and UKPDS in patients with T2DM.

30. **What are the criteria for diagnosis of diabetes in children?**

The diagnostic criteria for diabetes in children are same as in adults. However, the dose of glucose for performing OGTT is 1.75 g/kg of anhydrous glucose, but not exceeding 75 g. Further, HbA1c is a poor tool for the diagnosis of T1DM, as the rapidity of rise in blood glucose does not commensurate with glycation of hemoglobin. Nevertheless, HbA1c cutoff is the same in children as in adults.

31. **What are the treatment targets in patients with T1DM?**

The treatment targets in children and adolescents with T1DM are less stringent as compared to adults with T1DM. This is because of higher susceptibility to hypoglycemia in children due to unpredictable food intake and physical activity. The recommended HbA1c in children and adolescents (<18 years) with T1DM is <7.5%, while in adults it is <7%. However, the targets should be individualized based on patient's circumstances.

32. **What are the treatment modalities available for T1DM?**

The available treatment modalities for T1DM are summarized in the table given below.

Modality	Remarks
Basal-bolus insulin therapy	Most commonly practiced High glycemic variability as compared to CSII
Insulin pumps (CSII)	Expensive Risk of DKA in the event of mechanical failure

Modality	Remarks
DPP4 inhibitors, GLP-1 agonists (in addition to insulin)	Experimental Reduces glycemic variability and/or improves hypoglycemic unawareness
SGLT2 inhibitors (in addition to insulin)	Experimental No risk of hypoglycemia Action is insulin-independent Increased risk of urogenital infections
Pancreatic islet transplantation	Potentially curative therapy Insulin-independence progressively declines Risks associated with immunosuppressive therapy Limited availability of pancreatic islets Expensive
Immunomodulatory therapy	Serious adverse events Poor efficacy

33. **What are the disadvantages of regular insulin?**

In normal individuals, the first phase of insulin secretion starts immediately after food intake and lasts for 10–15 min and is due to release of preformed insulin granules. This is followed by second phase of insulin secretion which lasts for 90–120 min and is due to biosynthesis of insulin. The first phase of insulin secretion is responsible for suppression of hepatic glucose output, while the second phase regulates the entry of glucose into insulin-dependent target sites including muscle and adipocytes. On the contrary, regular insulin has onset of action in 30–60 min, exerts its peak effect at 2–4 h and its action lasts for 6–8 h. The delayed onset of action of regular insulin mandates its administration at least 30 min prior to meal, and the delay in peak effect results in early postprandial hyperglycemia. In addition, the prolonged duration of action of regular insulin results in late postprandial hypoglycemia, leading to inter-prandial snacking. Further, regular insulin has marked intra- and interindividual variations in absorption (up to 20–50%), thereby resulting in increased risk of hypo- or hyperglycemia, even with the same dose.

34. **What are the advantages with short-acting insulin analogues?**

Short-acting insulin analogues have an onset of action within 15 min and exert its peak effect at 1 h, and the action lasts for 3–4 h. Because of its rapid onset of action, it is convenient for the patient to administer insulin immediately before a meal, or sometimes immediately after a meal. This may be especially useful in children, elderly, and in patients with gastroparesis. The early peak effect results in better postprandial glycemic control, and short duration of action prevents the risk of late postprandial hypoglycemia. However, shorter duration of action can lead to late postprandial hyperglycemia. Despite these advantages of short-acting insulin analogues, the reduction in HbA1c is similar to that achieved with regular insulin.

35. **What are the demerits of Neutral Protamine Hagedorn insulin?**

Neutral Protamine Hagedorn (NPH) insulin is a crystalline suspension of insulin with protamine and zinc and is the oldest basal insulin available. The action of NPH starts within 1–3 h, peaks at 6–8 h, and lasts for 12–16 h. As the action of NPH lasts only for 12–16 h, it has to be administered twice daily in majority of patients. Further, the plasma level of NPH shows peak and trough, thereby leading to increased risk of hypo- and hyperglycemia, respectively. In addition, NPH shows marked intra- and interindividual variations in absorption (up to 30–50%), leading to wide swings in blood glucose levels.

36. **What are the advantages of newer long-acting insulin analogues?**

Newer long-acting insulin analogues include glargine, detemir, and degludec. These are peakless insulins with duration of action of approximately 18–36 h, have less intra- and interindividual variability in absorption and decreased risk of nocturnal hypoglycemia.

Parameter	Detemir	Glargine	Degludec
No of amino acid	50	53	50
Fatty acid chain	Present (myristic acid)	No	Present (hexadecanedioic acid)
pH	Neutral	Acidic	Neutral
Mechanism of prolonged duration of action	Binding to albumin in circulation	Precipitation at neutral pH in subcutaneous tissue	Multihexamer chain formation in subcutaneous tissue
Onset of action	1 h	1 h	1–1.5 h
Peak effect	3–9 h	No peak	No peak
Duration	6–23 h	11–24 h	40 h
Intra-/interindividual variation	Low	High	Lowest
Nocturnal hypoglycemia	Low	Low	Lowest
Binding affinity to IGF-1 receptor (as compared to regular insulin)	18-fold	641-fold	2-fold
Miscibility with short-acting analogue	No	No	Yes
Miscibility with GLP-1 receptor agonists	No	Yes	Yes

37. **What are the peculiarities of newer long-acting basal insulins?**

Insulin detemir is weight neutral as compared to other insulins, and this effect is possibly mediated by a direct effect on satiety center. In addition, detemir is more hepato-selective in its action because of greater availability of albumin-bound detemir to liver as compared to peripheral tissues, thereby resulting in reduced lipogenesis. Majority of patients require twice daily injection of detemir as its duration of action varies from 6 to 23 h.

Insulin glargine is the only insulin which has acidic pH. Its long duration of action allows once daily dosing in majority of patients. However, there is a concern for mitogenic potential due to its high affinity for IGF-1 receptors, although this has been refuted.

Insulin degludec offers an advantage of flexibility in dose schedule and can be administered between 8 and 36 h. In addition, as it is a truly peakless insulin, it is associated with the lowest incidence of nocturnal hypoglycemia among the basal insulins. Administration of degludec results in very high plasma insulin levels, and degludec has been shown to be associated with higher incidence of cardiovascular events.

38. **Why is fixed-dose premixed insulin not preferred in patients with T1DM?**

Premixed insulin consists of short-acting and intermediate-acting insulin in a fixed ratio, in order to provide prandial and basal insulin together to minimize the number of injections, thereby making it convenient to the patient. Patients with T1DM have absolute insulin deficiency, and administration of premixed insulin twice a day can never mimic the normal physiology. Further, it does not provide adequate post-lunch or pre-dinner insulin coverage. Therefore, it is difficult to achieve glycemic targets with the use of fixed-dose premixed insulin. The other limitation of fixed-dose premixed insulin include the inability to adjust the dose of regular and NPH insulins independently due to fixed formulation. Therefore, multiple subcutaneous injections (basal-bolus) is the ideal insulin regimen for the management of patients with T1DM. This was evidenced in DCCT, where patients aimed for intensive glycemic control received multiple subcutaneous injections and could achieve an HbA1c <7%.

39. **What are the adverse consequences of intensive insulin therapy?**

The adverse consequences of intensive insulin therapy are increased risk of hypoglycemia, peripheral edema, weight gain, initial worsening of retinopathy (including macular edema) and insulin neuritis. In addition, rapid reduction of blood glucose associated with initiation of intensive insulin therapy may result in change in refractory index of lens (hypermetropia), as a result of intraocular osmotic disequilibrium. The initial worsening of retinopathy after the initiation of intensive insulin therapy is a result of increased breakdown of blood-retinal barrier (consequent to upregulation of VEGF and HIF-1α), retinal ischemia due to loss of glucose-mediated retinal vasodilatation and increased angiogenesis due to elevated IGF-1 consequent to hyperinsulinemia. The clinical implication of this observation is that patients with proliferative retinopathy should be effectively treated for eye disease, prior to institution of intensive glycemic control.

40. **What is insulin lipodystrophy?**

Insulin lipodystrophy refers to localized hypertrophy or atrophy of adipose tissue at the injection site. Lipoatrophy was common with use of insulin derived from animal sources and is rare with the use of human insulin. However, lipohypertrophy is common with all insulin preparations, including analogues. The mechanism of lipohypertrophy is insulin-mediated lipogenesis through activation of lipoprotein lipase, whereas lipoatrophy is attributed to localized production of cytokines (TNFα) in response to immunological reaction against insulin (acting as hapten). Lipohypertrophy is managed by changing the site of insulin administration and, rarely, surgical excision. Lipoatrophy may respond to local steroids. Recently, insulin-induced amyloidosis has also been reported at the site of insulin administration. This clinically mimics lipohypertrophy, but has firm to hard nodular consistency as opposed to the soft consistency of lipohypertrophy.

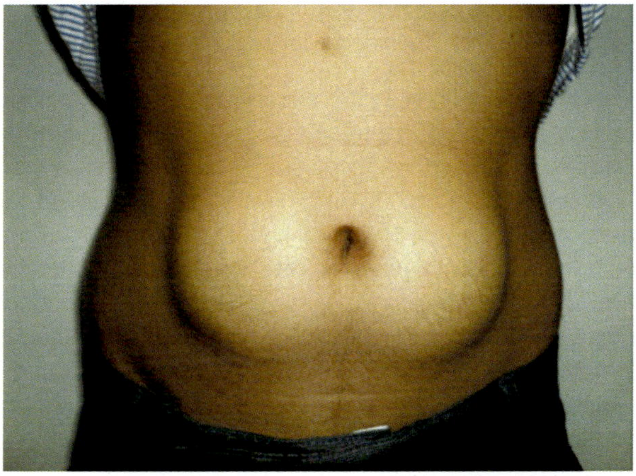

Fig. 16.1 Lipohypertrophy at injection site in a patient with T1DM

41. **What are the causes of failure to achieve target HbA1c despite intensive insulin therapy in a patient with T1DM?**

    Improper storage of insulin, incorrect technique of insulin administration, and inappropriate site of insulin injection are the common causes for failure to achieve glycemic targets despite intensive insulin therapy. Absolute insulin deficiency and marked intra- and inter-individual variability in the absorption of exogenous insulin are also major reasons for failure to achieve glycemic targets. In addition, gastroparesis, celiac disease, and autonomic neuropathy are associated with wide swings in blood glucose due to mismatch between nutrient absorption and insulin action, resulting in poor glycemic control. Further, noncompliance to therapy is common, especially in adolescents, who are known to have erratic eating habits resulting in meal–insulin mismatch. It is also difficult to achieve glycemic targets in children during peripubertal period despite intensive insulin therapy due to surge of growth hormone and gonadal steroids.

42. **Why do patients of T1DM with poor glycemic control have short stature?**

    Uncontrolled diabetes is a catabolic state and is associated with poor linear growth. This is because of limited availability of nutrients required for optimal growth and development and high circulating levels of cytokines which interfere with anabolism. Further, decreased portal vein insulin concentration impairs GH-mediated IGF1 and IGFBP3 generation by modulating GH receptor expression and post-receptor signaling at hepatocytes. Therefore, decreased level of serum IGF1 results in poor linear growth in patients with uncontrolled T1DM despite high circulating level of GH. In addition, concurrent presence of celiac disease, hypothyroidism, and hypogonadism may also contribute to poor growth. Early intensive glycemic control in patients with T1DM reverses the alterations in GH-IGF1-IGFBP3 axis, thereby resulting in normal linear growth.

43. **Why do patients with T1DM with poor glycemic control have delayed puberty?**

The delay in onset of puberty is not uncommon in patients with uncontrolled T1DM; however progression of pubertal events after initiation is usually normal. This may be attributed to catabolism associated with hyperglycemia and increased levels of cytokines (IL-6, TNF-α). The decrease in fat mass due to catabolic state results in low levels of leptin and thereby failure to stimulate kisspeptin–GnRH–gonadotropin axis, resulting in delayed puberty. In addition high levels of cytokines, hypercortisolemia, and hyperprolactinemia also contribute to delay in initiation of puberty. Further, coexisting untreated celiac disease and hypothyroidism also result in the delay in activation of GnRH pulse generator activity. Intensive glycemic control helps in restoration of hypothalamo–pituitary–gonadal axis and results in normal pubertal events as in healthy individuals.

44. **Why do patients with T1DM have wide fluctuations in blood glucose?**

Wide swings in blood glucose in patients with T1DM is due to absolute insulin deficiency, uninhibited α-cell activity, meal–insulin mismatch, and intra- and interindividual variability in absorption of insulin.

45. **Why are patients with T1DM at a higher risk for hypoglycemia as compared to those with T2DM?**

Patients with T1DM have approximately two episodes of symptomatic hypoglycemia per week and one episode of severe disabling hypoglycemia per year. The risk of hypoglycemia is increased in patients with T1DM due to absolute insulin deficiency, impaired "glucose–glucagon axis," and possibly, autonomic neuropathy. In normal individuals, the first-line defense mechanism against hypoglycemia is the decrease in insulin secretion, while the second-line defense mechanism is the release of glucagon from α-cells in response to decrease in intra-islet insulin (Δ change in intra-islet insulin). Because of absolute insulin deficiency, patients with T1DM have impaired first- as well as second-line defense mechanism against hypoglycemia. However, patients with T2DM have some endogenous β-cell reserve with intact first- and second-defense mechanisms against hypoglycemia. In addition, glucose–glucagon axis is severely impaired in patients with T1DM. Normally, rising glucose levels result in suppression of glucagon secretion, whereas declining glucose levels stimulate glucagon secretion. Impairment of glucose–glucagon axis during hypoglycemia in patients with T1DM occurs due to failure of upregulation of glucose receptors on α-cells despite reduced glucose levels. Further, with advanced duration of disease, concurrent presence of autonomic neuropathy predisposes to hypoglycemia as appropriate glucagon secretory response during hypoglycemia requires the presence of catecholamines and intact intra-islet nerves.

46. **What is Somogyi phenomenon?**

Somogyi phenomenon is defined as "post-hypoglycemic hyperglycemia". A hypoglycemic episode is followed by release of counter-regulatory hormones, i.e., catecholamines, glucagon, GH, and cortisol resulting in hyperglycemia. It is not uncommon and has an incidence of 12.6–67%. It usually manifests as early morning hyperglycemia, but can happen at any time of day as it is a consequence of mismatch between insulin administration, food intake, and physical activity. It is more likely to occur in those with advanced duration of diabetes, autonomic neuropathy, renal failure, hypothyroidism, and β-blocker therapy. Somogyi phenomenon should be suspected in patients with diabetes who have unexplained fasting hyperglycemia or wide swings in blood glucose. Estimation of plasma glucose on multiple occasions or continuous glucose monitoring system (CGMS) is helpful in the diagnosis. Treatment strategies include administration of interprandial/bedtime snacks, adjustment in insulin dose, and use of insulin analogues or continuous subcutaneous insulin infusion (insulin pump).

47. **What is "dawn" phenomenon?**

Dawn phenomenon is a physiological event characterized by early morning rise in blood glucose. It is attributed to nocturnal GH surge and early morning rise in cortisol and catecholamines, resulting in increased hepatic glucose output. This is exaggerated in patient with diabetes. The incidence of dawn phenomenon in patients with diabetes is 55%. Dawn phenomenon should be differentiated from Somogyi phenomenon by estimation of blood glucose between 3 and 5 a.m. or continuous glucose monitoring system. Fasting hyperglycemia due to Somogyi phenomenon requires reduction in insulin doses, while exaggerated dawn phenomenon needs an increase in insulin doses. The other measures include increased physical activity in the evening hours, reduced intake of carbohydrates in the last meal, or switching to long-acting insulin analogues instead of NPH.

48. **What is the "honeymoon" phase in T1DM?**

The "honeymoon" phase is defined as transient remission of diabetes characterized by decreased/no insulin requirement with maintenance of good glycemic control. However, the definition of "decrease in insulin requirement" is not well defined, but usually in clinical practice the reduction in doses of insulin to

<0.2IU/kg/day is considered as the "honeymoon" phase of T1DM. The differential diagnosis for the honeymoon phase is "ketosis-prone diabetes" that initially behaves like T1DM and subsequently as T2DM. The predictors of the honeymoon phase are older age at onset (5–12 years), male gender, duration of symptoms of hyperglycemia <2 weeks, absence of ketosis/ketoacidosis, mild hyperglycemia (HbA1c <8%), measurable β-cell function at presentation (fasting C-peptide levels), early initiation of treatment, and intensive glycemic control. This phase may last from weeks to years (1 month to 13 years). "β-cell rest," reduced gluco-lipotoxicity, decreased "β-cell antigen leak" (with suppression of immuno-inflammatory damage) and reduced oxidative stress after intensive insulin therapy are the probable mechanisms for the honeymoon phase. DHEAS, nicotinamide, and cyclosporine have been explored as options to prolong the honeymoon phase without success. As honeymoon phase is usually transient, regular surveillance is required to detect the resurgence of hyperglycemia.

49. **Why is insulin requirement higher before breakfast than before dinner, despite of heavy meal at dinner than breakfast?**

In healthy individuals, peak and area under curve for glucose achieved after breakfast is higher than after dinner despite similar amount of carbohydrate intake. This is attributed to early morning rise in cortisol, catecholamine, and delayed effect of nocturnal GH surge which continues to maintain hepatic glucose output in fasting state. However, in the dusk hours, falling levels of counter-regulatory hormones lead to lesser glucose peak and area under curve despite heavy dinner. Therefore, requirement of insulin is higher in the morning hours than before dinner.

50. **Who are the candidates for insulin pump therapy?**

Patients with T1DM who have wide swings in blood glucose, recurrent hypoglycemia, and hypoglycemic unawareness are potential candidates for insulin pump therapy. In addition, patients who fail to achieve target HbA1c <8.5% despite multiple insulin injections can also be benefitted with insulin pump therapy.

51. **What are the pros and cons of insulin pump therapy?**

Insulin pump delivers insulin continuously at a preset basal rate with preprandial bolus when required, thereby mimicking near-normal physiological insulin release. However, euglycemia can be maintained only for 62% time of the day with hyperglycemia for 30% and hypoglycemia for 8% time of the day. The advantages and disadvantages are summarized in the table given below.

Advantages	**Disadvantages**
Decreased frequency and severity of hypoglycemia	Technical failure with risk of DKA
Reduced glycemic variability	Cost
Avoidance of multiple daily injections	Increased unhealthy eating

Advantages	Disadvantages
Precise insulin dosing	Requires frequent blood glucose testing
Administration of basal insulin at different rates over 24 h (circadian variation)	Requires intensive education and motivation
Reduction in insulin requirement by 10–20%	Equipment needs to be carried throughout
Better glycemic control	Change of needle twice a week
Flexibility of lifestyle	
Improved quality of life	

52. **Why is the glycemic control better with insulin pump than with basal-bolus insulin therapy in patients with T1DM?**

    Multiple insulin injections are aimed to mimic near-physiological delivery of insulin in a patient with absolute/severe insulin deficiency; however, erratic absorption and action of subcutaneously administered insulin results in wide swings in blood glucose levels and increased risk of hypoglycemia. This is further complicated by increased inter-prandial snacking due to fear of hypoglycemia, resulting in worsening of glycemic control. In addition, the rate of delivery of long-acting insulin cannot be modulated to provide varying quantity of basal insulin at different points of time, once it is administered. This is particularly important to counteract fasting hyperglycemia (dawn phenomenon), when the requirement of basal insulin is higher as compared to rest of the day. Therefore, insulin pump therapy may be a good option to overcome these deficits. The intra-individual variation in the absorption of insulin when delivered as small doses through pump is only 3%, as opposed to 50% with a large dose of subcutaneously administered NPH insulin. Therefore, smooth and sustained delivery of insulin through pump ameliorates glycemic variability and decreases the risk of hypoglycemia. Further, the rate of delivery of basal insulin can be modified to deliver insulin at different quantities at various times of the day, particularly to target fasting hyperglycemia and inter-prandial glucose peaks. The flexibility of prandial insulin administration also helps in attainment of target HbA1c. However, some patients continue to have hypo- or hyperglycemia despite use of insulin pump.

53. **Which is the preferred insulin for CSII therapy?**

    CSII aims to deliver insulin at a continuous rate to provide basal insulin (for regulated hepatic glucose output) and boluses to target postprandial hyperglycemia. As the insulin delivery is continuous, long-acting insulin analogues have no place in CSII. Therefore, the preferred insulin is regular or rapid-acting analogues. Between these two insulins, rapid-acting analogues are preferred as they are monomeric and have favorable pharmacokinetic profile (less intra- and interindividual variation in absorption, rapid absorption, and short duration of action), resulting in better glycemic control.

54. **What are the available insulin pumps?**

Three types of insulin pumps are commercially available for delivery of insulin through CSII. Earlier models were equipped to deliver insulin; however, they did not have provision for integrated continuous glucose monitoring system (CGMS). The next-generation pumps are integrated with CGMS for real-time blood glucose monitoring, in addition to continuous delivery of insulin. This allows regular display of blood glucose levels at defined time intervals along with safety alarm and thus provides an opportunity to modulate the dose of insulin periodically (sensor augmented pumps). The current generation insulin pumps, in addition, have provision for suspending insulin delivery in the event of hypoglycemia (sensor augmented pumps with threshold suspension).

55. **What is the difference between "open-loop" and "closed-loop" insulin pumps?**

Insulin can be administered via an insulin pump either as an "open-loop" or a "closed-loop" system. The "open-loop" system delivers insulin at a preset rate and the insulin delivery rate has to be adjusted manually. Conventional insulin pumps, sensor augmented pumps, and sensor augmented pumps with threshold suspension represent "open-loop" insulin delivery systems. The "closed-loop" system has a provision for automated adjustment in the rate of insulin delivery depending on the ambient blood glucose level. The recently introduced "bionic pancreas" is an example of "closed-loop" insulin delivery system.

56. **What are the non-insulin therapies used in patients with T1DM?**

Besides insulin, drugs that have been explored in the management of patients with T1DM are metformin, pioglitazone, α-glucosidase inhibitors, dipeptidyl peptidase-4 (DPP4) inhibitors, glucagon-like peptide-1 (GLP-1) analogues, and pramlintide. These drugs are not a primary modality of treatment in T1DM and have been used as an adjunctive therapy with modest success. Insulin sensitizers (metformin, pioglitazone) can be used particularly in obese T1DM or during peripubertal period to overcome insulin resistance. The mechanism of action of DPP4 inhibitors/GLP-1 analogues in T1DM is to decrease the glucagon secretion from α-cells and to delay intestinal absorption of glucose. In addition, the use of DPP4 inhibitors may improve response to hypoglycemia by sensitizing α-cells to circulating glucose and GIP. Recently, SGLT2 inhibitors have also been tried in patients with T1DM as their action is independent of insulin action and duration of disease.

57. **How does GLP-1 inhibit glucagon?**

T1DM is characterized by absolute insulin deficiency and relative hyperglucagonemia. Addition of GLP-1 receptor agonists/DPP4 inhibitors along with insulin therapy may help to reduce glycemic variability in these patients by suppressing glucagon. The mechanisms involved in suppression of glucagon secretion by GLP-1 include direct inhibition of α-cells, restoration of "glucose–glucagon axis," and increased somatostatin secretion.

58. **What is the Edmonton protocol?**

The Edmonton protocol is a steroid-sparing immuno-suppressive protocol used in patients with T1DM who undergo islet transplantation. This includes administration of sirolimus, tacrolimus, and daclizumab, thereby avoiding the adverse effects associated with the use glucocorticoids, i.e., glucotoxicity, cardiovascular risk, and osteoporosis. Though complete and partial insulin independence was achieved in 72% of the patients at the end of 1 year, it could be sustained only in 31% at the end of 2 years after islet transplantation following the Edmonton protocol.

59. **When to assess a child with T1DM for diabetes-related microvascular complications?**

Screening should only be considered in children with T1DM who have duration of disease >3–5 years. Even in these children, screening should be commenced only if the child is >10 years of age or has entered puberty, whichever is earlier. For example, a child with onset of T1DM at age 3 years should be considered for screening at 6–8 years of age (duration of disease >3–5 years) only if he/she has entered into puberty. Otherwise, screening should commence after 10 years of age.

60. **When to initiate ACEI/ARBs in patients with T1DM?**

Screening for diabetic kidney disease should be commenced after 5 years of diagnosis in patients with T1DM. The presence of hypertension or albuminuria mandates initiation of therapy with ACEIs, and if intolerant to ACEIs, ARBs may be considered. ACEIs are considered as first-line drugs rather than ARBs, because of lack of data with ARBs in patients with T1DM. The target BP is <140/90 mmHg in adults with T1DM and below 95th percentile in children.

61. **When should statins be initiated in patients with T1DM?**

Children with T1DM aged 10–21 years should have a fasting lipid profile once in 3–5 years, while adults with T1DM should be screened yearly. In children (10–21 years), statins may be considered in those with LDL cholesterol (LDL-C) ≥100 mg/dl, while they are recommended if LDL-C ≥160 mg/dl, with a target LDL-C <100 mg/dl and non-HDL-C <130 mg/dl. However, in adults without cardiovascular disease (CVD), statins are recommended if LDL-C is >100 mg/dl, and in those with CVD if LDL-C >70 mg/dl, with LDL-C targets being <100 mg/dl and <70 mg/dl, respectively. Statins are not recommended below the age of 10 years in patients with T1DM, irrespective of the duration of disease, possibly because of paucity of data. The threshold for initiation of statins are set higher in children (10–21 years), because of the weak association of LDL-C and cardiovascular events in patients with T1DM.

62. **What are the diagnostic criteria for diabetic ketoacidosis?**

The criteria for diagnosis of diabetic ketoacidosis include blood glucose >250 mg/dl, ketonemia/ketonuria (plasma β-hydroxybutyrate >3 mmol/l or plasma acetone/acetoacetate positive in 1:2 dilution or urine ketones ≥3+), and pH <7.3 or serum bicarbonate <15 mEq/L. In a patient with diabetes, presence of hyperglycemia and ketosis in the absence of acidosis is consistent with a diagnosis of diabetic ketosis. The presence of ketosis and acidosis in a diabetic patient with blood glucose <250 mg/dl is termed euglycemic diabetic ketoacidosis. The causes include pregnancy, starvation, and suboptimal treatment with insulin.

63. **What are the causes of abdominal pain in a patient with diabetic ketoacidosis?**

The causes of abdominal pain in a patient with diabetic ketoacidosis are gastric dilatation, hypokalemia, acidemia, mesenteric ischemia, dysautonomia, and pancreatitis.

64. **Which is the key metabolite in the genesis of hyperglycemia in diabetic ketoacidosis?**

The key metabolite in the genesis of hyperglycemia in diabetic ketoacidosis is fructose-2,6-biphosphate (F-2,6-P2) and is synthesized from fructose-6-phosphate by the enzyme phosphofuctokinase-2 (PFK2). F-2,6-P2 allosterically stimulates the enzyme phsophofructokinase-1 (PFK1) and inhibits fructose-1,6-bisphosphatase, thereby resulting in stimulation of glycolysis and inhibition of gluconeogenesis, respectively. However, in the presence of high glucagon/insulin ratio, the levels of fructose-2,6-biphosphate are decreased which results in suppression of glycolysis and promotion of gluconeogenesis.

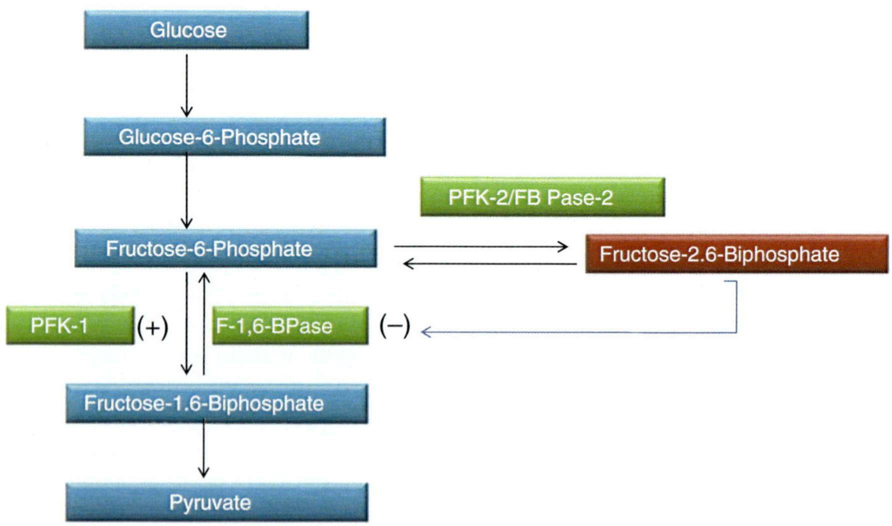

Fig. 16.2 The role of fructose-2,6-biphosphate in glucose homeostasis

65. **What are ketone bodies?**

Ketone bodies include acetone, acetoacetate, and β-hydroxybutyrate. Oxidation of free fatty acids (FFAs) leads to synthesis of acetyl-CoA and two molecules of acetyl-CoA combine to form acetoacetate. This is further converted to either β-hydroxybutyrate or acetone. Acetoacetate is excreted through urine and acetone through lungs, while β-hydroxybutyrate is converted to acetoacetate. However a small quantity of β-hydroxybutyrate is excreted in urine and can be measured, but the assays are not readily available. In the physiological state, the ratio of acetoacetate to β-hydroxybutyrate in blood is 1:3, and it may increase up to 1:8 in severe DKA, hypotension, and fasting state, because the conversion of acetoacetate to β-hydroxybutyrate is accelerated due to excess NADH. However, with the reversal of these states, β-hydroxybutyrate is converted back into acetoacetate.

66. **Are ketone bodies present in healthy individuals?**

Yes. Healthy individuals can have serum β-hydroxybutyrate level up to 0.6 mmol/l. Normally, in the late postprandial state, insulin secretion declines and glucagon rises, resulting in lipolysis and elevated levels of circulating free fatty acids (FFAs). In the liver, FFAs are converted to ketone bodies, which can be utilized by the brain in the event of decreased hepatic glucose output. In the physiological state, ketone body production is regulated because fasting state does not last beyond 8–10 h. Further, modestly elevated FFA and ketones stimulate insulin release, thereby preventing the development of ketosis.

67. **Why is ketone body production unabated in patients with DKA?**

In patients with T1DM, severe insulin deficiency and hyperglucagonemia result in accelerated lipolysis leading to elevated levels of circulating FFAs. Further, high glucagon/insulin ratio also results in increased hepatic carnitine content and decreased malonyl-CoA levels, which in turn activates carnitine palmitoylacyltransferase-1 (CPT1), thereby facilitating the transport of FFAs into mitochondria. Subsequently, FFAs are oxidized to acetyl-CoA in mitochondria (β-oxidation). In normal physiology, acetyl-CoA can enter into TCA cycle or can be utilized for triglyceride or ketone body synthesis. However, in patients with T1DM, acetyl-CoA cannot enter into TCA cycle due to non-availability of oxaloacetate, which is diverted to gluconeogenesis (due to increased glucagon/insulin ratio). Further, severe insulin deficiency does not allow acetyl-CoA to enter into triglyceride synthesis pathway. Therefore, acetyl-CoA is predominantly shunted to ketone body formation in the mitochondria. This is illustrated in the figure given below.

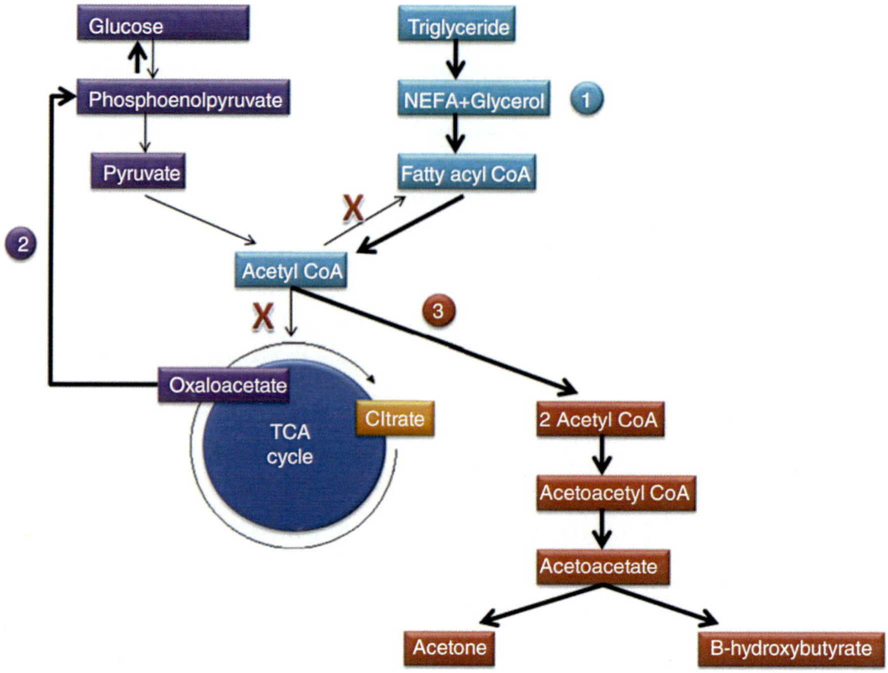

Fig. 16.3 Pathophysiology of ketogenesis in DKA. (*1*) Accelerated lipolysis due to severe insulin deficiency and excess glucagon, resulting in formation of acetyl-CoA. (*2*) Acetyl-CoA cannot enter into TCA cycle due to non-availability of oxaloacetate, which is diverted to gluconeogenic pathway as a consequence of insulin deficiency. (*3*) Acetyl-CoA is shunted to ketogenic pathway

68. **How to estimate ketone bodies?**

Ketone bodies can be estimated in blood or urine. The most widely used tests include nitroprusside test and enzymatic method (β-hydroxybutyrate dehydrogenase). Nitroprusside test can be used for estimation of ketones in urine as well as in blood; however, it detects only acetoacetate and acetone, but not β-hydroxybutyrate. The enzymatic method (β-hydroxybutyrate dehydrogenase) specifically measures β-hydroxybutyrate in blood.

69. **Can a patient with diabetic ketoacidosis have ketonemia without ketonuria?**

Yes. β-hydroxybutyrate is the predominant ketone body in patients with severe DKA as acetoacetate is preferentially converted to β-hydroxybutyrate. Therefore, urine ketones can be negative as nitroprusside test estimates only acetoacetate and acetone. Hence, when severe DKA is suspected, it is imperative to measure serum β-hydroxybutyrate by enzymatic method. Other causes of false-negative nitroprusside test include intake of ascorbic acid, urosepsis, and sample collection in an open container (because acetone is volatile).

70. **Is leukocytosis a reliable predictor of infection in patients with DKA?**

No. Patient with DKA can have leukocytosis due to stress-induced hypercortisolemia and catecholamine surge, hemoconcentration, or ketosis; however, this does not exceed beyond 25,000/mm^3 and fever is absent. In addition, precipitating factors for DKA like pancreatitis or myocardial infarction may also be associated with leukocytosis. However, the presence of fever and/or total leukocyte count >25, 000/mm^3 should raise a suspicion of infection. But the most reliable marker for infection in a patient with DKA is the presence of > 10% band forms of neutrophil (sensitivity 100%, specificity 80%).

71. **A 13-year-old boy presented with osmotic symptoms and BP 100/60 mmHg. On evaluation, his blood glucose was 600 mg/dl and had ketoacidosis. What should be initiated first, insulin or intravenous fluids?**

In patients with DKA, administration of intravenous saline should precede insulin therapy. Patients with DKA are commonly fluid depleted with a fluid deficit of 3–6 liters depending on the severity of DKA, and administration of insulin without prior fluid replacement can result in hypotension. This is due to insulin-mediated rapid shift of fluid from intravascular to interstitial compartment and its vasodilatory effect. Therefore, i.v. fluids are the first-line therapy in a patient, irrespective of blood glucose levels. Rehydration not only restores intravascular volume, but also dilutes circulating level of ketones and glucagon. Rehydration results in lowering of blood glucose by up to 23% as a result of hemodilution and increased renal perfusion and consequently, glucosuria.

72. **What are the biochemical parameters to be monitored in a patient with DKA?**

Biochemical parameters which are to be monitored in a patient with DKA include blood glucose, pH, serum anion gap, serum potassium, and phosphate. Frequent monitoring of blood glucose (hourly) helps in the assessment of response to treatment and titration of rate of insulin infusion. When blood glucose falls to <200 mg/dl, 5% dextrose should be added to prevent hypoglycemia, and insulin infusion should not be discontinued. Arterial pH and serum anion gap should be monitored 4–6 hourly to assess the efficacy of treatment. The recovery from DKA is heralded by progressive decrease in anion gap and increase in serum pH. Failure to improvement in these parameters suggests suboptimal hydration, inadequate insulin therapy, or other causes of metabolic acidosis (lactic/uremic). In addition, serum electrolytes including potassium and phosphate should be monitored at a frequency of 4–6 h.

73. **What are the electrolyte abnormalities present in a patient with DKA?**

The common electrolyte abnormalities in patients with DKA pertain to potassium, phosphate, magnesium, sodium, and chloride. Patients with DKA have severe depletion of body stores of potassium; however, serum potassium levels are usually normal at presentation. This occurs due to transcellular shift of potassium from intracellular to extracellular compartments as a result of acidosis and insulin deficiency. However, patients who have severe vomiting may have hypokalemia at presentation. In these patients, potassium supplementation should be initiated and insulin therapy should be withheld till serum potassium is >3.3 mEq/L. Initiation of insulin therapy can induce or worsen hypokalemia, and it is recommended to add potassium to i.v. fluids in all patients with DKA unless the patient is oliguric after rehydration or serum potassium >5.5 mEq/L. Patients with DKA are also phosphate depleted, and insulin therapy may further worsen it by promoting its transcellular shift. However, no benefit of phosphate administration has been demonstrated in clinical studies. Serum sodium levels are usually low in patients with DKA due to dilutional hyponatremia, and this is consequent to osmotic effects of glucose. Normal serum sodium in the presence of hyperglycemia denotes severe dehydration. Hyperchloremic metabolic acidosis may occur during therapy due to overzealous saline administration, and this entity should be considered in the presence of metabolic acidosis despite resolution of ketonemia. Hypomagnesemia in DKA is a result of urinary loss of magnesium and may require supplementation.

74. **When should bicarbonate be administered in a patient with DKA?**

Bicarbonate replacement in a patient with DKA is detrimental because it may worsen tissue hypoxia by shifting oxygen dissociation curve to the left, precipitate hypokalemia, impair cardiac contractility, induce paradoxical CNS acidosis, and cause rebound metabolic alkalosis. Hence, bicarbonate therapy is recommended only in patients with severe acidosis (pH <6.9), those with hemodynamic instability with pH<7.1, or in presence of hyperkalemia with ECG changes. The recommended dose is 1 mEq/kg body weight, and it has to be infused slowly over 30–60 min.

75. **When to discontinue insulin infusion in a patient recovering from DKA?**

Although the criteria for resolution of DKA include blood glucose <200 mg/dl, serum bicarbonate >18 mEq/L and pH >7.3, the decision to discontinue insulin infusion should be considered only after the patient starts accepting orally. Short-acting and intermediate-/long-acting insulin should be administered 30–45 min prior to discontinuation of insulin infusion to prevent the resurgence of counter-regulatory hormones and consequently, hyperglycemia and ketoacidosis.

76. **Why to encourage timely initiation of oral feeds in patients recovering from DKA?**

Patients with DKA usually have poor oral intake due to abdominal pain, nausea, vomiting, or concurrent illness. Timely initiation of oral feeds helps in repletion of hepatic glycogen stores due to attainment of higher portal vein glucose concentration, which cannot be achieved with parenteral dextrose. In addition, it also helps in the restoration of gut flora, repletion of trace elements (e.g., magnesium, phosphate) and prevents complications associated with prolonged i.v. fluid therapy.

77. **Despite recovery from DKA, what is the cause of persistent ketonuria?**

Ketone bodies, being lipophilic, accumulate in adipose tissue. The slow release of ketone bodies into circulation from adipose tissue explains the persistence of ketonemia/ketonuria even after recovery from DKA. In addition, during the recovery phase of DKA, β-hydroxybutyrate is converted to acetoacetate and rising level of acetoacetate (nitroprusside test) gives a false impression of worsening of disease. This "paradox" is usually seen in patients who had severe DKA with hemodynamic instability.

78. **What are the possibilities to be considered if a patient deteriorates after initial recovery from DKA?**

The possibilities which are to be considered in a patient who deteriorates after showing initial recovery from DKA include development of cerebral edema, cerebrovascular accident, rhino–orbito–cerebral mucormycosis (ROCM), occult infections, hospital-acquired sepsis, and acute kidney injury. Cerebral edema is commonly seen in children and is a result of rapid lowering of blood glucose which causes osmotic dysequilibrium, and is consequent to development of idiogenic osmoles, disturbances in water and sodium balance, increased blood–brain permeability, and probably a direct effect of insulin. Early recognition and intensive management with mannitol and/or dexamethasone may improve outcome.

79. **Why are patients with DKA predisposed to rhino–orbito–cerebral mucormycosis?**

The rhizopus fungi *Mucor* is characteristically ferrophilic and angioinvasive. Patients with DKA are predisposed for rhino–orbito–cerebral mucormycosis (ROCM) as acidosis increases the availability of free iron in circulation due to decreased binding with transferrin. In addition, presence of hyperglycemia further enhances the risk in these patients. The propensity of *Mucor* to invade blood vessels (angioinvasive) is responsible for the devastating complications associated with ROCM. The diagnosis should be suspected in a patient with DKA who manifests ptosis, vision loss, epistaxis, blackish eschar (nasal concha or hard palate), or hemiplegia. The presence of isodense or hyperdense lesions in ethmoid and/or paranasal sinuses on CT and aseptate, right-angled hyphae on cytology confirms the diagnosis of mucormyosis. Rapid initiation of therapy with amphotericin B along with aggressive surgical debridement is curative in majority of patients.

80. **When to suspect non-ketotic causes for altered sensorium in a patient with DKA?**

The causes of altered sensorium in DKA include cerebral intracellular dehydration, acidemia, and dyselectrolytemia (hypo- and hypernatremia). Hyperglycemia-related altered sensorium is classically associated with serum osmolality >320 mOsm/kg. However, if a patient with DKA has altered sensorium with serum osmolality <320 mOsm/kg, alternative causes for altered sensorium like meningitis, cortical vein thrombosis, stroke, and cerebral mucormycosis should be actively sought.

Suggested Reading

1. American Diabetes Association. Standards of medical care in diabetes—2014. Diabetes Care. 2014;37 Suppl 1:S14–80.
2. Jameson JL, De Groot LJ. Endocrinology: adult and pediatric. Philadelphia: Elsevier Health Sciences; 2010.
3. Longo D, Fauci A, Kasper D, Hauser S, Jameson J, Loscalzo J. Harrison's principles of internal medicine 18E EB. New York: McGraw Hill Professional; 2012.
4. Melmed S, Polonsky KS, Reed Larsen P, Kronenberg HM. Williams textbook of endocrinology: expert consult. London: Elsevier Health Sciences; 2011.

17 Type 2 Diabetes Mellitus

17.1 Clinical Rounds

1. **Why is there a global concern for diabetes?**

   There is an increasing prevalence of diabetes worldwide with 382 million people in 2013 and this is likely to increase to 592 million by 2035. Almost half of this population is unaware of their disease. Majority of people with diabetes are in the age group of 40–59 years. About three-fourth of people with diabetes live in low- and middle-income countries. The rise in prevalence of diabetes is attributed to population growth, increasing life span, sedentary lifestyle, consumption of calorie-dense food, and increasing prevalence of obesity.

2. **What is ICMR–INDIAB study?**

   The ICMR–INDIAB study is an all India initiative to assess the prevalence of type 2 diabetes and prediabetes. In its first stage, it covered three states (Maharashtra, Tamil Nadu, and Jharkhand) and one union territory (Chandigarh). This study demonstrated that the prevalence of diabetes is highest in Chandigarh (13.6%) and lowest in Jharkhand (5.3%), with an estimated burden of 62.4 million people with type 2 diabetes and 77.2 million with prediabetes all over the country.

3. **How is type 2 diabetes different in the Indian population?**

   The prevalence of diabetes peaks at 45–55 years of age in Indians, nearly a decade earlier as compared to the Western population, with a progressive decline beyond 65 years of age. Contrary to the Western world, the prevalence is higher in men as compared to women. Increased visceral fat (central obesity),

A. Bhansali, Y. Gogate, *Clinical Rounds in Endocrinology: Volume I - Adult Endocrinology*, DOI 10.1007/978-81-322-2398-6_17

greater consumption of carbohydrate-rich diet, and high prevalence of sedentary lifestyle predispose Indian population to diabetes. India was the "diabetes capital of the world," but currently China houses 114 million people with diabetes as opposed to 67 million in India.

4. **What are the two characteristic defects in type 2 diabetes?**

   Type 2 diabetes (T2DM) is characterized by two defects, namely, insulin resistance and insulin deficiency. However, insulin resistance alone cannot produce T2DM as long as β-cells are able to compensate for increasing insulin resistance. The failure of β-cells eventually leads to onset of hyperglycemia.

5. **What is insulin resistance?**

   Insulin resistance is defined as subnormal biological response to optimal levels of insulin. Insulin resistance is associated with altered carbohydrate, fat, and protein metabolism; however, in clinical context, it is usually considered in relation to carbohydrate metabolism, which manifests as hyperinsulinemia with or without dysglycemia. Some degree of insulin resistance is inbuilt in every healthy individual, as it protects from hypoglycemia. With advancing age, insulin resistance progressively increases as a result of increasing adiposity and adaptation to sedentary lifestyle. However, the slope of rise in insulin resistance is steeper during early and middle age as compared to older age.

6. **Can insulin resistance be organ specific?**

   The prime sites of insulin resistance are the liver, skeletal muscle, and adipose tissue. The insulin resistance may be organ specific, limited only to liver, muscle or adipose tissue. The clinical implication of this observation is that patients with fasting hyperglycemia predominantly have hepatic insulin resistance, while those with postprandial hyperglycemia predominantly have skeletal muscle and adipose tissue insulin resistance.

7. **What are the clinical markers of insulin resistance?**

   The clinical markers of insulin resistance are obesity (central/generalized), acanthosis nigricans, skin tags, double chin, lipodystrophy, and in women, features of androgen excess (alopecia, hirsutism, oligomenorrhea). The body mass index (>23 kg/m^2, as per Asian criteria) and waist circumference (>80 cm in women and >90 cm in men, as per Asian criteria) are also markers of insulin resistance. The abnormally high requirement of insulin (>2–3 IU/kg of body weight) for optimal glycemic control also suggests the presence of insulin resistance.

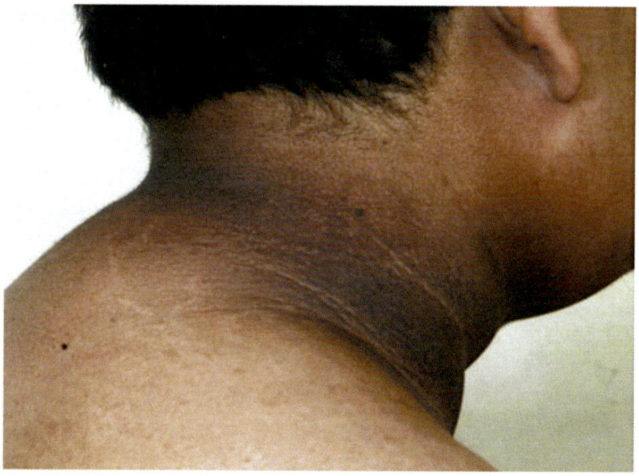

Fig. 17.1 Acanthosis nigricans in a patient with T2DM

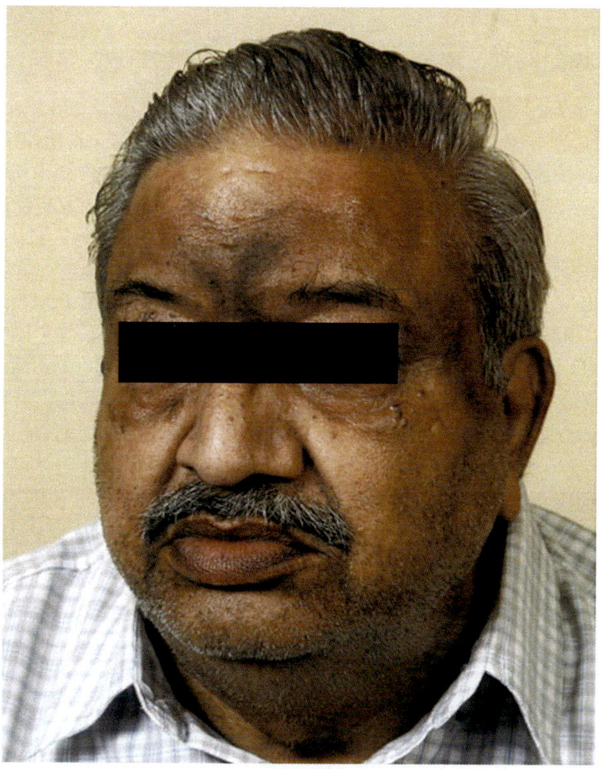

Fig. 17.2 Acanthosis nigricans at an atypical site (forehead) and double chin in a patient with T2DM

8. **Which is the best test to assess insulin resistance?**

   The hyperinsulinemic-euglycemic clamp is the "gold standard" for detection of insulin resistance/sensitivity. It is a direct measure of insulin sensitivity to assess the insulin-mediated glucose disposal into the skeletal muscle. The insulin suppression test is another direct measure of insulin sensitivity which involves use of somatostatin to inhibit endogenous insulin secretion, followed by insulin–glucose infusion.

9. **What are the other tests to assess insulin resistance?**

   The indirect measures of insulin sensitivity include frequently sampled intravenous glucose tolerance test (FSIVGTT) and short insulin tolerance test. The advantage of FSIVGTT as compared to hyperinsulinemic-euglycemic clamp study is that it is simple and also measures β-cell function. The other surrogate indices of insulin resistance are fasting plasma insulin, glucose/insulin ratio, homeostasis model assessment-insulin resistance (HOMA-IR), quantitative insulin sensitivity check index (QUICKI), and Matsuda insulin sensitivity index.

10. **What are the β-cell defects in the evolution of T2DM?**

    Insulin is secreted in rapid bursts at a frequency of 4 min and ultradian oscillations every 15–20 min, which maintains basal levels of insulin to regulate hepatic glucose output. The meal-related first phase of insulin secretion is due to the release of preformed granules and is responsible for knocking down hepatic glucose output in the immediate postprandial period. The second phase of insulin secretion is responsible for postprandial glucose disposal to skeletal muscle and is due to insulin biosynthesis. The earliest abnormality in type 2 diabetes is the loss of pulsatile insulin secretion, followed by loss of glucose-induced first phase insulin secretion and subsequently, delayed and prolonged second phase of insulin secretion. The loss of pulsatile secretion is responsible for fasting hyperglycemia, and loss of first phase and delayed and prolonged second phase of insulin secretion contributes to postprandial hyperglycemia. The concurrent presence of incretin deficiency/resistance contributes further to β-cell dysfunction and impaired crosstalk between α and β-cell, thereby resulting in worsening of hyperglycemia.

11. **How to assess β-cell function?**

    The β-cell function can be assessed by measurement of fasting C-peptide, stimulated C-peptide in response to glucagon/mixed meal, homeostasis assessment model-β (HOMA-β), and hyperglycemic insulin clamp (gold standard). The surrogate indices for assessment of β-cell function include oral glucose tolerance test, frequently sampled intravenous glucose tolerance test (FSIVGTT), and glucose/insulin ratio. The β-cell function progressively declines with age; it is lost by 50% at diagnosis of T2DM and by 90% at onset of T1DM.

12. **What are incretins?**

Incretins are peptides secreted by enteroendocrine cells in response to oral glucose or nutrients and potentiate glucose-mediated insulin secretion. The insulin secretion in response to incretin is glucose-dependent. The major incretins are glucagon-like peptide-1 (GLP1) and glucose-dependent insulinotropic polypeptide (GIP) and contribute to about 60% of the prandial insulin release. GLP1 is mainly produced by L cells in the distal intestine, and GIP is secreted by K cells from the duodenum.

13. **What is the role of GLP1 in glucose homeostasis?**

GLP1 plays an important role in glucose homeostasis through its effect on postprandial hyperglycemia by delaying gastric emptying and stimulating insulin release. However, GLP1 does not directly stimulate β-cell, but only potentiates the effect of glucose on insulin secretion. Further, GLP1 also inhibits glucagon secretion which results in decreased hepatic glucose output, and consequently, leads to reduction in fasting hyperglycemia. In addition, GLP1 also increases satiety and improves glycemic profile by reducing glycemic excursions.

14. **What is the incretin status in T2DM?**

Initially, it was believed that type 2 diabetes is a GLP1-deficient and GIP-resistant state. But, the recent data shows GLP1 levels to be variable, either low (GLP1 deficiency) or normal (GLP1 resistance) in patients with type 2 diabetes. The probable causes for GLP1 deficiency are asymptomatic gastroparesis (which is not uncommon in type 2 diabetes) and L-cell glucotoxicity. GLP1 resistance may be due to glucotoxicity at β-cell, which may be restored to normal with glycemic control. The variability in the GLP1 level in different studies has been attributed to the different assays used and type of GLP1 (total/intact) measured. Despite these conflicting data, patients with T2DM respond to DPP4 inhibitors and GLP1 analogues.

15. **What is glucose–glucagon axis?**

In a healthy individual, rising glucose level suppresses glucagon, and declining glucose level stimulates glucagon. The suppression of glucagon during hyperglycemia may be a direct effect of glucose on α-cell or a paracrine effect of β-cell through intra-islet insulin which is stimulated by GLP1 or may be a direct inhibitory effect of GLP1 on α-cell. During hypoglycemia, glucagon secretion is stimulated by GIP. This tightly regulated phenomenon responsible for the maintenance of glucose homeostasis is called "glucose–glucagon axis." Patients with T2DM have an impaired glucose–glucagon axis, and this can be improved with the use of GLP1 analogue/DPP4 inhibitors.

16. **What is "Starling curve of pancreas"?**

The term "Starling curve" is commonly used in cardiac physiology. In addition, this term is also used to describe β-cell response to rising blood glucose. Starling curve of pancreas states that there is an initial increase in insulin secretion in response to rising blood glucose (150 mg/dl), followed by subsequent decline in insulin secretion. It represents the natural history of hyperglycemia in type 2 diabetes and can be partially reversed by correcting glucotoxicity.

17. **What is glucotoxicity?**

Glucotoxicity is a metabolic phenomenon characterized by impaired insulin secretion (β-cell) and/or impaired insulin action (skeletal muscle, liver, and adipocytes) due to toxic effects of worsening hyperglycemia. The β-cell dysfunction is characterized by impaired glucose-stimulated insulin secretion as a consequence of decreased GLUT2 expression, oxidative stress, endoplasmic reticulum stress, hypoxia, and cytokine-induced apoptosis. Similar mechanisms operate at the skeletal muscle (reduced GLUT4 expression), liver, and adipocytes.

18. **What is lipotoxicity?**

Lipotoxicity is defined as the deleterious effects of increased free fatty acid (FFA) on β-cell (insulin secretion) and insulin target sites (muscle, liver, and adipocytes). Increased free fatty acid is due to enhanced lipolysis as a consequence of insulin resistance at adipocytes. The mechanism of FFA-mediated lipotoxicity is akin to glucotoxicity; hence, some prefer using the term gluco-lipotoxicity.

19. **What is the clinical relevance of gluco-lipotoxicity?**

The clinical implication of gluco-lipotoxicity is that early intensive treatment of hyperglycemia may reverse gluco-lipotoxicity and can lead to improvement in β-cell function and insulin sensitivity. This reversibility suggests that gluco-lipotoxicity causes functional abnormalities of β-cell and skeletal muscle, rather than structural defects. However, persistent gluco-lipotoxicity result in structural defects in these organs. Hence, early intensive treatment of hyperglycemia is beneficial for the preservation of β-cell function and results in a good "legacy effect" (metabolic memory).

20. **What is the ominous octet in T2DM?**

The ominous octet describes the organs/tissues involved in pathogenesis of T2DM and includes defects at β-cell, muscle, liver, adipocyte, gastrointestinal tract, α-cell, kidney, and central nervous system.

21. **What is thrifty genotype hypothesis?**

The thrifty genotype hypothesis was proposed by James Neel. According to this hypothesis, certain genes involved in insulin release and consequently fat storage, were naturally selected during the period of nutrient excess to provide survival advantage at the time of nutrient scarcity. But in the present scenario, with sustained availability of food, these putative genes have an adverse impact leading to obesity, insulin resistance and diabetes.

22. **What is thrifty phenotype hypothesis?**

The thrifty phenotype hypothesis was proposed by David Barker and is also called as "fetal origin of adult diseases." It states that intrauterine malnutrition leads not only to poor fetal growth but also to defective metabolic programming. This altered metabolic programming is a consequence of epigenetic and oxidative stress during intrauterine life leading to increased visceral fat, overactive counter-regulatory hormones and insulin resistance. The intrauterine malnutrition if combined with postnatal nutritional excess predisposes to obesity and metabolic syndrome. This stresses the role of optimal maternal nutrition during gestation, and children born small for gestational age should not be overfed.

23. **What are the animal models of T2DM?**

The animal models of T2DM combine two pathophysiologic features, namely, obesity-associated insulin resistance and β-cell dysfunction. The common animal models for obesity-associated insulin resistance and T2DM include agouti mouse, leptin and leptin receptor mutant mice, New Zealand obese mice, and Zucker diabetic fatty rats, whereas the animal models having predominantly β-cell dysfunction include AKITA mice and GK rat.

24. **What are the monogenic forms of diabetes associated with insulin resistance?**

The monogenic forms of diabetes associated with insulin resistance include disorders associated with either insulin receptor abnormalities or defect in adipogenesis. The causes include leprechaunism, Rabson–Mendenhall syndrome, congenital partial lipoatrophy (the Dunnigan or Kobberling–Dunnigan syndrome), congenital generalized lipoatrophy (Seip–Berardinelli syndrome), and mutation in peroxisome proliferator-activated receptor-γ (PPAR-γ).

25. **What are the monogenic forms of diabetes associated with defective insulin secretion?**

The monogenic forms of diabetes associated with defective insulin secretion include maturity-onset diabetes of the young (pancreatic transcription factor defects, β-cell enzyme defects), mitochondrial diabetes (mitochondrial dysfunction) and mutant insulin syndromes (mutation in insulin/proinsulin gene).

26. **What are the candidate genes for T2DM?**

T2DM is a polygenic disease, and multiple gene defects combined with environmental factors contribute to the development of the disease. The defects may be in insulin biosynthesis, insulin secretion, insulin receptor, post-receptor signaling pathway, or adipogenesis. The common putative genes are calpain-10, Kir6.2, peroxisome proliferator-activated receptor-γ, hepatocyte nuclear factor-4α, FTO, and transcription factor 7-Like 2 (TCF7L2). The TCF7L2 involved in insulin secretion is the most common implicated gene. These genes were identified by genome-wide association studies (GWAS). However, the contribution of these genes to the risk of developing diabetes is meagre.

27. **How to diagnose diabetes?**

The specific cutoffs to diagnose diabetes include fasting plasma glucose (FPG) ≥126 mg/dl (after 8–10 h of overnight fast) or random plasma glucose (RPG) ≥200 mg/dl with presence of symptoms (polyuria, polydipsia, and weight loss) or 2-h PG post-glucose load ≥200 mg/dl or HbA1c ≥6.5%. These values need to be confirmed subsequently, if equivocal except in those who are having symptoms/hyperglycemic crisis with random plasma glucose ≥200 mg/dl. However, the time frame for reconfirmation is not clear. Among FPG, RPG and 2h-PG post glucose load, fasting plasma glucose is most reproducible as it depends on hepatic glucose output which is fairly constant in an individual. 2-h PG post-glucose load is considered as the "gold standard" for the diagnosis; however, it is cumbersome. The random plasma glucose has diagnostic value only in the presence of symptoms as it is influenced by physical activity and meal constituents.

28. **What is the rationale for specific cutoffs of blood glucose to diagnose diabetes?**

The specific cutoffs of fasting plasma glucose and 2 h PG post-glucose load for the diagnosis of diabetes are based on the risk of development of diabetes-specific complication, diabetic retinopathy, in genetically predisposed individuals (Pima Indians, Hispanics, and Egyptian population). Furthermore, 2h PG post-glucose load ≥200 mg/dl has been shown to corroborate with an increased risk of cardiovascular events in various epidemiological and observational studies.

29. **Why is retina believed to be "mirror of diabetes"?**

Among all micro- and macrovascular complications of diabetes, diabetic retinopathy is considered to be the "mirror of diabetes". This is because the retinal changes associated with diabetes are unique to diabetes and not caused by any other disorders. Further, it can be easily diagnosed by ophthalmoscopy. Diabetic nephropathy is a also a diabetes-specific complication; however, non-diabetic renal disease commonly contribute to renal dysfunction in patients with diabetes. Hence, renal biopsy is required for the confirmation of diabetic nephropathy. Neuropathy is not considered as a specific complication of diabetes as multiple factors can contribute to its development including age, nutritional factors, and alcohol. Although macrovascular complications, especially cardiovascular diseases, are the major cause for morbidity and mortality in patients with type 2 diabetes, they are the manifestation of extensive and accelerated atherosclerosis which is contributed not only by hyperglycemia but also by other risk factors including hypertension, dyslipidemia, and aging.

30. **What is the utility of HbA1c in the diagnosis of diabetes?**

An HbA1c ≥6.5% is used to establish a diagnosis of diabetes. Estimation of HbA1c has numerous advantages over blood glucose for the diagnosis of diabetes. It is a marker of chronic hyperglycemia, has greater pre-analytical stability and does not require fasting or administration of glucose load. In addition, a single blood sample which can be taken at any time of day adds to convenience. The disadvantages of HbA1c are lower diagnostic sensitivity (44%), increased cost, limited utility in the presence of hemoglobinopathies, anemia, azotemia and pregnancy, and ethnic variability due to varying rate of glycation of hemoglobin. Further, the HbA1c assay also needs standardization according to the DCCT/UKPDS standards.

31. **When HbA1c should not be used for the diagnosis of diabetes?**

HbA1c is less reliable for the diagnosis of diabetes in patients with short duration of hyperglycemia (e.g. type 1 diabetes), anemia, azotemia and hemoglobinopathies and in pregnant women.

32. **Which test is considered as the reference standard for the diagnosis of diabetes?**

The 2-h PG post-glucose load >200mg/dl is considered as the reference standard for the diagnosis of diabetes because it best correlates with diabetic retinopathy, macrovascular disease, and HbA1c. However, it is cumbersome, has poor reproducibility and is used mainly for research purposes. The sensitivity and specificity of fasting plasma glucose and HbA1c as compared to the reference standard (2-h plasma glucose post-glucose load) for the diagnosis of diabetes are summarized in the table given below.

Tests	Sensitivity (%)	Specificity (%)
Fasting plasma glucose	50	95
HbA1c cutoff ≥6.5%	44	79

33. **A 45-year-old man was incidentally detected to have FPG of 128 mg/dl. On evaluation, his HbA1c was 6.2%. How to interpret?**

An HbA1c cutoff of 6.5% has a sensitivity of 44% to establish the diagnosis of diabetes, while FPG has a sensitivity of 50% in relation to the standard reference test of 2-h PG post-glucose load. In such discrepant situations, a repeat FPG and HbA1c should be performed. His repeat FPG was 130 mg/dl and

HbA1c was 6.3%. Therefore, in the index case, the diagnosis of diabetes should be considered as 2 values of FPG are >126 mg/dl. The lower sensitivity of HbA1c for the diagnosis of diabetes may be because of its inability to reflect minor swings in blood glucose in early diabetes.

34. **Who should be screened for diabetes?**

    Screening for type 2 diabetes is recommended in all adults who are overweight (BMI ≥23kg/m^2 for Asians or ≥25kg/m$_2$ for other races) and have one additional risk factor like sedentary life style, dyslipidemia, hypertension, cardiovascular disease and family history of diabetes. It is also recommended in women with previous history of gestational diabetes, macrosomia or in those with history of polycystic ovarian disease. Screening for diabetes is also indicated in all adults >45 years of age, irrespective of risk factors. Those with a normal screening test should be rescreened at an interval of 3 years.

35. **Why to screen for T2DM?**

    Screening for T2DM is cost-effective as treating diabetes is less expensive than treating its complications. Nearly 50% of patients with T2DM are asymptomatic at the time of diagnosis, and screening helps to identify these individuals. Screening also helps to identify subjects with prediabetes, and thereby provides an opportunity to intervene for the prevention of diabetes and diabetes-related complications.

36. **Why estimation of blood glucose by glucometer is not preferred for the diagnosis of diabetes?**

    Glucometers estimate capillary blood glucose and results are corrected to venous plasma glucose. However, high variability in glucose results between different glucometers and poor precision precludes their use for the diagnosis of diabetes mellitus.

37. **What is the difference between whole venous blood and venous plasma glucose?**

    The whole venous blood glucose is approximately 10–15% lower than venous plasma glucose. This is because 20% of blood volume constituted by proteins (4.8% plasma proteins and 15.2% RBC proteins) is inaccessible to glucose. Therefore, if blood water has a glucose concentration of 90mg/dl, the whole venous blood will have a glucose concentration of 72 mg/dl (as it consists of both plasma protein and RBC protein), and whole venous plasma will have a glucose concentration of 83mg/dl (as it consists of only plasma protein). Both WHO and ADA recommends the use of plasma glucose for the diagnosis of diabetes.

38. **When to suspect MODY?**

MODY should be suspected in those individuals with onset of diabetes <25 years of age with strong family history of diabetes particularly in three successive generations with onset of disease <40 years of age. In addition, absence of ketosis, lack of features of insulin resistance, and response to sulfonylureas for initial 2 years also supports a diagnosis of MODY in a patient with young onset diabetes. MODY must be differentiated from T1DM and young onset T2DM. The presence of ketosis/ketoacidosis, requirement of insulin since the diagnosis, lack of family history of diabetes, undetectable C peptide, and islet antibody positivity supports a diagnosis of T1DM, whereas the presence of obesity, features of insulin resistance, family history of diabetes and response to metformin suggests T2DM. Although there are thirteen forms of MODY, the common six types with their characteristics are summarized in the table given below.

Type	Genetic defect	Phenotype	Treatment
1	Hepatocyte nuclear factor-4α	Macrosomia Transient neonatal hypoglycemia, Hypotriglyceridemia, raised HDL-C	Sulfonylurea
2	Glucokinase gene	Mild hyperglycemia, Non-progressive	Life style modifications
3	Hepatocyte nuclear factor-1α	Most common	Sulfonylurea
4	Insulin promoter factor 1 (IPF/PDX1)	Pancreatic agenesis	Insulin
5	Hepatocyte nuclear factor-1β	Pancreatic atrophy, Urogenital anomalies	Insulin
6	Neurogenic differentiation factor-1	Very rare	Insulin

39. **Why maturity-onset diabetes in the young, despite having defect in β-cell, does not present with ketosis/ketoacidosis? Why patients with MODY do not manifest ketosis/ketoacidosis, despite defects in β-cell function?**

MODY, the most common form of monogenic diabetes is due to mutations in the genes involved in pancreatic embryogenesis, β-cell function, or glucose sensing. Despite this, patients with MODY do not manifest ketosis/ketoacidosis as they do not have absolute insulin deficiency. However, there are anecdotal case reports of ketosis/ketoacidosis in patients with MODY, particularly in those with advanced duration of disease.

40. **Why is it important to diagnose MODY?**

Maturity-onset diabetes in the young occurs due to defect in insulin secretion rather than insulin resistance. Hence, these patients respond well to therapy with sulfonylureas/insulin, and insulin sensitizers like metformin and pioglitazone are less effective. The risk of developing both microvascular and macrovascular complications is possibly simliar to patients with T2DM, except in MODY2 (glucokinase gene defect), where mild hyperglycemia poses lesser risk. Further, diagnosis of MODY is important in genetic counseling.

41. **Why do some patients with prediabetes/early diabetes present with postprandial hypoglycemia?**

The earliest abnormality in T2DM is impaired pulsatile insulin secretion, followed by loss of glucose-mediated first phase insulin secretion and subsequently, delayed and prolonged second phase insulin secretion. This delayed and prolonged second phase of insulin secretion may result in relative hyperinsulinemia which can manifest as postprandial hypoglycemia.

42. **What are the pitfalls in ADA/EASD guidelines for the management of T2DM?**

Guidelines by ADA/EASD are helpful in the comprehensive management of patients with T2DM in a systematic manner; however, they are fraught with several limitations. The guidelines fail to address strategies aimed at preservation of β-cell function/mass or maintenance of glycemic durability. The strong recommendation of metformin as a first-line drug is based on data from limited number of patients in UKPDS. Further, there is no specific recommendation for add-on therapy to metformin in the second tier. The recommendation to include SGLT2 inhibitors in the second tier appears to be less justified due to lack of long term safety data.

43. **A 44-year-old obese male, was incidentally detected to have T2DM with fasting blood glucose 150 mg/dl and HbA1c 8%. He had no diabetes-related complications. He insists on avoiding medications. How to manage?**

Lifestyle modification (LSM) is an integral part of management of T2DM, and includes medical nutritional therapy and physical activity. Lifestyle modification is effective in reducing HbA1c by 1–2% and is effective irrespective of duration of diabetes; however, it is difficult to sustain. The medical nutrition therapy focuses on limited intake of carbohydrate, trans fats, and saturated fat (<7%) and promotes high fiber intake. Recommended physical activity includes at least 150 min/week of moderate aerobic exercise, and twice weekly resistance training. In the index patient, a trial of lifestyle modification can be advised with estimation of HbA1c after 12 weeks. However, it needs to be emphasized that early institution of metformin is associated with improved glycemic control over time and reduced long-term complications.

44. **What is the use of artificial sweeteners in the management of diabetes?**

Artificial sweeteners are low-calorie substitutes for sucrose and helps in weight reduction and management of hypertriglyceridemia in patients with T2DM.

The commonly available FDA approved non-nutritive sweeteners are saccharin, aspartame and sucralose. Saccharin was the first non nutritive sweetener which was FDA approved; however, there have been concerns about bladder carcinogenesis in rats with its use. Aspartame consists of two amino acids, aspartic acid and phenylalanine and is 180 times as sweet as sucrose. However, it cannot be used for baking or cooking as it is heat labile. Sucralose, a potent natural sweetener, is approximately 1,000 times as sweet as sucrose. However, its use is associated with alteration in gut flora. The other FDA-approved non-nutritive sweeteners include acesulfame, neotame and advantame.

45. **Can exercise improve insulin sensitivity without weight loss?**

Yes. Exercise does improve insulin sensitivity even without weight loss. The immediate effect of exercise on glucose uptake is predominantly mediated through insulin-independent mechanisms like NO-mediated enhanced muscle blood flow, and increased intracellular AMP. The increase in intracellular AMP activates AMP kinase which promotes GLUT4 translocation. Long-term exercise training is associated with increase in type IIa muscle fiber, increased capillary density, mitochondrial number, and GLUT4 expression and translocation which results in improvement in insulin sensitivity.

46. **How to advice a patient with T2DM regarding exercise?**

Before recommending an exercise program to a patient with T2DM a detailed history and examination should be performed to evaluate for loss of protective sensations, diabetic retinopathy, and cardiac function. A combination of both aerobic exercise (e.g. walking, cycling and swimming) and resistance training (e.g. weight bearing exercise) is advocated as aerobic exercise improves hepatic and peripheral insulin resistance, while resistance training improves hepatic insulin resistance and lean muscle mass. The exercise program is said to be effective if the performer achieves 70% of the target heart rate, i.e., [(220-age) × 70%] or sweats during exercise.

47. **Why is metformin considered as the first-line drug for the management of patients with T2DM?**

An ideal drug for the management of T2DM should target the pathophysiology, achieve good glycemic control with durability, have minimal side effects, long-term safety data, and should be inexpensive. Metformin fulfills many of these criteria as it targets insulin resistance, reduces HbA1c by 1.5–2%, is weight neutral with virtually no risk of hypoglycemia, has long-term safety data including cardiovascular safety, and is inexpensive. Metformin increases the activity of adenosine monophosphate (AMP) kinase in the liver and muscle. The activated AMP kinase in the liver inhibits acetyl-CoA carboxylase (ACC) and sterol regulatory element-binding protein (SREBP-1c) decreasing lipolysis, hepatic steatosis, and hepatic insulin resistance, thereby reducing hepatic glucose output. It also increases muscle glucose transport through the activation of muscle AMP kinase. Metformin decreases the intestinal absorption of glucose and promotes peripheral glucose utilization through anaerobic glycolysis. The cardioprotective effect of metformin, as demonstrated in UKPDS, is mediated through improved lipid profile, decreased plasminogen activator inhibitor type 1 activity, and reduced hyperinsulinemia.

48. **Why metformin therapy is not associated with increased risk of hypoglycemia?**

    Metformin therapy is associated with minimal risk of hypoglycemia as it reduces circulating insulin levels because of improved insulin sensitivity. In addition, metformin has also been shown to increase glucagon in non-diabetic subjects; however, this effect may be less pronounced in individuals with T2DM.

49. **A 52-year-old obese male with type 2 diabetes for 5 years is on therapy with metformin 500 mg twice a day, with fasting blood glucose 100 mg/dl, HbA1c 7.1% and serum creatinine of 1.6 mg/dl. Should metformin be discontinued?**

    Metformin is excreted unchanged exclusively through the kidney. Use of metformin per se is not associated with worsening of renal function but may increase the risk of lactic acidosis in those with preexisting renal dysfunction. It may also increase the risk of renal dysfunction in patients who are dehydrated or undergoing radiocontrast study. Metformin is contraindicated when serum creatinine >1.5 mg/dl in men and >1.4 mg/dl in women. However, some recent literature demonstrates that the risk of lactic acidosis is very low even in patients with mild to moderate renal dysfunction. NICE guideline advocates continuation of full dose of metformin in patients with an estimated glomerular filtration rate (eGFR) of up to 45 ml/min, reduction in dose by 50% in those with eGFR between 45 and 30 ml/min, and discontinuation in those with eGFR <30 ml/min. In the index patient, his eGFR is 46 ml/min and hence can continue with metformin.

50. **A 62-year-old postmenopausal female with type 2 diabetes for 3 years, is on therapy with metformin 2 g/day, has HbA1c of 7.8%. She is skeptical of using sulfonylureas because of a previous hypoglycemic event. What to do next?**

    The available options for the management of the index patient include pioglitazone, DPP4 inhibitors, SGLT2 inhibitors and α-glucosidase inhibitors. Pioglitazone is a thiazolidinedione derivative with PPAR-ϒ (peroxisome proliferator-activated receptor-ϒ) agonist activity. It effectively reduces HbA1c by 1–1.5%, does not cause hypoglycemia, and preserves β-cell function. However, it increases the risk of atypical fracture (involving the distal fibula, tibia, and radius), particularly in postmenopausal women, due to its effect on the preferential diversion of primitive mesenchymal stem cells to adipocytes, rather than to osteoblast; hence, it should be avoided in the index patient. The preferred drugs, in the given patient, are DPP4 inhibitors, SGLT2 inhibitors or α-glucosidase inhibitors.

51. **A 58-year-old male with T2DM for 3 years, is on therapy with metformin 2 g/day, has HbA1c of 8.7%. He has congestive heart failure and is fearful of insulin. What to do next?**

    The available options include sulfonylureas, DPP4 inhibitors/GLP1 analogues, SGLT2 inhibitors and α-glucosidase inhibitors. Pioglitazone is contraindicated as it worsens heart failure due to fluid retention by stimulating sodium reabsorption from the collecting duct. The DPP4 inhibitor, saxagliptin, has been shown to increase the risk of heart failure whereas sitagliptin does not. GLP1 analogues have been shown to have a cardiovascular benefit, but limited data exists. Although α-glucosidase inhibitors are safe in patients with heart failure, their efficacy is modest. Limited data is available regarding the use of SGLT2 inhibitors in patients with heart failure. Hence, in this situation sulfonylureas or GLP1 analogues are the preferred drugs.

52. **What is the dosing schedule and time of administration of sulfonylureas?**

    The dosing schedule and time of administration of sulfonylureas is depicted in the table given below.

Sulfonylureas	Optimal doses (mg)	Maximal doses (mg)	Frequency of administration	Time of administration
Glibenclamide	10	20	OD/BD	30 min prior to meal
Glipizide	20	40	BD	30 min prior to meal
Gliclazide	160	320	BD	30 min prior to meal
Glimepiride	4	8	OD/BD	30 min prior to meal

53. **What should be the time of administration of antidiabetic drugs?**

    The time of administration of oral antidiabetic drugs and insulin is shown in the table given below.

Drugs	Time of administration
Sulfonylureas	30 min prior to meal
Metformin	With or after meals
Acarbose/voglibose	Just before major meals
Pioglitazone	Before meals but at fixed time
DPP4 inhibitors	Prior to meal
GLP1 agonists	Prior to meal
Regular insulin	30 min prior to meal
Short-acting insulin analogues	5 min prior to meal
Long-acting insulin analogues	
Glargine	Fixed time of day (8 am or 10 pm)
Degludec	Flexible (between 8 and 40 h)

54. **What is the HbA1c-reducing efficacy of various treatment modalities in the management of diabetes?**

The HbA1c-reducing efficacy of various treatment modalities in the management of T2DM is shown in the table given below.

Mode	HbA1c reduction
Lifestyle modification	1–2%
Sulfonylureas(SU)	1–1.5%
Metformin	1–1.5%
SU+metformin	1–1.5%
Pioglitazone	1–1.2%
DPP4 inhibitors	0.6–0.8%
GLP1 agonists	1–1.3%
Insulin	Unlimited

55. **A 52-year-old male well controlled (HbA1c 7.1%) with metformin, sulfonylurea, and pioglitazone presented with a history of sudden worsening of vision. What are the probabilities?**

Pioglitazone is associated with worsening of macular edema due to its fluid retention effect, and this can present with sudden worsening of vision. The probability of macular edema is higher in those with peripheral edema. Therapy includes discontinuation of pioglitazone and addition of spironolactone, which is more effective than loop diuretics in reducing macular edema. Other possibilities include retinal detachment, vitreous hemorrhage and central retinal artery/vein occlusion.

56. **Is the risk for bladder cancer with pioglitazone real?**

A possible association between bladder cancer and use of pioglitazone was first shown by the Prospective Pioglitazone Clinical Trial In Macrovascular Events (PROactive) trial. The French Caisse Nationale d'Assurance Maladie des Travailleurs Salaries (CNMTS) and US FDA adverse event reporting system showed an increased risk of bladder cancer with use of pioglitazone. The risk of bladder cancer was higher in those with a cumulative dose >28g and duration of use >2 years. Furthermore, animal studies also showed an increased risk of bladder cancer with high doses of pioglitazone. However, the Kaiser Permanente Northern California study and Taiwan National insurance database did not reveal an increased risk with the use of pioglitazone. Majority of patients who had bladder cancer developed it within 2 years of initiation of pioglitazone therapy, and this points to the role of pioglitazone in unmasking the disease rather than causing it. The proposed mechanisms for pioglitazone-induced bladder cancer in animals include chronic irritation of bladder mucosa due to abnormal urinary solidification and direct cytoproliferative effects of PPAR-ϒ receptors on urothelial cells. In the present clinical context, pioglitazone is to be avoided in those with a history of bladder cancer; however, more studies are required to evaluate the cause and effect relationship between use of pioglitazone and bladder cancer.

57. **What are the differences between GLP1 agonist and DPP4 inhibitors?**

Dipeptidyl-peptidase type 4 (DPP4) is an enzyme which is responsible for the degradation of endogenous incretins. DPP4 inhibitors prevent the degradation and increase the circulating level of endogenous incretins. GLP1 agonists are synthetic analogues of a naturally occurring GLP1, with longer duration of action and are resistant to degradation by DPP4. The differences between GLP1 agonist and DPP4 inhibitors are summarized in the table given below.

Properties	GLP1 agonist	DPP4 inhibitors
Mode of administration	Injectable	Oral
Increase in GLP1 level	10 fold	2–3 fold
Effect on satiety	Increased	None
Effect on weight	Weight loss (2–5 kg)	Weight neutral
HbA1c reduction	1–1.3%	0.6–0.8%
Gastric emptying	Delayed	No effect
Glycemic durability	Pronounced	Modest
Cardiovascular safety	Yes	Possibly safe

58. **How is the insulin secretion stimulated by DPP4 inhibitors different from sulfonylureas?**

Parameters	DPP4 inhibitors	Sulfonylureas
Insulin secretion	Glucose-dependent	Glucose-independent
Insulin biosynthesis	Increases	No effect
Risk of hypoglycemia	Mild	Severe
Proinsulin–insulin ratio	Favors insulin	Favors proinsulin
Inhibition of gllucagon secretion	Moderate	Mild
α-cell sensitivity to glucose	Restores	No effect
Improvement in β-cell mass	Possible	No
Effect on body weight	Neutral	Usually weight gain

59. **Why is therapy with DPP4 inhibitors/GLP1 analogues associated with low risk of hypoglycemia in patients with T2DM?**

Both DPP4 inhibitors and GLP1 analogues potentiate glucose-mediated insulin secretion, and as the blood glucose is reduced to 72 mg/dl, insulin secretion is suppressed. In addition, DPP-4 inhibitors restore α-cell sensitivity to glucose by increasing the level of GIP during hypoglycemia. Hence, therapy with these agents are associated with low risk of hypoglycemia.

60. **What are the differences between short-acting and long-acting GLP1 analogues?**

Short-acting GLP1 analogues have predominant effect on postprandial hyperglycemia through its effect on gastric emptying, while long-acting GLP1 analogues have predominant effects on fasting plasma glucose by inhibition of glucagon secretion. The short-acting analogues need to be administered twice daily, while long-acting GLP1 analogues can be given once daily to once weekly.

61. **What are the nondiabetic benefits of GLP1 analogues?**

GLP1 agonists have been used in patients with morbid obesity and polycystic ovarian disease. In addition, its potential role has been explored in numerous disorders including hypoglycemia after bariatric surgery, congestive cardiac failure, acute coronary syndrome, and osteoporosis. GLP1 causes weight loss by increasing satiety. The cardiac benefits of GLP1 agonists are mediated through improved lipid profile, decreased systolic blood pressure (as a result of increased atrial natriuretic peptide, vasodilatation), and reduced infarct size.

62. **Why incretin-mediated insulin secretion is glucose-dependent?**

Incretins act through G protein-coupled receptors (GPCR) present on β-cell and the downstream signaling pathway requires the presence of cyclic AMP for augmentation of glucose-mediated insulin secretion. The source of cyclic AMP (adenosine monophosphate) is intracellular ATP (adenosine triphosphate), which is generated following the entry of glucose into β-cell. When the blood glucose decreases to approximately 72mg/dl, glucose entry into β-cell is suppressed and ATP generation is inhibited, thereby restraining insulin secretion.

63. **Is there a risk of pancreatitis with incretin-based therapy?**

Patients with T2DM have an increased risk of pancreatitis. There are anecdotal case reports of pancreatitis with the use of DPP4 inhibitors and GLP1 agonists. However, the cause and effect relationship between pancreatitis and incretin-based therapies is not established. Recently, an autopsy study showed pancreatic ductal and periductal cell hyperplasia resulting in canalicular obstruction in patients who received incretin-based therapies. This observation may explain the occurrence of pancreatitis in patients receiving incretin-based therapies. However, this study had several limitations like small number of patients (n = 8), heterogeneity in age of study population, and presence of confounding variable like hypoxia, which per se may cause islet proliferation. Therefore, more data is required to make conclusive remarks about the risk of pancreatitis with the use of DPP4 inhibitors and GLP1 agonists.

64. **Is there a risk of pancreatic tumors with incretin therapy?**

GLP1 receptor has been demonstrated on both endocrine and exocrine pancreatic tissue. DPP4 inhibitors and GLP1 agonists have been shown to promote β-cell proliferation in rodent models. Theoretically, the long-term use of incretin-based therapy may induce β-cell proliferation and tumorigenesis in humans. A recent study showed the occurrence of pancreatic neuroendocrine tumor and glucagonoma in patients who received incretin-based therapies. However, these data require further substantiation.

65. **What is the rationale of combining GLP1 agonists and basal insulin?**

The rationale of combining GLP1 agonists and basal insulin is summarized in the table given below.

Characters	Basal insulin	GLP1 agonist
Targets	Insulin deficiency β-cell dysfunction	Incretin defect ? β-cell dysfunction/mass
FPG	Reduced ↓Hepatic glucose output	Reduced ↓Glucagon
PPG	Reduced ↑glucose uptake Skeletal muscle Adipocyte	Reduced ↑Glucose-dependent insulin secretion ↓Glucose-dependent glucagon secretion ↓Gastric emptying
Body weight	3–5 kg gain ↑Appetite ↑Adipogenesis	2–3 kg loss ↓Appetite ↑Satiety Delayed gastric emptying
Risk of hypoglycemia	Increased	Decreased Glucose-dependent insulin secretion Restoration of glucose–glucagon axis
Cardiovascular safety	Possibly neutral	Cardioprotective Decrease in SBP Favorable lipid profile

66. **What are SGLT2 inhibitors?**

Approximately 98% of the filtered glucose is reabsorbed in proximal convoluted tubule (PCT), while the rest is reabsorbed in the distal convoluted tubule and collecting ducts. SGLT2 (sodium-dependent glucose co-transporter 2) mediates 90% of the glucose reabsorbed in the S1 segment of PCT, while SGLT1 mediates 10% of glucose reabsorption in the S2 and S3 segment of PCT. It has been shown that SGLT2 is upregulated in patients with diabetes, and this has been included as one of the components of "ominous octet" in the pathogenesis of T2DM. SGLT2 inhibitors are a new class of drugs which suppresses 30–40% of glucose reabsorption in PCT, thereby resulting in glycosuria with loss of 300 Kcal (~75 g glucose) per day. The reduction in HbA1c achieved by this class of drug is around 0.6–0.9%. However, these drugs are less effective if eGFR is <45 ml/min or if baseline HbA1c is <7.7%, as this level of HbA1c corresponds with a blood glucose of 160–180 mg/dl which is equivalent to transport maximum (T_{max}) for glucose.

67. **What are the characteristics of SGLT2 inhibitors?**

SGLT2 inhibitors are unique antidiabetic drugs which selectively act on renal tubule, do not require the presence of insulin for their action and are effective irrespective of duration of diabetes. In addition, these drugs have a low risk of hypoglycemia, induce weight loss (2–3 kg), and can be combined with other classes of drugs like DPP4 inhibitors and metformin. Further, there is a reduction in the systolic blood pressure of 3–4 mmHg and diastolic BP of 2 mmHg.

68. **What are the concerns with SGLT2 inhibitors?**

Glycosuria promoted by SGLT2 inhibitors predisposes to genital fungal infections and urinary tract infections, and the risk is four-fold higher as compared to those who do not use SGLT2 inhibitors. There is also an increased incidence of falls and stroke in the elderly, possibly due to reduction in intravascular volume. There have been concerns for bladder carcinoma with the use of SGLT2 inhibitors, although the cause and effect relationship is not established. Further, it has been shown that in response to glucosuria there is a compensatory increase in hepatic glucose output, possibly due to elevated glucagon levels. In addition, modest increase in LDL cholesterol is also a concern with the use of SGLT2 inhibitors.

69. **What are the unique features of insulin glargine?**

Glargine is a "peakless" long-acting insulin analogue. The substitution of amino acid asparagine with glycine and the addition of two arginine molecules to the carboxyl-terminus of B-chain differentiate it from human insulin. Of the currently available insulins, it is the only insulin which has an acidic pH of 4 as against all others which have a neutral pH of 7. When insulin glargine is administered subcutaneously, it makes micro-precipitates in the alkaline pH of subcutaneous tissue, and insulin is released slowly into circulation. If insulin glargine is inadvertently administered intravenously, it will act like short-acting insulin, as it will not form micro-precipitates. Because of its acidic pH, it cannot be mixed with other insulins. It has duration of action of approximately 18–24 h, which allows a single daily dose; however, 10% of patients may require twice daily administration. Insulin glargine is usually used as basal insulin during night time to normalize fasting hyperglycemia. However, if it causes nocturnal hypoglycemia, it should be administered in the morning.

70. **What are the concerns with the use of insulin glargine?**

Many observational studies demonstrated an increased risk of cancer with the use of insulin glargine in patients with diabetes. This was further supported by in vitro data, which showed a higher mitogenic potential of insulin glargine as compared to human insulin, because of its higher affinity (10 times) for IGF1 receptors. However, this association was not supported by most meta-analysis and ORIGIN study. It was further shown that the insulin glargine is converted into two metabolites, M1 and M2, which has much lesser affinity for IGF1 receptor as compared to human insulin. Similarly, there was a fear of progression of diabetic retinopathy with insulin glargine due to its increased IGF1 receptor binding; however, this risk has been refuted.

71. **Which insulin is weight neutral?**

Insulin therapy is associated with weight gain as it promotes calorie retention (reduces glucosuria), adipogenesis, and sodium and water retention. However, insulin detemir is weight neutral possibly because of its direct effect on satiety center or a preferential action at hepatocytes than adipocytes. The use of insulin glargine is associated with lesser weight gain as compared to NPH insulin because of decreased risk of hypoglycemia, and consequently reduced inter-prandial snacking.

72. **What are the characteristics of insulin detemir?**

Insulin detemir is a long-acting insulin analogue with peak effects at 6–8 h and duration of action lasting 8–24 h. It differs from human insulin that amino acid at the 30th position is removed and a 14-carbon aliphatic fatty acid is added at the 29th position of B-chain of insulin. This modification increases the binding with albumin in circulation and prolongs its duration of action. In addition, minimal intra- and inter individual variability in absorption kinetics, absence of weight gain and low risk of hypoglycemia are other distinctive features of insulin detemir. Detemir has to be administered twice daily and ideally should not be mixed with other insulins.

73. **How does insulin degludec differ from glargine?**

Degludec a long-acting insulin analogue with deletion of last amino acid from the B-chain and addition of hexadecanedioic fatty acid at 29th position. However, it differs from glargine in that it has ultra long duration of action of nearly 40 h, is truly "peakless," has a neutral pH, flexibility of administration during anytime of the day between 8 and 40 h, and can be mixed with other insulins. Although the overall risk of nocturnal hypoglycemia is lesser with insulin degludec as compared to insulin glargine, the efficacy in terms of HbA1c reduction is similar. In addition, some studies suggest a relative increase in cardiovascular events with the use of degludec as compared to glargine. This was attributed to hyperinsulinemia due to degludec rather than intensive glycemic control.

74. **Why is insulin degludec long acting?**

The modification of an insulin molecule with deletion of last amino acid from B-chain and addition of hexadecanedioic fatty acid at 29th position creates dihexamers in the presence of phenol and zinc. When injected, phenol diffuses away, and this dihexamer is reorganized to multihexamer which prolongs the resident time of insulin in subcutaneous tissue. Further, with gradual diffusion of zinc, these multihexamers slowly dissociate into readily absorbable monomers.

75. **What is an ideal basal insulin?**

An ideal basal insulin should be able to provide a peakless and stable insulin levels for at least 24 hours, with minimal intra- and inter-individual variability, and minimal/no risk of hypoglycemia, weight gain and mitogenic potential.

76. **What is the utility of premixed insulin in the management of T2DM?**

Premixed insulin consists of short-acting and intermediate-acting insulin in a fixed ratio, which reduces the number of injections and increases patient's convenience. Premixed insulin therapy is less complex than basal-bolus regimen and provides both basal and pre-prandial insulin as a single injection. It is useful in patients with both fasting and post-prandial hyperglycemia, particularly in those with some residual endogenous β-cell reserve. Premixed insulin should be avoided in patients with T1DM, advanced duration of T2DM and in those with "brittle" diabetes as it leads to wide glycemic excursions in these patients. Premixed insulin analogues may be better than conventional premixed insulin for postprandial glucose control with reduced risk of hypoglycemia.

77. **When to initiate insulin in patients with type 2 diabetes at diagnosis?**

In patients with T2DM, insulin should be initiated at diagnosis in those with HbA1c >9%, osmotic symptoms, significant weight loss, fasting plasma glucose >200–250 mg/dl, ketosis/ketoacidosis, and in the presence of complications like infections, and acute coronary syndrome and significant hepatic or renal dysfunction.

78. **What is Monnier's hypothesis?**

Monnier's hypothesis dissects the contribution of fasting and postprandial hyperglycemia at different levels of HbA1C. At an HbA1C <7.3%, approximately 70% of the glycemic burden is contributed by post-prandial hyperglycemia, and the rest by fasting hyperglycemia, whereas at an HbA1C >10.2% approximately 70% of the glycemic burden is contributed by fasting hyperglycemia and the rest by post-prandial hyperglycemia. Both fasting and post-prandial hyperglycemia contributes equally to the glycemic burden in those with HbA1C between 7.3 and 10.2%.

79. **What should be targeted first in a patient with diabetes who have both fasting and postprandial hyperglycemia?**

In a patient with T2DM who has both fasting and post-prandial hyperglycemia, the HbA1c is likely to be >8% and at this level of glycemia, the contribution of fasting hyperglycemia is approximately 50% to the overall glycemic burden and it progressively increases with rising HbA1c. Hence, in these patients fasting plasma glucose should be targeted first. In addition, normalization of fasting plasma glucose also results in reduction of postprandial hyperglycemia as a "carryover" effect. In case of failure to control post-prandial hyperglycemia despite normalization of fasting plasma glucose, additional therapies are required to control post-prandial hyperglycemia. If post-prandial hyperglycemia is targeted first in patients with both fasting and post-prandial hyperglycemia, subsequent addition of therapy aimed to target fasting hyperglycemia may result in increased risk of post-prandial hypoglycemia.

80. **A 52-year-old man with type 2 DM of 8 year duration had FPG 170 mg/dl and HbA1c 8.9%. He is on metformin 2 g per day and glimepiride 4 mg per day. What to do next?**

This patient with long-standing T2DM is unable to achieve a target HbA1c <7% despite therapy with optimal doses of metformin and sulfonylureas. Failure to achieve glycemic control with advancing disease suggests progressive and inexorable nature of β-cell failure in patients with T2DM. The available options for the management of index patient includes increasing the doses of sulfonylurea/metformin, or addition of pioglitazone, DPP4 inhibitors, SGLT2 inhibitors, α-glucosidase inhibitors, GLP1 agonists or basal insulin. However, further increase in doses of sulfonylurea (glimepiride >4mg/day) or metformin (>2000 mg/day) has only modest effects on glycemia. The addition of DPP4 inhibitors, SGLT2 inhibitors or α-glucosidase inhibitors will decrease HbA1c only by 0.5–0.8%. Pioglitazone may be an option; however it may not help to achieve target HbA1c in this individual. Therefore, the addition of basal insulin, or long acting GLP-1 agonist will be the most appropriate measure to normalize fasting plasma glucose and HbA1c.

81. **When to add basal insulin?**

It is ideal to add basal insulin as early as possible because T2DM is also an insulin-deficient state. Various studies have demonstrated that use of insulin in newly diagnosed patients with T2DM even for 2–4 weeks resulted in early attainment of target HbA1c, stable glycemic control, and preservation of β-cell function over the next few years. In clinical practice, basal insulin is added either in second tier or third tier to control fasting hyperglycemia, especially if HbA1c is >8.5%.

82. **Who are the candidates for self-monitoring of blood glucose?**

Self-monitoring of blood glucose is an integral part of diabetes management and allows the participation of patient in diabetes care, helps to guide treatment decisions and response to therapy. Glycemic excursions can also be detected by the effective use of SMBG. All patients with T1DM or T2DM who are on intensive insulin therapy are advised SMBG before and after meals, bedtime, prior to exercise or driving and on suspicion of hypoglycemia. In addition patients with type 2 diabetes who are on less intensive insulin therapy are also candidates for SMBG, although the frequency of SMBG is not well defined. All women with gestational diabetes should also undergo SMBG.

83. **A 65-year-old male known diabetic for 10 years presented with urosepsis. On evaluation he had spot blood glucose of 360 mg/dl and HbA1C of 10.2%. How to manage hyperglycemia in this patient?**

In the index patient, a detailed evaluation should be performed to assess hemodynamic stability, sensorium, hydration status and complications of diabetes. Biochemical evaluation include blood glucose, renal function test, electrolytes, serum ketones, and arterial blood gas analysis. If the patient who is hemodynamically stable and is accepting orally, basal-bolus insulin regimen should be initiated, whereas patient who have hypotension/altered sensorium/ recurrent vomiting should be managed with insulin infusion. A good glycemic control helps in early recovery, and the targets of blood glucose in a non-critically ill patient are pre-meal values <140 mg/dl and random blood glucose <180 mg/dl. Use of sliding scale regimen with short-acting insulin alone should be discouraged as this regimen is invariably associated with marked swings in blood glucose profile. This patient was managed with basal-bolus insulin regimen, i.v. fluids, and parenteral antibiotics.

84. **How to manage hyperglycemia in a critically ill patient?**

Insulin is the preferred therapy for the management of critically ill patients with hyperglycemia. Although good glycemic control is important for early recovery, critically ill patients are at a higher risk of hypoglycemia when insulin therapy is initiated. Therefore, the recommended blood glucose target in this population is 140–180mg/dl. This can be accomplished by administration of intravenous insulin therapy in patients who are not allowed orally/not accepting orally. Addition of basal insulin (subcutaneous) to intravenous insulin regimen minimizes the swings in blood glucose, smoothens glycemic control and reduces the risk of hypokalemia. In patients who are on naso-gastric feed, hyperglycemia can be managed with basal-bolus regimen, preferably comprising of insulin analogues.

Suggested Reading

1. American Diabetes Association. Standards of medical care in diabetes—2014. Diabetes Care. 2014;37 Suppl 1:S14–80.
2. American Diabetes Association. Diagnosis and classification of diabetes mellitus. Diabetes Care. 2014;37 Suppl 1:S81–90.
3. Jameson JL, De Groot LJ. Endocrinology: adult and pediatric. Philadelphia: Elsevier Health Sciences; 2010.
4. Longo D, Fauci A, Kasper D, Hauser S, Jameson J, Loscalzo J. Harrison's principles of internal medicine. 18th ed. New York: McGraw Hill Professional; 2012.
5. Melmed S, Polonsky KS, Larsen PR, Kronenberg HM. Williams textbook of endocrinology: expert consult. London: Elsevier Health Sciences; 2011.
6. Rodbard HW, Jellinger PS, Davidson JA, Einhorn D, Garber AJ, Grunberger G, Handelsman Y, et al. Statement by an American Association of Clinical Endocrinologists/American College of Endocrinology consensus panel on type 2 diabetes mellitus: an algorithm for glycemic control. Endocr Pract. 2009;15(6):540–59.

Diabetes-Related Complications-I

18

18.1 Clinical Rounds

1. **What are the microvascular complications of diabetes?**

   Microvascular complications of diabetes include retinopathy, nephropathy, and neuropathy. These complications occur due to involvement of vessels which are <10 μm in size, hence the name "microvascular." Glucose entry in these tissues is insulin independent, and therefore these organs are predisposed for the deleterious effects of hyperglycemia. Microvascular complications are a function of duration of diabetes, and the risk is continuous at all levels of hyperglycemia. These complications do occur even in subjects with prediabetes, although at a much lower frequency (3–10%), as opposed to 50–90% of patients with diabetes.

2. **How does hyperglycemia induce microvascular damage?**

   Chronic hyperglycemia results in initiation of a cascade of events that eventually leads to microvascular damage. The details of these events are depicted in the figure given below.

A. Bhansali, Y. Gogate, *Clinical Rounds in Endocrinology: Volume I - Adult Endocrinology*, DOI 10.1007/978-81-322-2398-6_18

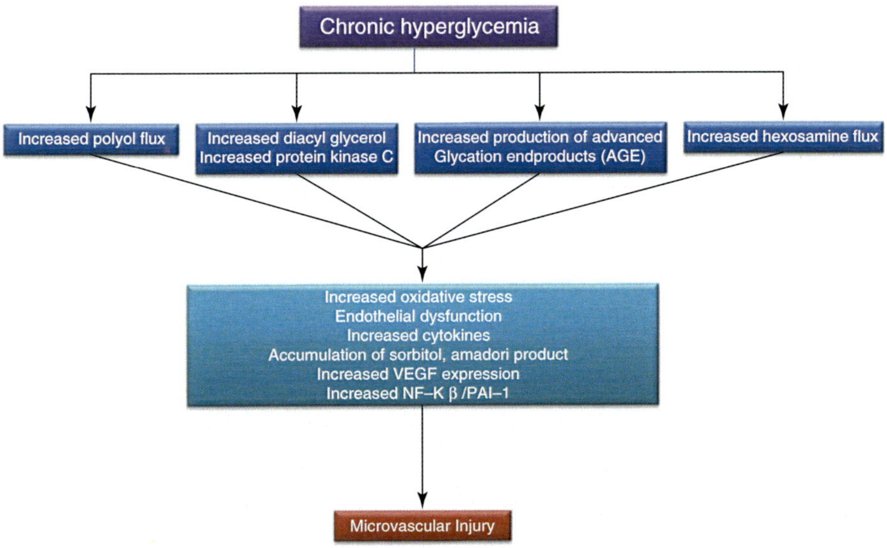

Fig. 18.1 Pathophysiology of hyperglycemia-mediated microvascular complications

3. **What are advanced glycosylation end products?**

   Advanced glycosylation end products are the result of nonenzymatic glycosylation of glucose with amino group of intra- and extracellular proteins or lipids. Early nonenzymatic glycosylation products (Schiff's base) are reversible; however, with chronic hyperglycemia, these products undergo Amadori rearrangement and finally lead to the formation of advanced glycosylation end products (AGEs). AGEs have been shown to interfere with cross-linking of proteins, reduce NO synthase, impair endothelial function, disrupt extracellular matrix composition and structure, and alter gene expression. These events eventually result in the onset and progression of diabetic micro- and macrovascular complications.

4. **Which is the most specific diabetes-related complication?**

   The most specific diabetes-related complication is diabetic retinopathy. It is considered as a mirror of hyperglycemic damage. The onset and severity of retinopathy directly correlates with duration and degree of hyperglycemia, as opposed to other microvascular complications like neuropathy and nephropathy, which are also influenced by non-glycemic factors. The incidence of diabetic retinopathy progressively increases from an HbA1c of 7 to 10% and plateau thereafter.

5. **What are the modalities useful in evaluation of diabetic retinopathy?**

   Ophthalmoscopic fundus examination with dilated pupil is the simplest and inexpensive initial workup. Fundus photography may be used for documentation and monitoring of diabetic retinopathy. Fluorescein angiography is indicated in patients with macular ischemia, painless loss of vision and for guiding treatment of clinically significant macular edema. Optical coherence tomography (OCT) is to be performed in those who have suspicion of macular edema.

6. **How to assess the severity of diabetic retinopathy?**

The severity of diabetic retinopathy is classified by Early Treatment Diabetic Retinopathy Study scale (ETDRS)/International Classification of Diabetic Retinopathy and Diabetic Macular Edema, after a detailed fundus examination with a dilated pupil. The presence of microaneurysm, soft exudates, intraretinal microvascular abnormalities, and venous beading constitutes non-proliferative diabetic retinopathy (NPDR). Proliferative diabetic retinopathy (PDR) is characterized by neovascularization (at disk or elsewhere), vitreous hemorrhage, and retinal detachment. Clinically significant macular edema (CSME) is characterized by retinal thickening and/or hard exudates within 500 μm from center of macula. CSME can occur with any stage of NPDR or PDR.

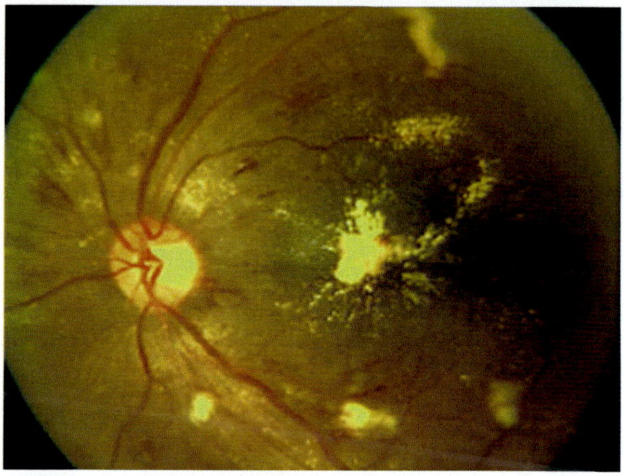

Fig. 18.2 Fundus photograph showing NPDR with CSME—multiple cotton-wool spots, retinal hemorrhages, and extensive hard exudates

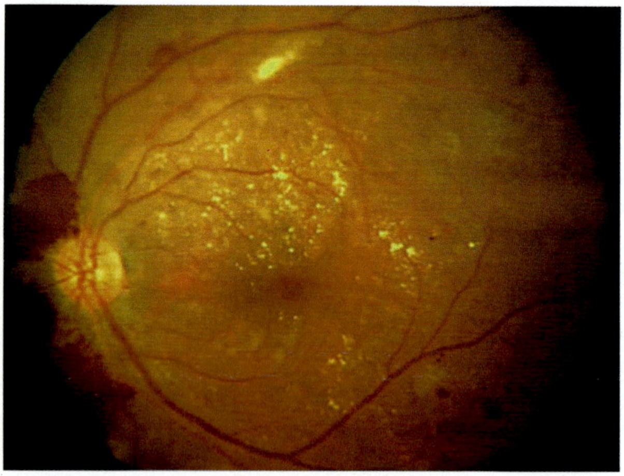

Fig. 18.3 Fundus photograph showing PDR with neovascularization of the disk (NVD) and preretinal hemorrhages

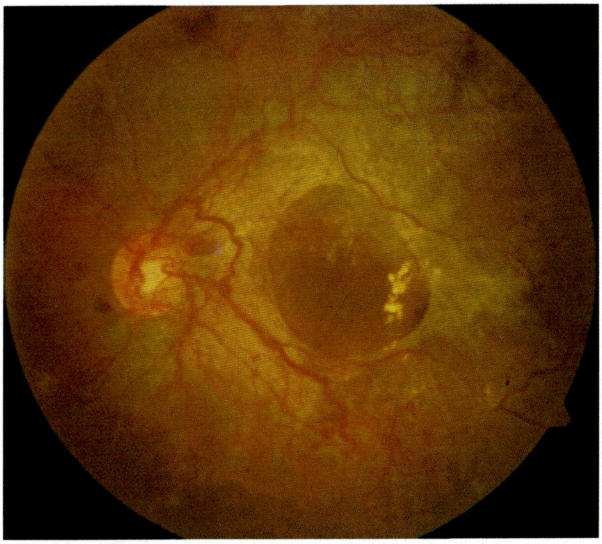

Fig. 18.4 Fundus photograph showing PDR with extensive fibrovascular proliferation and tractional retinal detachment (TRD)

7. **What are the nondiabetic causes of microaneurysm?**

   Microaneurysm is a result of outpouching of retinal vessel wall resulting from loss of pericytes, the supporting cells for retinal endothelial cells. The presence of >2 microaneurysm is considered as significant. Nondiabetic causes of microaneurysm include hypertension, iron deficiency anemia, sickle-cell anemia, leukemia, subacute bacterial endocarditis, systemic lupus erythematosus, and retinoblastoma. Microaneurysms are not only present in retina but also in the heart and kidney.

8. **What are the causes of painless loss of vision in a patient with diabetes?**

   Clinically significant macular edema (CSME), central retinal artery or vein occlusion, vitreous hemorrhage, and tractional retinal detachment are the causes of acute-onset painless loss of vision in a patient with diabetes. Cataract and chronic glaucoma are associated with gradual loss of vision.

9. **What are the differential diagnoses of ptosis in a patient with diabetes?**

   Ptosis in a patient with diabetes may be due to cranial mononeuropathy involving IIIrd nerve, cavernous sinus thrombosis (as a consequence of rhino-orbital mucormycosis), or rarely myasthenia gravis. Oculomotor nerve palsy in diabetes is associated with pupillary sparing due to preservation of peripherally placed pupillary nerve fibers, as opposed to their involvement in compressive lesions.

10. **What are the risk factors for progression of diabetic retinopathy?**

    The risk factors that contribute to progression of diabetic retinopathy are prolonged duration of hyperglycemia, hypertension, dyslipidemia, puberty, and pregnancy. Myopia is protective against the development of diabetic retinopathy. Vigorous exercise in a patient with severe NPDR or PDR may increase the risk of vitreous hemorrhage and retinal detachment.

11. **A 60-year-old male presented with acute coronary syndrome and is planned for thrombolytic therapy. He is a known diabetic for 15 years and has proliferative diabetic retinopathy. Is thrombolytic therapy contraindicated?**

    Neither thrombolytic therapy (streptokinase) nor antiplatelet treatment (aspirin) increases the risk of vitreous hemorrhage in patients with diabetic retinopathy. Hence, thrombolytic therapy can be safely administered in the index patient.

12. **What is the comprehensive therapy for diabetic retinopathy?**

    The specific treatment of diabetic retinopathy is photocoagulation; however, comprehensive management of diabetes is important to halt the progression of retinopathy. A good glycemic control (HbA1c <7%), optimal blood pressure control (140/90 mmHg, JNC VIII), correction of anemia, and use of statins and fenofibrate (can help in resolution of hard exudates), with appropriate focal photocoagulation in CSME or pan-retinal photocoagulation in severe NPDR/PDR, prevent the progression of diabetic retinopathy. ACE inhibitors/ARBs not only controls blood pressure but have an independent protective effect on diabetic retinopathy due to existence of local renin–angiotensin–aldosterone system in retina. A good comprehensive diabetes management has shown to reduce/eliminate the need for photocoagulation in 20–30% of patients with CSME.

13. **What is the role of anti-VEGF antibody in diabetic retinopathy?**

    Vascular endothelial growth factor (VEGF) is overexpressed in retinal microvasculature in patients with uncontrolled blood glucose and is responsible for neovascularization. Anti-VEGF antibodies like bevacizumab and ranibizumab have been shown to be useful in CSME and in selected patients with PDR.

14. **What are the antidiabetic medications to be avoided in patients with CSME?**

    Pioglitazone can worsen macular edema in patients with diabetes and hence should be avoided. In addition, intensive insulin therapy can also lead to worsening of CSME; therefore, aggressive glycemic control with insulin should be avoided in these patients.

15. **Why is there initial worsening of diabetic retinopathy with intensive glycemic control?**

    Intensive glycemic control is associated with initial worsening of diabetic retinopathy followed by stabilization and improvement. This initial worsening has been attributed to retinal hypoxia due to loss of glucose-mediated retinal vasodilatation and increased angiogenesis due to elevated IGF1 consequent to hyperinsulinemia.

16. **What is diabetic neuropathy?**

    Diabetic neuropathy is defined as any symptom and/or sign of nerve dysfunction in a patient with diabetes, after exclusion of other causes. This includes dysfunction of peripheral, cranial, or autonomic nerves.

17. **How to classify diabetic neuropathy ?**

    Diabetic neuropathy can be classified as generalized or focal/multifocal. Generalized symmetrical neuropathy is predominantly a result of hyperglycemia, while focal and multifocal neuropathies (except entrapment syndromes) are vascular in origin. The classification of diabetic neuropathy is summarized in the table given below.

Generalized symmetrical polyneuropathy

Acute sensory neuropathy
Chronic sensorimotor neuropathy (diabetic polyneuropathy)
  Small-fiber neuropathy
  Large-fiber neuropathy
Autonomic neuropathy

Focal and multifocal neuropathies
Focal-limb neuropathy—includes mononeuropathy and entrapment syndromes Cranial neuropathy Proximal-motor neuropathy (amyotrophy) Truncal radiculoneuropathy Coexisting chronic inflammatory demyelinating neuropathy

18. **What is large fiber neuropathy?**

    Large fibers are thick, myelinated nerve fibers comprising of Aα and Aβ fibers. Aα fibers innervate muscles and are involved in motor control, while Aα and Aβ accomplish sensory functions like touch, vibration, and proprioception. Involvement of large nerve fibers in diabetic neuropathy results in deep-seated gnawing pain, numbness, unsteadiness of gait, atrophy of intrinsic muscles of feet which manifests as foot deformities and slippage of footwear. As large fiber neuropathy is associated with loss of proprioception, it predisposes to foot ulceration.

19. **What is small fiber neuropathy?**

    Small fibers are thin, unmyelinated, or sparsely myelinated nerve fibers and comprise of Aδ and C fibers. Aδ fibers transmit pain and cold sensation, while

C fibers carry pain and warm sensation and regulate autonomic functions. Involvement of these fibers manifests as severe burning pain, paresthesia, allodynia, hyperalgesia, followed by loss of pain and temperature sensation, and autonomic dysfunction.

20. **What is aldose reductase?**

    Aldose reductase is the rate-limiting enzyme of polyol pathway, in which glucose is reduced to sorbitol by aldose reductase and sorbitol is further oxidized to fructose by sorbitol dehydrogenase. Aldose reductase activity is upregulated by hyperglycemia, resulting in depletion of intracellular NADPH and NAD^+. Depletion of NADPH results in decreased synthesis of reduced glutathione, nitric oxide, and myoinositol, while increased $NADH/NAD^+$ ratio leads to formation of AGEs and activation of protein kinase C pathway. All these events contribute to tissue damage by free radical injury. Intensive treatment with insulin normalizes blood glucose, thereby decreasing aldose reductase activity. Aldose reductase inhibitors have been tried in the management of diabetic retinopathy and neuropathy, without much success.

21. **Is diabetic neuropathy reversible?**

    Cranial mononeuropathies (III, IV, VI, and VII) and diabetic amyotrophy are reversible, as they are vascular in origin. In addition, truncal radiculoneuropathy also resolves spontaneously within 4–6 months. Further, neuropathy associated with acute metabolic decompensation like severe hyperglycemia or hypoglycemia (insulin neuritis) is also reversible.

22. **What is diabetic amyotrophy?**

    Diabetic amyotrophy is a misnomer as it is not a primary muscle disease; rather it is a lumbosacral radiculoplexopathy. Classically, it involves middle-aged men with long-standing diabetes and poor glycemic control. Patients present with severe pain in thigh, which is commonly unilateral (but may also be bilateral) and asymmetrical proximal muscle weakness of lower limb, followed by muscle atrophy. It is usually accompanied with weight loss. Nerve conduction study shows axonopathy, while electromyography is suggestive of denervation. Nerve histology demonstrates epineural vasculitis. Intensive glycemic control and physiotherapy may hasten recovery. Methylprednisolone, intravenous immunoglobulins and plamsapharesis have been tried. These immunomodulatory therapies may help in relieving pain and sensory symptoms; however, do not result in early recovery. The disorder is self-limiting, but the recovery is usually incomplete.

23. **Why is there glove and stocking pattern of sensory involvement in diabetic neuropathy?**

    Chronic sensorimotor neuropathy is the most common form of diabetic neuropathy and is characterized by distal and symmetrical involvement, also called as glove and stocking pattern. This is due to length-dependent involvement of nerve fibers, where longest nerve fibers are predominantly involved. This also explains the development of neuropathic signs and symptoms in lower limbs earlier than in upper limbs. The differential diagnosis of chronic sensorimotor neuropathy includes B_1, and B_{12} deficiency, toxin intake (e.g., alcohol, B_6 overdose), and paraproteinemia.

24. **What are the tests to assess diabetic peripheral neuropathy?**

    Ankle reflex, tuning fork, and monofilament test are simple bedside tests for the assessment of large fiber neuropathy, whereas testing for pain, touch, and temperature sensation is used for small fiber neuropathy. Ankle reflex has good sensitivity, but poor specificity for the diagnosis of large fiber neuropathy. The 10-g monofilament (Semmes–Weinstein) is a good tool to identify the foot at risk for ulceration with a sensitivity of 86–100%. Quantitative assessment of large fiber neuropathy can be performed by vibration perception threshold whereas pain and thermal perception thresholds is used for small fiber neuropathy. Vibration perception threshold (VPT) is sensitive modality for the diagnosis of large fiber neuropathy. A vibration perception threshold >25 V is considered as abnormal and is the strongest predictor of foot ulceration.

25. **How to detect early diabetic neuropathy?**

    Quantitative sensory tests for vibration (VPT), pain and temperature can diagnose even subclinical neuropathy. In addition, corneal confocal microscopy and skin biopsy with PGP 9.5 immunostaining can also help in detection of early small-fiber neuropathy in patients with diabetes.

26. **When to perform nerve conduction study in a patient with diabetes?**

    Nerve conduction study (NCS) is not indicated for the routine diagnosis of diabetic sensorimotor neuropathy. However, NCS can be helpful in detecting subclinical neuropathy, non-diabetic neuropathy superimposed on diabetic neuropathy (e.g., chronic inflammatory demyelinating polyneuropathy), and focal neuropathies, which include diabetic amyotrophy and entrapment neuropathies. In addition, NCS may be useful in quantifying and monitoring the progression of disease in clinical trials.

27. **What is insulin neuritis?**

    Insulin neuritis is a severe painful neuropathy seen in patients with uncontrolled type1 or type 2 diabetes, after intensive glycemic control. This usually occurs after initiation of insulin, although it has also been described with oral antidiabetic drugs. "Insulin neuritis" is usually reversible. The proposed mechanisms include endoneurial ischemia (as a part of steal phenomenon), hypoglycemia-induced microvascular neuronal damage, and abnormal discharges from the regenerating nerves.

28. **Why is diabetic neuropathy painful?**

    Painful neuropathy is present in 10% of patients with diabetes. Painful neuropathy can be classified based on duration of symptoms as acute (<6 months) or chronic (>6 months). Pain associated with diabetic neuropathy is due to hyperglycemia-mediated injury to afferent nerve fibers which result in formation of abnormal pulse generator that dysrhythmically discharge impulses, even in the absence of stimuli. Increased concentration of sodium channels is partly responsible for the abnormal firing of these neurons. In addition, damaged afferent nerves also become sensitive to norepinephrine. There is also decreased pain threshold in patients with diabetes due to disinhibition of central nociceptive neurons and decreased opioid tone due to hyperglycemia.

29. **How to treat painful diabetic neuropathy?**

Pain associated with diabetic neuropathy is mediated through Aδ and C nerve fibers and is modulated at the level of spinal cord and cortex. Drugs which target C fiber-mediated pain include capsaicin and clonidine. Capsaicin depletes axonal substance P, while clonidine inhibits norepinephrine-mediated impulse generation in C fibers. Pregabalin, other anticonvulsants, and tricyclic antidepressants (e.g., amitriptyline) target Aδ fibers by modulating Na^+ channels, thereby inhibiting impulse conduction. Selective serotonin reuptake inhibitors (e.g., fluoxetine) and serotonin and norepinephrine reuptake inhibitors (e.g., duloxetine) act at cortical level and enhance central pain inhibitory system. Tramadol increases central opioid tone and is useful in reducing pain. In addition, good glycemic control should be aimed to reduce the severity of pain and to target the pathogenic mechanism. The role of α-lipoic acid and other antioxidants is limited.

30. **What is the role of C-peptide in diabetic peripheral neuropathy?**

Neuropathy is more severe in patients with T1DM than in T2DM, at similar levels of hyperglycemia. This suggests a role of C-peptide in the pathogenesis of diabetic peripheral neuropathy. C-peptide treatment in diabetic BB rat resulted in improved nerve conduction velocity, axo-glial function, and normalization of para-nodal demyelination. However, data in humans are limited.

31. **What are the clinical implications of cardiac autonomic neuropathy?**

Resting tachycardia (heart rate 90/min), impaired exercise tolerance, and orthostatic hypotension suggest the presence of cardiac autonomic neuropathy in a patient with diabetes. Patients with cardiac autonomic neuropathy are at an increased risk for ventricular arrhythmias, diabetic cardiomyopathy and have higher perioperative morbidity and mortality. In addition, these patients are predisposed for sudden death.

32. **How does clonidine help in the management of orthostatic hypotension?**

Clonidine acts on central presynaptic α-2 adrenergic receptors and inhibits central sympathetic tone, thereby leading to reduction in blood pressure. In periphery, clonidine acts on postsynaptic α-2 adrenergic receptors and causes vasoconstriction and increases venous return. As the central action predominates, clonidine is used as an antihypertensive agent. In patients with autonomic neuropathy, as central sympathetic outflow is inhibited, the peripheral action of clonidine predominates, thereby resulting in improvement in orthostatic hypotension.

33. **When to clinically suspect gastroparesis?**

A diabetic patient presenting with postprandial fullness, early satiety, nausea/vomiting, and wide fluctuations in blood glucose should be suspected to have diabetic gastroparesis. The most common cause of gastroparesis is autonomic neuropathy. In addition, uncontrolled blood glucose, ketosis, dyselectrolytemia, and use of drugs like tricyclic antidepressants, calcium channel blockers, and DPP4 inhibitors/GLP1 agonists may also cause transient gastroparesis. Treatment includes small frequent meals and use of prokinetic agents (e.g., dopamine antagonists and motilin agonists).

34. **What are the characteristics of diabetic diarrhea?**

Diarrhea is not an uncommon complication in patients with long-standing uncontrolled diabetes. Diabetic diarrhea is typically painless and intermittent, may alternate with constipation, occurs more frequently at night ("nocturnal diarrhea"), and may be accompanied with fecal incontinence. The stools are watery and voluminous, and may be accompanied with steatorrhoea. Despite frequent bowel movements, weight loss is not a feature of diabetic diarrhea, unless accompanied with steatorrhoea. The pathogenic mechanisms implicated in diabetic diarrhea include autonomic neuropathy, bacterial overgrowth, bile acid malabsorption, pancreatic exocrine insufficiency, and possibly altered gut-hormone secretion, e.g., motilin and cholecystokinin. The other causes of diarrhea in a patient with diabetes include celiac disease and drugs like metformin and acarbose.

35. **How does clonidine help in the management of diabetic diarrhea?**

Clonidine is an α-2 adrenergic receptor agonist. It is helpful in the management of diabetic diarrhea due to autonomic neuropathy. α-2 adrenergic receptors regulates water and electrolyte reabsorption and secretion in small intestine; in normal individuals the net balance is in favor of absorption. However, in patients with long-standing diabetes with autonomic neuropathy, secretion exceeds the absorption because of the loss of adrenergic tone. Clonidine restores adrenergic tone, and this results in net absorption of water and electrolytes, thereby decreasing stool frequency.

36. **What are the manifestations of diabetic cystopathy?**

The earliest symptom of diabetic cystopathy is decrease in frequency of urination due to impaired bladder sensations. In addition, urinary retention, overflow incontinence, and recurrent urinary tract infections may be the presenting manifestation. Post-void residual volume (>150 ml) suggests cystopathy. Cystometry and voiding cystometrogram are useful for the confirmation of diagnosis. Treatment includes frequent voiding, acetylcholine receptor agonist (e.g., bethanechol), or α-blocker (e.g., doxazosin).

37. **What is diabetic foot?**

Diabetic foot can be defined as abnormalities of peripheral nerves, vessels, bones, joints, or soft tissues of foot, due to persistent hyperglycemia, with or without infection or breach in continuity of skin in a patient with diabetes. This definition also encompasses the foot at risk.

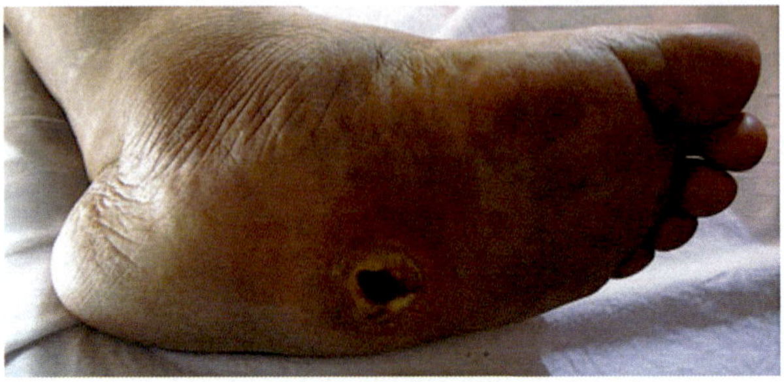

Fig. 18.5 Rocker bottom deformity with a neuropathic ulcer

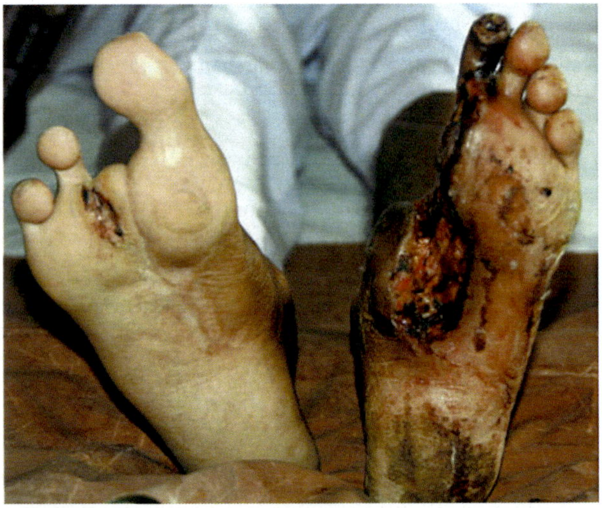

Fig. 18.6 Left foot with nonhealing ulcer and digital gangrene, predominantly of vascular etiology. Small ulcer below the base of fourth toe and a callosity over the head of first metatarsal in right foot, suggestive of neuropathic etiology. Note amputation of two toes

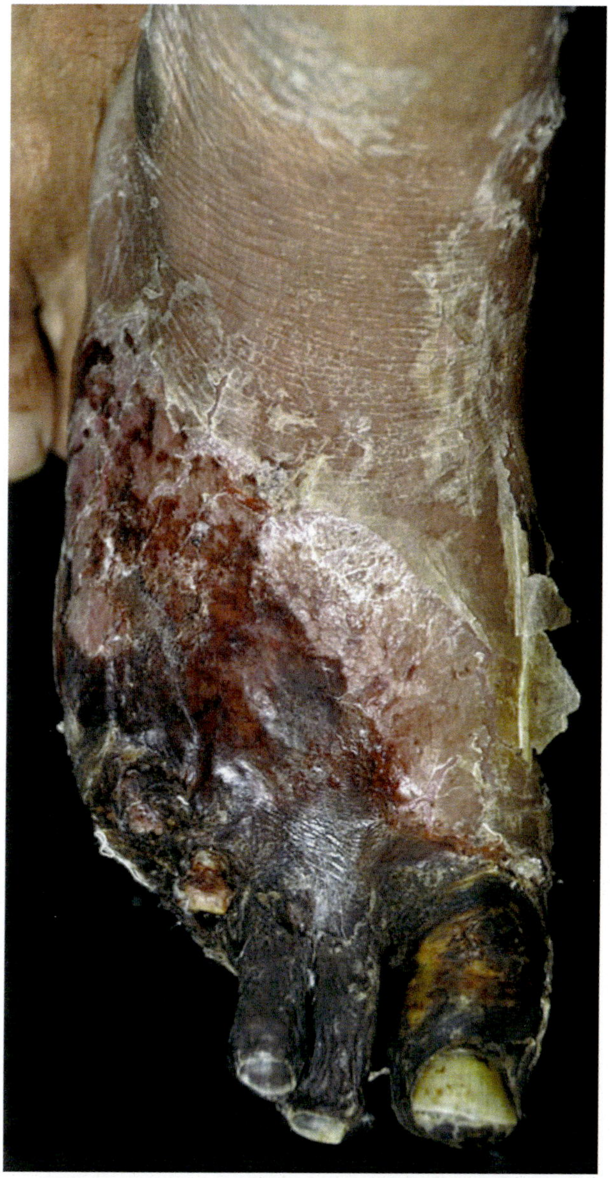

Fig. 18.7 Forefoot gangrene in a diabetic patient with peripheral arterial disease

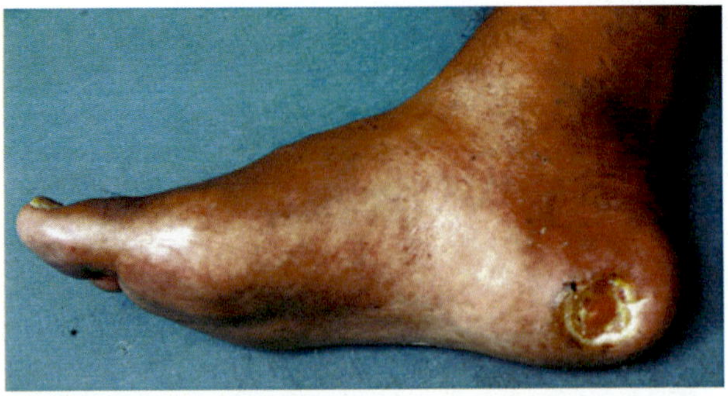

Fig. 18.8 Ulcer in the medial aspect of heel suggestive of an ischemic ulcer due to posterior tibial artery involvement

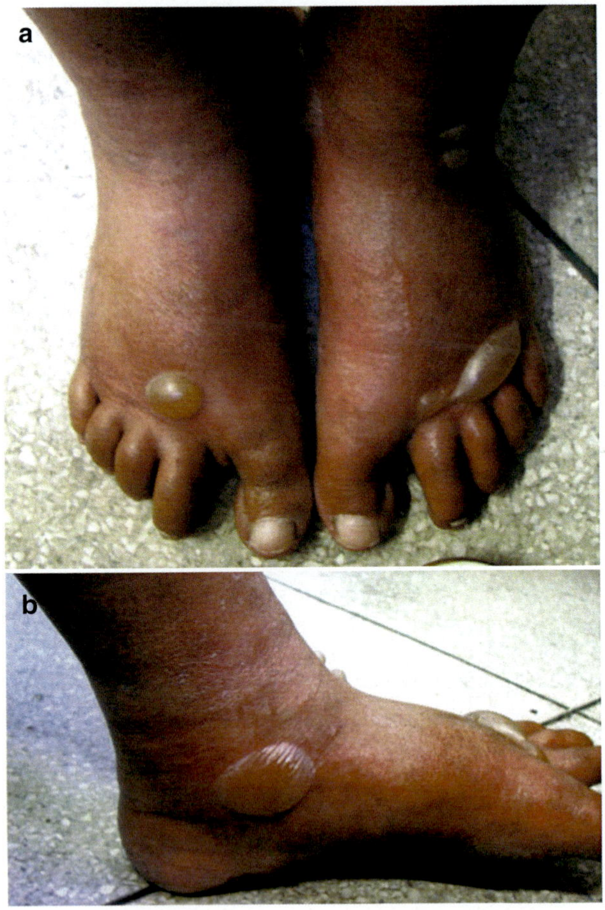

Fig. 18.9 (**a**, **b**) Diabetic bullopathy

38. **What is acute Charcot's foot?**

Acute Charcot's foot is characterized by the presence of signs of inflammation (warmth, erythema, and swelling) in a foot with loss of protective sensations, without breach in continuity of skin. A temperature difference of more than 2 °C between two feet (by infrared thermometer) is the most important clinical sign to diagnose acute Charcot's foot. Cellulitis closely mimics acute Charcot's foot and must be excluded, as treatment strategies are different for these two disorders. X-ray foot is usually normal in acute Charcot's foot. However, MRI and triple phase bone scan helps in clinching the diagnosis. The characteristic MRI features of acute Charcot's foot include periarticular focal bone marrow edema, preservation of periarticular subcutaneous fat, and absent sinus tracts or soft tissue fluid collections. Triple phase bone scan shows increased osteoblastic activity in all three phases.

39. **What is chronic Charcot's foot?**

Chronic Charcot's foot is characterized by disorganization or destruction of a joint or bone of foot with loss of protective sensations without breach in continuity of skin. Osteomyelitis closely mimics chronic Charcot's and needs to be excluded as treatment strategies are different for these disorders; however, they

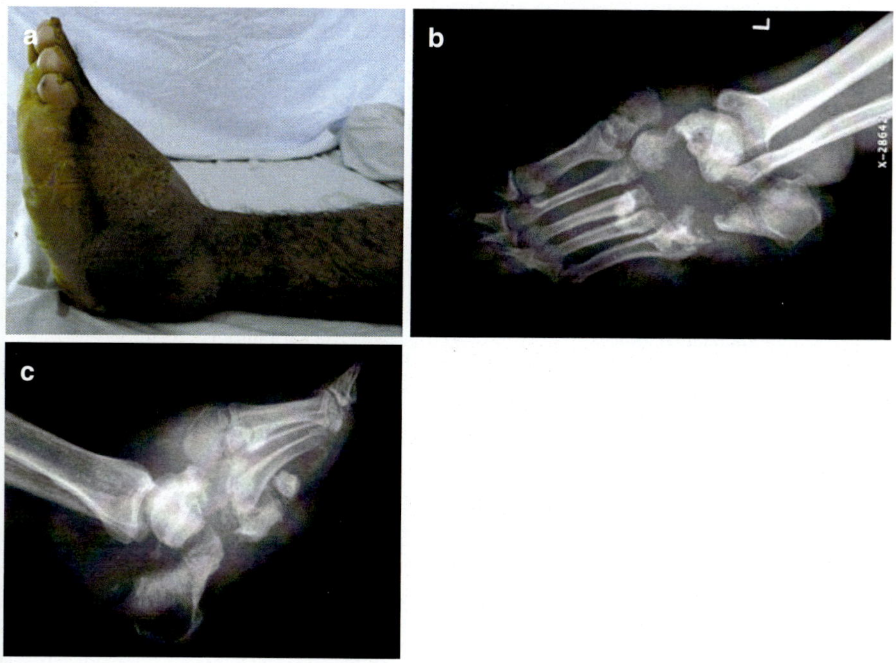

Fig. 18.10 (**a**) Rocker bottom deformity with soft tissue swelling of foot and dry skin in a patient with T2DM suggestive of Charcot's neuroarthropathy. (**b**, **c**) X-ray foot of the same patient showing extensive destruction of tarsal bones and tibiotalar joint

often coexist. Diabetes is the most common cause of Charcot's neuroarthropathy; other causes include syphilis, leprosy, chronic alcoholism, and spinal cord injury.

40. **How to differentiate chronic Charcot's foot from osteomyelitis?**

The differences between chronic Charcot's foot and osteomyelitis are summarized in the table given below.

Parameters	Chronic Charcot's foot	Osteomyelitis
Site	Commonly midfoot	Weight bearing areas—toes and metatarsal heads
Distribution	Multiple bones/joints	Focal
Deformity	Present	Absent
Soft tissue changes	Subcutaneous tissue edema	Sinus tract, abscess
Bone marrow edema	Periarticular	Diffuse involvement of a single bone
Bone marrow signal	Normal or low signal intensity on T1 and T2	Low signal intensity on T1 and high signal intensity on T2

41. **How to classify Charcot's foot?**

Charcot's foot can be classified as acute or chronic depending on clinical characteristics. Chronic Charcot's foot can be objectively classified based on radiology. The Eichenholtz classification has three stages, namely, stage of development, coalescence, and remodeling. Sanders–Frykberg is an anatomical classification according to the site of involvement of foot and is depicted in the table given below.

Pattern	Location	Specific features
I	Forefoot	Atrophic destruction of bones, plantar ulceration
II	Tarsometatarsal joint	Rocker bottom deformity Plantar ulceration
III	Talonavicular, calcaneocuboid, and naviculocuneiform joint	Rocker bottom deformity
IV	Ankle joint	Extensive joint destruction Gait instability
V	Calcaneum	Calcaneal avulsion fracture

42. **How to classify diabetic foot ulcer?**

The various classifications proposed for diabetic foot ulcer are Wagner–Meggitt, University of Texas, and PEDIS (perfusion, extent, depth, infection, and sensation). The merits and demerits of these classifications are summarized in the table given below.

Characters	Wagner	Texas	PEDIS
Classification	6 grades	4 stages 4 grades	Scoring system
Etiological considerations			
Infection	No	Yes	Yes
Neuropathy	No	No	Yes
Vascularity	No	Yes	Yes
Depth of wound	Yes	Yes	Yes
Extent of wound	No	No	Yes
Guidance for treatment	No	Yes	Yes

Wagner's classification is commonly used in clinical practice as it is simple and convenient. It is based on depth of ulcer, but it neither addresses the etiopathogenesis (neuropathic/ischemic) nor the size of the ulcer. Although the Texas classification distinguishes between infected and ischemic ulcer, it does not take neuropathy or gangrene into account. The PEDIS classification differentiates between a limb-threatening and life-threatening diabetic foot ulcer and thus helps in guiding the treatment.

43. **What are the prerequisites for the healing of a diabetic foot ulcer?**

The prerequisites for healing of a diabetic foot ulcer can be summarized by the acronym "AVOID."

A—**A**dequate glycemic control
V— restoration of **V**ascularity
O—strict **O**ff-loading
I—**I**nfection control
D—thorough **D**ebridement

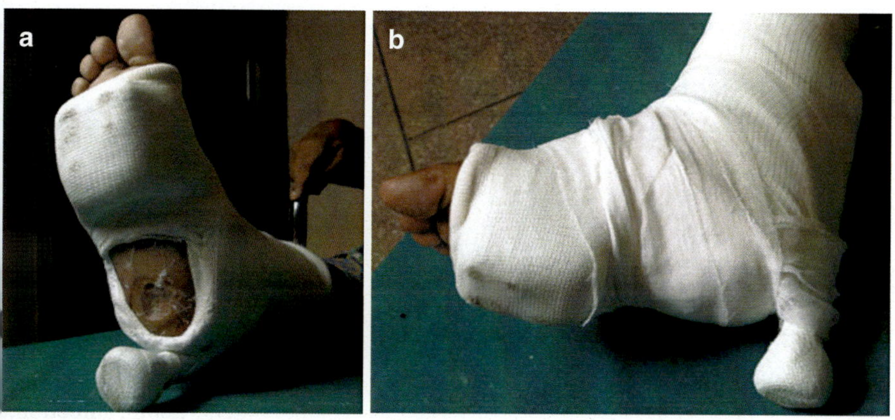

Fig. 18.11 (**a**, **b**) Modified partial contact cast with an open window for off-loading of a hind foot ulcer

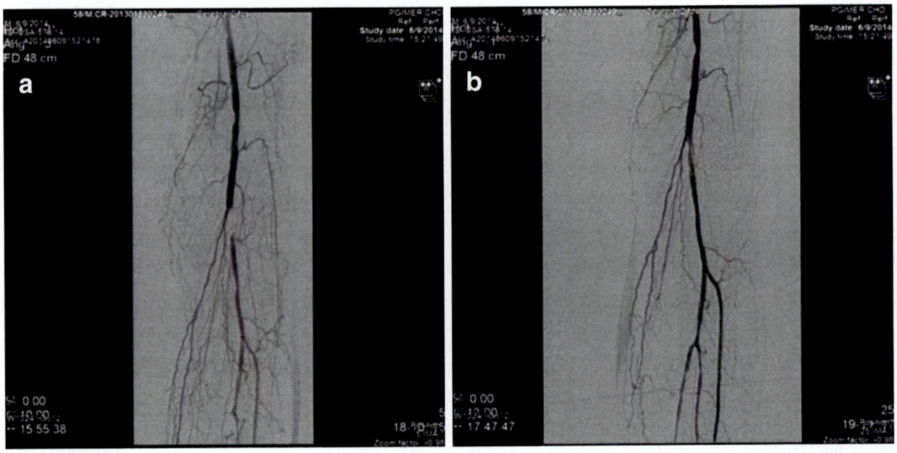

Fig. 18.12 (**a**) DSA image showing severe stenosis of popliteal artery with reduced distal flow. (**b**) Post angioplasty DSA image showing improved luminal caliber with good distal flow

44. **What are the clinical implications of a chronic diabetic foot ulcer?**

    Chronicity of a diabetic foot ulcer denies the possibility of significant vascular insufficiency and suggests that the wound is likely to be neuropathic or neuro-infective in etiology. The common causes of nonhealing diabetic foot ulcer are ineffective off-loading, incomplete debridement, presence of osteomyelitis, and inappropriate antibiotic therapy. In addition, inadvertent presence of foreign body and infections by atypical microorganisms like mycobacterium or fungi should also be considered in a patient with nonhealing ulcer. The clues for presence of osteomyelitis include exposed bone, persistent discharging sinus, ulcer >2 cm^2, or a positive probe test.

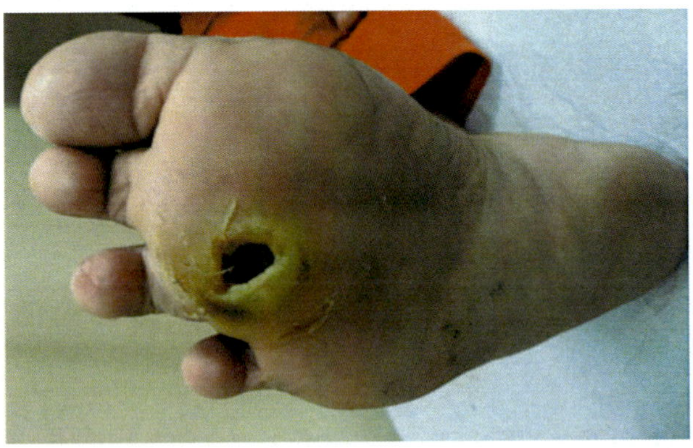

Fig. 18.13 Nonhealing punched-out ulcer with surrounding callosity. This patient had a digit amputation 3 years earlier. Chronicity of the ulcer suggests a neuropathic etiology

45. **What is the role of bisphosphonates in Charcot's foot?**

Charcot's foot is characterized by aseptic inflammation and/or disorganization or destruction of joints or bones of foot. Increased vascularity due to autonomic neuropathy, repeated unnoticed trauma because of loss of protective sensation, increased cytokines (TNF-α, IL-6), and decreased secretion of calcitonin gene-related peptide (CGRP) contributes to progressive joint and bone destruction. TNF-α and IL-6 enhance osteoclast-mediated bone resorption, and this is further facilitated by decreased CGRP, which increases the ratio of receptor activator of nuclear factor kappa-B ligand (RANKL) to osteoprotegerin (OPG) in favor of RANKL, thereby inducing osteoclastogenesis. Bisphosphonates are potent osteoclast inhibitors and are helpful in the management of acute Charcot's neuroarthropathy. However, they do not modulate the subsequent course of disease. In patients with chronic Charcot's foot, bisphosphonates are not useful, and the treatment strategies include immobilization, customized footwear, arthrodesis, or reconstructive surgery.

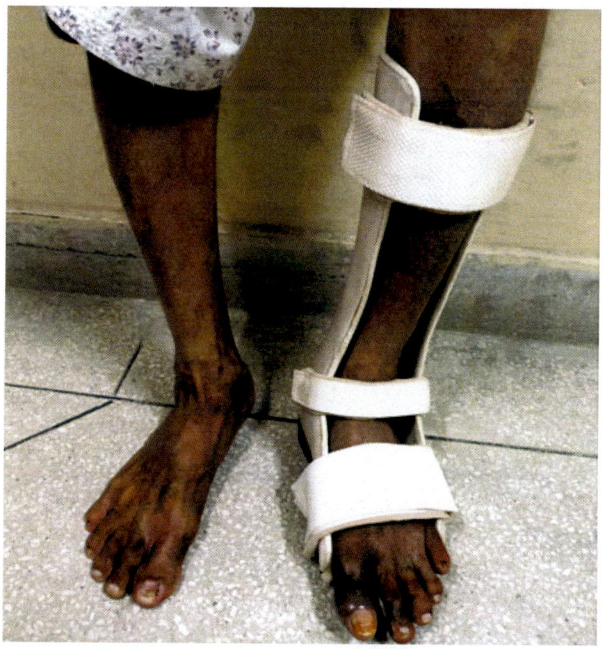

Fig. 18.14 Customized footwear for a patient with Charcot's neuroarthropathy predominantly involving hind foot. The footwear is aimed to immobilize ankle joint

46. **What are the causes of exuberant granulation tissue in a patient with diabetic foot ulcer?**

The presence of exuberant granulation tissue in a patient with diabetic foot ulcer denies the possibility of significant vascular insufficiency and infection. The causes of exuberant granulation tissue include intensive insulin therapy (via facilitation of IGF1 generation), topical application of growth factors (e.g., platelet-derived growth factor), and morbid obesity (due to hyperinsulinemia and increased IGF1). The presence of exuberant granulation tissue prevents the apposition of ulcer margins and results in nonhealing of ulcer despite optimal therapy. Therefore, appropriate debridement of granulation tissue is essential to allow healing of the ulcer.

47. **What is "diabetic hand"?**

Soft tissue changes or infection in the hand are not uncommon in patients with diabetes. The soft tissue changes in the hand include limited joint mobility, Dupuytren's contracture, carpal tunnel syndrome, and stenosing flexor tenosynovitis (FTS) or trigger finger.

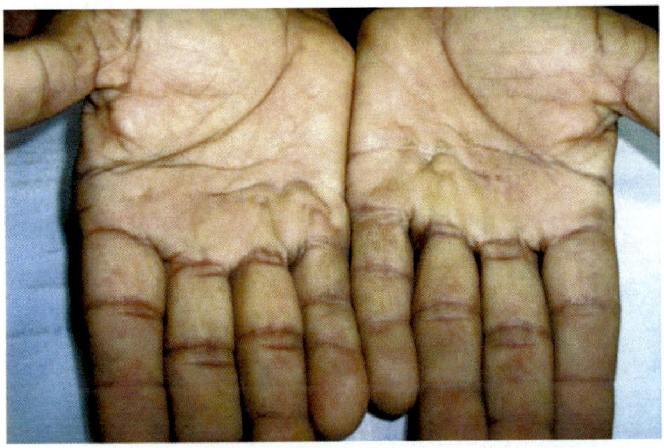

Fig. 18.15 Bilateral Dupuytren's contracture with nodularity in patient with long-standing T2DM

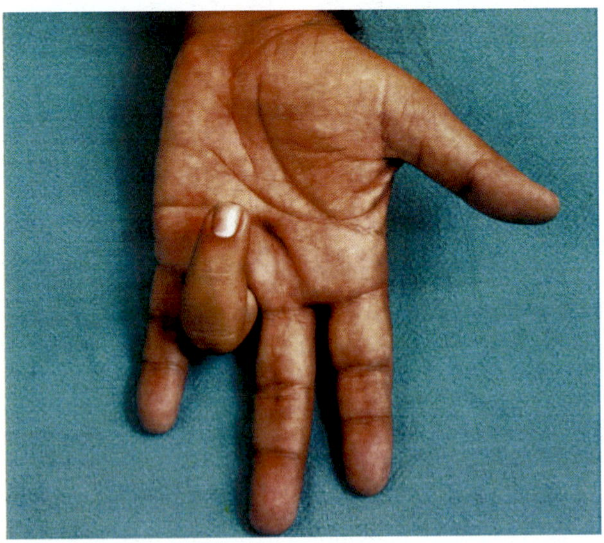

Fig. 18.16 Stenosing flexor tenosynovitis (*trigger finger*)

48. **What is "limited joint mobility"?**

Limited joint mobility (LJM), a disorder of soft tissue of hand, is characterized by restriction of movement of interphalangeal, metatarso-phalangeal, and rarely, wrist joint. LJM can be assessed either by prayer sign or table test. The severity of LJM is staged by Brink–Starkman classification. LJM is result of abnormal cross-linking of collagen fibers due to advanced glycosylation end products. As LJM is more common in patients with T1DM, autoimmune mechanism have also been implicated in its pathogenesis. LJM usually correlates with duration of diabetes and microvascular complications.

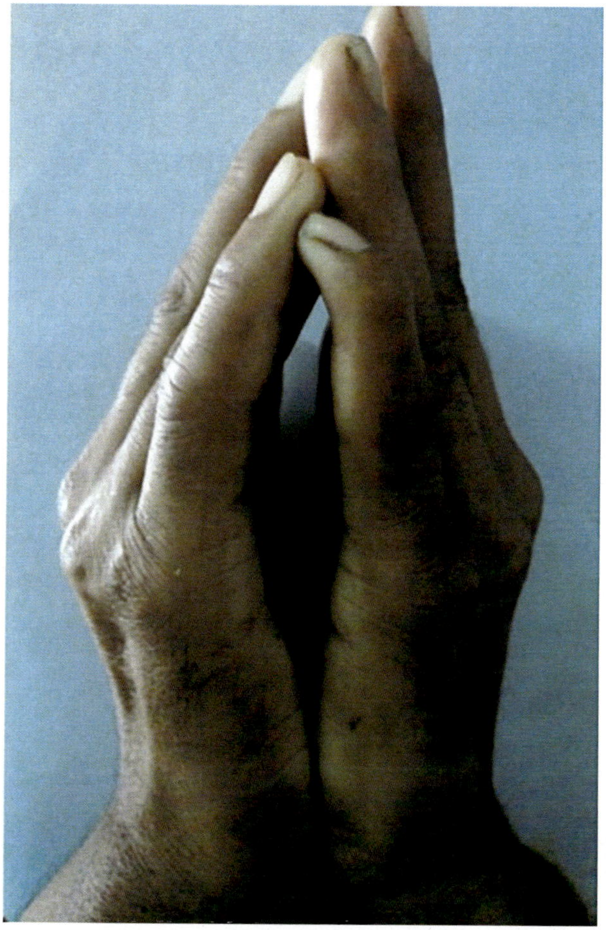

Fig. 18.17 Prayer sign denoting limited jointed mobility

49. **What is Brink–Starkman classification?**

Brink–Starkman classification system comprises of five stages to define the severity of limited joint mobility.
Stage 0—No abnormality
Stage I—Skin thickening with no contractures
Stage II—Bilateral fifth-finger contractures
Stage III—Other fingers involved bilaterally
Stage IV—Bilateral finger and wrist involvement
Stage V—Bilateral finger, wrist, and other joint involvement

Suggested Reading

1. Jameson JL, De Groot LJ. Endocrinology: adult and pediatric. Philadelphia: Elsevier Health Sciences; 2010.
2. Longo D, Fauci A, Kasper D, Hauser S, Jameson J, Loscalzo J. Harrison's principles of internal medicine. 18th ed. New York: McGraw Hill Professional; 2012.
3. Melmed S, Polonsky KS, Larsen PR, Kronenberg HM. Williams textbook of endocrinology: expert consult. London: Elsevier Health Sciences; 2011.

Diabetes-Related Complications II

19

19.1 Clinical Rounds

1. **What is diabetic kidney disease**?

   Renal disease specific to diabetes is called diabetic nephropathy. The characteristic features of diabetic nephropathy are albuminuria and progressive decline in glomerular filtration rate. However, recently the term diabetic kidney disease (DKD) has been suggested instead of diabetic nephropathy. This is because diabetic nephropathy is a histopathological diagnosis, and renal biopsy is routinely not indicated in patients with diabetes and renal dysfunction.

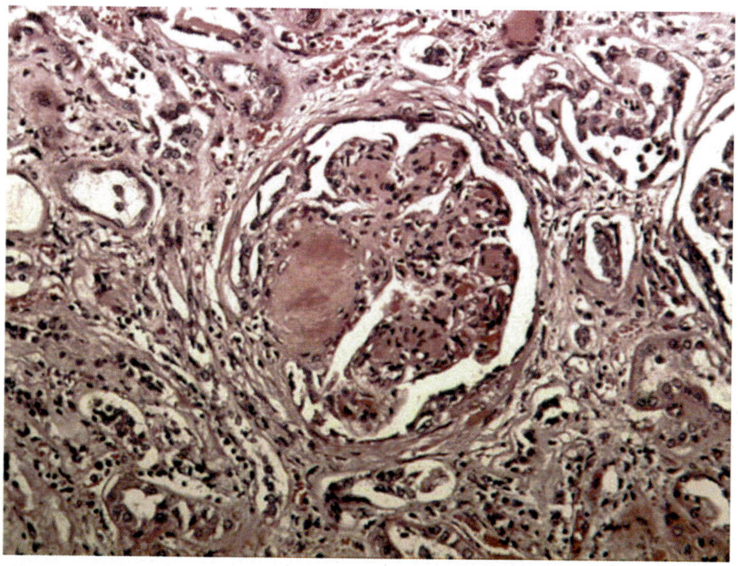

Fig. 19.1 Microphotograph showing nodular Kimmelstiel–Wilson lesion with increased mesangial cellularity, characteristic of diabetic kidney disease (H&E 20×)

A. Bhansali, Y. Gogate, *Clinical Rounds in Endocrinology: Volume I - Adult Endocrinology*, DOI 10.1007/978-81-322-2398-6_19

2. **Do all patients with diabetes develop DKD**?

No. Approximately 5–40% of patients with T2DM develop DKD; 20% of these individuals have DKD at diagnosis and 30–40% at 10 years. However, 25–40% of patients with T1DM develop DKD after 5 years of duration of disease.

3. **What is the normal urinary protein excretion**?

In a healthy adult, 24-h urinary protein excretion is <150 mg/day. Of the total protein excreted, approximately 20% is contributed by albumin, while the rest by tubular protein (Tamm–Horsfall protein). Therefore, the 24-h urinary albumin excretion is <30 mg/day in healthy individuals.

4. **What is microalbuminuria**?

Microalbuminuria is defined as 24-h urinary albumin excretion of 30–299 mg/day or urinary albumin excretion rate of 20–199 μg/min or spot urinary albumin/creatinine ratio of 30–299 mg/g of creatinine. As compared to 24-h urine collection, spot albumin to creatinine ratio is a convenient test to assess albuminuria. Currently, the term microalbuminuria has been replaced with "albuminuria" as there is no "micro"-albumin.

5. **What are the nondiabetic causes of microalbuminuria**?

Non-diabetic causes of microalbuminuria include fever, exercise, hypertension, congestive heart failure, urinary tract infections, pregnancy, and drugs like captopril and tolbutamide. Uncontrolled hyperglycemia per se can also lead to increased urinary albumin excretion.

6. **What is persistent microalbuminuria**?

Persistent microalbuminuria is defined as presence of albuminuria in the range of 30–299 mg/day on two occasions, at least 1 month apart, over a period of 3–6 months. It is important to confirm persistence of microalbuminuria as patients with diabetes may have transient albuminuria due to fever, exercise, and uncontrolled blood glucose per se.

7. **What is dipstick proteinuria**?

The presence of dipstick proteinuria denotes 24-h urinary protein excretion of ≥500 mg. This corresponds to urinary albumin of 300 mg, as 60% of urinary protein is contributed by albumin in macroproteinuric states. Therefore, urinary protein excretion of ≥500 mg/day or albumin excretion of ≥300 mg/day is considered as macroproteinuria/macroalbuminuria, respectively. Currently, the preferred term for macroalbuminuria is high albuminuria.

A scheme for evaluation of proteinuria in a patient with diabetes is depicted in the figure given below.

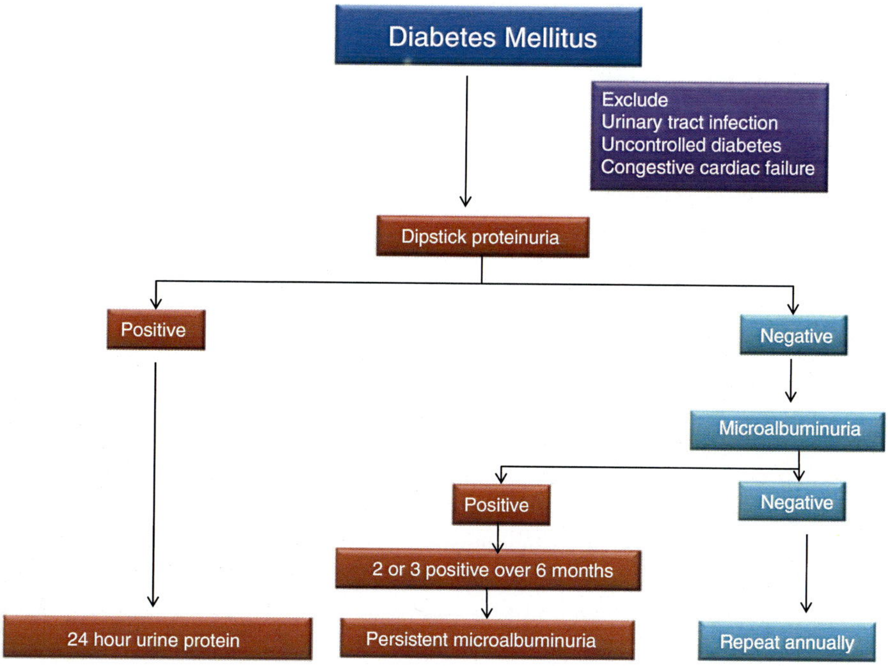

Fig. 19.2 Evaluation for proteinuria in a patient with diabetes

8. **What is the significance of persistent microalbuminuria?**

Forty percent of patients with T1DM develop microalbuminuria after 5–10 years of disease. Among these patients, 40% have spontaneous remission of albuminuria, 30–40% do not progress, while 20–30% develop macroalbuminuria. On the contrary, microalbuminuria is present in 7% of patients with T2DM at diagnosis and in 18% at 5 years after the diagnosis of diabetes; one-third of these patients progress to macroalbuminuria, one-third have stable disease, and the rest have resolution of albuminuria. Persistent microalbuminuria is a marker of early-stage DKD and is a predictor of future cardiovascular events.

9. **Can there be DKD without albuminuria?**

Although albuminuria is a classical manifestation of DKD, 20–30% of patients with histologically proven diabetic nephropathy may not have albuminuria. The only abnormality in these patients is progressive decline in glomerular filtration rate. Therefore, renal function should be estimated periodically in all patients with diabetes.

10. **Why do patients with DKD have proteinuria?**

Proteinuria in patients with DKD is due to intrarenal hemodynamic alterations and glomerulotubular structural abnormalities. Intraglomerular hypertension, loss of negative charge on glomerular basement membrane, and altered podocyte function with increase in glomerular pore size (normal 10 to 35°A) result in proteinuria.

11. **What is intraglomerular hypertension**?

Normal intraglomerular pressure is 30–50 mmHg, and this is required for optimal filtration across the glomerular basement membrane. Intraglomerular hypertension is the earliest abnormality in the pathogenesis of diabetic nephropathy and is caused by increased renal plasma flow (hyperperfusion), exaggerated differential efferent arteriolar constriction, and mesangial proliferation. The consequence of intraglomerular hypertension is hyperfiltration.

- Increased renal plasma flow is due to hyperglycemia and elevated levels of GH/IGF1, glucagon, angiotensin II, and nitric oxide.
- Differential efferent arteriolar constriction is a physiological phenomenon due to increased expression of AT_1 receptors on efferent arteriole as compared to afferent arteriole. However, activation of renal RAAS results in increased levels of local angiotensin II, leading to increased intraglomerular pressure.
- In addition, mesangial proliferation due to cytokines like TGF-β and VEGF-A leads to increase in extracellular matrix deposition and also contributes to intraglomerular hypertension.

12. **What are the structural abnormalities that result in proteinuria in patients with DKD**?

Podocytopathy, thickening of glomerular basement membrane (GBM), and mesangial proliferation are the early structural abnormalities associated with proteinuria in patients with DKD.

- Podocytes are the visceral epithelial cells present in Bowman's space and determine the size of the filtration slit. Local increase in angiotensin II causes podocyte injury (effacement of podocytes and detachment) and apoptosis, resulting in increased size of filtration slit and consequently proteinuria. In addition, nephrin, a key protein required for podocyte integrity is downregulated by angiotensin II. Further, overexpression of VEGF-A in podocytes increases vascular permeability and worsens proteinuria.
- Increased expression of angiotensin II leads to reduced expression of heparan sulfate proteoglycans in GBM. This result in loss of negative charge on GBM, facilitating free passage of negatively charged albumin across GBM (selective proteinuria). Further, there is thickening of GBM due to increased protein synthesis (collagen IV) and impaired protein degradation as a result of non-enzymatic glycation, and consequently leads to worsening of proteinuria and renal function.
- Increased angiotensin II leads to expression of various growth factors including TGF-β; this results in increased deposition of extracellular matrix (collagen IV and fibronectin) in mesangium and mesangial cell hypertrophy.

Mesangial proliferation results in intraglomerular hypertension and consequently proteinuria.

In later stages of DKD, tubulointerstitial inflammation, fibrosis, and atrophy result in further deterioration of renal function.

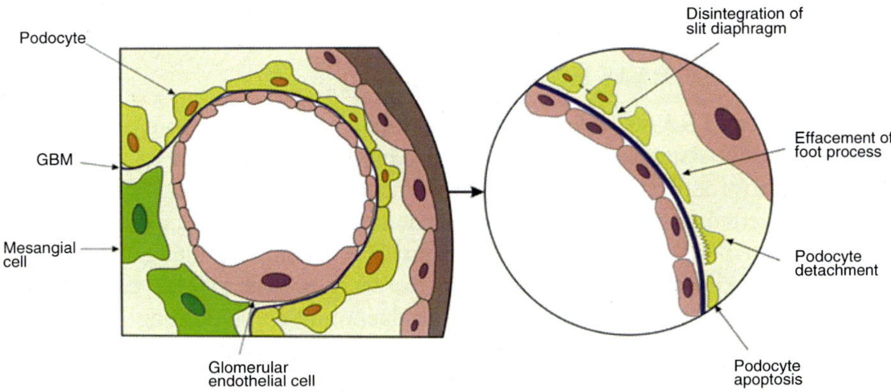

Fig. 19.3 Podocytopathy in diabetic kidney disease

13. **What are the markers of early diabetic nephropathy**?

Indicators of early diabetic nephropathy include increased glomerular filtration rate, increased serum prorenin (due to glycosylation of protease which converts prorenin to renin), augmented sodium–lithium counter-transport activity and the presence of exercise-induced microalbuminuria. In addition, urinary biomarkers like cystatin C, nephrin, and transferrin have been explored to predict DKD.

14. **When to suspect nondiabetic kidney disease in a patient with diabetes**?

Non-diabetic kidney disease (NDKD) is more prevalent in patients with T2DM than in T1DM. The clinical clues that suggest NDKD in patients with diabetes are short duration of illness, presence of active urinary sediments (RBC, WBC casts), absence of retinopathy, and rapid rise in serum creatinine. Further, patients with T2DM with rapid decline in eGFR should be suspected to have NDKD as rate of decline in GFR in patients with T2DM is approximately 0.5 ml/min/month as opposed to 0.96 ml/min/year in healthy individuals. The common causes of NDKD include pyelonephritis, renal abscess, cystitis, obstructive uropathy, and acute papillary necrosis.

15. **Why is diabetic nephropathy a "low renin" state**?

Hypertension in patients with diabetes is associated with normal renin activity in approximately 60%, low in 30%, and high in 10%. However, with onset of diabetic kidney disease (DKD), plasma renin activity is suppressed and DKD is characteristically a “low renin” state. This is attributed to increased sodium and water reabsorption in response to activation of local RAAS in proximal convoluted tubule and glomeruli. It should be noted that “local” RAAS is different from “systemic” RAAS. In addition, autonomic neuropathy, increased glycation of protease which impairs conversion of prorenin to renin, and decreased intrarenal PGI2 (prostacyclin) also contributes to “low renin” state.

16. **What is “local” RAAS in kidney**?

    The systemic RAAS is involved in regulation of blood pressure and sodium homeostasis. Angiotensinogen synthesized in liver is converted to angiotensin I by renin (produced from juxtaglomerular apparatus) in circulation. Angiotensin I is converted to angiotensin II in the endothelium of pulmonary capillaries by the enzyme ACE. Angiotensin II acts on AT_1 receptors resulting in vasoconstriction, aldosterone synthesis, and increased sodium and water reabsorption. However, the “local RAAS” involves production of angiotensinogen in proximal tubular cells, synthesis of renin by distal tubular and collecting duct cells, and expression of ACE activity in glomerulus and collecting duct cells and increased expression of AT_1 receptors. This “local RAAS” is upregulated in patients with diabetic kidney disease due to hyperglycemia, oxidative injury, and mechanical stress.

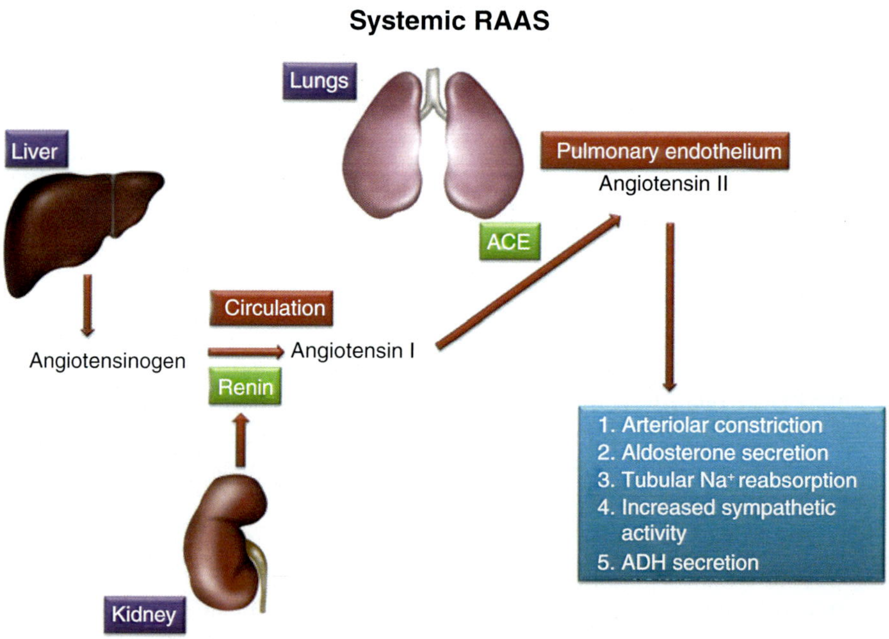

Fig. 19.4 Depiction of systemic renin–angiotensin–aldosterone system

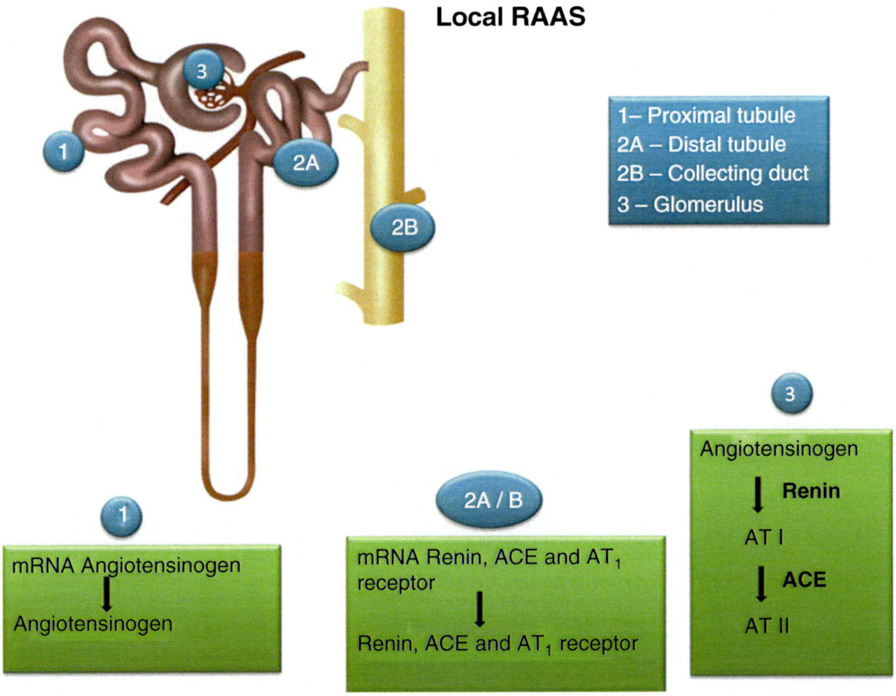

Fig. 19.5 Depiction of intrarenal renin–angiotensin–aldosterone system

17. **Why are ACEI/ARBs effective in "low renin" hypertension associated with DKD**?

    Despite the presence of "low renin" hypertension in patients with DKD, ACEIs and ARBs are effective in lowering arterial blood pressure. This is because of inhibition of local renal RAAS, leading to decreased angiotensin II formation and consequent inhibition of sodium and water reabsorption in proximal convoluted tubule. In "low renin" states, there is an activation of non-ACE pathways (chymase, cathepsin G, and chymostatin sensitive angiotensin II generating enzyme) leading to increased angiotensin II production (approximately 60–70%) and systemic hypertension. Administration of ARBs effectively blocks angiotensin II receptors type 1, thereby controlling blood pressure in "low renin" hypertension.

18. **How do ACEIs/ARBs reduce proteinuria**?

    Local existence of renin–angiotensin–aldosterone system (RAAS) in kidney is the pathophysiological basis of use of ACEIs/ARBs in DKD. Hyperglycemia-induced upregulation of local RAAS and consequently increased levels of renal angiotensin II result in intraglomerular hypertension, decreased synthesis of glomerular basement membrane proteoglycans and nephrin (leading to loss of negative charge of GBM), altered podocyte function, and increased pore size. These alterations result in proteinuria and progressive renal damage. Administration of ACEIs/ARBs inhibits local RAAS and thereby decrease proteinuria and prevents the progression of renal disease. Further, reduction in proteinuria is independent of decrease in systemic blood pressure.

19. **Is there a role for dual RAAS blockade in diabetic kidney disease**?

    Dual RAAS blockade has been tried in patients with macroalbuminuria. However, various studies have convincingly demonstrated that combined use of ACEIs and ARBs is associated with increased risk of hyperkalemia and worsening of eGFR. Therefore, dual RAAS blockade is not currently recommended in the management of DKD. Similarly, addition of direct renin inhibitor aliskiren to ACEIs or ARBs has no added advantage but increases the risk of hyperkalemia.

20. **A 45-year-old male, a known case of T2DM for the past 15 years presented with hyperkalemia (5.9 mEq/L) and serum creatinine of 1.5 mg/dl. He was not on therapy with ACEIs or ARBs. What is the likely possibility**?

    In patients with T2DM, hyperkalemia with near-normal serum creatinine in the absence of ACEI or ARB therapy is highly suggestive of hyporeninemic hypoaldosteronism (type IV renal tubular acidosis). This occurs due to renal parenchymal damage, decreased conversion of prorenin to renin, and impaired RAAS activity due to autonomic neuropathy. The use of ACEIs and ARBs should be avoided in patients with type IV renal tubular acidosis. Treatment includes loop diuretics for hyperkalemia and, rarely, fludrocortisone.

21. **What are the causes of rise in serum creatinine after initiation of ACEIs/ARBs therapy in patients with diabetes**?

    There may be a rise in serum creatinine of up to 30% within in 2–4 weeks after initiation of ACEIs/ARBs therapy. This is due to the effect of ACEIs/ARBs on efferent arteriole resulting in vasodilatation, thereby decreasing perfusion pressure. However, this rise in serum creatinine does not mandate discontinuation of therapy unless the rise is more than 30% or is associated with hyperkalemia. The other causes of worsening of renal function after initiation of ACEIs/ARBs include bilateral renal artery stenosis and overzealous use of diuretics. Further, accelerated hypertension and uncontrolled hyperglycemia may contribute to worsening of renal function despite continuation of ACEIs/ARBs.

22. **How does ACEIs or ARBs prevent diabetes**?

    Use of ACEIs/ARBs has been demonstrated to prevent new-onset diabetes. A meta-analysis of 13 trials showed risk reduction of new-onset diabetes by 24% with ACEIs and 23% with ARBs. This is attributed to increased skeletal muscle blood flow, upregulation of IRS-2 mRNA expression, and inhibition of adipocyte RAAS. Decreased levels/action of angiotensin II leads to skeletal muscle vasodilatation, thereby improving the delivery of insulin to muscle, the prime target of insulin action. Further, ACEIs/ARBs increase IRS-2 mRNA expression in adipocytes and muscle and facilitate insulin signaling pathway. In addition, inhibition of adipocyte RAAS by ACEIs/ARBs results in differentiation of preadipocyte to smaller adipocytes, which are more insulin sensitive as compared to larger adipocytes.

23. **A 60-year-old male with T2DM presented with acute-onset lumbar pain and haematuria. He also had history of passage of flakes in urine. What is the likely diagnosis**?

    The passage of flakes in urine indicates necrosed papilla, and the likely diagnosis in the index case is acute papillary necrosis. The common precipitating factors for papillary necrosis include urinary tract infections and drugs like NSAIDs. Renal papilla is predisposed for ischemic injury and consequent necrosis because it has a precarious blood supply as it lies in the "watershed" region. Renal angiotensin II has also been incriminated in the pathogenesis of acute papillary necrosis. Patients with diabetes are predisposed for papillary necrosis because of accelerated atherosclerosis, increased angiotensin II, and vulnerability to urinary tract infections. The presence of "signet ring" on intravenous pyelography is diagnostic of acute papillary necrosis.

24. **What are the modalities to preserve renal function in patients with DKD**?

    A good glycemic control (HbA1c <7%), optimal blood pressure control (140/90 mmHg-JNC VIII, and ADA), use of ACEIs or ARBs, use of statins, correction of anemia (target Hb 11 g/dl), metabolic acidosis, and secondary hyperparathyroidism halts/delays the progressive decline in eGFR and reduces proteinuria in patients with DKD. Prevention of urinary tract infection also helps to preserve renal function. In addition, drugs like pioglitazone, linagliptin, and statins have been demonstrated to have additional benefit in reducing proteinuria.

25. **What are the causes of hypertension in diabetes**?

    Almost 50% of patients with T2DM are hypertensive at diagnosis of diabetes, while 80–90% of diabetics become hypertensive with the development of proteinuria. On the contrary, in patients with T1DM, development of hypertension coincides with the onset of proteinuria. The cause of hypertension in majority of patients (80–90%) with T2DM is "essential" hypertension. In addition, hyperinsulinemia/insulin resistance, diabetic kidney disease, renal artery stenosis, and autonomic neuropathy also contribute to hypertension.

26. **How does insulin resistance cause hypertension**?

    Insulin resistance/hyperinsulinemia has been incriminated as one of the major pathogenetic mechanisms in the development of essential hypertension. The similar mechanism also operates in majority of patients with T2DM. Insulin resistance/hyperinsulinemia increases blood pressure by promoting sodium and water reabsorption in proximal convoluted tubule, increased sodium–lithium counter-transport activity (facilitating entry of sodium into cell), enhanced intracellular movement of calcium (increasing vascular tone), endothelial dysfunction, and loss of vasodilatory effect of insulin in insulin-resistant state.

27. **What is the drug of choice for the management of hypertension in patients with diabetes?**

    Diabetes is a state of resistant hypertension and majority of patients with T2DM require at least 2–3 antihypertensive medications for the achievement of target blood pressure of <140/90 mmHg. The first-line drug for hypertension in patients with diabetes is ACEIs/ARBs. Low doses of ACEIs/ARBs, which is commonly used in clinical practice, may control blood pressure, but may not yield optimal cardiac or renal benefits. Therefore, 10–20 mg of ramipril or 80 mg of telmisartan should be used to obtain these benefits. Failure to achieve target BP with ACEIs/ARBs requires add-on therapy with calcium channel blockers or diuretics or β-blockers. Those with coronary artery disease should receive β-blockers, and their use should not be refrained because of risk of hypoglycemia. It is advised to start treatment with combination of two antihypertensive drugs in individuals with BP >150/100 mmHg. The combination of ACEIs and ARBs should be avoided as it may result in worsening of renal function and hyperkalemia.

28. **What is the surrogate link between micro- and macrovascular complications**?

    Microalbuminuria is regarded as a surrogate link between micro- and macrovascular complications. Microalbuminuria not only represents renal microangiopathy and glomerular leak, but also reflects presence of diffuse vascular damage ubiquitously. There is generalized increase in vascular permeability along with endothelial dysfunction which results in outpouring of proatherogenic molecules (e.g., oxidized LDL cholesterol and fibrinogen) into the subendothelial space, thereby accelerating the process of atherosclerosis. This is termed as Steno hypothesis.

29. **What is "ticking clock" hypothesis**?

    "Ticking clock" hypothesis states that the risk of macrovascular disease starts much earlier before the onset of overt diabetes, and this was demonstrated in the San Antonio Heart Study. The concurrent presence of multiple risk factors like obesity, insulin resistance/hyperinsulinemia, dyslipidemia, and hypertension in individuals with prediabetes results in increased risk for cardiovascular disease and future onset of diabetes.

30. **What are the risk factors for macrovascular complications in patients with diabetes?**

The risk factors for macrovascular complications in diabetes are age, poor glycemic control, hypertension, dyslipidemia, proteinuria, and smoking. Nevertheless, the data from United Kingdom Prospective Diabetes Study (UKPDS) demonstrated that vasculature at different sites respond differentially to various risk factors. High LDL cholesterol and smoking predispose for coronary artery disease, hypertension is associated with increased risk for stroke, whereas smoking and hyperglycemia are linked to increased risk for peripheral vascular disease and gangrene.

31. **Does intensive glycemic control improve cardiovascular outcome in patients with T2DM?**

Four large studies have evaluated the effect of intensive glycemic control on cardiovascular outcome in patients with T2DM. The United Kingdom Prospective Diabetes Study (UKPDS) demonstrated that intensive glycemic control reduced the risk for fatal and nonfatal myocardial infarction by 16%, as compared to conventional therapy. But, this difference was not statistically significant. However, the long-term follow-up of UKPDS cohort demonstrated the emergence of statistically significant relative risk reduction for myocardial infarction by 15%. This effect was attributed to "legacy effect" or "good metabolic memory." However, the recent Action to Control Cardiovascular Risk in Diabetes (ACCORD) study showed increased mortality with intensive glycemic control. The increased mortality in the study was attributed to severe hypoglycemia. Two other studies, Veterans Affairs Diabetes Trial (VADT) and Action in Diabetes and Vascular Disease: PreterAx and Diamicron MR Controlled Evaluation (ADVANCE), did not observe any improvement in cardiovascular outcome with intensive glycemic control. Unlike UKPDS which recruited newly diagnosed patients with T2DM (with a mean age of 53 years), these three studies involved patients with long duration of diabetes and cardiovascular comorbidities. This suggests that intensive glycemic control early in course of disease improves cardiovascular outcomes, while intensive glycemic control may be detrimental in patients with advanced duration of disease. The results of three large studies are summarized in the table given below.

Parameters	ACCORD	ADVANCE	VADT
Mean age (years)	62	66	60
Duration of diabetes (years)	10	8	11.5
History of CVD (%)	35	32	40
Baseline HbA1c (%)	8.1	7.2	9.4
HbA1c goal (%)	<6	≤6.5	<6.0
HbA1c achieved (%)	6.4	6.3	6.9
Severe hypoglycemia (%)	16.2 vs. 5.1[a]	2.7 vs. 1.5[a]	24.1 vs. 17.6[a]
HR for primary outcome	0.9 (0.78–1.04)	0.94 (0.84–1.06)	0.88 (0.74–1.05)
HR for mortality	1.22 (1.01–1.46)	0.93 (0.83–1.06)	1.07 (0.81–1.42)

[a]Intensive versus conventional group

32. **Is it justified to screen for coronary artery disease in asymptomatic patients with diabetes**?

    No. Although patients with diabetes have an increased risk of coronary artery disease (CAD), patients who are asymptomatic and have a normal ECG at rest do not require further evaluation. Detection of Ischemia in Asymptomatic Diabetics (DIAD) study did not demonstrate any benefits of screening for CAD in asymptomatic patients with diabetes. Further, Bypass Angioplasty Revascularization Investigation 2 Diabetes (BARI2D) study demonstrated that even in patients who have established CAD, treatment of cardiovascular risk factors like hypertension, dyslipidemia, and obesity was equally effective and comparable to revascularization procedures in preventing mortality and cardiovascular events. Therefore, every patient with diabetes should be screened for cardiovascular risk factors at least annually and if present should be treated aggressively.

33. **What are the treatment targets in patients with diabetic dyslipidemia**?

    Dyslipidemia in diabetes is characterized by high triglycerides, low HDL-C, and mildly increased or normal LDL-C. However, small, dense, LDL-C particles predominantly contribute to the LDL-C concentration. The primary target in the management of diabetic dyslipidemia is LDL cholesterol, as it has a strong correlation with increased cardiovascular events and mortality. Further, lowering LDL-C to defined targets has been shown to improve cardiovascular outcomes. As recommended by ADA, the target for LDL-C are <100 mg/dl in patients without CAD and <70 mg/dl in those with established CAD, and the drug of choice in treatment of dyslipidemia is statins. Fibrates are recommended if serum triglyceride is >500 mg/dl, after achieving optimal glycemic control. However, the use of fibrates does not have any additional impact on cardiovascular outcome, and when combined with statins, it may increase adverse events like transaminitis and myopathy. Targeting HDL-C has not been found to be rewarding in terms of prevention of cardiovascular events.

34. **Do all patients with T2DM require statins**?

    The indications for initiation of statin therapy are summarized in the table given below. ACC/AHA guidelines do not recommend targets for LDL-C, but suggest lowering of LDL-C by >50% or 30–50% from baseline by use of high-intensity or moderate-intensity statin therapy, respectively. High-intensity statin therapy includes use of atorvastatin 40–80 mg/day or rosuvastatin 20–40 mg/day with reduction of LDL-C >50% from baseline, while moderate-intensity statin therapy include the use of 10–20 mg/day of atorvastatin or rosuvastatin 5–10 mg/day and aims for 30–50% reduction in LDL-C. High-intensity statin therapy is indicated in patients with diabetes as the benefits in cardiovascular outcomes has been demonstrated with high-dose statins.

Further, use of low-dose statin therapy, which is very common in clinical practice, is not supported by RCTs.

	ACC/AHA guidelines	ADA guidelines
High-intensity statin therapy	Established CAD LDL-C >190 mg/dl Age 40–75 years with LDL-C between 70 and 189 mg/dl and have an estimated 10-year cardiovascular risk ≥7.5%	Established CAD Age 40–75 years with ≥1 CVD risk factor (LDL-C >100 mg/dl, hypertension, smoking, and overweight/obesity)
Moderate-intensity statin therapy	Age 40–75 years with LDL-C between 70 and 189 mg/dl and have an estimated 10-year cardiovascular risk <7.5%	Age 40–75 years, even without cardiovascular risk factors

In individuals <40 or >75 years of age with CVD risk factors, ADA recommends moderate- to high-intensity statin therapy, whereas ACC/AHA guidelines recommend individualization of statin therapy depending upon the presence of risk factors, side effect profile, and patient preference

35. **What are the pleiotropic effects of statins**?

    Statins are the most potent LDL-C lowering drugs. In addition, they have numerous pleiotropic effects including stabilization of coronary plaques, reduction in proteinuria, and resolution of retinal hard exudates, increase in bone mineral density, and have antioxidant/anti-inflammatory effects. Further, use of statin therapy is also associated with reduced risk of dementia.

36. **What is statin-induced myopathy**?

    Approximately 1.5–5% of patients who recieve statins have muscle-related symptoms. Statin-induced myopathy may present as myalgia which is associated with mild elevations of creatine phosphokinase (CPK) or myositis with CPK elevations >10 times of upper limit of normal. Rarely, rhabdomyolysis can occur with the use of statins, and this is associated with CPK >10,000 IU/l and rise in serum creatinine.

37. **What are the mechanisms for statin-induced myopathy**?

    The mechanism of statin-induced myopathy remains elusive; however, various theories have been proposed. Statins may result in mitochondrial dysfunction by reducing the levels of coenzyme Q10, which is a product in the mevalonate pathway. Isoprenoids, another end product in the same pathway, is also depleted with the use of statins, and this may promote muscle apoptosis. Statins may also decrease myocyte membrane cholesterol content, thereby impairing muscle membrane potential. In addition, statins also increases expression of atrogin1, an ubiquitin protein ligase, resulting in decreased MyoD which is critical for muscle protein synthesis.

38. **Who are at risk for statin-induced myopathy**?

Vitamin D deficiency, hypothyroidism, chronic alcoholism, older age (>80 years), strenuous physical activity, liver and renal disease, and concomitant use of drugs like fibrates, ketoconazole, or macrolide antibiotics increase the risk of statin-induced myopathy. Hypothyroidism is associated with reduced metabolism of statins, thereby predisposing for statin-induced myopathy. Vitamin D deficiency results in activation of myostatin-atrogin 1 cascade and low level of IGF-1, which leads to dysfunction of sarcolemmal T-tubular system and consequently muscle breakdown.

39. **How to manage statin-induced myopathy**?

Serum CPK, creatinine, T_4 and TSH, and 25-(OH)D should be estimated in patients who complain of muscle-related symptoms, while on statin therapy. If symptoms are mild and tolerable with CPK elevation <10-fold, statin therapy can be continued. If symptoms are intolerable and CPK elevation is <10-fold, switching to hydrophilic statins like rosuvastatin, pravastatin, or fluvastatin is recommended. Concurrent vitamin D deficiency and hypothyroidism if present, should be adequately treated. CPK elevation >10-fold or presence of rhabdomyolysis mandates discontinuation of statin therapy. Alternative therapies like ezetimibe can be tried but have not been shown to improve cardiovascular outcome.

40. **Does statins cause diabetes**?

Use of statins is associated with increased incidence of new-onset diabetes, with an estimated relative risk of 9%. The risk is dose dependent, greater in elderly individuals, and is a "class effect," although some studies using pravastatin have shown a decreased risk of diabetes. A recent meta-analysis showed that 255 patients need to be treated with statins for 4 years to cause one additional case of new-onset diabetes. However, this treatment also resulted in the prevention of 5.4 cardiovascular events. Therefore, the risk of developing diabetes with the use of statins is meager, and benefits outweigh the risk.

41. **How does statins cause diabetes**?

The underlying mechanisms for the development of statin-induced incident diabetes include decreased expression of GLUT2, reduced coenzyme Q10-mediated ATP production, and impaired calcium-mediated insulin secretion leading to β-cell secretory defects. Further, statin therapy may promote β-cell apoptosis. Statins have also been shown to induce insulin resistance by decreasing GLUT4 expression in adipocytes. These detrimental effects of statins are due to reduced availability of mevalonate and its downstream metabolites (e.g., isoprenoids).

42. **Are statins safe in renal failure**?

Use of statins is not associated with increased risk of renal insufficiency in patients with diabetes. However, those statins which are excreted through kidney require dose modification, and these include pravastatin (20% renal excretion), simvastatin (13%), and rosuvastatin (10%). In contrast, only 2% of atorvastatin is excreted through kidney; therefore, it does not require any dose modification. Statins have been shown to reduce albuminuria, although studies using rosuvastatin have yielded conflicting results.

43. **How to define hypoglycemia in a patient with diabetes**?

Hypoglycemia in a patient with diabetes is defined as blood glucose <70 mg/dl, with or without adrenergic or neuroglycopenic symptoms. The blood glucose threshold to define hypoglycemia is higher in patients with diabetes as compared to nondiabetic individuals, where the cutoff is 55 mg/dl. This is because the threshold for activation of defense mechanisms against hypoglycemia is set at a higher level in diabetic individuals and higher threshold also provides time to the patient for taking action to prevent progression into neuroglycopenia. In addition, it provides a safety margin while using glucose monitoring devices, as these devices have limited accuracy at low plasma glucose levels.

44. **What are the adaptive responses to hypoglycemia**?

The initial adaptive response to hypoglycemia is cessation of insulin secretion at blood glucose of approximately 80–85 mg/dl. This is followed by activation of counter-regulatory hormones including glucagon followed by catecholamines, cortisol, and GH at blood glucose of 65–70 mg/dl. Symptoms of hypoglycemia appear at blood glucose of 50–55 mg/dl, and cognitive dysfunction occurs at <50 mg/dl. These observations have been derived from hypoglycemic-hyperinsulinemic clamp studies in healthy individuals.

45. **Why do patients with advanced duration of T2DM have a higher risk of hypoglycemia**?

Patients with advanced duration of T2DM are at higher risk of developing hypoglycemia than those with newly diagnosed T2DM. This is because of severe endogenous insulin deficiency and impaired glucose–glucagon axis. The first line of defense against hypoglycemia is the decrease in insulin secretion with declining levels of glucose; however, this fails to occur in those with long-standing diabetes due to poor β-cell reserve. Further, in normal physiology, decrease in insulin secretion results in reduction of intra-islet insulin levels. This "Δ change" in intra-islet insulin is required for the stimulation of α-cells to secrete glucagon. This second line of defense is also lost in patients with long-standing T2DM as there is no further decline in intra-islet insulin levels due to profound endogenous insulin deficiency. The other mechanism for the development of hypoglycemia in these patients is impaired glucose–glucagon axis, i.e., decreased responsiveness of α-cells to hypoglycemia. This is due to defective glucose sensing at α-cells, inability of GIP to stimulate glucagon secretion, and increased level of somatostatin. Further, frequent episodes of hypoglycemia lead to sympathoadrenal failure (hypoglycemia-associated autonomic failure) resulting in defective epinephrine secretion (third line of defense against hypoglycemia), thereby predisposing a patient to recurrent and severe hypoglycemia.

46. **How to classify hypoglycemia in a patient with diabetes**?

Hypoglycemia is classified in patients with diabetes as **severe** (requiring assistance of another person), **documented symptomatic** (symptoms with spot glucose <70 mg/dl), **asymptomatic** (spot glucose <70 mg/dl without symptoms), **probable symptomatic** (symptoms without documentation of blood glucose), and **relative hypoglycemia** (symptoms with spot glucose >70 mg/dl). The importance of this classification is that it not only takes into account severe hypoglycemia, but also includes patients with a suspicion of hypoglycemia. In addition, it also helps to provide uniformity in defining hypoglycemia as an adverse event with antidiabetic drugs in scientific studies.

47. **How to manage hypoglycemia in diabetes**?

The treatment strategies for hypoglycemia should be individualized. Patients with hypoglycemia presenting only with adrenergic symptoms should be treated with oral glucose tablets or fruit juice or candy, irrespective of blood glucose levels. Blood glucose should be re-estimated after 15–20 min, and failure of normalization of blood glucose requires further administration of oral glucose/carbohydrates. Patients receiving basal insulin or long-acting sulfonylureas (glibenclamide or glimepiride) require close monitoring for at least 24–72 h. Patients with hypoglycemia along with cognitive dysfunction should be administrated 25 g of dextrose (25% dextrose, 100 ml) intravenously to rapidly normalize blood glucose and may require continuous administration of 5% dextrose, depending upon improvement in sensorium and antidiabetic treatment received. Blood glucose should not be allowed to overshoot >200 mg/dl, as rapidly rising blood glucose may lead to cerebral dehydration and further worsening of sensorium. Intravenous dextrose should be discontinued only when patient starts taking orally, as hepatic glycogen stores are repleted only with oral intake. After recovery from the episode, an active search should be made to explore the cause of hypoglycemia

48. **Does diabetes increase the risk of infection**?

Infections are more severe and aggressive in patients with diabetes; however, it is still debatable whether diabetes per se increases the risk of infections. Cutaneous candidiasis is the most common infection, followed by urinary tract infection and pneumonia. However, rhino-orbital-cerebral mucormyosis, malignant otitis externa, emphysematous pyelonephritis, and emphysematous cholecystitis are unusual but potentially fatal infections seen exclusively in patients with diabetes. Hyperglycemic milieu, altered leukocyte function, and increased oxidative stress contribute to more severe and aggressive infections in diabetes.

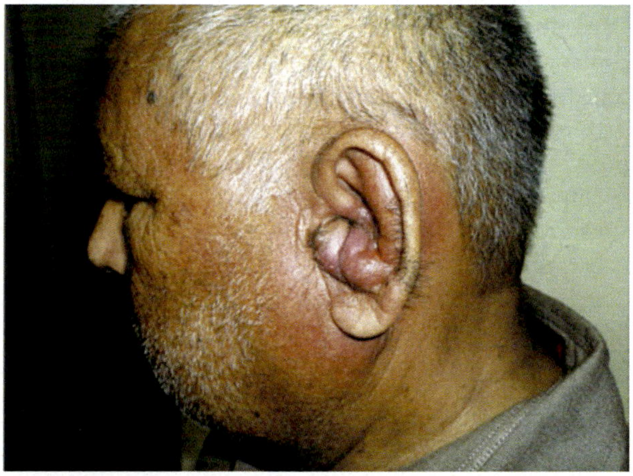

Fig. 19.6 Malignant otitis externa in a patient with T2DM

49. **Are microorganisms causing emphysematous pyelonephritis and emphysematous cholecystitis same**?

    Emphysematous pyelonephritis is caused by *E. coli*, *Pseudomonas*, or *Klebsiella*, organisms that produce carbon dioxide and methane from necrotic tissue by facultative anaerobic glycolysis. Emphysematous cholecystitis is caused by *Clostridia*, which is a commensal in the intestinal tract. However, it can also be caused by gram-negative organism like *E. coli* as a complication of septicemia.

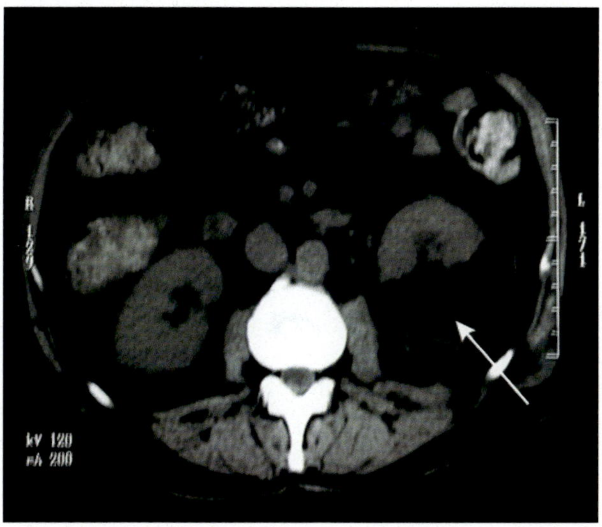

Fig. 19.7 Emphysematous pyelonephritis in a patient with T2DM

50. **What are the causes of anemia in diabetes**?

Anemia is not uncommon in patients with diabetes, and the causes include diabetic kidney disease (DKD), autonomic neuropathy-related gastroparesis, and blind-loop syndrome. Autonomic neuropathy is associated with impaired absorption of micronutrients from the gastrointestinal tract. In addition, drugs used in the management of T2DM like metformin and pioglitazone can also result in anemia. Metformin impairs calcium channel-mediated B_{12} absorption in distal small intestine and contribute to macrocytic anemia. Pioglitazone results in anemia due to hemodilution and preferential diversion of primitive mesenchymal stem cells to adipocytes rather than to erythropoietic stem cells. Further, chronic pancreatitis is more common in T2DM, which causes B_{12} and folic acid malabsorption. Occult gastrointestinal bleed is not uncommon in patients with diabetes as antiplatelet drugs are frequently used in these patients. Beside this, patients with T1DM are predisposed for celiac disease, pernicious anemia, and autoimmune thyroid disorders, which can also lead to anemia.

51. **What are the causes of abdominal pain and vomiting in a patient with diabetes**?

Abdominal pain and vomiting can occur in a patient with diabetes due to diabetic ketoacidosis, acute pancreatitis, acute cholecystitis, acute papillary necrosis, gastroparesis, and diabetic kidney disease. Further, acute coronary syndrome may mimic acute abdomen. Drugs like metformin, gliptins, and GLP1 analogues may also cause abdominal pain, nausea, and vomiting in these patients.

Suggested Reading

1. Jameson JL, De Groot LJ. Endocrinology: adult and pediatric. Philadelphia: Elsevier Health Sciences; 2010.
2. Longo D, Fauci A, Kasper D, Hauser S, Jameson J, Loscalzo J. Harrison's principles of internal medicine. 18th ed. New York: McGraw Hill Professional; 2012.
3. Melmed S, Polonsky KS, Larsen PR, Kronenberg HM. Williams textbook of endocrinology: expert consult. London: Elsevier Health Sciences; 2011.

Diabetes During Pregnancy

20

20.1 Clinical Rounds

1. **What is gestational diabetes mellitus?**
   Gestational diabetes mellitus (GDM) is defined as glucose intolerance of any severity with onset or first recognition during pregnancy.

2. **What are the lacunae of this definition?**

   This definition of GDM which entails glucose intolerance of any severity and first recognition during pregnancy has many limitations. Hyperglycemia due to pregnancy per se is mild, whereas hyperglycemia associated with preexisting diabetes is usually severe; therefore categorizing all these women as GDM may not be appropriate. Further, hyperglycemia due to pregnancy usually manifests at 24–28 weeks of gestation, while preexisting diabetes may manifest even during first trimester. Almost 10–20% of patients who are detected to have hyperglycemia at the first antenatal visit may have preexisting diabetes, and by definition these women will be classified as GDM. This differentiation is important as women with preexisting diabetes are more likely to have fetal malformations, need evaluation and monitoring for diabetes-specific complications. Moreover, some women with preexisting diabetes may even have type 1 diabetes, and these women may develop diabetic ketoacidosis, which is unusual in GDM. Therefore, the appropriate term should be "hyperglycemia during pregnancy" rather than GDM. In addition, this definition does not entail absolute numerical values of plasma glucose to define hyperglycemia during pregnancy as opposed to the diagnosis of diabetes in nonpregnant population.

A. Bhansali, Y. Gogate, *Clinical Rounds in Endocrinology: Volume I - Adult Endocrinology*, DOI 10.1007/978-81-322-2398-6_20

3. **What are the differences in a patient with preexisting diabetes and gestational diabetes?**

Parameters	Preexisting diabetes	Gestational diabetes
Onset	Preconceptional	Postconceptional
Type of DM	T2 DM/T1DM	Transient hyperglycemia
Degree of hyperglycemia	Moderate to severe	Mild
Diabetic complications	Microangiopathy, Macroangiopathy Placental vasculopathy	Uncommon
Comorbidities	Hypertension	Pregnancy induced hypertension
Outcome	Diabetic embryopathy Spontaneous abortion IUGR Intrauterine death	Macrosomia Difficult labor Maternal and neonatal risk for future T2DM

4. **What is "fuel-mediated teratogenesis"?**

Fuel-mediated teratogenesis refers to teratopathy occurring due to exposure of embryo or fetus to the unfavorable milieu of metabolic fuels such as high levels of glucose and ketones. Therefore, a pregnancy with diabetes is at risk for fuel-mediated teratogenesis. The type and severity of defects depend on the time of gestation at which the embryo/fetus has been exposed. If the exposure to high levels of glucose occurs during embryogenesis (<8 weeks of gestation), it results in diabetic embryopathy, as seen in patients with uncontrolled preexisting diabetes. However, if fetus (after 8 weeks of gestation) is exposed to this abnormal metabolic milieu, then anthropometric and metabolic abnormalities predominate the clinical picture, rather than embryopathy.

5. **What is diabetic embryopathy?**

Diabetic embryopathy is a result of peri-conceptional uncontrolled hyperglycemia which influences organogenesis during embryonic period. Therefore, diabetic embryopathy is a feature of preexisting diabetes and is not expected in patients with GDM. The congenital anomalies associated with diabetic embryopathy include neural tube defects, caudal regression syndrome, transposition of great vessels, ventricular septal defect, hypoplastic left heart syndrome, renal agenesis, duodenal atresia and hypoplastic femur. Out of these numerous anomalies, neural tube defects are the most common, while the diabetes-specific defect is caudal regression syndrome (sacral agenesis). The prime pathogenetic mechanism implicated in congenital malformation is the exposure of embryo to hyperglycemia, hyperketonemia (3 β-hydroxybutyrate), and metabolites like inositol, sorbitol, and arachidonic acid. In addition, altered folate metabolism and accumulation of reactive oxygen species (ROS) also contribute to it.

6. **What are the maternal risks associated with GDM?**

Women with GDM have an increased risk of preeclampsia, fetal loss, difficult labor, and future risk of developing T2DM.

7. **What are the fetal risks associated with GDM?**

Macrosomia (>4 kg), intrauterine death (if FPG >105 mg/dl), neonatal hypoglycemia, polycythemia (chronic fetal hypoxia due to lung immaturity), hypocalcemia (functional hypoparathyroidism due to hypomagnesemia), and hyperbilirubinemia (associated with polycythemia) are the immediate risks to the fetus. Further, these newborns are at future risk of developing obesity and T2DM.

8. **When to screen for hyperglycemia in pregnancy?**

Every pregnant woman should be screened for hyperglycemia as early as possible (first contact visit or preferably <12 weeks); if not, there is a probability of missing preexisting diabetes. With the current IADPSG guidelines, women with fasting plasma glucose of 92–125 mg/dl in the first trimester, which is currently categorized as GDM, will also remain undiagnosed. If the screening test is negative at first trimester, retesting is recommended in all women between 24 and 28 weeks of gestation. The retesting at 24–28 weeks is recommended as insulin resistance peaks at this time due to rising concentration of progesterone, human placental lactogen, prolactin, cortisol, and growth hormone.

9. **Who should be screened for hyperglycemia in the first trimester of pregnancy?**

The aim of screening at first trimester is to recognize those women with preexisting diabetes. According to ADA guidelines, individuals with a high risk of having type 2 diabetes require screening at the first trimester of pregnancy. Therefore, all adult women with a prepregnant BMI >25 kg/m^2 with one additional risk factor like hypertension or polycystic ovarian disease, ethnic group with high diabetes prevalence, the presence of family history of diabetes in the first-degree relatives, or personal history of abnormal glucose intolerance or bad obstetric outcome should be screened for hyperglycemia in the first trimester. However, the current IADPSG guidelines recommend universal screening for hyperglycemia during first trimester.

10. **Who should be screened for hyperglycemia at 24–28 weeks of gestation?**

All pregnant women require screening for hyperglycemia with oral glucose challenge test at 24–28 weeks of gestation except those who were diagnosed with overt diabetes (FPG ≥126 mg/dl, RPG ≥200 mg/dl, or HbA1c ≥6.5%) in the first trimester.

11. **How to screen for hyperglycemia at first trimester?**

    At first antenatal visit, a pregnant woman can be screened with fasting plasma glucose (FPG) or random plasma glucose (RPG) or HbA1c. FPG ≥126 mg/dl or RPG ≥200 mg/dl or HbA1c ≥6.5% confirms the diagnosis of preexisting diabetes; however, it requires confirmation on a subsequent day in case of equivocal hyperglycemia. A FPG value of 92–125 mg/dl establishes the diagnosis of GDM at the first trimester of pregnancy.

12. **How to screen for hyperglycemia at 24–28 weeks of gestation?**

    There are two approaches to screen for hyperglycemia at 24–28 weeks of gestation: a one-step approach or two-step approach. A one-step approach involves screening with a 75-g 2-h oral glucose tolerance test (OGTT). The two-step approach includes a 50-g oral glucose challenge test (GCT) irrespective of time of the day and meal intake, and if 1-h plasma glucose value ≥140 mg/dl, then a 100-g 3-h OGTT should be performed.

Parameters	**One-step approach**	**Two-step approach**
Recommendations	IADPSG	NIH
Time	24–28 weeks	24–28 weeks
Fasting	Required	*Step 1:* GCT—not required *Step 2:* GTT—required
Samples	Fasting, 1, 2 h	*Step 1:* GCT—1 h *Step 2:* GTT—fasting, 1, 2, 3 h
Dose of glucose load	75 g	*Step 1:* GCT—50 g *Step 2:* GTT—100 g
Diagnostic cutoffs (mg/dl)	Fasting ≥92[a] 1 h ≥180 2 h ≥153	*Step 1:* GCT—if 1 h ≥140, proceed to step 2 *Step 2:* GTT[b] Fasting ≥95 1 h ≥180 2 h ≥155 3 h ≥140
Remarks	Higher number of women diagnosed with GDM Benefits of intervention based on a single abnormal value are to be explored	*Step 1* Does not require fasting May underdiagnose GDM *Step 2* 4 samples required Requirement of two abnormal values improves diagnostic specificity

[a]Any one value should be abnormal
[b]Two values should be abnormal

13. **Why should the criteria of diagnosis of GDM be different from that of diabetes in nonpregnant individuals?**

Gestational diabetes mellitus (GDM) is a state of transient disruption in glucose–insulin homeostasis but is associated with adverse maternal and fetal outcomes. The risk to mother and fetus starts even at a fasting plasma glucose >75 mg/dl, 1-h plasma glucose >106 mg/dl and 2-h plasma glucose of >91 mg/dl after 75-g glucose load. Further, this risk is continuous with rising blood glucose level. Therefore, the diagnostic criteria should be stringent and are targeted to improve both fetal and maternal outcomes. In addition, hemodilution, increased RBC turnover, and accelerated fetal anabolism also influence the diagnostic criteria.

14. **What are the cutoffs to establish a diagnosis of GDM?**

The diagnostic criteria by different working groups are summarized in the table given below. These cutoffs have been derived with OGTT done between 24 and 28 weeks of gestation.

Plasma glucose (mg/dl)	O'Sullivan and Mahan[a] 100-g OGTT (1964)	Carpenter and Coustan[a] 100-g OGTT (1973)	DIPSI 75-g OGTT (2006)	IADPSG[b] 75-g OGTT (2010)	WHO[b] 75-g OGTT (2013)
Fasting (h)	≥105	≥95	–	92–125	92–125
1	≥190	≥180	–	≥180	≥180
2	≥165	≥155	140–199	153–199	153–199
3	≥145	≥140	–		

[a]Two values should be abnormal
[b]Any one value should be abnormal

However, any patient with FPG ≥126 mg/dl or 2-h PG post-glucose load ≥200 mg/dl should be diagnosed with overt diabetes (IADPSG).

15. **Can a diagnosis of GDM be made in the first trimester?**

Conventionally, the diagnosis of GDM was considered on the basis of OGTT performed between 24 and 28 weeks of gestation. However, the current guidelines (IADPSG) recommend estimation of FPG, RPG, or HbA1c during the first trimester, and if FPG is 92–125 mg/dl, then a diagnosis of GDM can be made, even during first trimester.

16. **What is the basis of diagnostic criteria for GDM?**

The earlier diagnostic criteria for GDM by O'Sullivan and Mahan and Carpenter and Coustan were based on the maternal risk of development of diabetes after delivery. However, these criteria did not consider the relationship between maternal hyperglycemia and maternal/neonatal outcomes. The HAPO study (2008) changed the concept for the diagnosis of GDM as it showed a continuous association between rising maternal plasma glucose levels and adverse neonatal and maternal outcomes. Subsequently, IADPSG revised the criteria for the diagnosis of GDM based on HAPO study.

17. **How were the IADPSG cutoffs for GDM derived?**

    HAPO study demonstrated continuous association of maternal plasma glucose with adverse maternal and neonatal outcomes, and there was no inflection point for these outcomes. However, to be of use in clinical practice, definite cutoffs are required for the diagnosis and management of GDM. International Association of Diabetes and Pregnancy Study Groups (IADPSG) defined the criteria for the diagnosis of GDM from the data available from the HAPO study. This was done by individual estimation of the mean FPG, 1- and 2-h glucose level for the entire HAPO cohort, and these were taken as a reference value with odds ratio of 1 for the occurrence of perinatal complications like birth weight >90th percentile, cord serum C-peptide >90th percentile, or percent infant body fat >90th percentile. The glucose levels at which the odds ratio for these complications reached a threshold of 1.75 were estimated, and these values were FPG ≥92, 1 h ≥180, and 2 h ≥153 mg/dl. Henceforth, the diagnostic criteria for GDM were derived.

18. **What are the glycemic targets in a patient with hyperglycemia during pregnancy?**

    The glycemic targets in patients with hyperglycemia during pregnancy, either GDM or overt diabetes, are similar. These include FPG <95 mg/dl (ideally <90 mg/dl), 1-h PPG ≤140 mg/dl, and 2-h PPG ≤120 mg/dl, provided these targets can be achieved without an undue risk of hypoglycemia. In addition, in women with overt diabetes, HbA1C should be maintained ≤6.5%.

19. **How to monitor glycemic control in a patient with hyperglycemia during pregnancy?**

    Self-monitoring of blood glucose (SMBG) is recommended in all women with hyperglycemia during pregnancy, and this includes fasting, premeal and post-meal (1 h or 2 h) and at 4 am. However, a practical approach is to reduce the frequency of monitoring to 4-point profile (fasting and post-meal) once the glycemic targets are achieved and sustained. Targeting fasting plasma glucose is important as FPG >90 mg/dl is associated with increased risk of macrosomia. Although 1-h or 2-h post-meal value is recommended for monitoring, targeting 1-h post-meal glucose value may be more rewarding. This is extrapolated from the HAPO study which showed that 1-h post-OGTT blood glucose level at diagnosis had higher odds ratio for adverse maternal and fetal outcomes as compared to 2-h glucose value. HbA1c is not recommended for monitoring of GDM because the data is scarce. However, in women with overt diabetes, HbA1C should be monitored and maintained ≤6.5%.

20. **How to initiate treatment in GDM?**

Medical nutrition therapy (MNT) is recommended for all women with GDM or overt diabetes with the aim to provide adequate nutrition for appropriate trimester-specific weight gain. One of the key components of MNT is to restrict the carbohydrate intake to 35–45% of total calories ingested. Pregnant women with normal preconceptional BMI should increase their caloric intake by 360 and 475 kcal/day during the second and third trimester, respectively. Obese women are recommended to restrict their calorie intake by one-third of their prepregnancy intake but should at least ensure intake of 1,600 kcal/day to prevent starvation ketosis. This should be complemented with moderate physical activity for 30 min a day comprising of aerobic and non-weight-bearing exercises. An initial trial of MNT and lifestyle modifications for 2 weeks is recommended in all patients with GDM, and if it fails to achieve FPG ≤95 mg/dl and 2-h PPG ≤120 mg/dl, then insulin therapy should be initiated. However, in patients with overt diabetes insulin therapy should be initiated along with MNT.

21. **How to initiate insulin therapy in GDM?**

Insulin is a category B drug (no risk of teratogenicity based on animal data), and at physiological levels, it does not cross the placenta. Therefore, it is the preferred treatment during pregnancy. Treatment should be tailor-made according to the requirements of the patient. If the patient has fasting hyperglycemia, NPH insulin/detemir should be initiated at a dose of 0.1–0.2 units/kg/day. In case of postprandial hyperglycemia, regular/lispro/aspart should be initiated at a dose of 0.1 units/kg preprandially to target the corresponding postprandial blood glucose level. However, patients with both fasting and postprandial hyperglycemia should be started on basal–bolus regimen. The dose of insulin should be titrated based on SMBG profile. Patients with overt diabetes may require higher doses of insulin, even at initiation. However, with advancing pregnancy, insulin requirement progressively increases both in women with GDM and overt diabetes.

22. **Do insulin analogues edge over conventional insulin in the management of hyperglycemia during pregnancy?**

The short-acting insulin analogues lispro and aspart and the long-acting analogue detemir have been approved for use in pregnancy. The safety data for glargine appears to be reassuring but is not yet FDA approved for the use in pregnancy. However, glargine may be continued in women who were receiving it preconceptionally. There is no data regarding the use of glulisine in pregnancy. Short-acting analogues have the advantage of flexibility in administration (no lag time required between insulin administration and meal intake), better control of early postprandial hyperglycemia, and avoidance of late prandial hypoglycemia, as compared to regular insulin. However, the efficacy of short-acting analogues is similar to regular insulin, and there is no difference in maternal or fetal outcomes in women treated with short-acting analogues versus regular insulin. Long-acting analogues (detemir and glargine) have the advantage of lesser nocturnal hypoglycemia as compared to NPH insulin. However, the insulin analogues are more expensive than conventional insulin.

23. **What is the role of continuous subcutaneous insulin infusion therapy in the management of hyperglycemia during pregnancy?**

    Patients with preexisting diabetes who are on continuous subcutaneous insulin infusion (CSII) therapy can be safely continued with it during pregnancy. However, initiation of CSII during pregnancy is not routinely recommended as precious time is lost in optimizing therapy with CSII. However, initiation of CSII may be considered in those women who are unable to achieve glycemic targets with basal–bolus insulin regimen or have wide fluctuations in blood glucose levels despite multiple injections. Nevertheless, there is a risk of keto-acidosis and neonatal hypoglycemia with the use of CSII during pregnancy.

24. **Is there a role for metformin in the management of GDM?**

    Metformin is a category B drug and 10–16% of drug crosses the placental barrier. Concerns with the use of metformin during pregnancy include increased incidence of preeclampsia and neonatal hypoglycemia. However, this was refuted by Metformin in Gestational diabetes study (MIG), and metformin was shown to be safe during pregnancy, although there was an increased incidence of preterm birth. In addition, almost 50% of women in the same study required supplemental insulin along with metformin for glycemic control. Therefore, patients with mild hyperglycemia who fail to attain glycemic targets with MNT and do not prefer to use insulin can be treated with metformin during second and third trimester.

25. **What is the role of metformin during first trimester of pregnancy?**

    Patients with polycystic ovarian disease who conceive on metformin were initially recommended to continue the drug during the first trimester to prevent fetal loss. In addition, the use of metformin during first trimester was thought to reduce the risk of GDM in women with PCOS. However, the available evidence does not support these benefits of metformin therapy during pregnancy, and the only indication for continuing metformin during first trimester in women with PCOS is the concurrent presence of T2DM. Follow-up data of infants born to mother treated with metformin (2.5 g/day) did not show any teratogenicity, or adverse effects on birth weight/birth length, or motor and social development.

26. **What is the status of oral antidiabetics in the management of GDM?**

    Among sulphonylureas, glibenclamide has been studied in patients with GDM as there is minimal fetal exposure due to its high degree of protein binding. It was found to be safe and effective with a favorable neonatal outcome with reduced incidence of macrosomia, neonatal hypoglycemia, and higher APGAR score. Glibenclamide may be an alternative in women with GDM with mild hyperglycemia (FPG <110 mg/dl) with onset after 25 weeks of gestation. The α-glucosidase inhibitor, acarbose has been tried in a few studies and was shown to be effective in improving postprandial glucose profile. However, the long-term safety data with OAD's are scarce and hence are not recommended at present.

27. **How to plan a pregnancy in a woman with preexisting diabetes?**

A woman with preexisting diabetes planning pregnancy should attain optimal glycemic control (HbA1c <6.5%) for at least 3–6 months prior to conception. Patients on oral antidiabetic drugs should be switched to insulin. Patients who are on premixed insulin should be initiated on basal–bolus regimen as this helps in achieving sustained and smooth glycemic control and provides greater flexibility to the patient. A thorough evaluation for retinopathy and nephropathy should be undertaken as these complications can worsen during pregnancy. In the presence of severe NPDR or PDR, conception should be deferred and LASER therapy should be instituted, if indicated. Estimation of renal function including creatinine clearance and proteinuria is mandatory as patients with eGFR <60 ml/min or macroproteinuria are at very high risk for adverse fetal and maternal outcomes. Blood pressure should be adequately controlled with labetalol, methyldopa, calcium channel blockers, and α-blockers. ACEI, ARBs, and diuretics should be stopped when pregnancy is planned. In addition, statins and fibrates should also be discontinued when pregnancy is planned. Patients with preexisting diabetes should be advised to take 5 mg of folic acid for at least 3 months prior to conception to reduce the incidence of neural tube defects. Further, evaluation of thyroid function tests should be done in all patients with preexisting type 1 and type 2 diabetes.

28. **What are the predictors of worsening of diabetic complications during pregnancy?**

Long duration of diabetes, poor glycemic control prior to conception, uncontrolled blood pressure, and coexisting anemia are the important determinants of progression of microvascular complications of diabetes during pregnancy. Patients with preexisting proliferative diabetic retinopathy or renal insufficiency may experience worsening of these complications.

29. **Why is monitoring with HbA1c not useful during pregnancy?**

HbA1c is a useful test in early pregnancy to differentiate GDM from preexisting diabetes. However, it is not an ideal test for either diagnosis or monitoring during pregnancy as it does not accurately reflect the true glycemic status during pregnancy due to hemodilution (falsely low), increased RBC turnover (falsely low), and concurrent iron deficiency (falsely high). Further, HbA1c takes long time (3 months) to reflect alterations in glycemic status, and therefore HbA1c cannot be used for optimizing glycemic control during pregnancy. Nevertheless, it is recommended that patients with preexisting diabetes should maintain their HbA1c ≤6.5%. Fructosamine (glycated albumin) is a better indicator of glycemic control during pregnancy as compared to HbA1c because it reflects the glycemic status over the preceding 3 weeks. However, it is not commonly available and is not well validated for outcomes.

30. **What are the limitations of IADPSG criteria for the diagnosis of GDM?**

    IADPSG was the first to define cutoffs for the diagnosis of GDM based on maternal and fetal outcomes. These criteria were derived from the data of HAPO study which was the first of its kind to show a continuous risk between maternal hyperglycemia and adverse perinatal outcomes even at FPG ≥75 mg/dl, 1-h glucose ≥106 mg/dl, and 2-h glucose ≥91 mg/dl, levels much lower than the diagnostic thresholds used earlier for the diagnosis of GDM. However, the major limitation is extrapolation of these data obtained between 24 and 28 weeks of pregnancy to define GDM in the first trimester as well (FPG 92–125 mg/dl). In addition, IADPSG recommends OGTT which requires fasting state and three samples over 2 h for the diagnosis of GDM. Further, the use of a single abnormal value to define GDM may result in overdiagnosis and consequently medicalization of many "normal" pregnancies.

31. **What is the sensitivity of fasting plasma glucose, 1-h PG, and 2-h PG for the diagnosis of GDM?**

    A single abnormal glucose value during 75-g OGTT defines GDM (FPG ≥92 mg/dl or 1-h PG ≥180 mg/dl or 2-h PG ≥153 mg/dl). However, FPG alone detects GDM in 51.5% of patients, while 1-h PG and 2-h PG identifies 35.4% and 13.1%, respectively. Therefore, in clinical practice, estimation of FPG alone is a useful tool to identify significant number of women with GDM.

32. **What are the limitations of DIPSI criteria for the diagnosis of GDM?**

    Diabetes in Pregnancy Study Group of India (DIPSI) provided guidelines for the diagnosis and management of GDM in pregnancy. DIPSI recommends universal screening of all pregnant women at 24–28 weeks of gestation by performing a 75-g OGTT, irrespective of meal status. A 2-h glucose value post-OGTT between 140–199 mg/dl is diagnostic of GDM, and a value ≥200 mg/dl is diagnostic of overt diabetes. In addition, a new category "decreased gestational glucose tolerance (DGGT)" was introduced in women who had 2-h PG level between 120 and 139 mg/dl. The limitations of the DIPSI criteria are lack of FPG measurement (which identifies 50% of patients with GDM) and 1-h PG estimation (strongly correlates with maternal and neonatal adverse outcomes) and lack of validation of these cutoffs in Indian population for maternal and neonatal outcomes.

33. **How to manage hyperglycemia during labor?**

    Patients with hyperglycemia during pregnancy require frequent blood glucose monitoring (every 1–2 hourly) at the onset of labor. OADs, if used, should be discontinued; adequate hydration must be ensured; and blood glucose be maintained between 72 and 126 mg/dl. Insulin infusion should be used to maintain these glycemic targets. Intravenous dextrose must be used along with insulin, to prevent hypoglycemia or starvation ketosis. Birth weight needs to be documented, and neonate has to be monitored for respiratory distress, hypoglycemia, hyperbilirubinemia, hypocalcemia, and hypomagnesemia.

34. **How to monitor a patient with hyperglycemia during pregnancy after delivery?**

    Patients with preexisting and overt diabetes should be continued on anti-hyperglycemic therapy. However, insulin doses may require modification after delivery based on glucose profile with target of FPG 90–130 mg/dl and 2-h post-meal glucose <180 mg/dl and many women can be managed on oral antidiabetic drugs. Glucose-lowering therapy (insulin/OADs) should be discontinued immediately after delivery in patients with GDM. Blood glucose (fasting and postprandial) should be monitored for 24–72 h in these women to assess the need for any anti-hyperglycemic therapy as some women diagnosed with GDM may have persistent hyperglycemia, possibly due to underlying type 2 diabetes. At 6–12 weeks postpartum, women who had GDM should be subjected to a 75-g OGTT to categorize them as normal, prediabetes, or diabetes, using the standard criteria for nonpregnant adults.

35. **How to manage diabetes during lactation?**

    The best treatment option to manage diabetes during lactation is possibly insulin. However, metformin and second-generation sulfonylureas (glibenclamide and glipizide) have been safely used in lactating women. Metformin is secreted into breast milk in the range of 0.28–1.08%, but this concentration is too low to have any detrimental effects on the infant. This is supported by the fact that the use of metformin had no adverse effect on infant growth and motor and social development during first 6 months of life. Glibenclamide and glipizide are extensively bound to circulating proteins and hence not secreted into breast milk. However, there is no data regarding the use of glimepiride or gliclazide during lactation.

Suggested Reading

1. American Diabetes Association. Standards of medical care in diabetes—2014. Diabetes Care. 2014;37 Suppl 1:S14–80.
2. Blumer I, Hadar E, Hadden DR. Diabetes and pregnancy: an endocrine society clinical practice guideline. Clin Endocrinol Metab. 2013;98:4227–49.
3. International Association of Diabetes and Pregnancy Study Groups Consensus Panel, Metzger BE, Gabbe SG, Persson B, et al. International Association of Diabetes and Pregnancy Study Groups recommendations on the diagnosis and classification of hyperglycemia in pregnancy. Diabetes Care. 2010;33:676–82.